Radiology of Infectious and Inflammatory Diseases - Volume 1

Hongjun Li • Jian Wang • Xuening Zhang
Editors

Radiology of Infectious and Inflammatory Diseases - Volume 1

Brain and Spinal Cord

Springer

Editors
Hongjun Li
Capital Medical University
Beijing You An Hospital
Beijing, China

Xuening Zhang
Department of Radiology
The Second Hospital of Tianjin Medical University
Tianjin, China

Jian Wang
Medical Imaging Center
First Affiliated Hospital of Xinjiang Medical University
Urumqi, China

Shanghai Universal Medical Imaging Diagnostic Center
Shanghai University
Shanghai, China

ISBN 978-981-99-0038-1 ISBN 978-981-99-0039-8 (eBook)
https://doi.org/10.1007/978-981-99-0039-8

Jointly published with Science Press
The print edition is not for sale in China (Mainland). Customers from China (Mainland) please order the print book from: Science Press.

This Springer imprint is published by the registered company Springer Nature Singapore Pte Ltd.
The registered company address is: 152 Beach Road, #21-01/04 Gateway East, Singapore 189721, Singapore

Preface

With the rapid development of modern society and economy, people's lifestyles and population mobility have changed, and the impact of infectious and inflammatory diseases on human survival and socio-economic development has become increasingly significant. The National Health Commission has issued a document emphasizing the need to establish infectious disease departments and infection control offices in hospitals above the second level nationwide, placing unprecedented emphasis on the danger of infectious diseases to human health. In the past 30 years, the development of medical imaging diagnosis and treatment technology has greatly contributed to the change of modern diagnosis and treatment mode. The high reliance of modern medicine on medical imaging technology has given the medical imaging profession an important mission in the field of diagnosis and differential diagnosis of infectious and inflammatory diseases.

In the course of long-term clinical practice and scientific research, my team and I realized that it had seriously affected the quality of patient care and outcomes, caused the misuse of clinical antibiotics, affected patient health and quality of life, and increased the economic burden on families and society because of the neglect and lack of research on the construction of a key disciplinary system, systematic theoretical system, and standardized guidelines for infection and inflammation diseases. Based on the above considerations, this book brings together the Infectious Diseases Group of the Radiology Branch of the Chinese Medical Association, the Infection Imaging Committee of the Radiologists Branch of the Chinese Medical Association, the Infection and Inflammation Radiology Committee of the Chinese Society of Research Hospitals, the Infection (Infectious Diseases) Imaging Working Committee of the Chinese Association for STD and AIDS Prevention and Control, the Infectious Diseases Imaging Group of the Infectious Diseases Hospital Branch of the Chinese Hospital Association, and the Beijing Technological Innovation Alliance for Imaging and Treatment. The book summarizes the imaging features and evolution of infectious and inflammatory diseases, reveals the pathological basis of infectious and inflammatory diseases, and presents the key points of imaging diagnosis and differential diagnosis of infectious and inflammatory diseases. I believe that the publication of this set of books will promote the prevention and control of infection and inflammatory diseases, rational drug use and academic development of radiological imaging diagnosis in China, and effectively serve the precise clinical treatment.

This set of books provides the first systematic theoretical treatment of the subject of infection and inflammatory radiology. There are a total of six volumes, including a cranial spinal cord volume, a head and neck volume, a cardiothoracic volume, an abdominopelvic volume, a skeletal muscle volume, and a pediatric volume. The content covers the four major groups of pathogenic (bacterial, fungal, viral, parasitic) infections associated with infectious diseases and inflammatory diseases such as autoimmune diseases.

This series of books features three main advantages: (1) close to the clinical setting, with a complete range of diseases, covering common, frequent, and rare clinical infections and inflammatory diseases; (2) the information is comprehensive, which emphasizes the objective basis of diagnosis, especially the completeness, representativeness, continuity, and authenticity of cases and images; (3) most of the information comes from the editor's clinical experience and accumulation, and several parts of the information are authorized by international colleagues, and the overall absorption and citation of the latest research results at home and abroad, as well as the layout and content of the books are innovative in nature.

For the successful publication of this set of books, we set up an advisory committee and an expert committee, with scientific design and systematic demonstration, and it took more than 1 year to design the outline and revise the manuscript. In addition to the Chinese version, Springer Publishing Group will publish the English version. The editorial committee attached great importance to the book and organized several training sessions for the editorial board members on writing standardization, explained the process of professional review and finalization, and assigned specialized personnel to organize review, revision, and supplementation. As the editor-in-chief of this book, I would like to express my sincere gratefulness for this. At the same time, I would like to express my sincere gratitude to the members of the national infectious disease imaging team who participated in the preparation of this book for their efforts.

In the face of the current critical situation in the prevention and treatment of infectious and inflammatory diseases, the publication of this monograph will serve as another powerful weapon in the war against infectious and inflammatory diseases, and will play an important role in improving the level of diagnosis and treatment of physicians, improving the quality of life of patients, and prolonging their lives.

The process of scientific development is also a process of gradual improvement of people's understanding, and deviations are inevitable, so I would appreciate your kind advice and look forward to its improvement!

Beijing, China
November 2019

Hongjun Li

Preface

As an "Old and Fashionable" topic, infectious diseases have been with human development since the era of plague and famine. In recent years, with the continued prevalence of diseases such as severe acute respiratory syndrome, avian influenza, and Ebola hemorrhagic fever, novel pathogens are being discovered and the spectrum of underlying diseases is being transformed and pathogen resistance has been increasing, and the risk of infectious diseases to humans continues to deteriorate. In the 1970s, some experts predicted that infectious diseases could be completely defeated in the near future, but now it seems that the cause of defeating infectious diseases is a long way off.

Being an emerging branch of the medical disease classification system, infectious and inflammatory diseases have seen various types of research flourish in various fields in recent years. Infectious diseases of the central nervous system are one of the common serious infectious diseases, and the diversity and complexity of their lesions make early diagnosis and accurate diagnosis very difficult, with rapid disease progression and high rates of death and sequelae. With the rapid development of imaging technology, medical imaging plays a pivotal role in the diagnosis of the disease, and its role in assessing the efficacy and prognosis cannot be ignored. At present, there are few monographs on nervous system infection, and the existing books in the field of imaging medicine are limited in their description of infectious and inflammatory diseases of the central nervous system, covering few diseases, inconsistent classification methods, and incomplete descriptions of new imaging techniques.

In this context, the book series "Infection and Inflammation Radiology" led by Prof. Li Hongjun from our infection imaging community was born. Radiology of Infection and Inflammation—Cranial, Cerebrospinal and Spinal Volumes is one of the volumes that takes care to draw on the proven national and international experience in recent years in infectious and inflammatory diseases of the central nervous system with due attention to clinical utility.

This book clearly differentiates the traditional classification of infectious and inflammatory diseases into those that are affiliated with infectious diseases and those that are not, clearly differentiating it from other similar books. Each disease in this book is described with a corresponding pathology, highlighting the contrast and causal relationship between pathology and imaging presentations. Each disease has individually distilled diagnostic points that are concise and easy to access. In addition, this book presents research advances in the imaging of infectious and inflammatory diseases of the central nervous system and discusses the value of a variety of new imaging techniques that are relatively well established in the diagnosis and differential diagnosis of various diseases or in guiding treatment and assessing prognosis, in conjunction with the most recent references.

With an excellent authoring team, this book is compiled by a number of renowned experts in the field of imaging of CNS infectious and inflammatory diseases in China, combining the latest domestic and international guidelines, research advances, and their own clinical practice experience. The book also brings together cases from more than a dozen large tertiary hospitals in China where these experts work, showing valuable images of multiple diseases, especially those of some rare diseases. It is a valuable reference book for imaging and other clinicians.

I would like to express my sincere gratitude to all the editorial board, the editorial staff, and colleagues who contributed cases to this book! With an eye to the current practical needs of the general reader for clinical work and extended learning, this book is an informative, concise, easy-to-read, efficient, and practical reference on infection imaging. Due to limited conditions, some rare diseases lack typical pictures, and we hope that colleagues will criticize and correct any shortcomings in this book.

Urumqi, China
February 2020

Jian Wang

Contents

Part III Special Infectious and Inflammatory Diseases of the Central Nervous System

About the Editors

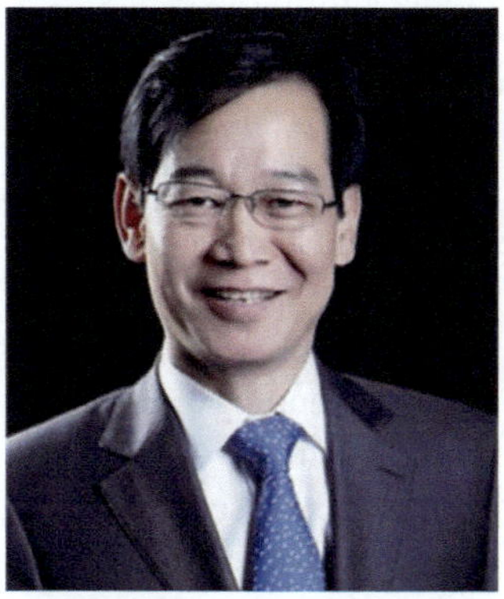

Hongjun Li, MD Chief Physician, Professor, Doctoral Supervisor. He is currently the Director of the Medical Imaging Center of Beijing Youan Hospital, Capital Medical University, and Deputy Director of the Department of Medical Imaging of Capital Medical University. He is one of the first cohorts of "Ten Hundred Thousand" health professionals in Beijing, and one of the first cohorts of "215" high-level health professionals in Beijing. He is an editor-in-chief of *Radiology of Infectious Diseases*, associate editor of *BMC*. He is an associate editor of *Neurology*. He is the chairman of Infectious Diseases Group of Chinese Radiology Branch, the chairman of Infection Imaging Committee of Radiologists Branch of Chinese Physicians Association, the chairman of Infection and Inflammation Radiology Committee of Chinese Research Hospital Society, the chairman of Infection (Infectious Diseases) Imaging Working Committee of Chinese STD and AIDS Prevention and Control Association, and the chairman of Beijing Technology Innovation Alliance of Imaging Diagnosis and Treatment.

Dr. Li is mainly engaged in diagnostic imaging of infection and inflammation and has supervised more than 20 doctoral and master's students. In recent years, Dr. Li has conducted more than 10 research projects, including 1 major project of National Science and Technology, 1 key and 2 general programs of National Natural Science Foundation of China. He has edited 2 textbooks, 28 monographs in English and Chinese, and 3 translations of monographs, and the total number of downloads of English monographs has reached 160,000. He also edited *Radiology of HIV/AIDS* and *Radiology of Infectious Diseases 1–2*, which were awarded the "Outstanding Book Award for Publication" in 2014 and 2015 respectively, and the "General Award" by the State Administration of Press, Publication, Radio, Film and Television in 2017. He has published more than 200 papers, including more than 60 SCI articles. He has obtained 2 national invention patents and 16 intellectual property registrations. He received 9 provincial and ministerial awards, including the Chinese Medical Science and Technology Award. He was awarded the title of "Master Teacher and Apprentice" by the Beijing Municipal Federation of Trade Unions, and his research team was awarded the title of "Scientific and Technological Innovation Cultivation Team" by the Beijing Municipal Hospital Administration and "Municipal

Staff Innovation Studio" by the Beijing Municipal Federation of Trade Unions and Beijing Municipal Science and Technology Commission.

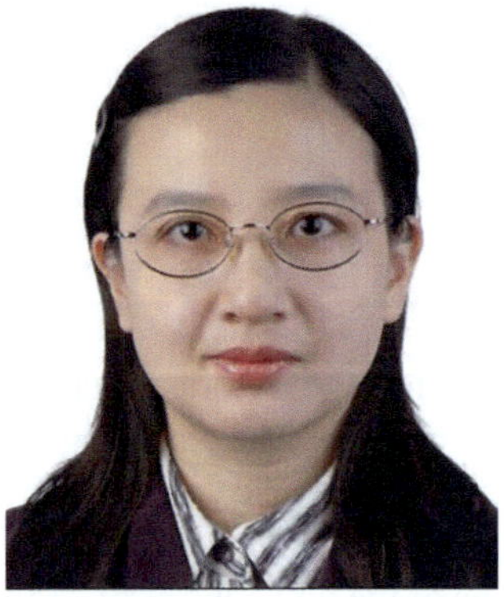

Jian Wang Deputy director of the Imaging Center of the First Affiliated Hospital of Xinjiang Medical University, Chief Physician, Professor, Doctoral Supervisor. She is the member of the Magnetic Resonance Imaging Group of the Radiology Branch of the Chinese Medical Association, member of the Neuroimaging Specialty Committee of the Radiologists Branch of the Chinese Medical Association, member of the Neurology Group of the Magnetic Resonance Imaging Specialty Committee of the Radiology Branch of the Chinese Medical Association, standing member of the Infection and Inflammation Radiology Specialty Committee of the Chinese Society of Research Hospitals, standing member of the Neurodegenerative Diseases Specialty Committee of the Chinese Society of Microcirculation, and standing member of the Magnetic Resonance Imaging Equipment and Technology Specialty Committee of the Chinese Medical Equipment Association. She is also the deputy director of the Infectious Disease Imaging Committee of Beijing Imaging and Diagnostic Technology Innovation Union, the executive member of Xinjiang Radiology Branch of Chinese Medical Association, the leader of Magnetic Resonance Group of Xinjiang Radiology Branch of Chinese Medical Association, the deputy director of Xinjiang Uygur Autonomous Region Diagnostic Radiology Quality Control Center, the member of Xinjiang Medical Association Medical Accident Technical Identification Expert Pool, the member of Xinjiang Uygur Autonomous Region Class B Large Medical Equipment Management Committee. She is also the member of the expert pool of medical equipment bidding expert pool of Xinjiang Uygur Autonomous Region Finance Department, and a natural science expert of Xinjiang. She is also an editorial board member of *Radiology of Infectious Diseases* and member of International Society for Magnetic Resonance in Medicine (ISMRM). Dr. Wang has received more than 10 grants from the National Natural Science Foundation of China and other scientific research funds, and won the second prize of the Science and Technology Progress Award of Xinjiang Uygur Autonomous Region (provincial level) in 2017. She has supervised 39 master's and PhD students (including 2 overseas students).

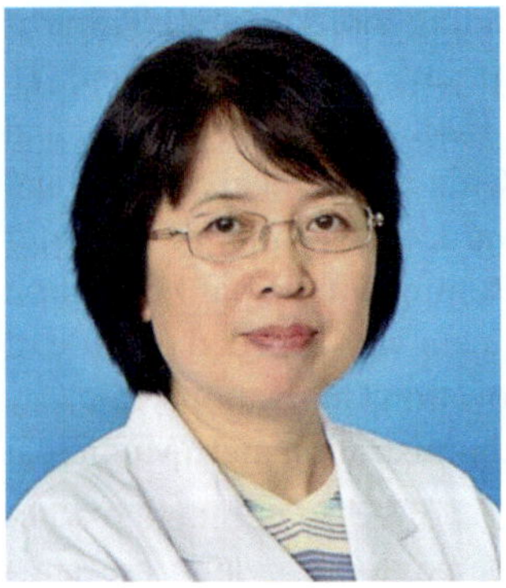

Xuening Zhang Chief of the Department of Medical Imaging, Second Hospital of Tianjin Medical University, Chief Physician, Professor, Doctoral Supervisor. She is a member of the Radiology Branch of the Chinese Medical Association, member of the Magnetic Resonance Committee of the Radiology Branch of the Chinese Medical. He is a member of the Radiology Branch of the Chinese Medical Association, and deputy director of the Magnetic Resonance Committee of the Radiology Branch of the Chinese Medical Association. She is also the member of the Standing Committee of the Radiology Committee of the China Healthcare International Exchange and Promotion Association, member of the Standing Committee of the Magnetic Resonance Imaging Equipment and Technology Committee of the China Medical Equipment Association, member of the Nanomedicine Committee of the Chinese Biomedical Engineering, member of the Board of Directors of the China Imaging Technology Research Society, deputy director of the Tianjin Radiology Branch, and vice president of the Radiology Society of the Tianjin Physicians Association.

Editors and Contributors

Associate Editors

Wenxiao Jia The First Affiliated Hospital of Xinjiang Medical University, Urumqi, China

Guihua Jiang Guangdong Second People's Hospital, Guangzhou, China

Hanqiu Liu Huashan Hospital, Fudan University, Shanghai, China

Shuang Xia Tianjin First Central Hospital, Tianjin, China

Li Li Beijing You'an Hospital, Capital Medical University, Beijing, China

Jun Liu The Second Xiangya Hospital of Central South University, Changsha, China

Chunhui Jiang The First Affiliated Hospital of Xinjiang Medical University, Urumqi, China

Yinhua Jin Xiamen Fifth Hospital, Xiamen, China

Longlin Yin Sichuan Provincial People's Hospital, Chengdu, China

Min Luo Zigong Fourth People's Hospital, Zigong, China

Kang Li Chongqing Hospital, University of Chinese Academy of Sciences, Chongqing, China

Contributors

Aniwar Ulam The Eight Affiliated Hospital of Xinjiang Medical University, Urumqi, China

Xiaoqing Cheng Eastern War Zone General Hospital, Nanjing, China

Hongyan Chen Beijing Tiantan Hospital, Capital Medical University, Beijing, China

Mi Chen The First Affiliated Hospital of Xinjiang Medical University, Urumqi, China

Mingquan Chen Huashan Hospital, Fudan University, Shanghai, China

Tingting Chen The Second Hospital of Harbin Medical University, Harbin, China

Pingfeng Dai The Second Affiliated Hospital of School of Medicine, Zhejiang University, Hangzhou, China

Dabiao Deng Guangdong Sanjiu Brain Hospital, Guangzhou, China

Shuang Ding Medical Imaging Center, First Affiliated Hospital of Xinjiang Medical University, Urumqi, China

Fei Dong The Second Affiliated Hospital of School of Medicine, Zhejiang University, Hangzhou, China

Wenhuan Du People's Hospital of Gaochang District, Turpan, Turpan, China

Xiaodan Du Zhuhai Hospital of Integrated Traditional Chinese and Western Medicine, Zhuhai, China

Yuanyuan Fang The First Affiliated Hospital of Xinjiang Medical University, Urumqi, China

Liwei Fu The Second Affiliated Hospital of School of Medicine, Zhejiang University, Harbin, China

Zi'ao Fu Teda International Cardiovascular Hospital, Tianjin, China

Lijuan Gao The First Affiliated Hospital of Xinjiang Medical University, Urumqi, China

Xin Gao Medical Imaging Center, First Affiliated Hospital of Xinjiang Medical University, Urumqi, China

Xin Gao Shanghai Universal Medical Imaging Diagnostic Center, Shanghai University, Shanghai, China

Jun Guo Guangdong Sanjiu Brain Hospital, Guangzhou, China

Yinglin Guo Harbin Daowai District Taiping People's Hospital, Harbin, China

Yulin He The First Affiliated Hospital of Nanchang University, Nanchang, China

Cong Huang The 926th Hospital of the Chinese People's Liberation Army Joint Logistics and Security Forces, Kaiyuan, China

Rui Huang Department of Radiology, Xijing Hospital, Air Force Military Medical University, Xi'an, China

Chunhui Jiang Medical Imaging Center, First Affiliated Hospital of Xinjiang Medical University, Urumqi, China

Guihua Jiang Guangdong Second People's Hospital, Guangzhou, China

Wenxiao Jia The First Affiliated Hospital of Xinjiang Medical University, Urumqi, China

Yinhua Jin Xiamen Fifth Hospital (Xiang'an Hospital of the First Affiliated Hospital of Xiamen University), Xiamen, China

Hong Li The Second Affiliated Hospital of School of Medicine, Zhejiang University, Hangzhou, China

Hongjun Li Capital Medical University, Beijing You An Hospital, Beijing, China

Huimin Li People's Hospital of Inner Mongolia Autonomous Region, Huhhot, China

Jin Li The First Affiliated Hospital of Xinjiang Medical University, Urumqi, China

Kang Li Chongqing Hospital, University of Chinese Academy of Sciences, Chongqing, China

Li Li Beijing You'an Hospital, Capital Medical University, Beijing, China

Qing Li Tianjin First Central Hospital, Tianjin, China

Bailu Liu The Second Hospital of Harbin Medical University, Harbin, China

Hanqiu Liu Huashan Hospital, Fudan University, Shanghai, China

Jun Liu The Second Xiangya Hospital of Central South University, Changsha, China

Jundi Liu The First Affiliated Hospital of Xinjiang Medical University, Urumqi, China

Lili Liu The Second Hospital of Harbin Medical University, Harbin, China

Lulu Liu Medical Imaging Center, First Affiliated Hospital of Xinjiang Medical University, Urumqi, China

Qiang Liu Shandong Provincial Hospital, Jinan, China

Xingbo Liu Xinjiang Bortala Mongolian Autonomous Prefecture People's Hospital, Bole, China

Yupeng Liu First Hospital of Qinhuangdao, Qinghuangdao, China

Xiaohong Li The First Affiliated Hospital of Xinjiang Medical University, Urumqi, China

Yanran Li The First Affiliated Hospital of Xinjiang Medical University, Urumqi, China

Yuehua Li The Sixth People's Hospital of Shanghai Jiao Tong University, Shanghai, China

Jun Lu Medical Imaging Center, First Affiliated Hospital of Xinjiang Medical University, Urumqi, China

Min Luo Zigong Fourth People's Hospital, Zigong, China

Zhehao Lv The First Hospital of Harbin Medical University, Harbin, China

Jianhua Ma The First Affiliated Hospital of Xinjiang Medical University, Urumqi, China

Nuerbiyemu Abulikemu The First Affiliated Hospital of Xinjiang Medical University, Urumqi, China

Liling Peng Shanghai Universal Medical Imaging Diagnostic Center, Shanghai University, Shanghai, China

Yongde Qin The First Affiliated Hospital of Xinjiang Medical University, Urumqi, China

Meiji Ren Beijing You'an Hospital, Capital Medical University, Beijing, China

Kai Shang Shanghai Sixth People's Hospital, Shanghai, China

Yunjin Song School of Medicine, Shanghai University, Shanghai, China

Jiaying Tang The First Affiliated Hospital of Xinjiang Medical University, Urumqi, China

Hui Tian The First Affiliated Hospital of Xinjiang Medical University, Urumqi, China

Chao Wang The Second Affiliated Hospital of School of Medicine, Zhejiang University, Hangzhou, China

Fei Wang The First Affiliated Hospital of Xinjiang Medical University, Urumqi, China

He Wang Institute of Brain-like Intelligence Science and Technology, Fudan University, Shanghai, China

Jian Wang Medical Imaging Center, First Affiliated Hospital of Xinjiang Medical University, Urumqi, China

Shanghai Universal Medical Imaging Diagnostic Center, Shanghai University, Shanghai, China

Jinying Wang Medical Imaging Center, First Affiliated Hospital of Xinjiang Medical University, Urumqi, China

Qianfeng Wang Fudan University, Shanghai, China

Shaozhou Wang Tianjin Third Central Hospital, Tianjin, China

Shifeng Wang Tianjin Panorama Medical Imaging Diagnostic Center, Tianjin, China

Shui Wang Beijing Children's Hospital Xinjiang Hospital, Beijing, China

Weiwei Wang Huashan Hospital, Fudan University, Shanghai, China

Wensheng Wang Guangdong Sanjiu Brain Hospital, Guangzhou, China

Yan Wang People's Hospital of Xinjiang Uygur Autonomous Region, Urumqi, China

Yan Wang The Second Affiliated Hospital of Xiamen Medical School, Xiamen, China

Yunling Wang The First Affiliated Hospital of Xinjiang Medical University, Urumqi, China

Ling Wu Medical Imaging Center, First Affiliated Hospital of Xinjiang Medical University, Urumqi, China

Shuang Xia Tianjin First Central Hospital, Tianjin, China

Hui Xing The First Affiliated Hospital of Xinjiang Medical University, Urumqi, China

Jingjing Xu The Second Affiliated Hospital of School of Medicine, Zhejiang University, Hangzhou, China

Ning Xu Jinan first people's Hospital, Jinan, China

Zhiqiang Xu Zhengzhou Central Hospital, Zhengzhou, China

Jing Yang The First Affiliated Hospital of Xinjiang Medical University, Urumqi, China

Junle Yang Journal of Practical Radiology, Xian, China

Yuxin Yang The Sixth People's Hospital of Xinjiang Uygur Autonomous Region, Urumqi, China

Yibanu Medical Imaging Center, First Affiliated Hospital of Xinjiang Medical University, Urumqi, China

Longlin Yin Sichuan Provincial People's Hospital, Chengdu, China

Luolin Yin Beijing You'an Hospital, Capital Medical University, Beijing, China

Xiaoping Yin The Affiliated Hospital of Hebei University, Baoding, China

Yongxiao You Beijing Shunyi Maternal and Child Health Hospital, Beijing, China

Dan Zhang Medical Imaging Center, First Affiliated Hospital of Xinjiang Medical University, Urumqi, China

Jian Zhang Hangzhou Panorama Medical Imaging Diagnostic Center, Hangzhou, China

Jianping Zhang Tianshui Xin Tiantan Trauma and Orthopaedic Hospital, Tianshui, China

Xuening Zhang Department of Radiology, The Second Hospital of Tianjin Medical University, Tianjin, China

Zhiqiang Zhang General Hospital of Eastern Theater Command, Nanjing, China

Zongjun Zhang Jiangsu Provincial Hospital of Integrated Traditional Chinese and Western Medicine, Nanjing, China

Yanling Zhou Xiaolan People's Hospital, Southern Medical University, Zhongshan, China

Mingwang Zhu Capital Medical University Sanbo Brain Hospital, Beijing, China

Part I

General Introduction to Infectious and Inflammatory Diseases of the Central Nervous System

1 Introduction to Imaging Methods

Bailu Liu, Yuehua Li, Kai Shang, Jian Zhang, He Wang, Qianfeng Wang, Jiaying Tang, Yongde Qin, Xiaohong Li, and Xin Gao

Central nervous system infections remain relatively high in morbidity and mortality worldwide; many of the known pathogens that can cause infectious diseases include broad-spectrum bacteria, viruses, fungi, mycobacteria, and parasites. In 1971, Omran [1] proposed a theory of epidemiological transition in developing countries, describing the mortality changes and disease patterns of CNS infections in these countries, which consisted of three phases, namely, the "era of plague and famine," the "era of pandemics," and the "era of degeneration and human-made diseases." A recent annual mortality rate published in the United States and data from the World Health Organization reflect a decline in mortality associated with infectious diseases and a gradual evolution of infectious diseases to chronic diseases. CNS infection is common clinical serious infectious conditions, which are mainly meningitis and encephalitis syndrome, etc. CNS diseases such as intracranial tumor, cerebral hemorrhage, and craniocerebral trauma can be treated effectively by surgery, but the rate of postoperative infection is still on the rise. The progression of CNS infections is often very rapid in nature and is characterized by a high mortality rate and a high incidence of sequelae.

Multimodal medical imaging has played a prominent role in the diagnosis, treatment, follow-up, and assessment of prognosis of various CNS diseases. Present examinations used for CNS infectious diseases include cranial radiographs, computed tomography (CT), magnetic resonance imaging (MRI), nuclear imaging, and functional and molecular imaging, all of which have their own advantages and limitations. Innovative new imaging technologies have greatly expanded the applications of imaging in central nervous system diseases. This chapter focuses on the various imaging techniques of the central nervous system and advancements in new imaging techniques.

CNS infections and inflammatory diseases that are not diagnosed in a timely manner and given diagnostic treatment may lead to a certain mortality rate at times. When a suspected CNS infectious disease is encountered, imaging physicians who can provide relatively complete diagnostic and differential diagnostic information may offer clinicians objective information which is crucial to the treatment of the disease.

1.1 X-Ray Imaging Techniques

Bailu Liu, Yuehua Li, and Kai Shang

1.1.1 X-Ray Imaging Principle

The X-ray image is an image formed directly by X-ray transmitted through the human body. It is a direct analog gray-scale image, consisting of images of different shades of gray

B. Liu
The Second Hospital of Harbin Medical University, Harbin, China

Y. Li (✉)
The Sixth People's Hospital of Shanghai Jiao Tong University, Shanghai, China

K. Shang
Shanghai Sixth People's Hospital, Shanghai, China

J. Zhang
Hangzhou Panorama Medical Imaging Diagnostic Center, Hangzhou, China

H. Wang
Institute of Brain-like Intelligence Science and Technology, Fudan University, Shanghai, China
e-mail: hewang@fudan.edu.cn

Q. Wang
Fudan University, Shanghai, China
e-mail: qianfengwang@fudan.edu.cn

J. Tang · Y. Qin · X. Li
The First Affiliated Hospital of Xinjiang Medical University, Urumqi, China

X. Gao
Shanghai Universal Medical Imaging Diagnostic Center, Shanghai University, Shanghai, China

H. Li et al. (eds.), *Radiology of Infectious and Inflammatory Diseases - Volume 1*,
https://doi.org/10.1007/978-981-99-0039-8_1

from black to white, which reflects the anatomical and pathological conditions of human tissue and structures through the density of the image and its variations, which is mainly acquired by digital X-ray imaging equipment. There are three conditions that must be present for X-rays to be produced: (1) a population of freely moving electrons, (2) a high-voltage electric field that causes electrons to move at high speed under vacuum conditions, and (3) a target surface that prevents fast-moving electrons. Therefore, two essential pieces of equipment are necessary for X-ray imaging, namely, an X-ray bulb and a high-voltage generator. The penetration, fluorescence, and photoreceptor effects of X-rays are the basis for their application in diagnostic imaging. In addition, there are differences in the absorption of X-rays due to different densities of human tissues and different structures of pathological tissues, which result in a black and white contrasted image on the fluoroscope or photograph. The extent to which X-rays are absorbed through different tissues in the body and other substances can be influenced by the following factors: (1) the density of the substance, (2) the thickness of the substance, and (3) the wavelength of the X-ray.

1.1.2 X-Ray Imaging Method

Digital X-ray imaging equipment is an X-ray device that digitizes X-ray transmission images and processes them for conversion into analog images for display. Depending on the imaging mechanism, it can be divided into computed radiography (CR) devices and digitized radiography (DR) devices [2].

CR records X-ray images using an image plate (IP) and then converts the stored signal into an optical signal by laser scanning, and the optical signal is converted into an electrical signal by a photomultiplier tube, which is then input to a computer for processing by analog/digital (A/D) conversion to form a high-quality digital image. CR utilizes IP as a planar radiation detector, which mainly includes information acquisition, information conversion, information processing, information storage, and recording components:

1. Information acquisition: Instead of traditional film, IP is used to record X-ray images in the form of latent images. The X-ray photons injected into the IP are absorbed by the photo-stimulated luminescent (PSL) fluorescent material within the fluorescent layer, releasing electrons, some of which are scattered within the fluorescent material in a semi-stable state, forming the latent image. The semi-stable electrons are converted to fluorescence (PSL phenomenon) when the IP with latent image is scanned linearly with the laser beam, and the intensity of this fluorescence is proportional to the intensity of the X-rays at the time of the first excitation.
2. Information conversion: The conversion is realized by the image reading device, which completes the photoelectric conversion and A/D conversion of the fluorescent image, and finally converts it into a digital image signal.
3. Information processing: This is executed by computer, which performs various post-processing on digital images, such as enlargement, grayscale processing, subtraction processing, etc.
4. Information storage and recording: Laser printer film is the conventional way of recording. The CR image can also be displayed directly on the computer monitor.

Based on different detector structure types and imaging technologies, DR can be divided into direct digital X-ray imaging (amorphous selenium), indirect digital X-ray imaging (amorphous silicon), CCD X-ray imaging, and multiwire proportional chamber (MWPC) imaging. Amorphous selenium and amorphous silicon are presently mostly used for imaging [3]. The X-ray photons will react with cesium iodide (CsI) to generate fluorescence when they pass through the amorphous silicon flat panel detector. These fluorescent photons will be converted into the corresponding electrical signals by the photodiode. Studies have shown that the quantum capture efficiency of amorphous silicon flat panel detectors is significantly improved, which means that the X-ray dose can be significantly reduced without compromising image quality. The X-ray will interact with the amorphous selenium semiconductor to produce positive and negative electron pairs when they pass through the amorphous selenium detector, generating the corresponding electrical signals. The process does not involve significant information conversion with minimal information loss while obtaining clear, high-quality images.

The emergence of digital X-ray devices such as CR and DR has replaced traditional film, which can be connected to the picture archiving and communication system (PACS) for sharing over the network; facilitating storage, transmission, and remote diagnosis; and contributing to the development of teleradiology. DR devices have higher spatial resolution and signal-to-noise ratio than CR devices [4], have shorter imaging times, and require lower X-ray doses, but CR devices are less expensive and can be used in conjunction with original X-ray machines. Both devices have advantages over conventional screen-and-slice photography in terms of X-ray dose, image resolution, and post-processing.

1.1.3 X-Ray Imaging Methods Commonly Used in the Brain and Spinal Cord

A cranial X-ray is the most commonly used X radiographic method for craniospinal imaging. Anterior-posterior and lateral view is commonly used, while axial, tangential, and mento-vertical view may sometimes be used as needed. The anterior-posterior view shows images of symmetrical shape and size of the two orbits, with the outer edges of the two orbits shown equidistant from the outer edge of the skull. The skull is properly laid out in the X-ray radiograph, and the image quality is considered satisfactory when the petrosa does not overlap with the supraorbital rim. The lateral view of the skull clearly shows the edge of the sella turcica, and the image quality is considered satisfactory when the anterior-posterior pterygoid process overlaps without bilateral display. The axial view is used to present a symmetrical skull base image of the ambilateral petrous bone and zygomatic bone. The image quality is satisfied when the mandible's coronoid process is equidistant from the outer edge of the skull on both sides, the inferior dentition overlaps with the interbrow, the odontoid process is anterior to the middle of the foramen magnum of the occipital bone but does not overlap with the anterior edge of the atlas, and the foramen ovale and foramen spinosum of the middle cranial fossa are clearly displayed. The mento-vertical position (skull base position) allows observation of the skull base; the frontal-occipital position (Towne's) shows the occipital bone, petrosal bone, and internal auditory canal; the orbital position visualizes the orbit, supraorbital fissure, and wings of sphenoid bone; the 45° axio-anterior oblique posterior (Stenver's) view visualizes the petrosal bone, internal auditory canal, and inner ear structures; and the local tangential view reveals details of the local skull. In addition, tomography can be used to detect bone and calcium plaques at the base of the skull; stereography can be used to detect intracranial calcium plaques or foreign bodies in relation to the spatial location of the cranial cavity; and magnification photography can show details of local bone structures.

The cranial X-ray radiographs usually could not provide a definitive diagnosis for infectious diseases of the central nervous system, but only indirect signs suggest intracranial lesions without specificity, for instance, intracranial septic infections and intracranial tuberculosis may show intracranial hypertension, mainly with widening of the cranial suture, increased pressure traces in the cerebral gyrus, bone resorption in the sella turcica, and enlargement and deformation of the sella turcica. Further CT and MRI should be performed when the cranial X-ray radiographs suggest abnormalities.

Pneumoencephalography, ventriculography and cisternography were once commonly used to diagnose cranial diseases; however, they have been abandoned as they are invasive techniques that can cause serious complications such as intracranial infection, intracranial hemorrhage, and cerebral edema.

1.2 CT Imaging Techniques

Yuehua Li, Jian Zhang, and Kai Shang

1.2.1 CT Imaging Principle

CT is the acronym for computed tomography. CT images are digitally converted reconstructed analog images, which are composed of a certain number of pixels of different gray scale from black to white aligned in an intrinsic matrix. The gray scale of the pixel reflects the X-ray absorption coefficient of the corresponding voxel. The basic imaging process is as follows: The X-ray is first emitted from the X-ray bulb, which is adjusted into an X-ray beam by the collimator and then penetrates a section of the human body before reaching the detector, where it is received and A/D converted to obtain an X-ray absorption profile of that section of the human body in a certain direction. This information is then stored in the computer, and the X-ray tube is rotated around the section to obtain a 360° X-ray absorption profile. This data is also input into the computer, and the display processor performs an inverse projection or analytical calculation of the absorption profile data in each direction to obtain the X-ray absorption values of the voxels at each spatial location within the section. These data are matrixed by spatial coordinates and displayed on the monitor in different resolution gray scales to obtain an anatomical image of the human section. The CT image also reflects the degree of absorption of X-ray by organs and tissues in gray scale. Where black shadows indicate low-absorption areas, i.e., low-density areas, such as lung tissue containing air, gray shadows indicate moderate-absorption areas, i.e., medium-density areas, such as muscles or organs of soft tissue, and white shadows indicate high-absorption areas, i.e., high-density areas, such as bone tissue containing high amounts of calcium. CT images have relatively high-density resolution and can be used for quantitative density analysis. In order to achieve the most optimal display of the tissue structures and lesions to be observed on CT images, it is necessary to employ different windowing techniques according to their range of CT values, which mainly include window level and window width [5]. The window width (W) is the range of the gray scale being displayed, and its middle value is called the window level (C). By increasing the window level, the image displayed on the fluorescent screen becomes black; by decreasing the window level, the image turns white. By increasing the window width, the number of layers on the image increases and the contrast between tissues decreases; by decreasing the window width, the number of layers on the image decreases and the contrast between tissues increases.

1.2.2 CT Imaging Post-processing Techniques

The CT image is a tomographic image and can be subjected to various post-processing. CT image post-processing techniques involve a variety of 2D display techniques, 3D display techniques, and a multitude of other techniques for analysis, processing, and display. The two-dimensional display technologies consist of multiplanar reformation (MPR) and curved planar reformation (CPR); three-dimensional display technologies include volume rendering (VR), maximum intensity projection (MIP), minimum intensity projection (minIP), etc. The development and application of these analytical display techniques has greatly expanded the application areas of CT and significantly increased its diagnostic value.

1.2.3 CT Imaging Methods Commonly Used in the Brain and Spinal Cord

CT examination provides high diagnostic power for central nervous system diseases and has been commonly used. However, CT examinations use X-rays, and the radiation dose is significantly higher than that of conventional X-rays, which to a certain extent limits the application of CT, especially for the detection of specific lesions in obstetrics and gynecology and pediatric patients. In addition, there are still limitations in the etiologic diagnosis of disease with CT.

1. *CT plain scan and contrast-enhanced scan.* CT plain scan is a CT examination without contrast (an iodine agent which is impervious to X-ray), while CT contrast-enhanced scan is performed with intravenous injection of contrast to improve the contrast between the layers of tissue, thereby increasing the resolution of the CT examination.

   CT plain scan can show the location and extent of brain parenchymal lesions in CNS infection and inflammatory diseases and promptly detect the presence of edema, calcification, hemorrhage, and changes in the cerebrospinal fluid circulation system in the lesion area; enhanced scan is effective in showing the condition of endyma, blood-brain barrier, meningeal lesions, envelope of brain abscess, etc. A larger dose of enhanced scan is more helpful to visualize some small lesions. In some cases of CNS infectious diseases, CT scan is usually negative on the first to third day of onset, whereas enhanced scan can improve the detection rate of lesions, facilitate early diagnosis and treatment, improve clinical symptoms, and reduce mortality [6]. Therefore, enhanced CT scan should be performed promptly if there is a high suspicion of intracranial infection, and CT review should be performed in the recent future. However, for some patients with intracranial infections, there is the phenomenon of different diseases with mimicking images, and their CT findings are relatively similar, which cannot determine the specific pathogen by CT examination alone and requires analysis and comparison with other imaging examinations, laboratory tests, and clinical features to continuously improve the diagnostic accuracy. Figure 1.1 shows a patient with a brain abscess in which the CT scan image shows only a slightly hypodense foci next to the right lateral ventricle, and the extent of the lesion is blurred, while the boundary and extent of the lesion can be clearly shown after enhancement.
2. *CT angiography (CTA).* CTA is a noninvasive vascular imaging technique, the basic principle of which is to inject contrast agent through a vein, and the original tomographic image can be obtained by rapid scanning with multilayer spiral CT when the concentration of contrast agent in the target vessel reaches a threshold, and the three-dimensional structure of the vessel can be displayed by post-processing techniques such as VR and MIP. CTA is safe, convenient, and rapid for the diagnosis of cerebrovascular lesions. It also characterizes and locates the lesion and can be used as a screening method for cerebrovascular diseases such as cerebral aneurysms. Some people may experience adverse reactions to contrast agents, including facial flushing, headache, nausea, vomiting, hives, and conjunctival congestion in mild cases, or respiratory distress, unconsciousness, shock, cardiac arrhythmia, or cardiac arrest in severe cases, which require immediate emergency measures such as tracheotomy and cardiopulmonary resuscitation. CTA and magnetic resonance angiography (MRA) are primarily used to show the structure and course of arteries, while CT venous angiography and magnetic resonance venous angiography are more effective in the venous phase.

   There are four main techniques for cranial CTA, namely, general CTA, digital subtraction CTA, dual-energy CTA, and time-resolved CTA.

   (a) Conventional CTA: The basic principle is to inject contrast intravenously and acquire continuous volume during the peak filling period of the target vessel using spiral CT and then reconstruct the image of the target vessel in 2D or 3D or even 4D by using the post-processing function of computer. The conventional CTA in the general sense is a non-debridement CTA technique, which is more difficult to visualize lesions in the skull base segment of the internal carotid artery due to the overlapping of the skull base bones.

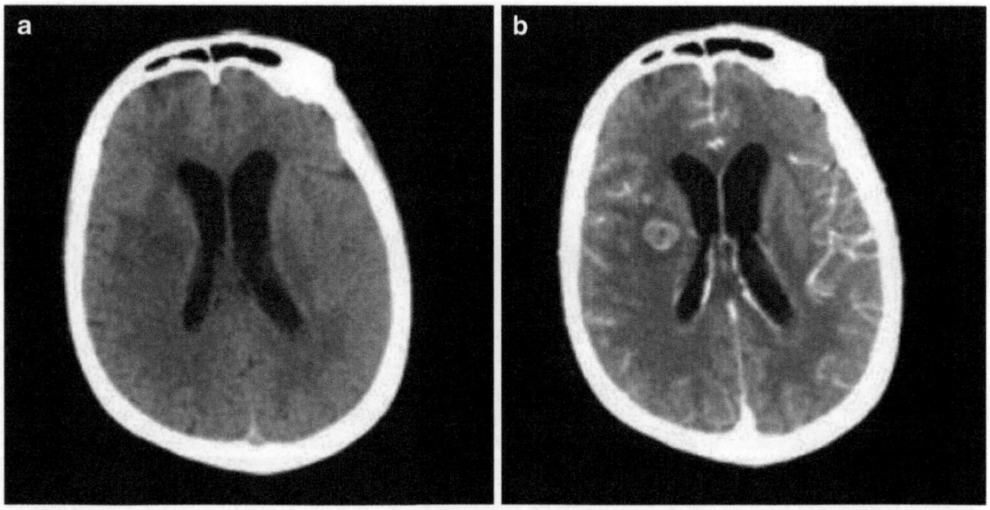

Fig. 1.1 Right paraventricular brain abscess. (**a**) CT plain scan shows a slightly hypodense lesion next to the right lateral ventricle, with slight compression of the right lateral ventricle; (**b**) enhanced CT can demonstrate the location, extent, and enhancement of the lesion more clearly

(b) Digital subtraction CTA: It is an automated bone subtraction CTA, which can better display lesions in the skull base segment of the internal carotid artery and improve the detection rate of internal carotid aneurysms in the skull base segment. Digital subtraction CTA uses the principles of digital subtraction angiography (DSA) to perform phase subtraction after two volume scans of plain and enhanced, and the subtracted data obtained is reconstructed in different ways to show the anatomy and lesions of the target vessels. Commonly used post-processing methods are VR, MIP, and MRP. VR takes different peaks of the pixel density histogram in the scanned volume to represent different tissues and then calculates on different tissue percentages for each pixel and converts them into different gray scales, displaying all sorts of structures in the volume in three dimensions with different gray scales and different transparency, which observes the vascular situation primarily through three dimensions. MIP is to superimpose the scanned 3D data and project the highest density voxels in the 3D data into the 2D data at the angle selected by the operator as the projection direction, and the remaining voxels are deleted in that projection direction. MIP can be projected from any angle, mainly to observe vascular calcification. MPR is a process of tomographic image reconstruction in any direction using three-dimensional reconstruction technique for data obtained from CT sampling, including planar reconstruction and curved surface reformation, which is mainly used to observe the relationship between the vicinity of blood vessels and to display tortuous vessels on the image. The technique is now routinely applied in clinical settings.

It should be noted that this technique requires that the bulb exposure angles should remain synchronized during the two subvolume scans. Low-tube voltage and low-tube current techniques should be used in plain scan to reduce the radiation dose received by the patient. Although radiation dose reduction measures have been used in the plain scan, it still increases the radiation dose received by the patient to some extent because of the requirement for two volumetric scans, plain and enhanced. Poor image alignment can occur in critically ill or poorly coordinated patients, where post-processing of the image is necessary with enhanced volumetric CT data, and this process is similar with the conventional CTA. During the digital subtraction CTA scan, the patient should be advised not to swallow and to remain still during the examination and to remove any metal ornaments from the head to avoid artifacts. The image quality is also related to the injection velocity of the autoinjector, which generally reaches 4.5–5.0 ml/s to obtain high-quality cranial CTA images. However, in elderly patients with poor vascular elasticity, high injection speed may cause leakage of contrast agent outside the blood vessels, and therefore it is often necessary to reduce the injection speed appropriately. Figure 1.2 shows a set of images obtained after digital subtraction CTA post-processing of the head and neck vessels.

(c) Dual-energy CTA: It is a method to remove bony structures (including vascular hard plaques) based on the difference in X-ray attenuation rates between the iodine component and the calcified or bony component of blood at different energy X-rays, whereby blood vessels in complex structures can be directly separated using dual-energy mode scanning and algorithmic processing. Presently, the dual-source and dual-energy CT technology is more than sophisticated. This technique allows for the acquisition of a

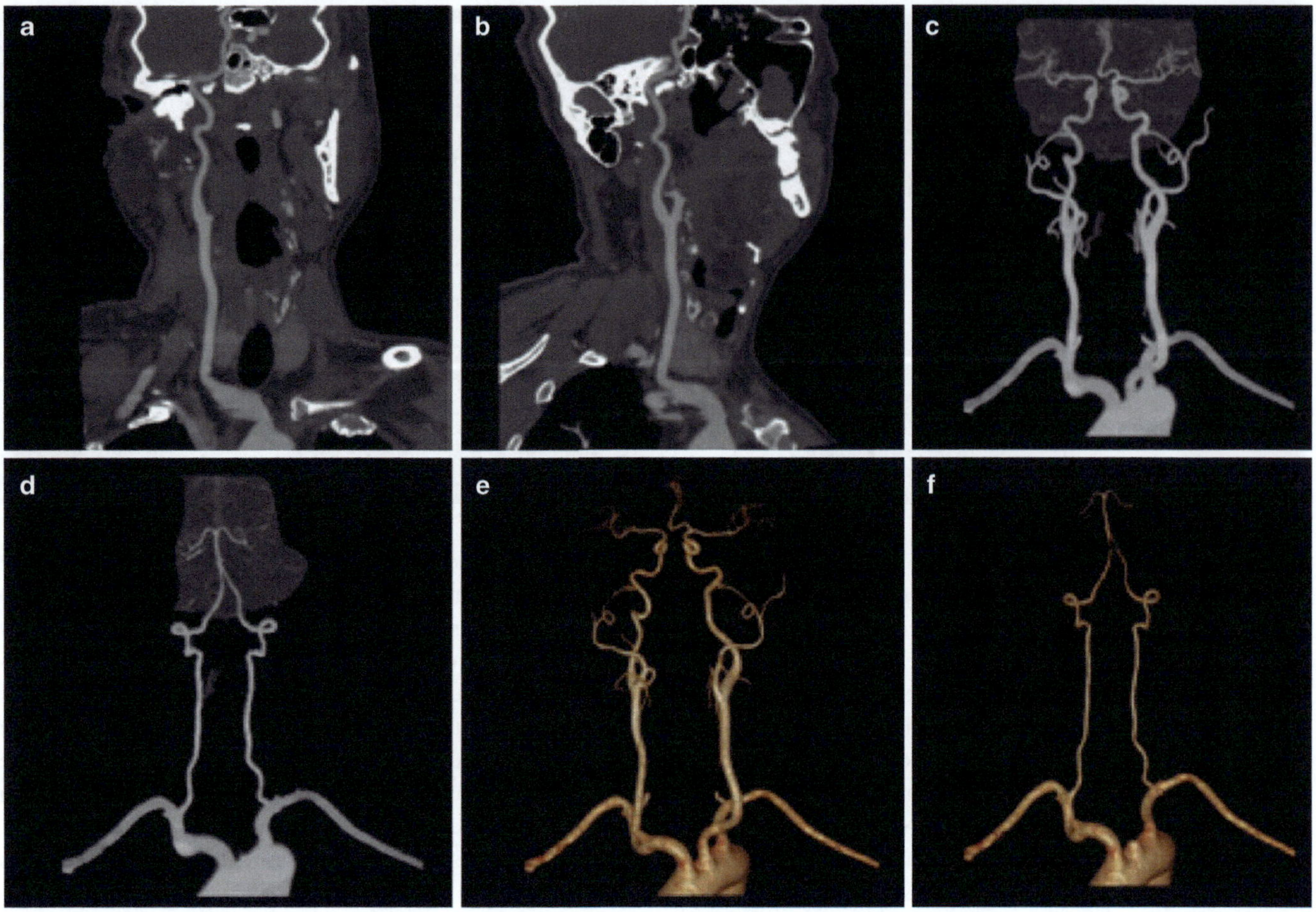

Fig. 1.2 Display of head and neck vessels by different CT post-processing techniques. (**a**, **b**) Curved surface reformation images of the head and neck arteries; (**c**, **d**) maximum density projection images of the intracranial anterior and posterior circulation; (**e**, **f**) volume reproduction images of the intracranial anterior and posterior circulation with bone removed

bone-depleted CTA image and a virtual cranial scan image to meet diagnostic needs with only one dual-energy enhanced CT scan and special dual-energy post-processing software, reducing the radiation dose to the patient and reducing the probability of poor image alignment. It has the same high diagnostic accuracy as digital subtraction CTA in the diagnosis of intracranial aneurysms.

(d) Time-resolved CTA: It is the technique of acquiring volumetric data of target vessels using multilayer spiral CT perfusion imaging, and then reconstructing the image with dynamic three-dimensional effect by post-processing software. It can be used not only for 3D imaging of cerebral vessels but also for providing functional parameters such as morphological changes of target vessels, which is a further expansion of the conventional concept of CT perfusion imaging technology and is mainly used for the diagnosis of cerebral ischemic lesions and vascular malformations.

3. *Energy spectrum CT* is a CT that uses the different absorption attenuation coefficients produced by substances at different energy X-rays to provide more image information than conventional CT. It has changed the conventional CT imaging method in which a single CT value is the standard and achieved high-resolution and high-definition images at ultralow doses, which has greatly improved CT imaging technology. The energy spectrum CT can conduct single-energy imaging, energy spectrum curve analysis, material separation and quantitative analysis, and effective atomic number calculation.

(a) Single-energy imaging: The energy spectrum CT can acquire 101 single-energy images in the range of 40–140 keV by the single-bulb dual-energy instantaneous switching isotropic acquisition technique, which is clearly different from the conventional CT using mixed-energy radiography. The corresponding CT values are obtained by calculating the absorption attenuation coefficients of the X-rays for different energies of the tissue, and thus the corresponding energy spectrum curves can be obtained. The differences in the energy profiles between substances are more pronounced in the lower-energy bands, and the corresponding differences in the CT values are the largest. The best single-energy image can be obtained when the target tissue has the greatest difference in attenuation from the adjacent parenchymal organs at a certain energy level with minimal image noise, which is the optimal kiloelectron volt (keV) value for imaging that tissue. The image quality, signal-to-noise ratio, and contrast-to-noise ratio of single-energy images are superior to those of conventional CT and can also significantly reduce metallic artifacts, hardening artifacts of high-density contrast agents, hardening artifacts of dense bone edges, etc.

(b) Energy spectrum curve analysis: Substances exhibit different absorption and attenuation abilities with the change of X-ray energy, which enables to obtain the characteristic energy spectrum curve of a substance. The different energy spectrum curves suggest variations in their histological structures and pathological types.

(c) Substance separation and quantitative analysis: The photoelectric effect and the Compton effect produced by X-rays passing through substances collectively determine the attenuation curve of the substance, while any substance has its own specific attenuation curve. The attenuation curves of the substances are linear, and two substances can be selected as substrates; the spatial distribution and density of the target substance can be calculated by converting one substance into the density of two substrates that produce the same attenuation, and then the spatial distribution and density of the target substance can be calculated based on the known attenuation coefficients of the substrates, thus realizing the separation and quantitative analysis of the substance. It is important to note that substance composition analysis is not determining the substance composition but rather producing the same attenuation effect by the given two substrates. Consequently, the substrates chosen for the separation of substances are not static, but the most used are aqueous and iodine with different attenuation coefficients.

(d) Effective atomic number calculation: Every substance has a characteristic attenuation curve. The atomic number of an element is the effective atomic number of a substance when the X-ray absorption coefficient of that element is the same as the absorption attenuation coefficient of that substance, which can be used clinically for substance detection and identification.

The energy spectrum CT has outstanding advantages in angiography. Conventional CTA with mixed-energy X-ray has been found to be less effective in showing small arteries with a diameter of 1.5–3.0 mm due to sclerotic beam artifacts and a lower signal-to-noise ratio. However, energy spectrum CT allows scanning with lower-energy single-energy X-rays, which reduces sclerotic beam artifacts and increases contrast between tissues, highlighting small blood supply arteries injected with iodine-containing contrast agents and improving image quality. Meanwhile, the optimal single-energy imaging technique of energy spectrum CT can control the image noise in the proper range, further optimizing the display of small blood supply arteries of the lesion.

The energy spectrum scan requires high tube voltage, and the bulb is prone to overheat, which makes the energy spectrum scan unsuitable for a longtime, wide-range, and small-pitch uninterrupted scanning for the protection of the tube. In addition, the amount of data obtained from the energy spectrum scan is about five times larger than that of conventional CT, which takes a longer time for reading and post-processing of the images [7–9].

1.3 MRI Imaging Techniques

He Wang, Qianfeng Wang, and Jiaying Tang

1.3.1 Basic Principles and Image Characteristics of MR

The MR image, like CT image, is a digitally simulated grayscale image that can be displayed using windowing techniques and is capable of various image post-processing. However, the gray scale on MR images does not indicate the density of the tissue and lesion but rather represents the MR signal intensity, reflecting the length of the relaxation time and the magnitude of the proton density, which differs from CT.

Compared to CT examinations, which provide single density parameter imaging, MRI examinations can provide multiparameter imaging, such as T_1 values reflecting T_1 relaxation time and T_2 values reflecting T_2 relaxation time. Imaging that primarily reflects the difference in T_1 values between tissues is referred to as T_1-weighted imaging (T_1WI). Imaging that primarily reflects the difference in T_2 values between tissues is referred to as T_2-weighted imaging (T_2WI). Imaging that primarily reflects the difference in proton density between tissues is termed proton density-weighted imaging (PDWI). Cranial tissues and their lesions have different T_1 values, T_2 values, and proton densities, so T_1WI, T_2WI, and PDWI produce different signal intensities, which are manifested as different grayscale values. MRI examinations provide a diagnosis of craniocerebral diseases based on these grayscale changes. In general, the stronger the tissue signal, the brighter the corresponding part of the image; the weaker the tissue signal, the darker the corresponding part of the image.

However, it should be noted that the relationship between the length of the relaxation time T_1 and T_2 values and the signal intensity differs on T_1WI and T_2WI images. Short T_1 values are high signal, such as fat tissue; long T_1 values are low signal, such as cerebrospinal fluid; short T_2 values are low signal, such as bone cortex; and long T_2 values are high signal, such as cerebrospinal fluid. MRI examinations can also be performed by administering an intravenous contrast agent to artificially alter the contrast between the T_1 or T_2 values of the tissue and the lesion, in other words, the signal intensity of the T_1WI, or T_2WI images, to facilitate the detection and diagnosis of the lesion.

MRI examinations can be performed in multiple sequences, of which the most commonly used are spin echo (SE) sequences for T_1WI; turbo SE (TSE) or fast SE (FSE) sequences for T_2WI and PDWI and gradient echo (GRE) sequences are mainly used to acquire T_1WI, and T_2^*WI; inversion recovery (IR) sequences include short-time IR sequences for fat suppression and long-time IR sequences for free water suppression, i.e., fluid-attenuated inversion recovery (FLAIR) sequences; echo planar imaging (EPI) sequences are a fast imaging sequence mainly used for diffusion-weighted imaging (DWI), perfusion-weighted imaging (PWI), and functional imaging.

MR also allows for multidirectional tomography. In the clinical application of cranial diseases, MRI examinations routinely acquire axial, coronal, and sagittal tomographic images. Sometimes tomography of the inclined plane can also be performed according to diagnostic needs. The combination of multidirectional images can clearly demonstrate the anatomical relationship of tissue structures and help to clarify the origin and extent of the lesion.

Another outstanding advantage of MR images in terms of high soft tissue resolution is to facilitate the identification of normal structures and tissue types of lesions. In addition, some specific imaging sequences and imaging methods facilitate further confirmation of the histological features of the lesion. For example, subacute hemorrhage and fat tissue present similar hyperintense on T_1WI and T_2WI; however, when frequency-selective fat suppression technique is applied, the fat tissue is suppressed to low signal, while subacute hemorrhage remains high signal. Another example is that calcification and hemosiderin both present hypointense on T_2WI, which is difficult to distinguish from each other, but can be differentiated by applying GRE sequences or susceptibility weighted imaging (SWI), which show different signal intensities due to their different magnetization rates. The different imaging sequences and methods of MRI can facilitate the identification and diagnosis of lesions by accurately identifying the different histological types of normal structures and lesions.

In addition, MRI enables a variety of specific structural and functional imaging, which can reflect information on structural and functional aspects of the brain and structural and functional changes resulting from lesions. These special imaging methods include cerebral angiography, DWI, diffusion tensor imaging (DTI), PWI, magnetic resonance spectroscopy (MRS), SWI, and functional magnetic resonance imaging (fMRI).

1.3.2 Commonly Used MR Examinations for Infectious and Inflammatory Diseases of the Brain and Spinal Cord

1. *MRI plain and enhanced scans*: MRI plain scan is performed for patients without contrast injection. Presently, the majority of routine clinical examinations are MRI plain scans. However, when there is a large overlap between the relaxation times of normal and abnormal tissues, the MR signal of the lesioned tissue is similar to that of the normal tissue, and the lesioned tissue cannot be effectively distinguished on plain scan, or when the lesion can be detected on plain scan but the edges and internal structures of the lesioned tissue are not well visualized, it is necessary to inject contrast agent for the patient to increase the contrast, which is enhanced MR scan.

   Enhanced MR scan can help detect lesions that cannot be identified on plain scan and have an important role in the examination of many diseases. When contrast agent is injected intravenously into the patient, the distribution concentration of contrast agent varies among different tissues, and the contrast agent also affects the relaxation time of the tissues, which makes the difference between the images of normal and diseased tissues more pronounced and makes it easy to distinguish the lesions from the normal tissues. As an example, gadolinium-based contrast agents are the most widely used MRI contrast agents in clinical practice due to their strong paramagnetic effect. Gadolinium-based contrast agents achieve signal enhancement by altering the microenvironment of the lesion area, shortening the T_1 relaxation time, and accentuating the high signal on the T_1WI image.
2. *MRA*: Refers to a magnetic resonance imaging technique that uses the characteristics of blood flow to contrast the MR signal difference between blood flow and surrounding relatively stationary tissue [10]. MRA is widely used for clinical measurement of blood flow velocity, examination of lesions in blood vessels and surrounding tissues, etc., and is generally imaged using the GRE sequence. The MRA can be divided into two main categories, black blood and bright blood, based on the black and white of the blood displayed. Bright blood techniques can be fur-

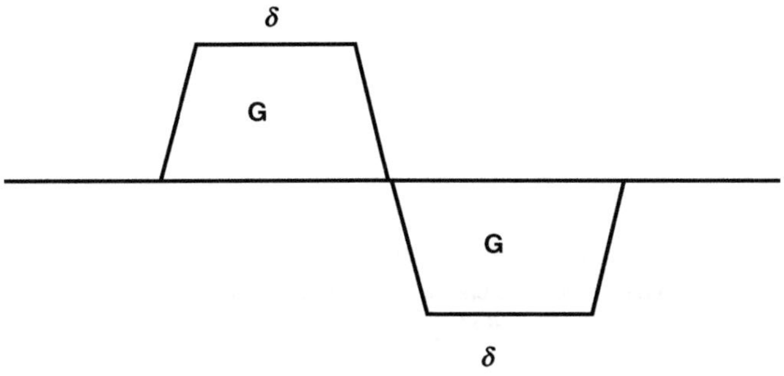

Fig. 1.3 Symmetric gradients applied in PCA imaging. *G* represents the gradient strength; δ represents the length of the gradient

ther divided into those with and without contrast enhancement [11].

The common methods of bright blood MRA examination are time-of-flight (TOF) and phase-contrast angiography (PCA) [12]. TOF is the most commonly used non-enhanced angiography method, which primarily utilizes RF pulses to saturate the tissues at the imaging site. These tissues appear as hypointense on the image because they are saturated, while the blood inside the vessel flows into the imaging site due to its flow characteristics, so that the blood inside the vessel appears as hyperintense on the image, thus enabling the differentiation between the vessel and the surrounding tissues. Two-dimensional TOF and three-dimensional TOF are commonly used in clinical practice. Two-dimensional TOF has a wide range of applications in angiography at sites where the direction of blood flow is perpendicular to the imaging plane, such as carotid arteries and peripheral vessels. Three-dimensional TOF is widely used in intracranial vascular imaging because of its ability to obtain high signal-to-noise ratio and spatial resolution.

PCA is achieved by applying two symmetrical gradients to the imaging site (Fig. 1.3; the gradients have the same amplitude and duration and opposite polarity). For stationary tissues, the positive and negative gradients produce equal scattering and regrouping phases, and their total phase change is zero; for flowing tissues, the positive and negative gradients produce a nonzero phase change due to their flow effects, so that the vessels and stationary tissues produce phase contrast. The strength of the phase is proportional to the velocity of blood flow in the vessel, and the direction of blood flow can also be determined from the positive and negative phases.

Balanced steady-state free precession (bSSFP)-MRA is another contrast-free angiography [13], in which the image contrast is determined by T_2/T_1 value. BSSFP sequence keeps the corresponding balance in each gradient direction, reduces the signal loss caused by blood flow, and can image in any blood flow direction. On bSSFP-MRA images, the arteries and veins both show hyperintensity, which is suitable for the imaging of thoracic aorta and coronary artery.

Black blood MRA suppresses the blood signal flowing in the blood vessel and retains the signal of surrounding static tissue, so that the blood on the blood vessel image displays hypointensity. The black blood signal can be achieved by accelerating the flow dispersion phase (fast spin echo sequence) or according to the T_1 value and T_2 value of blood and tissue (inversion recovery sequence).

Bright blood MRA can be divided into contrast-enhanced angiography and non-contrast-enhanced angiography. Arterial spin labeling (ASL)-MRA, bSSFP-MRA, TOF, and PC are all contrast-free-enhanced angiography [14].

Contrast-enhanced MR angiography (CE-MRA) is performed by high-pressure injection of a contrast-enhancing agent (e.g., gadolinium preparation), which is used to shorten the T_1 and T_2 relaxation times of the blood, thereby revealing the vasculature of the diseased tissue [15]. The advantages of CE-MRA over contrast-free MRA (e.g., time-of-flight and phase-contrast methods) are shorter acquisition times, improved imaging range, and reduced magnetization rate artifacts caused by blood flow and pulsation.

Magnetic resonance venography (MRV) refers to the technique of imaging the veins, which is usually performed using contrast injection or phase contrast. MRV is an important method for evaluating the intracranial venous system and diseases [16].

3. *Structural MRI*: It refers to the structural image that is scanned at high resolution in MRI, usually three-dimensional high-resolution T_1WI. Taking structural images of the human brain as an example, on the one hand, structural images have good gray-white matter contrast, which can be used to examine abnormal changes in tissue structure and even to quantify the volume of white or gray matter in specific brain regions; on the other hand, the clear gray-white matter contrast of structural images of the brain can be used to provide accurate localization for subsequent examinations, such as the positioning of the spectrum of the scan and the alignment of the anterior-posterior association during functional image scanning. In addition, structural images can be useful for post-processing of data, e.g., in functional brain data analysis, structural images are used to segment and align to stan-

dard brain templates, enabling more accurate alignment and analysis of functional images.

1.4 DSA Imaging Technique

Yuehua Li, Jian Zhang, and Kai Shang

1.4.1 Principle of DSA Imaging

DSA is a new examination method that combines computer and conventional X-ray angiography and was first developed by the Mistretta group at the University of Wisconsin and the Nadelman group at the University of Arizona in the 1980s. The basic content of subtraction technique is to subtract two frames of the same part of the human body, so as to obtain their difference part; the image without contrast agent is called mask image or mask, and the image obtained after injecting contrast agent is called contrast image or filled image. The image signal following subtraction is correlated with the absorption coefficient of the contrast agent and blood vessels, proportional to the thickness of the contrast agent and independent of the background. In subtracted images, background images such as bones and soft tissues are eliminated, leaving only images of blood vessels containing contrast (Fig. 1.4) [17].

The DSA imaging system consists of five components by function and structure: (1) X-ray machine with stable radiation quality; (2) fast image processing device; (3) X-ray positioning system and frame; (4) system control component; and (5) external equipment such as image display, storage, and network transmission component.

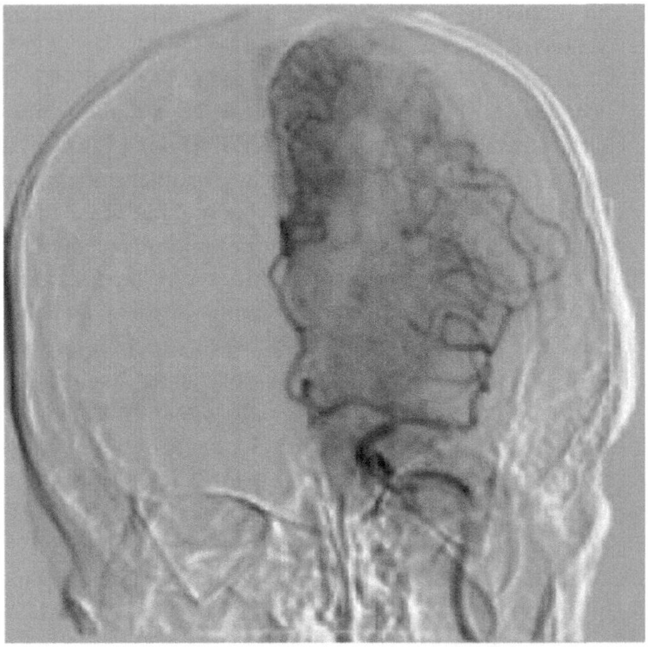

Fig. 1.4 Cranial DSA examination technique. Left internal carotid artery angiography

1.4.2 DSA Imaging Methods Commonly Used for Infectious and Inflammatory Diseases of the Brain and Spinal Cord

1. *The pulsed image mode*: Utilizes intermittent X-ray pulses to acquire the mask image when the contrast agent is not flowing into the vessel of interest, and the X-ray image is acquired and subtracted during the process of gradual diffusion of the contrast agent to obtain a series of continuous and interval subtracted images, with a large interval between each subtracted image frame and a high signal-to-noise ratio of the acquired images which are suitable for such areas as cerebral vessels, carotid arteries, hepatic arteries, and arteries of the extremities where the activity is slow.
2. *The super-pulsed method*: It performs X-ray pulse photography at a rate of 6–30 frames/s, followed by high-speed repeated subtraction frame by frame, enabling continuous observation of X-ray digital images or subtracted images at the speed of real-time video, with high dynamic clarity. It is suitable for fast-moving parts such as pulmonary arteries, coronary arteries, and heart.
3. *The continuous image mode*: The X-ray used can be either continuous or pulsed X-rays, obtaining a continuous image with a frequency of 25 or 30 frames/s synchronized with the camera, showing fast-moving parts with high temporal resolution.

With the development of technology, DSA systems also feature some specialized functions, such as rotational DSA, three-dimensional DSA, real-time smoothed mask (RSM) DSA, etc. Rotational DSA is an examination method to achieve dynamic observation by injecting contrast agent for exposure acquisition during the rotation of the C-arm, which can obtain angiographic images from different angles, increasing the observation angle and showing diseased vessels with more advantages. Three-dimensional DSA is a product of the combination of rotational angiography, DSA technology, and computerized three-dimensional image processing technology, which can display three-dimensional images of blood vessels through post-processing such as VR and surface-shaded display (SSD) by workstations. It has overcome the problem of overlapping vascular structures, to provide more anatomical details and cerebral blood flow information for the observation of vascular lesions and localization measurement as well as diagnosis of vascular stenosis, offering the necessary conditions for various interventions [18, 19]. RSM-DSA is an alternative subtraction method for DSA. It allows the acquisition of subtraction images in a single motion after contrast injection, avoiding the tedious process of two motion acquisitions and the possibility of subtraction failure due to patient movement between acquisitions.

Cerebral angiography can be divided into whole brain angiography, selective cerebral angiography, and superselective cerebral angiography. During the operation, the femoral artery is often punctured and cannulated, bilateral vertebral arteries and common carotid arteries are imaged separately, and superselective angiography is performed according to the condition. DSA shows the full-time course of cerebral circulation and blood flow compensation, which has obvious advantages in the diagnosis and interventional treatment of intracranial vascular diseases. In cerebral vasculitis, DSA can clearly show the inflammatory changes in blood vessels caused by various reasons, such as stenosis or occlusion of blood vessels in different areas, tortuosity and stiffness of blood vessel travel, a few arterial dilatation or aneurysm caused by inflammation damaging the middle layer of the arterial wall, etc. It is the gold standard for the diagnosis of various vascular inflammatory diseases. However, the diagnosis of vascular inflammatory diseases requires a combination of clinical manifestations and laboratory findings, as some of the vascular changes in cerebrovascular inflammatory diseases are nonspecific and may even be negative. DSA can also be used for long-term follow-up observation of structural damage to the patient's blood vessels.

However, DSA has some limitation. First, its main contraindications are as follows [5]: (1) those with severe bleeding tendency; (2) those with severe cardiac, hepatic, or renal insufficiency; and (3) those with contrast allergy. Second, DSA imaging has certain limitations, mainly including the following: (1) The patient needs to be highly cooperative during the imaging and avoid all random movements; (2) although DSA is good for displaying small arterial branches, it cannot yet display tiny vessels with a diameter of <0.2 mm; (3) involuntary movements (such as swallowing, breathing, and gastrointestinal peristalsis) can produce artifacts and affect image clarity.

1.5 Radionuclide Imaging Techniques

Yongde Qin, Xiaohong Li, and Xin Gao

1.5.1 Principles of Positron Emission Computed Tomography

Positron emission computed tomography (PET) is the use of positronium nuclides to label or synthesize the corresponding imaging agent, which is introduced into the body and localized in the target organ. These nuclides emit positrons during the decay process, which, after a short distance in the tissue, interact with the negative electrons in the surrounding material, resulting in annihilation radiation and the emission of two photons with opposite directions and equal energy (511 keV). PET employs a series of detectors arranged in pairs at 180° to each other and connected to a conformal line to detect annihilating radiation photons, thereby obtaining a tomographic distribution of positronium in the body and the location, morphology, size, metabolism, and function of the lesion to diagnose the disease. Since PET utilizes positron emitter markers such as ^{11}C, ^{13}N, ^{15}O, and ^{18}F (similar to the biological behavior of H), which are essential elements in the normal tissue structure of the human body, as imaging agents and uses drugs such as deoxyglucose, amino acids, choline, thymine, ligands of receptors, and blood flow imaging agents as tracers, it can display the metabolism, function, blood flow, cell proliferation, and receptor distribution of the body and focal tissue cells at the molecular level, providing more physiological and pathological diagnostic information for clinical purposes [20].

1.5.2 Positron Emission Computed Tomography Methods Commonly Used in Infectious and Inflammatory Diseases of the Brain and Spinal Cord

1. *PET brain metabolic imaging*: The human brain is very metabolically active, and its functional activity is extremely complex. Brain metabolic imaging is of great importance in studying the changing patterns of functional metabolic activities of the central nervous system and in exploring brain diseases. Glucose is almost the only energy substance for brain tissue, and changes in the rate of glucose metabolism in the brain can reflect the functional activity of the brain. Fluorodeoxyglucose (^{18}F-FDG) is a glucose analog with the same cellular transport and hexokinase phosphorylation process as glucose but remains in brain cells after conversion to ^{18}F-FDG-6-P, which is no longer involved in further glucose metabolism. Observations and measurements of the distribution of ^{18}F-FDG in the brain will provide insight into the state of glucose metabolism in the brain. Its clinical applications mainly include localization and diagnosis of epileptic foci; diagnosis and condition assessment of Alzheimer's disease; differentiation, staging, and grading of benign and malignant brain tumors; determination of efficacy and prognosis; and diagnosis of recurrent and residual lesions. Most active foci of infection demonstrate high uptake of ^{18}F-FDG, which can therefore be utilized to detect foci of infection, respond to the glucose metabolic activity of infected lesions, and allow assessment of treatment efficacy. For PET/MRI, FDG uptake is corroborated by MRI findings.

   In addition to glucose metabolic imaging, there are also oxygen metabolic imaging (^{15}O), amino acid metabolic imaging (^{11}C-MET, ^{18}F-FET), nucleic acid metabolic imaging (^{18}F-FLT), lack of oxygen metabolic imaging (^{18}F-FMISO), and choline metabolic imaging (^{11}C-CHO). Cerebral metabolic imaging allows to obtain cerebral oxygen metabolic rate and oxygen extraction fraction, which are important indicators of the level of cerebral oxygen metabolism. Amino acid metabolic imaging mainly reflects the level of protein anabolism in the brain, while neuronal cells in the normal adult brain are mostly mature cells; hence, there is no significant protein synthesis. The tumor cells show high amino acid uptake in conjunction with high glucose metabolism and accelerated amino acid transport to meet the demand of cell growth and proliferation, which therefore manifests as high amino acid uptake, coupled with very low amino acid uptake by normal brain cells, thus accentuating the lesion. Amino acid metabolic imaging (^{11}C-MET, ^{18}F-FET) has a low background in the brain, and infectious lesions show mild to moderate metabolic elevation. It is presently used for the differential diagnosis of infectious lesions, demyelinating lesions, and tumors. Choline metabolism is the entry of ^{11}C-CHO into the cell through specific transporters, and after intracellular metabolism, the end product phosphatidylcholine is integrated into the cell membrane. The rate of choline uptake by cells reflects the rate of cell membrane synthesis, and thus it can be used as an indicator of tumor cell proliferation and division, which is a direct or indirect tracer of tumor cell proliferation and division [21].

2. *PET neuroreceptor imaging*: Neuroreceptor imaging is designed to obtain parameters such as receptor distribution, density, and affinity of receptors by PET, which is based on receptor-ligand-specific binding through the use of positron emitting radionuclides to label specific ligands in the living human brain. The synthesis, release, binding to postsynaptic membrane receptors, and reuptake of specific central neurotransmitters can be observed using radionuclide-labeled precursors of synthetic neurotransmitters, which is called neurotransmitter imaging. The quantitative or semiquantitative parameters of central neurotransmitters or receptors can be obtained through physiological mathematical models, allowing for diagnosis, treatment decisions, efficacy assessment, and prognosis of certain neurotransmitter- or receptor-related diseases. The main neuroreceptors that are presently being studied and applied are the dopamine receptor (dopamine receptor), the acetylcholine receptor, 5-serotonin receptor, benzodiazepine receptor, opioid receptor, etc. [22].
3. *PET/MR brain imaging*:

   PET/MR is a large functional metabolic and molecular imaging diagnostic device that combines positron emission tomography and magnetic resonance imaging technology. Compared with other examinations, PET/MR is highly sensitive and accurate, especially for early detection, early diagnosis, and accurate assessment of neurodegenerative diseases without obvious structural changes, such as Alzheimer's disease, epilepsy, and Parkinson's disease. In addition, it has incomparable advantages for the identification of benign and malignant intracranial malignant tumors, the determination of malignant glioma borders, the identification of posttreatment radiation necrosis and recurrence of tumors, and the accurate selection of tumor biopsy sites by other imaging means [23].

References

1. Omran AR. The epidemiologic transition: a theory of the epidemiology of population change. Milbank Mem Fund Q. 2005;83(4):731–57.
2. Wang K, Xiao J. Analysis of the principles and applications of digital X-ray technology. Med Equip. 2015;28(1):23–4.
3. Ahluwalia GK. Applications of chalcogenides: S, Se and Te. Cham: Springer; 2017.
4. Salvini E, Pedroli G, Montanari G. Digital storage phosphor radiography. Doses and image quality. Radiol Med. 1994;87(6):847–51.
5. Bai R, Zhang X. Medical imageology. 3rd ed. Beijing: People's Medical Publishing House; 2010.
6. Zhang H, Yu HL, Hu ML. Value of CT scanning methods in diagnosis of patients with intracranial infections. Chin J Nosocomiol. 2018;28(5):715–7, 725.
7. Shi M, Gao J. Clinical application of spectrum CT in angiography. Chin Med Dev. 2016;31(7):6–8.
8. Ren QG, Sli Y, Li JY. The basic principle and clinical applications of CT spectral imaging. Int J Med Radiol. 2011;34(6):559–63.
9. Huang R, Li Y. Clinical applications and research advances in energy spectrum CT. Radiol Pract. 2015;30(1):81–3.
10. Hartung MP, Grist TM, Francois CJ. Magnetic resonance angiography: current status and future directions. J Cardiovasc Magn Reson. 2011;13:19.
11. Wheaton AJ, Miyazaki M. Non-contrast enhanced MR angiography: physical principles. J Magn Reson Imaging. 2012;36:286–304.
12. Saloner D. The AAPM/RSNA physics tutorial for residents. An introduction to MR angiography. Radiographics. 1995;15(2):453–65.
13. Miyazaki M, Lee VS. Nonenhanced MR angiography. Radiology. 2008;248:20–43.
14. Moran PR. A flow velocity zeugmatographic interlace for NMR imaging in human. Magn Reson Imaging. 1982;1:197–203.
15. Moran PR, Moran RA, Karstaedt N. Verification and evaluation of internal flow and motion. True magnetic resonance imaging by the phase gradient modulation method. Radiology. 1985;154:433–41.
16. Bryant DJ, Payne JA, Firmin DN, et al. Measurement of flow with NMR imaging using a gradient pulse and phase difference technique. J Comput Assist Tomogr. 1984;8:588–93.
17. Ai M, Ruan X, Wang Y, et al. The history, current status and future trends of digital subtraction. Med Equip. 2000;13(6):1–6.
18. Gailloud P, Oishi S, Carpenter J, et al. Three-dimensional digital angiography: new tool for simultaneous three-dimensional rendering of vascular and osseous information during rotational angiography. Am J Neuroradiol. 2004;4(4):571–3.
19. Abe T, Hirohata M, Tanaka N. Clinical benefits of rotational 3D angiography in endovascular treatment of ruptured cerebral aneurysm. Am J Neuroradiol. 2002;23(4):686–8.
20. Santiago JFY. Positron emission tomography with computed tomography (PET/CT). New York: Springer; 2015.
21. Christian PE, Waterstram-Rich KM. Nuclear medicine and PET/CT. 7th ed. Amsterdam: Elsevier; 2011.
22. Wang H, Zuo C, Huang Z, et al. 11C-CFT brain PET clinical application of imaging in the diagnosis of early Parkinson's disease. Chin J Clin Med Imaging. 2010;21(4):229–32.
23. Wu Y, Sun X, Lin S, Bao Z. Application of combined PET/MR imaging. Radiol Pract. 2015;13(6):104–6.

2 Functional and Molecular Imaging Techniques

He Wang, Qianfeng Wang, Yongde Qin, Xin Gao, Chunhui Jiang, and Liling Peng

Conventional imaging is able to show all aspects of human anatomy; however, it is incapable of visualizing the physiological and pathophysiological processes of the human body. With the rapid advancement of imaging technology, functional and molecular imaging is gradually moving from experimental studies to clinical applications, providing dynamic and functional information of the human body and developing to analyze the pathogeny for diseases at the cellular and molecular levels.

2.1 Functional Imaging

He Wang, Qianfeng Wang, and Yongde Qin

With the gradual improvement of modern imaging technology, functional imaging has shown excellent ability in diagnosis and differential diagnosis of diseases, and emerged innovative techniques can more accurately and safely present the functional state of tissues and organs. The more established functional imaging methods in clinical practice include CT perfusion imaging (CTP), perfusion-weighted imaging (PWI), diffusion-weighted imaging (DWI), diffusion tensor imaging (DTI), blood oxygenation level-dependent (BOLD) magnetic resonance imaging (MRI), susceptibility-weighted imaging (SWI), and dynamic contrast-enhanced magnetic resonance imaging (DCE-MRI).

2.1.1 CT Functional Imaging

CTP consists of multiple successive isotropic scans of selected layers, while contrast is injected intravenously. The interval between each scan is 0.5–1 s. The time-density curve is obtained for each pixel in the level, and the horizontal coordinate of the curve is the time, and the vertical coordinate is the increased CT value after contrast injection, which shows the change of contrast concentration in the organ and consequently indirectly reflects the change of blood perfusion in the tissue and organ. In cranial perfusion, parameters such as cerebral blood flow (CBF), cerebral blood volume (CBV), mean transit time (MTT), time to peak (TTP), and capillary permeability (PS), which are calculated based on time-density curves, can be obtained after image reconstruction and pseudocolor staining, reflecting the perfusion status of brain tissue. CBF is the blood flow flowing through a certain amount of cerebral vascular in unit time, in mL/(min · 100 g). CBV is the total volume of blood present in a certain amount of vascular structures of brain tissue, measured in mL/100 g. MTT is the average time it takes for blood to pass through specific brain tissues via different pathways, which is the time it takes for blood to circulate from the arterial terminal to the venous terminal, usually measured in seconds (s). TTP is the time, in seconds, from the initiation of the contrast agent to its peak on the time-density curve. PS is the rate of unidirectional leakage of contrast agent from the endovascular to the tissue interstitial space, measured in mL/(min · 100 g). Alterations in microcirculation of local cerebral tissue blood flow are suggestive for the detection of lesions.

The theoretical basis of CTP is the radiotracer dilution principle and the central volume law of nuclear medicine:

H. Wang (✉)
Institute of Brain-like Intelligence Science and Technology, Fudan University, Shanghai, China
e-mail: hewang@fudan.edu.cn

Q. Wang
Fudan University, Shanghai, China
e-mail: qianfengwang@fudan.edu.cn

Y. Qin · C. Jiang
The First Affiliated Hospital of Xinjiang Medical University, Urumqi, China

X. Gao · L. Peng
Shanghai Universal Medical Imaging Diagnostic Center, Shanghai University, Shanghai, China

H. Li et al. (eds.), *Radiology of Infectious and Inflammatory Diseases - Volume 1*,
https://doi.org/10.1007/978-981-99-0039-8_2

BF = BV/MTT. The principles of nuclear medicine perfusion imaging are also applicable to CT perfusion in that the iodine-containing contrast agent essentially meets the requirements of a non-diffusive tracer.

There are two main algorithms for CTP: non-deconvolution and deconvolution. The non-deconvolution algorithm is simpler by neglecting the effect of intravenous outflow of the contrast agent, and assuming that there is no extravasation and recirculation of the contrast agent, i.e., the first-pass effect of the contrast agent is used to calculate each parameter. This algorithm tends to underestimate CBF and requires a large injection rate for contrast injection, which increases the difficulty and risk of the operation, although it is simple. The deconvolution algorithm, although complex, does not need to make some artificial assumptions about the hemodynamic situation of tissues and organs in advance, and it only takes into account the inflow of blood into the arteries and outflow of veins for mathematical calculation processing based on the actual situation, which reflects more realistically the amount of contrast agent accumulated in tissues and organs over time, and the calculation deviation is small and closer to the actual blood perfusion situation. In addition, the contrast agent injection rate requirement is relatively low (generally 4–5 mL/s), so the application prospect is wider. Figure 2.1 shows the brain CT perfusion image obtained using the deconvolution algorithm, which is a hemispheric perfusion image of a normal human with essentially the same perfusion in both hemispheres.

The quality of CT perfusion images is affected by several factors, including the total amount and rate of contrast agent injection and the cardiac function of the patient. Because of the short circulation time (3–5 s) and low relative CBV, it is essential to obtain high-quality images by injecting the appropriate amount of contrast agent as soon as possible to

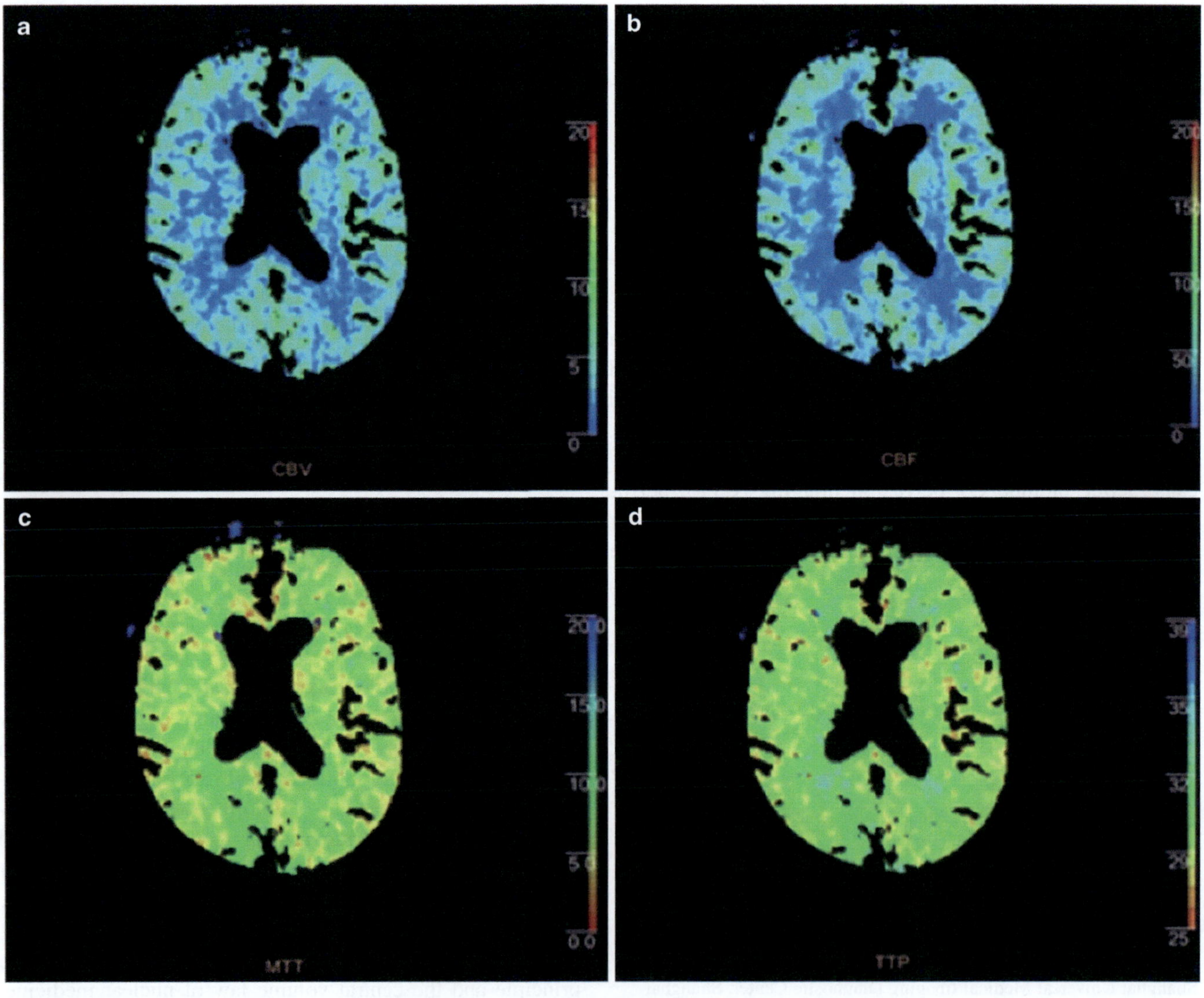

Fig. 2.1 Brain CT perfusion images. (**a**) CBV; (**b**) CBF; (**c**) MTT; (**d**) TTP

ensure that it is in the brain tissue and not escaping from the venous system before the data are acquired and the time-density curve peaks. If the injection rate is too low, the contrast agent may flow out of the tissue from the vein before it reaches its peak, and the CT values obtained at this time may not truly reflect the perfusion of the brain tissue, and the resulting peak time-density curve may be low and the TTP will be increased.

2.1.2 MR Functional Imaging

1. **DWI**. Diffusion is the random motion (Brownian motion) of water molecules within tissues due to thermal energy. The free motion of water molecules is affected by the presence of some obstacles such as cell membranes, organelles, and biomolecules, and thus the diffusion of water molecules varies from tissue to tissue, and this diffusion contrast is highlighted by DWI with magnetic resonance through specific motion sensitive sequences.

   Magnetic resonance DWI offers different contrast of different tissues than conventional MRI images, and it is very sensitive in showing the identification of acute cerebral infarction and other acute brain lesions, which also play a very important role in the identification of most tumors in various parts of the body, and has become an important supplement to conventional MRI examinations. However, the importance of DWI in the field of magnetic resonance is not only its prominence in qualitative analysis, but, more importantly, DWI offers a new set of quantitative parameters that are primarily dependent on the motion of water molecules rather than on the proton density, T_1 or T_2 values of the tissue. With the continuous development of DWI technology and the establishment of different models, DWI quantification parameters are continuously enlarged.

   The most basic sequence of DWI is the Stejskal-Tanner spin-echo (SE) diffusion sequence [1] (Fig. 2.2), in which two symmetrical diffusion-sensitive gradients are added before and after the 180° pulse of the SE sequence; for stationary (weakly diffused) water molecules, the proton spin scattered by the first gradient pulse will be reconverged by the second gradient pulse, and the signal will not be degraded. While for the moving (strongly diffused) water molecules, the scattered phase proton caused by first gradient pulse spin left the original position, the first gradient field is not the same gradient field due to the second gradient puls and the phase can no longer be fully reunited and the signal is reduced. The time required for diffusion imaging with conventional SE sequences is considerable, while slight movements of the subject can produce more pronounced motion artifacts. With the development of gradient technology, the SE-EPI DWI sequence is now the most commonly used in clinical practice, which can significantly reduce imaging time, reduce motion artifacts, and increase sensitivity to changes in signal intensity due to molecular motion.

   The apparent diffusion coefficient (ADC) is the most commonly used quantitative parameter of diffusion in clinical practice, which can characterize the diffusion of water molecules in tissues in a relatively simple way, and its mathematical model is a single exponential model, calculated as:

$$S(b)/S_0 = \exp(-b \times \mathrm{ADC}) \tag{2.1}$$

   where $S(b)$ is the signal strength when b takes a certain value, S_0 is the signal intensity when there is no diffusion weighting, and b can be calculated from a standard rectangular gradient pulse pair.

$$b = \gamma^2 G^2 \delta^2 (\Delta - \delta/3) \tag{2.2}$$

   where γ is the spin-to-magnetic ratio (H, 42.58 MHz/T), G is the intensity of the diffusion gradient magnetic field (motion probing gradients, MPG), δ is the duration of one MPG pulse, and Δ is the interval between the leading edges of two MPG pulses.

   According to Fick's law, true diffusion is the net motion of molecules due to concentration gradients. In

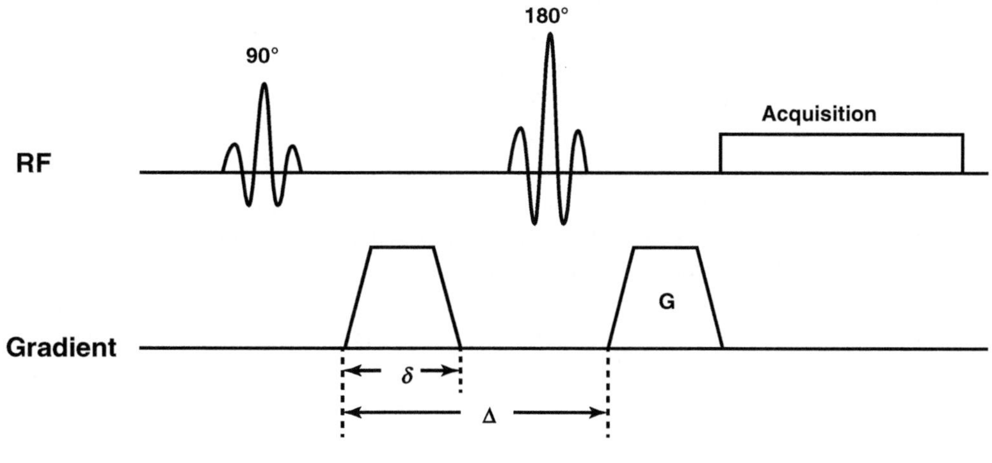

Fig. 2.2 Stejskal-Tanner SE diffusion sequence

MR imaging, the molecular motion due to concentration differences is indistinguishable from the blood flow motion within the vessel and therefore can only be termed the ADC, not the diffusion coefficient.

2. **DTI**. Under ideal conditions, the diffusion of water molecules is isotropic, i.e., the diffusion coefficient is identical in all directions; however, this is not the case in many tissues (e.g., white matter of the brain) in practical applications. To study the anisotropic diffusion of water molecules, a new technique, DTI, was developed based on conventional DWI, a concept originally proposed by Basser et al. [2].

   DTI can quantitatively characterize the direction of diffusive motion of water molecules in tissues in three dimensions. The most important concepts in DTI are the three eigenvectors and eigenvalues, which correspond to the direction and length of the three axes of the diffusion ellipsoid. Fractional anisotropy (FA) is the proportion of anisotropic components of water molecules to the total diffusion tensor with values ranging from 0 to 1. For isotropic media, the eigenvalues in the three directions are equal, and the FA value is 0. For columnar anisotropic media, the eigenvalues along the long axis of the column are much larger than those in the other two directions, and the FA value is close to 1. The known eigenvalues also allow the calculation of parameters such as relative anisotropy (RA) and volume ratio (VR), which are more commonly used in clinical applications for FA. Since there are six independent variables in the elements of the 3 × 3 matrix describing the DTI tensor, at least six directional diffusion images need to be acquired to calculate the eigenvalues. With the use of specific algorithms, DTI can provide anatomical and functional information about the brain and reconstruct the white matter fiber tracts of the brain that is not feasible with other imaging methods. DTI has significant implications for the diagnosis of cerebral white matter disease and cerebrovascular disease, the localization of lesions prior to neurosurgery, and the determination of the adjacent relationship between lesions and fiber tracts.

3. **Diffusion kurtosis imaging** (DKI) was originally proposed by Jensen et al. [3] in 2005 as an extension of DTI. The kurtosis is a quantity used to describe the characteristics of the curve, as shown in Fig. 2.3, where the kurtosis is 0; the curve has a Gaussian distribution, so in the field of diffusion, the kurtosis is used to characterize the extent to which the diffusion of water molecules deviates from the Gaussian distribution. With the introduction of kurtosis, the MR signal can be expressed as:

$$\ln\left[S(b)\right] = \ln\left[S(0)\right] - bD_{\text{app}} + \frac{1}{6}b^2 D_{\text{app}}^2 K_{\text{app}} + O\left(b^3\right) \quad (2.3)$$

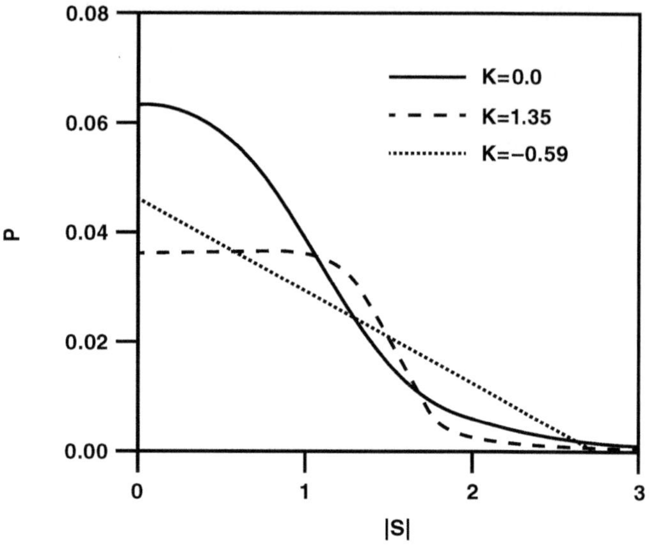

Fig. 2.3 Kurtosis (*K*) reflects the degree of deviation from the Gaussian line pattern

where K_{app} is the kurtosis and the higher order term $O(b^3)$ can usually be ignored. DKI data acquisition, like DTI, requires multiple directions. In addition, it is necessary to combine multiple *b* value acquisition to calculate the kurtosis, which makes the acquisition time longer than that of conventional DTI. However, the advantages of DKI over DTI are still evident, such as the absence of values for FA values at the intersection of gray and white matter fibrils in the brain, where DTI is unable to evaluate the lesion, while DKI is able to do so. DKI is now being increasingly used and has evolved from applications in the cerebral nervous system to other sites.

4. **Intravoxel Incoherent Motion (IVIM) Imaging**

   Both conventional DWI and DTI assume that the diffusion-weighted signal decays in a monoexponential manner as the *b* value increases, which is actually not valid in many cases, especially when the *b* value is high. The IVIM biexponential model can better describe this multi-exponential signal decay than the monoexponential model [4]. The double exponential model considers both fast diffusion proton pools and slow diffusion proton pools coexisting within each voxel, which is calculated as:

$$\frac{S(b)}{S_0} = f \times \exp\left(-bD_1\right) + \left(1 - f\right) \times \exp\left(-bD_2\right) \quad (2.4)$$

f and $(1 - f)$ are the volume rates of fast diffusing protons and slow diffusing protons, respectively; D_1 and D_2 are the corresponding ADC values. In practical situations, there are at least two typical cases of such fast and slow diffusion proton pools (Fig. 2.4).

In order to solve the (2.3) equation, multiple *b* value acquisitions are required for diffusion image acquisition,

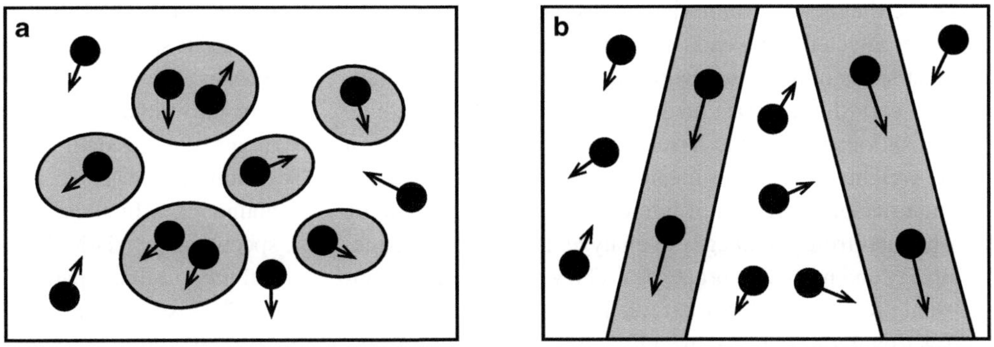

Fig. 2.4 Fast and slow diffusion proton pool. (**a**) Intracellular water molecules (fast diffusion) and extracellular water molecules (slow diffusion); (**b**) intravascular water molecules (fast diffusion, i.e., blood perfusion) and extravascular water molecules (slow diffusion)

and the number and size of b need to be determined depending on the actual situation (e.g., the site examined and the patient's condition). When solving, the more commonly used is the Marquardt-Levenberg algorithm; using this algorithm requires pre-set initial values, and inappropriate initial values can lead to a failure of the fit or fall into a local minimum and get the wrong result. In addition, the more variables that need to be fitted, the more difficult it is to set the initial values. To make the results more stable, there are some simplifications in certain applications, such as in this biexponential model of diffusion and perfusion in Fig. 2.4b, where it can be assumed that there is an order of magnitude difference in the diffusion and perfusion ADC, so that at high b values (e.g., $b > 200$), the fast diffusion component has decayed sufficiently, so that the curve for the high b value part can be considered as a monoexponential decay, and a simple linear fit gives the slow diffusion ADC and the volume rate, leaving the only unknown, and the fast diffusion ADC is also easily obtained. Another simplification is to fix the unimportant parameters and fit the remaining two parameters.

5. **Perfusion Imaging Technique**

Magnetic resonance perfusion imaging is a MRI technique that reflects tissue microvascular distribution and blood perfusion and can provide information on hemodynamic aspects [5]. Perfusion imaging is generally used to diagnose diseases by continuously scanning tracers within the blood vessels or injected into the body to reflect the hemodynamic characteristics of local blood flow according to the changes in the local signal [6]. Magnetic resonance perfusion imaging has been widely used for the qualitative and differential diagnosis of intracranial neoplastic lesions, tumor grading, and prognostic rating.

Commonly used perfusion imaging methods are dynamic magnetization rate contrast (DSC), dynamic contrast enhanced (DCE), and arterial spin labeling (ASL) [7]. Both DSC and DCE require intravenous contrast enhancement, while ASL does not require intravenous contrast injection. DSC is also known as MR PWI. DSC features high temporal resolution and no radioactivity and has been widely used in clinical practice. The parameters commonly used in DSC are CBV, relative cerebral blood volume (rCBV), and MTT.

DSC perfusion imaging requires intravenous injection of a paramagnetic contrast agent (e.g., gadolinium contrast), and images are typically acquired using T_2^*-weighted fast gradient echo (GRE) or planar echo sequences (EPI). Since contrast agents are generally paramagnetic or superparamagnetic, the influx of contrast agents into the capillary bed may increase the energy exchange between hydrogen protons and the external environment, accelerate the recovery of hydrogen protons from the excited state to the equilibrium state, and shorten the longitudinal relaxation time (T_1) on the one hand; on the other hand, the contrast agents that enter the vessels will generate additional fields, increase the local field inhomogeneity around the vessels, and, together with the diffusion of contrast agents among the tissues, increase the scattered phase of protons, thus shortening the transverse relaxation time (T_2) and quasi-transverse relaxation time (T_2^*) of the tissues. The blood-brain barrier of normal brain tissue prevents the outward penetration of the intravascular contrast agent, which results in a significant difference in magnetization rate inside and outside the vessel, and the difference in magnetization rate causes changes in the magnetic field of the vascular appendage, resulting in a decrease in the transverse relaxation time of the extravascular tissue protons. The DSC perfusion method reflects the microvascular perfusion characteristics by continuous measurement of the blood flow signal over time when the contrast agent first enters the capillary, and generally 1–2 min is sufficient to complete the data acquisition. Long TR is generally used for DSC perfusion imaging, which minimizes the effect of T_1 weighting in the image signal.

DCE, like DSC, requires injection of exogenous contrast agent to reflect the microcirculatory characteristics before, during, and after blood inflow into organs or tissues and can quantitatively or semi-quantitatively measure changes in tissue hemodynamics and is widely used in the diagnosis of tumorigenic lesions [8]. The contrast agent injected intravenously accumulates in the extracellular space of the tissue by perfusion through the capillaries, and the contrast agent shortens the longitudinal relaxation time of the tissue. Repeated scanning of fast T_1-weighted sequences means that the curve of the signal intensity of the region of interest (ROI) over time can be obtained from the images to analyze the capillary permeability and perfusion properties. The volume transfer constant (K_{trans}), fractional extracellular space volume (V_e), fractional plasma volume (V_p) and the interstitium-to-plasma rate constant (K_{ep}) are commonly used quantitative parameters for DCE.

ASL perfusion imaging does not require an exogenous contrast agent but instead uses the patient's own water molecules to act as an endogenous tracer, which is clinically easy to perform and relatively safe [9]. ASL can be classified as continuous arterial spin labeling (CASL), pulsed arterial spin labeling (PASL), and pseudo continuous arterial spin labeling (pCASL) according to the way of labeling arterial blood [10]. ASL is mainly used for perfusion imaging of the skull and brain, labeling the protons in the internal carotid artery, requiring two acquisitions of labeled and unlabeled images. Saturation pulses and 180° pulse flips can be used to label protons. The 180° pulse flip method has a 2× signal dynamic range and a higher signal-to-noise ratio in the image. With a 180° flip pulse, blood protons upstream of the imaging site, i.e., in the internal carotid artery, are flipped (labeled), and the image acquisition begins when the labeled protons flow into the area contained in the FOV, resulting in a labeled image. The unmarked image is generally achieved by applying two successive 180° flip pulses so that the magnetization vector of the protons in the internal carotid artery corresponds to a return to the original position. Finally, the non-labeled image is subtracted from the labeled image to obtain the perfusion image of the cranial vasculature.

6. **Magnetic Resonance Spectroscopy (MRS) Imaging**

It is theoretically metabolic imaging and belongs to the same molecular level of imaging as DWI, so it is presented here together. MRS is presently the only technique for noninvasive detection of chemical properties of metabolites in living tissues which can provide important information in the diagnosis of tumors and quantification of metabolites in psychiatric diseases, making it an important tool for clinical measurement of metabolites and study of tissue lesions [11].

The commonly used magnetic resonance spectra include ^{1}H spectrum, ^{13}C spectrum, ^{19}F spectrum, ^{31}P spectrum, ^{15}N spectrum, etc. The signal intensity of magnetic resonance spectra is related to the abundance of nuclei and their content in living tissues. Generally, the signals of nuclei with low content in living tissues, such as ^{13}C spectrum, ^{19}F spectrum, ^{31}P spectrum, ^{15}N spectrum, etc., are weaker. The measurement of low content nuclei is generally only done in scientific research and animal experiments due to their low signal-to-noise ratio and long scanning time. The content of water in living organisms is abundant, which is why magnetic resonance hydrogen spectroscopy (^{1}H-MRS) is the most commonly used spectral measurement parameter in clinical practice [12].

The tissues contain different components and are in different chemical environments. The resonance frequencies of the hydrogen protons in the tissues are different due to the effect of electron shielding, which are in different magnetic environments, and this change in frequency is represented by the chemical shift δ in the wave spectrum:

$$\delta = \frac{\omega - \omega_{ref}}{\omega_{ref}} \tag{2.5}$$

The chemical shifts expressed in this way are independent of the strength of the external magnetic field. The chemical shifts are expressed in parts per million (ppm).

The goal of in vivo MRS is the noninvasive quantification of metabolic compounds in living tissue. The area of the spectral peak obtained by MRS is proportional to the number of nuclei in the selected VOI, and therefore the concentration of metabolites can be quantified by measuring the area of the spectral peak. Depending on the VOI selection method, two heavily used spectral sequences, point-resolved spectroscopy (PRESS) and stimulated-echo acquisition mode (STEAM), are used for monomeric spectroscopy [13].

PRESS uses two 180° repolymerization pulses after the first 90° pulse, and the gradient of the selected layer is added in three orthogonal directions (Fig. 2.5), and the method of localizing VOI using the PRESS technique is also known as the double SE method [14]. In contrast, the STEAM method for locating VOI is similar to PRESS (Fig. 2.6), except that STEAM uses three 90° pulses for excitation of the selected layers, and the signal intensity of the obtained spectrum is half of that of the PRESS signal with the same parameters [15].

MRS is generally a signal acquisition for a specific tissue region with relatively weak signal strength, and the signal-to-noise ratio of the spectrum can be improved by increasing the averaging times. MRS also requires high homogeneity of the magnetic field, and it is important to effectively homogenize the field in the ROI prior to data acquisition. In the case of hydrogen spectrum, for example, the water content in human tissues is much higher than that of metabolites, so the water peak (at 4.7 ppm) in the hydrogen spectrum is much higher than

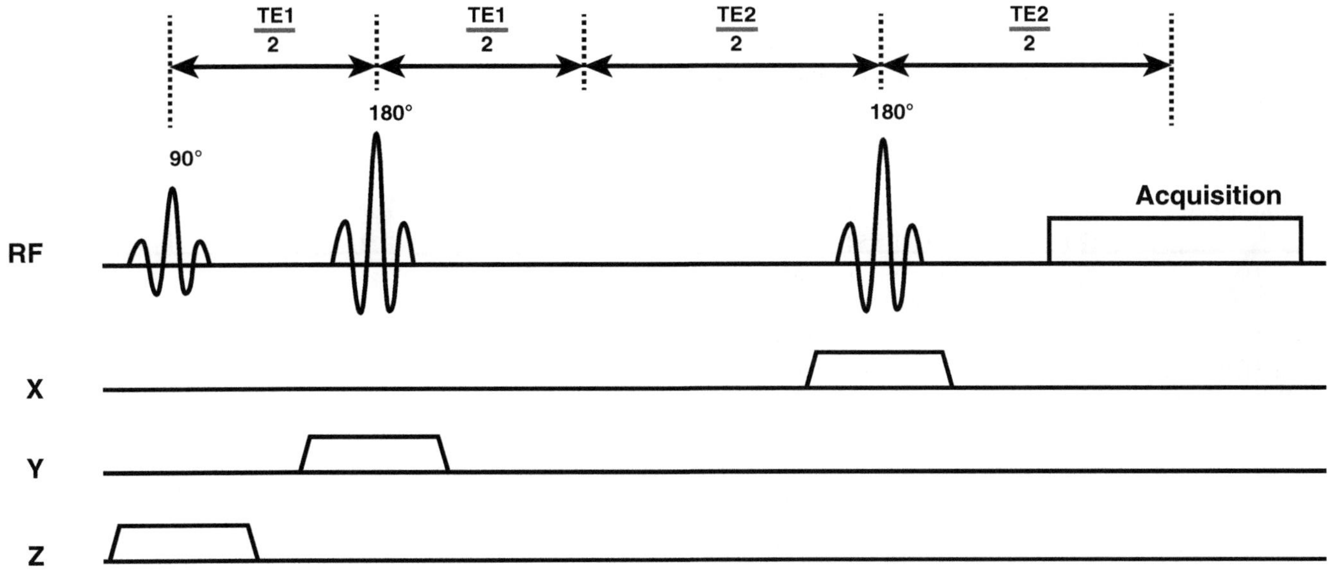

Fig. 2.5 PRESS sequence timing diagram

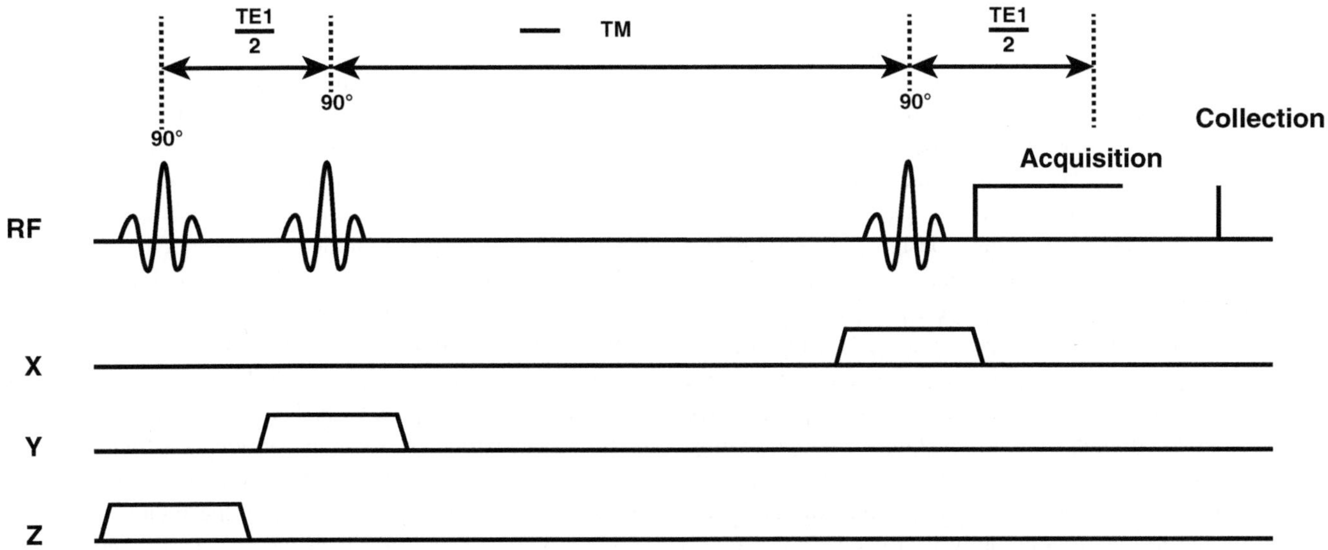

Fig. 2.6 STEAM sequence timing diagram

that of metabolites, and the water peak will drive the fluctuation of the baseline. So it is necessary to suppress the water peak when collecting MRS data. Chemical shift selective saturation (CHESS) is a commonly used method to suppress water peaks [16]. CHESS suppresses the water peaks by applying pulses of longer duration (better frequency selectivity) to flip the water peaks to the *XY* plane and then dropping the magnetization vector using a very strong gradient scattering. The effectiveness of CHESS in suppressing water peaks is generally improved by a combination of three or more pulses and gradients.

7. **Functional magnetic resonance imaging (fMRI)**. It emerged in the 1990s. The fMRI reflects changes in the magnetic resonance signal of the brain caused by blood oxygen metabolism during neural activity [17]. Over the past 30 years, fMRI has developed rapidly and has become an important research tool in the fields of psycho-cognition, psychiatry, and neurobiology.

   The mechanism of fMRI is BOLD, which was originally proposed by Ogawa et al. [18] in 1990. The cerebral vasculature contains two types of hemoglobin, deoxyhemoglobin and oxygenated hemoglobin, which are antimagnetic (no unpaired electrons, no magnetic moment)

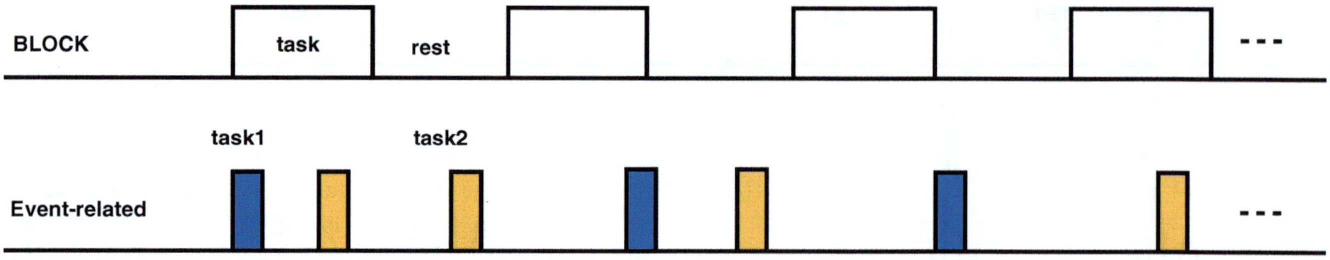

Fig. 2.7 Block- and event-related experimental design

and paramagnetic (unpaired electrons, magnetic moment). While the neurons start to be active, the ratio of deoxyhemoglobin to oxygenated hemoglobin decreases, the local magnetization decreases, the T_2^* of the tissue increases, and the cerebral cortex associated with neural activity exhibits an enhanced signal on the MRI image.

To detect neural activity in the brain, which is relatively transient, requires the use of a fast sequence sensitive to magnetic field changes to record changes in the BOLD signal. The most widely used sequence for fMRI experiments is the gradient echo and echo-planar imaging (GRE-EPI) sequence [19], which typically acquires images of the whole brain in about 2 s.

The fMRI experiments are generally divided into block experimental designs and event-related experimental designs (Fig. 2.7). The group block experimental design alternated between task and resting state intervals, whereas the event-related experimental design was randomized between stimulus presentation and resting conditions.

SPM, FSL, Brain Voyager, etc., are the most commonly used software for processing fMRI data. The preprocessing steps generally include interlayer time correction, head motion alignment, image alignment, tissue segmentation, spatial normalization, and smoothing. Following pretreatment, general linear model (GLM) analysis and group analysis at the individual level were performed to obtain brain activation results corresponding to the experimental task (Fig. 2.8).

A GLM is a linear combination of single or multiple variables to represent the time series signal acquired by MRI:

$$Y = X\beta + \varepsilon \tag{2.6}$$

where Y is the measured block time series signal, X is the design matrix, β is the parameter matrix, ε is the error variable (with mean 0), and the covariance is σ^2 In (In is the n-dimensional unit matrix). The GLM for each pixel of the functional image time series can be solved using the least squares method to obtain the parameter β estimates, and the t and p values can be obtained by statistical tests on the parameter estimates.

Spontaneous neural activity refers to the pattern of neural activity in the brain in the absence of specific external stimuli and cognitive task states [20, 21]. It has been found that the spontaneous activity of the human brain consumes 90% or more of the total energy consumed by the brain, and the study of spontaneous neural activity is an important topic in neuroscience. In 1995, Biswal et al. [22] found a significant correlation between low-frequency (0.1 Hz) signal fluctuations in the bilateral cerebral motor cortex during the no-task state. This functional imaging method of acquiring magnetic resonance signals from the brain in a stimulation-free task, awake and relaxed state, to study spontaneous neural activity and functional connectivity (FC) of brain regions is the rest-state fMRI. The resting state data acquisition time is generally about 8 min, and its data preprocessing method is similar to the task state. The resting state is generally concerned with the low frequency range of 0.01–0.1 Hz, and band-pass filtering is required for data preprocessing.

There are several more commonly used parameters for the resting state, namely, amplitude of low frequency fluctuation (ALFF), regional homogeneity (ReHo), and FC [23–25]. ALFF is the average amplitude at low frequencies (generally 0.01–0.1 Hz), which reflects the strength of spontaneous brain nerve activity in the resting state. ReHo is the correlation of the signal between adjacent voxels over time and is characterized by calculating the Kendall harmony coefficient for all voxels in a region. FC refers to the correlation between different brain regions spatially. Generally, the region of interest (ROI) is selected first and then the correlation between the whole brain and the time series signal of this ROI is calculated. The region with high correlation is functionally relevant. The default network, auditory network, visual network, attention network, and sensorimotor network are a few of the more common brain networks.

2.1.3 PET Cerebral Perfusion Imaging

PET cerebral perfusion imaging is an important part of neuro-nuclear medicine, which can assess the cerebral perfusion status of various diseases and quantitatively measure CBF, and provides high value for the diagnosis of transient ischemic attack and reversible ischemic encephalopathy, diagnosis of cerebral infarction, diagnosis and differential diagnosis of Alzheimer's disease, localization and diagnosis of epileptic foci, differential diagnosis of recurrence and

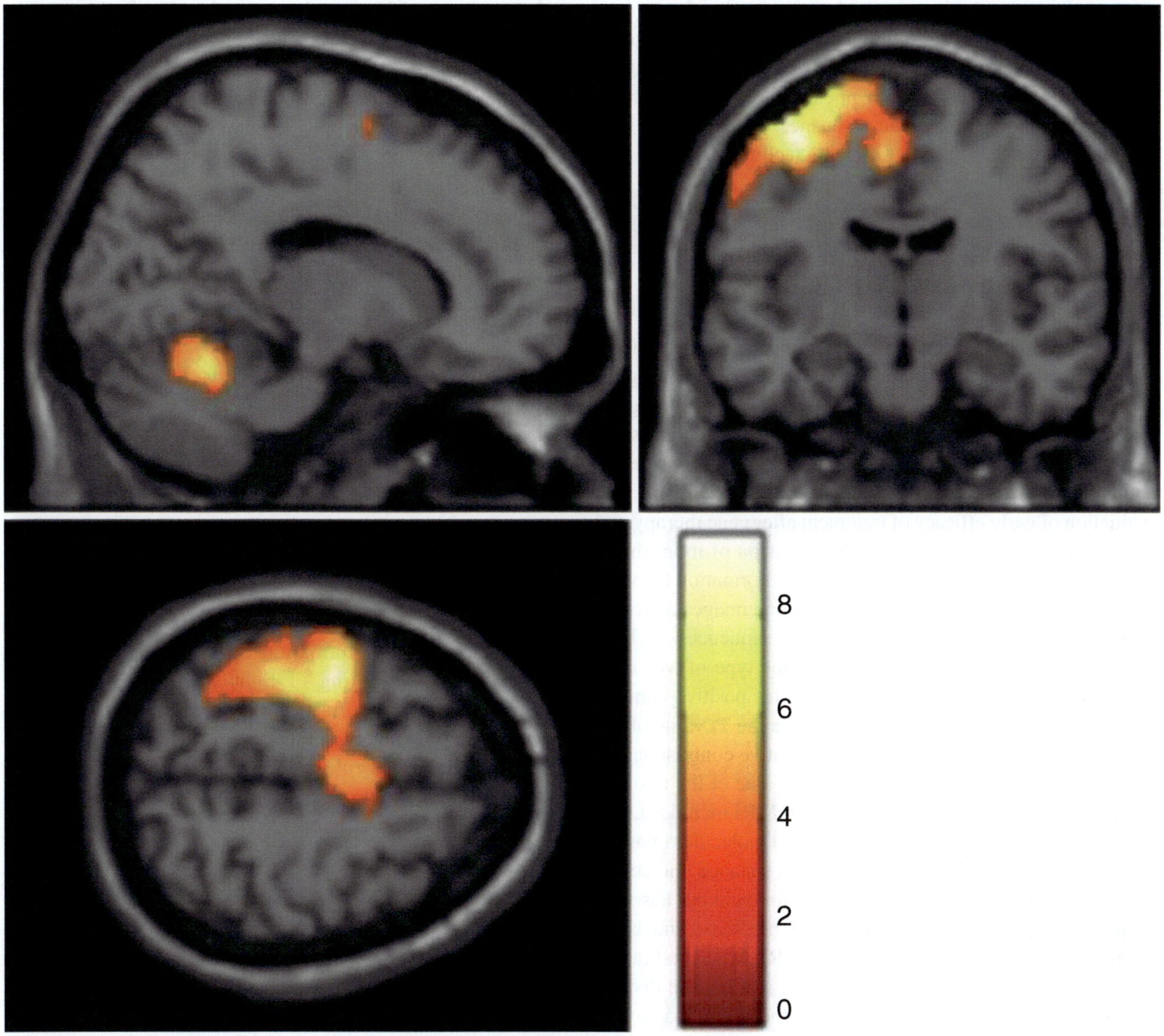

Fig. 2.8 Motor cortical activation induced by right finger movements

necrosis after brain tumor surgery and radiotherapy, and brain function research. The commonly used imaging agents are $^{15}O\text{-}H_2O$, $^{13}N\text{-}NH_3{\cdot}H_2O$, etc.

2.2 Molecular Imaging

Xin Gao, Chunhui Jiang, and Liling Peng

2.2.1 Overview

In 1999, Weissleder [26] of Harvard University first introduced the concept of molecular imaging, a science that uses imaging to show specific molecules at the tissue, cellular, and subcellular levels, to reflect changes at the molecular level in the living body, and to study their biological behavior qualitatively and quantitatively in imaging [27]. While classical diagnostic imaging techniques mainly show diseases with anatomical alterations, molecular imaging has an important role in disease gene therapy, disease progression assessment, drug therapy aid selection, and new drug development, especially in oncology, through the development of new tools, reagents, and methods to probe for abnormalities in disease processes at the cellular and molecular levels and to detect abnormalities before they appear. Molecular imaging is the product of combining molecular biology technology and modern medical imaging, which is the hot spot of medical imaging research and an important direction of development at present. It is generally accepted that there are three main elements to molecular imaging techniques: molecular probes, signal amplification, and high-sensitivity detection techniques. The main clinical applications of molecular imaging techniques can be divided into nuclear medicine molecular imaging techniques, magnetic resonance molecular imaging techniques, optical molecular imaging techniques, etc.

2.2.2 Molecular Magnetic Resonance Imaging (mMRI) Techniques

mMRI is a technique that allows for the qualitative and/or quantitative study of physiological processes such as gene expression, metabolic activity, and intracellular biological activity in biological tissues, using specific molecules as the basis for imaging. This enables the monitoring of lesion development in vivo, the study of pathological mechanisms, the evaluation of early efficacy of treatment after gene therapy and before phenotypic changes, and the provision of more three-dimensional and rapid three-dimensional information than traditional histological examination. The tissue images are often acquired using the appropriate imaging sequences such as T_1WI, T_2WI, and T_2^*WI, depending on the type of MR contrast [28]. This is the case, for example, for positive contrast agents based on gadolinium agents, where the T_1 value of the tissue is primarily measured, and for negative contrast agents based on iron oxide, where the T_2 or T_2^* value of the tissue is commonly measured. The broad scope of MRI includes DWI, PWI, and MRS in addition to marker target molecular imaging and reporter gene imaging. Magnetic resonance molecular imaging is still in the early stage of development but has very promising applications in both clinical medicine and basic research. The combined application of MRI, MRS, and radionuclide imaging allows for more specific and precise display of pathophysiological processes. MR microscopic imaging technology utilizes small high-field and ultrahigh-field magnetic resonance devices for imaging that can show living metabolic processes and is now available as a PET/MRI fusion model, which will likely be the most challenging molecular imaging device in the future [29].

MRI has become an important method and technique in molecular imaging because of its high resolution, no radiological damage, and no tissue depth restriction, which is incomparable to other imaging techniques in molecular imaging applications [30]. At present, MR molecular imaging has been applied to basic and clinical medical research fields and achieved significant breakthroughs, which is still mainly limited to preclinical research, and a few trials in the clinic can be used for apoptosis imaging, tumor angiogenesis, neurotransmitter delivery, stem cell transplantation detection, etc. It has good prospects for early diagnosis of multisystem diseases, metabolic imaging, cell tracing, gene analysis, and metabolic imaging.

2.2.3 Optical Molecular Imaging Techniques

Optical imaging is a technique that uses bioluminescence and fluorescence for in vivo imaging of living animals. Bioluminescence is the phenomenon of labeling cells with a luciferase gene and using the protease it produces to react biochemically with the corresponding substrate, ultimately producing an optical signal. Fluorescence imaging uses fluorescent reporter genes (GFP, RFP), fluorescent dyes (Cyt, dyes), quantum dots (QD) and rare earth upconversion nanoparticles to label the nucleic acids or specific proteins in cells [31]. Both technologies require sensitive optical detection systems to directly monitor genetic and cellular changes in living organisms and to observe the dynamic processes of tumor growth, invasion, and metastasis. Optical molecular imaging, as an important part of molecular imaging, has been widely used in recent years in several fields, such as drug development and clinical practice.

Optical molecular imaging has the advantages of being noninvasive, radiation-free, and highly sensitive; can be imaged in real time, with high resolution for superficial soft tissues; and can identify different components and obtain functional imaging information by virtue of the different absorption and scattering of light waves by soft tissues. Fluorescence imaging functions as real-time, noninvasive, and specific tracking and detection in early tumor diagnosis and has an important role in tumor treatment research, such as adjuvant tumor therapy, intraoperative tumor imaging, and tumor-targeted drug delivery, as well as imaging to reflect the degree of tumor invasiveness, to accurately assess patient prognosis, and to detect tumor recurrence; however, due to the low tissue penetration ability, it is presently primarily utilized in molecular imaging studies in small animals to evaluate antigen and antibody binding, transgenesis, and gene expression [32].

2.2.4 Magnetic Particle Imaging (MPI)

MPI is a novel radiological imaging method that provides radiation-free molecular imaging. The technology generates three-dimensional images by probing magnetic iron oxide nanoparticles in vivo and has the ability to acquire high-temporal-resolution images in just milliseconds, using its high temporal resolution to solve problems that are beyond the reach of many existing imaging techniques. Magnetic nanoparticles (MNP) have their own unique advantages in biomedical applications: (1) the particle size can be controlled from 2 to 20 nm, and the optimized particle size and properties can be easily matched to biomolecular studies; (2) nanoparticles can be controlled by an applied magnetic field and have many advantages for in vivo and in vitro applications; (3) MNP play an important role in MRI image contrast enhancers.

In recent years, MNP have been applied in MRI, as drug carriers, and as thermal therapy media for cancer thermal therapy and near-infrared spectrum photothermal therapy due to the above properties. It is possible to detect diseases by noninvasive MRI due to their magnetic characteristics. Combined with some advanced properties such as specific targeting, multimodality, and delivery of chemotherapeutic agents, the imaging effectiveness and applicability of MNP are expanded with promising applications [33].

2.2.5 Nuclear Medicine Molecular Imaging Techniques

Nuclear medicine molecular imaging (NMI) is an imaging technique in which radionuclides are labeled with specific substrates (such as glucose, purines or pyrimidines, fatty acids, amino acids, etc.), ligands of specific antibodies or receptors, or oligonucleotides that are required for human activities, to make specific probes, which can be used to visualize the distribution, metabolism, excretion, and other dynamic changes in the body over a certain period of time by introducing these probes into the human body.

The most important feature of nuclear medicine imaging is to reflect the specific functional and metabolic state of an organ or tissue by using its selective uptake of certain imaging agents and to understand its location, morphology, size, and other anatomical structures. Nuclear medicine molecular imaging primarily provides information about cellular signal transduction, gene expression, biochemical metabolism, etc. It can provide molecular information about diseases before the morphological and structural changes occur, which helps to achieve early diagnosis of diseases, and the results obtained are closer to the real situation, hence enabling a new level of understanding, diagnosis, and treatment of diseases [34]. PET, in particular, is not only used to identify the benignity and malignancy of tumors, determine the staging and grading, assess treatment effects, and judge prognosis but also has a unique value in the determination and revision of tumor treatment plans.

2.2.6 Ultrasound Molecular Imaging Techniques

The application of ultrasound molecular imaging refers to the use of microbubble contrast agent to access the target tissue through the vascular pathway, and observe the target area at the tissue, cellular, and subcellular levels in order to reflect the changes in the molecular basis of the lesioned tissue, cellular, and subcellular levels, in order to reflect the changes in the molecular basis of the lesioned tissue. A molecular probe is a complex consisting of a substance that binds specifically to a target tissue in combination with a substance that produces an imaging signal. High-resolution imaging systems can detect amplified signal changes with the use of molecular probes (i.e., microsphere contrast agents attached to specific ligands or antibodies) to indirectly reflect information about targeted tissue molecules or genes. Ultrasonic microbubble contrast agents possess promising development prospects in molecular imaging and also demonstrate great application space due to the maturation of microbubble preparation technology and the development of ultrasound contrast detection technology in recent years. Instead of being limited to obtaining information about blood perfusion within tissues, present ultrasonography is increasingly being applied to specific ultrasound molecular imaging techniques. By intravenous injection, a specific ligand is attached to the surface of an ultrasound microbubble contrast agent with a diameter smaller than that of red blood cells, and in vivo, through the tight binding of the ligand to the receptor, the microbubble contrast agent can stay accurately and for a longer period of time in the target tissue to observe the biological changes at the molecular level inside the living target tissue for specific ultrasound molecular imaging in vitro [35]. Ultrasound molecular imaging technology has been the hot spot of clinical research by using in vivo simulated immunohistochemistry or in situ hybridization to highlight the pathological changes in the diseased tissues by targeting biomolecules, thereby reflecting the genuine pathogenesis and significantly improving the sensitivity and accuracy of diagnostic imaging.

The advent of ultrasound molecular imaging has provided the prerequisite for early diagnosis and specific treatment of patients with malignant tumors, and certain research results have been achieved. Ultrasound molecular imaging will play a greater role in the diagnosis and treatment of malignant tumors with the further development of molecular biology; the integration with physics, chemistry, and materials science (nanotechnology, etc.); and the continuous improvement of new contrast preparation materials and methods.

References

1. Stejskal EO, Tanner JE. Spin diffusion measurements: spin echoes in the presence of time-dependent field gradient. Chem Phys. 1965;42:288–92.
2. Basser PJ, Mattiello J, Le Bihan D. Estimation of the effective self-diffusion tensor from the NMR spin echo. J Magn Reson B. 1994;B103:247–54.
3. Jensen JH, Helpern JA, Kaczynski K. Diffusional kurtosis imaging: the quantification of non-Gaussian water diffusion by means of magnetic resonance imaging. Magn Reson Med. 2005;53:1432–40.
4. Luciani A, Vignaud A, Cavet M, et al. Liver cirrhosis: intravoxel incoherent motion MR imaging—pilot study. Radiology. 2008;249:891–9.
5. Cuenod CA, Balvay D. Perfusion and vascular permeability: basic concepts and measurement in DCE-CT and DCE-MRI. Diagn Interv Imaging. 2013;94:1187–204.

6. Salerno M, Beller GA. Noninvasive assessment of myocardial perfusion. Circ Cardiovasc Imaging. 2009;2:412–24.
7. Jahng GH, Li KL, Ostergaard L, et al. Perfusion magnetic resonance imaging: a comprehensive update on principles and techniques. Korean J Radiol. 2014;15:554–77.
8. Tofts PS. T1-weighted DCE imaging concepts: modelling, acquisition and analysis. Magnetom Flash. 2010;3:30–5.
9. Borogovac A, Asllani I. Arterial spin labeling (ASL) fMRI: advantages, theoretical constrains and experimental challenges in neurosciences. Int J Biomed Imaging. 2012;6:658101.
10. Ferre JC, Bannier E, Raoult H, et al. Arterial spin labeling (ASL) perfusion: techniques and clinical use. Diagn Interv Imaging. 2013;94:1211–23.
11. Arnold JT, Dharmati S, Packard ME. Chemical effects on nuclear induction signals from organic compounds. J Chem Phys. 1951;19:507.
12. Harris RK, Becker ED, de Menezes SMC, et al. NMR nomenclature. Nuclear spin properties and conventions for chemical shifts (IUPAC recommendations 2001). Pure Appl Chem. 2001;73:1795–818.
13. Moonen CT, von Kienlin M, van Zijl PC, et al. Comparison of single-shot localization methods (STEAM and PRESS) for in vivo proton NMR spectroscopy. NMR Biomed. 1989;2:201–7.
14. Klose U. Measurement sequences for single voxel proton MR spectroscopy. Eur J Radiol. 2008;67:194–201.
15. Frahm J, Merboldt KD, Hänicke W. Localized proton spectroscopy using stimulated echoes. J Magn Reson. 1987;72:502–8.
16. Haase A, Frahm J, Hanicke W, et al. 1H-NMR chemical-shift selective (CHESS)imaging. Phys Med Biol. 1985;30:341–4.
17. Belliveau JW, Kennedy DN, McKinstry RC, et al. Functional mapping of the human visual cortex by magnetic resonance imaging. Science. 1991;254:716–9.
18. Ogawa S, Tank DW, Menon R, et al. Intrinsic signal changes accompanying sensory stimulation: functional brain mapping with magnetic resonance imaging. Proc Natl Acad Sci U S A. 1992;89:5951–5.
19. Bandettini PA, Wong EC, Hinks RS, et al. Time course EPI of human brain function during task activation. Magn Reson Med. 1992;25:390–7.
20. Barkhof F, Haller S, Rombouts SARB. Resting-state functional MR imaging: a new window to the brain. Radiology. 2014;272:29–49.
21. Brown GG, Perthen JE, Liu TT, et al. A primer on functional magnetic resonance imaging. Neuorpsychol Rev. 2007;17:107–25.
22. Biswal B, Yetkin FZ, Haughton VM, et al. Functional connectivity in the motor cortex of resting human brain using echo-planar MRI. Magn Reson Med. 1995;34:537–41.
23. Cox RW. AFNI: software for analysis and visualization of functional magnetic resonance neuroimages. Comput Biomed Res. 1996;29:162.
24. Lowe MJ, Mock BJ, Sorenson JA. Resting state fMRI signal correlations in multi-slice EPI. Neuroimage. 1996;3:S257.
25. Zang Y, Jiang T, Lu Y, et al. Regional homogeneity approach to fMRI data analysis. Neuroimage. 2004;22:394–400.
26. Weissleder R. Molecular imaging: exploring the next frontier. Radiology. 1999;212(3):609–14.
27. Toczek J, Sadeghi MM. Molecular imaging concepts. J Nucl Cardiol. 2016;23(2):271–3.
28. James ML, Gambhir SS. A molecular imaging primer: modalities, imaging agents, and applications. Physiol Rev. 2012;92(2):897–965.
29. Huang G. Chinese clinical medical imaging -PET and molecular imaging subseries. Beijing: Peking University Medical Press; 2015.
30. Aime S, Cabella C, Colombatto S, et al. Insights into the use of paramagnetic Gd (III) complexes in MR-molecular imaging investigations. J Magn Reson Imaging. 2002;16(4):394–406.
31. Fazel J, Rötzer S, Seidl C, et al. Fractionated intravesical radioimmunotherapy with (213) Bi-anti-EGFR-MAb is effective without toxic side-effects in a nude mouse model of advanced human bladder carcinoma. Cancer Biol Ther. 2015;16(10):1526–34.
32. Cheng H, Chi C, Shang W, et al. Precise integrin-targeting near-infrared imaging-guided surgical method increases surgical qualification of peritoneal carcinomatosis from gastric cancer in mice. Oncotarget. 2017;8(4):6258–72.
33. Fazel J, Rtzer S, Seidl C, et al. Fractionated intravesical radioimmunotherapy with 213Bi-anti-EGFR-MAb is effective without toxic side effects in a nude mouse model of advanced human bladder carcinoma. Cancer Biol Ther. 2015;16(10):1526–34.
34. Qingyu R, Xing Y, Yanhua Z. Advances in molecular imaging research in nuclear medicine. Mod Med Oncol. 2012;20(12):2658–60.
35. Liu J, Zhang P, Liu P, et al. Endothelial adhesion of targeted microbubbles in both small and great vessels using ultrasound radiation force. Mol Imaging. 2012;11(1):58–66.

3 Application of Imaging Techniques in Craniospinal Infection and Inflammatory Diseases

Yunling Wang, Jing Yang, and Chunhui Jiang

Infectious diseases are a very specific group of diseases caused mainly by pathogens such as bacteria, viruses, fungi, and parasites. Pathogenic microorganisms can come from either outside the body or from normal microorganisms in the body. Therefore, the classification of CNS infectious diseases according to pathogenic microorganisms is the most common and basic method of classification (Table 3.1).

Imaging techniques, especially CT and MRI, often play an important role in the diagnosis of infectious diseases of the central nervous system. Despite the low specificity of the imaging manifestations of most intracranial infectious diseases, imaging techniques are still important auxiliary examinations, which can be integrated with medical history, clinical symptoms and signs, and laboratory tests to make an accurate diagnosis.

Table 3.1 Classification of infectious diseases of the central nervous system

Classification	Pathogenic microorganisms
Bacterial infection	
Gram-stain-positive bacterial infections	*Staphylococcus* infections, *Streptococcus pneumoniae* infections, group B and A *Streptococcus* infections, *Mycobacterium tuberculosis* infections, listeriosis
Gram-stain-negative bacterial infections	*Neisseria meningitidis* infection, *Escherichia coli* infection, *Pseudomonas aeruginosa* infection, *Klebsiella pneumoniae* infection, etc.
Viral infection	
Herpesvirus	Herpes simplex virus infection, varicella-zoster varicella-zoster virus infection, EB virus infection, cytomegalovirus infection, human herpesvirus 6 infection, etc.
Enterovirus infections	Enterovirus infections, poliovirus infections, etc.
Paramyxovirus infections	Measles virus infections, mumps virus infections, etc.
Flavivirus infection	Japanese encephalitis virus infection, dengue virus infection, forest encephalitis virus infection, yellow fever virus infection, West Nile virus infection and Murray Valley virus infection, etc.
Other viral infections	Rabies virus infection, human immunodeficiency virus infection, rubella virus infection, lentivirus infection, etc.
Fungal infections	*Cryptococcus*/*Novel Cryptococcus* infections, *Aspergillus* infections, *Mucor* infections, *Candida albicans* infections, *Coccidioides* infections, *Actinomyces* infections, *Histoplasma* infections, etc.
Parasitic infections	Cerebral cysticercosis, cerebral echinococciasis, cerebral schistosomiasis, cerebral schistosomiasis larvae, cerebral malaria, cerebral amoebiasis, etc.
Other special types of infections	Lyme disease, neurosyphilis, rickettsial infections, infectious proteins including Creutzfeldt-Jakob disease, novel Creutzfeldt-Jakob disease, etc.

Y. Wang (✉) · J. Yang · C. Jiang
The First Affiliated Hospital of Xinjiang Medical University, Urumqi, China

H. Li et al. (eds.), *Radiology of Infectious and Inflammatory Diseases - Volume 1*,
https://doi.org/10.1007/978-981-99-0039-8_3

3.1 Bacterial Infection

3.1.1 Significance of Imaging in Bacterial Infections of the Brain and Spinal Cord

The clinical symptoms of craniospinal bacterial infections are usually obvious and severe, which necessitates early detection, diagnosis, and treatment to prevent fatal complications. Imaging techniques can provide important information for the early diagnosis of disease. Lumbar puncture is often required to evaluate the condition and confirm the diagnosis in patients with suspected encephalitis or meningitis, but imaging should still be preferred in patients with neurologic deficits, immunodeficiency, or unconsciousness.

3.1.2 Conventional Imaging Techniques in Craniospinal Bacterial Infections

Common pathogens of intracranial septic infections include *S. meningitidis*, *S. pneumoniae*, *S. staphylococcus*, *H. influenzae*, *S. pyogenes*, and *Escherichia coli.* Pathological changes include septic meningitis, brain abscess, ventriculitis, and ventricular effusion. The imaging performance varies in different parts of involvement and in different stages of lesions. The imaging performance can serve as auxiliary diagnosis and localization, while the qualitative diagnosis mainly relies on history, physical signs, laboratory tests of cerebrospinal fluid, etc. Cerebral abscesses have a more typical imaging presentation and are easily diagnosed.

1. **X-rays:** It is often inconclusive but can occasionally show calcification of the abscess envelope, pneumatization or fluid levels within the abscess when applied to septic encephalitis and brain abscesses of bacterial infection of the central nervous system, and can help to localize the primary lesion of the abscess.
2. **Angiography:** In the acute phase of encephalitis, angiography reveals widely distributed segmental stenosis of cerebral artery branches, which is mainly caused by arterial spasm due to inflammatory stimulation, and in the abscess formation phase, signs such as abscess occupancy, vascular invasion, and increased blood flow are seen.
3. **CT and MRI:** It is often normal in the early stages of encephalitis, or focal, fuzzy, hypodense foci with significant occupancy effects are seen. However, CT scan may show mild dilatation of the ventricular system and subarachnoid space with diffuse brain swelling once the infection has progressively progressed. In approximately half of the cases in the abscess formation stage, a regular or irregular isodense or slightly dense ring can be seen around the hypodense foci as a fibrous envelope layer, and enhanced scans show that the abscess remains hypodense within the abscess and that the abscess wall is mildly enhanced.

MRI may appear normal in the early stages of acute bacterial meningitis or may show mild dilatation of the ventricular system and subarachnoid space with diffuse brain swelling. Early MRI is more sensitive than CT in detecting abnormal meningeal enhancement in the basal cistern, lateral fissure, and deep corticothalamic sulcus, with enhancement distributed along the cerebellar vermis, falx, and convexity of the brain. Both MRI and CT can reveal many comorbid manifestations of meningitis, such as ventriculitis, hydrocephalus, subdural effusion, subdural pus, and epidural abscess.

Ventriculitis manifests as ventricular canal thickening and intensification, ventricular enlargement, and fluid accumulation, and ventricular pus accumulation may manifest as circumferential intensification of pus cavities within the ventricles.

3.1.3 Application of New Imaging Techniques in Craniospinal Bacterial Infections

DWI offers significant value in differentiating brain abscesses from necrotizing brain tumors. The pus of bacterial brain abscess is a viscous fluid composed of a variety of inflammatory cells, bacteria, necrotic tissue, and proteins, with increased cellular viscosity, markedly restricted diffusion of water molecules, reduced ADC values, and a characteristic DWI sequence showing significant high signal.

PWI can also be used in the differential diagnosis of tumors versus abscesses, where the mean relative cerebral blood volume is significantly higher in solid areas of brain tumors than in the cystic wall of brain abscesses.

^{1}H-MRS can be used as an important complementary imaging method to conventional MRI and DWI for the characteristic presentation of abscess cavities in untreated brain abscesses: absence of N-acetylaspartate (NAA), choline (Cho) and creatinine (Cr) peaks, and elevated levels of amino acids (AA, 0.9 ppm) and lactic acid (Lac, 1.3 ppm) with or without elevated levels of acetic acid (1.9 ppm) and succinic acid (2.4 ppm). Amino acids are considered to be characteristic markers of septic abscesses and are the result of protein hydrolysis by polymorphonuclear leukocytes in the pus.

Magnetization transfer (MT) imaging shows abnormally reinforced meninges better than CT, with high signal on plain T_1WI, MT sequences and significant enhancement on early scan T_1WI, MT sequences. In addition, MT helps to determine the etiology of meningitis. Tuberculous meningitis has a significantly higher magnetization transmission rate than viral meningitis, and fungal meningitis and septic meningitis exhibit a higher magnetization transmission rate compared to tuberculous meningitis.

DTI is a relatively new magnetic resonance imaging technique that provides information on the fine structure of tissues. The common metrics of DTI are fractional anisotropy (FA) and mean diffusivity (MD). Inflammatory cells in the subarachnoid space are aligned in a certain direction due to the upregulation of the body's immune response in meningitis, causing an increase in FA values. FA is increased in both enhanced and non-enhanced cortical regions in septic meningitis, in both neonates and adults, and in both enhanced and non-enhanced cortical regions, suggesting that FA is more meaningful and that quantitative analysis provides more valuable information for the diagnosis and assessment of prognosis of infectious diseases of the central nervous system [1].

3.1.4 Comparison of the Diagnostic Value of Imaging Techniques

Bacterial infections of the cranial spinal cord are examined primarily by CT and MRI. X-rays are of limited value for the diagnosis of specific intracranial lesions. DSA is the gold standard for diagnosing vascular lesions. Bacterial septic infection or *Mycobacterium tuberculosis* infection can lead to vasculitis secondary to cerebral infarction. DSA provides a visualization of the vasculature; however, it has been partially replaced by noninvasive tests such as CTA and MRA. CT has a wide range of applications in disease screening because of its fast-scanning speed and low cost. In addition, CT is superior to MRI in showing microcalcifications and cortical destruction. However, MRI has a high resolution of soft tissue, and the diagnostic accuracy is significantly higher than that of CT. Its multi-series, multi-modality examination can provide more information for the localization, characterization, and even quantitative diagnosis of bacterial infections in the cranial spinal cord. With the emergence of several new MR techniques and the gradual popularization of clinical applications in recent years, MRI offers promising applications for diagnosis, differential diagnosis, and posttreatment follow-up of diseases.

3.2 Viral Infection

3.2.1 Significance of Imaging in Viral Infections of the Brain and Spinal Cord

Clinically, the diagnosis of viral encephalitis is relatively common; however, viral encephalitis has become a "waste basket" of various similar diseases because of the difficulty in obtaining etiologic evidence. For encephalitis that is genuinely caused by viruses, it is often generalized or simplified due to the absence of either etiologic or specific laboratory findings. Imaging examinations can provide important information for the diagnosis and differential diagnosis of the disease in view of the different aggressiveness and virulence and the different sites and shapes of lesions caused by different viruses.

3.2.2 Conventional Imaging Techniques in Craniospinal Viral Infections

The severity of each viral infection varies greatly, and the imaging manifestations are diverse in nature, with most lacking specificity, while some viral infections do not have positive imaging. Viral infection may manifest as diffuse brain parenchymal involvement, with lesions prevalent in the frontal lobe, parietal lobe, basal ganglia, and thalamus, but also involving the brainstem, cerebellum, and corona radiata. Both gray and white matter can be involved, and the affected brain tissue may present changes such as edema, inflammatory cell infiltration, neuronal cell degeneration, necrosis, and glial cell proliferation. X-ray plain films have limited diagnostic value for craniospinal virus infection, and the main imaging methods for diagnosis are CT and MRI, which can provide guidance for stereotactic localization and help evaluate prognosis and outcome.

Herpes simplex encephalitis, for example, appears on MRI as a unilateral or bilateral asymmetric temporal, frontal, or insula-like lesion with blurred margins, mostly involving the cortex and subcortical white matter, with some occupying effect, which has a low signal on T_1WI, high signal on T_2WI, and high signal on FLAIR. The differential diagnosis includes glioma, Rasmussen's encephalitis, abscess, limbic lobe encephalitis, and paraneoplastic syndrome. Varicella-zoster virus is more common to cause white matter ischemia/infarction, especially at the gray-white matter junction, while gray matter is less commonly involved but may have abnormal enhancement. The differential diagnosis includes metastases, embolism (cardiogenic), and CNS vasculitis. Lesions due to vasculitis are usually small and mostly do not appear in the gray-white matter junction area. MRI of JC viral infection (i.e., progressive multifocal leukoencephalopathy) may show typical multifocal or fused subcortical white matter non-enhancing lesions, which may also involve the gray matter. The differential diagnosis includes CNS lymphoma, glioma, disseminated encephalomyelitis, and sarcoidosis, and if the lesions are confined to the white matter, post-chemotherapy and post-radiotherapy changes need to be excluded; acute disseminated encephalomyelitis after viral infection may show subcortical white matter lesions, most of which include U fibers [2].

3.2.3 Application of New Imaging Techniques in Craniospinal Viral Infections

At this stage, the application of new imaging techniques in craniospinal viral infections is relatively limited, and some of the lesions may show restricted diffusion on DWI, but they are not specific. Other techniques still need to be further investigated for the diagnosis, differential diagnosis, prognosis, and assessment of treatment effects. Confirmation of diagnosis depends on the detection of virus-specific IgM and IgG antibodies in laboratory tests or the detection of viral RNA by reverse transcription polymerase chain reaction (RT-PCR) amplification.

3.2.4 Comparison of the Diagnostic Value of Imaging Techniques

The main imaging methods for craniocerebrospinal virus infection are CT and MRI. MRI demonstrates the viral infection lesions more clearly than CT, especially in revealing the location and extent of lesion involvement, while CT is better than MRI in revealing microcalcifications. The diagnosis is difficult in most cases due to the lack of specificity in clinical symptoms and imaging manifestations caused by viral infection and the overlap between them. A few viruses invade specific areas and may be suggestive for a qualitative diagnosis.

3.3 Fungal Infection

3.3.1 Significance of Imaging in Fungal Infections of the Brain and Spinal Cord

Imaging plays an important role in the diagnosis of intracranial fungal infections. Although the qualitative diagnosis of craniocerebrospinal fungal infection may primarily rely on the history of fungal infection, physical signs, and laboratory examination of cerebrospinal fluid, the imaging manifestations are nonspecific; still, some imaging signs caused by fungal infection are suggestive for the diagnosis, and imaging examination can be used as one of the important auxiliary diagnostic tools.

3.3.2 Conventional Imaging Techniques in Craniospinal Fungal Infections

The two main groups of common causative agents of intracranial fungal infections include the following: One group is usually the pathogenic fungi that infect immunodeficient or immunosuppressed individuals, such as *Candida*, *Aspergillus*, and *Trichoderma*; the other group is the pathogenic fungi that infect normal immunocompetent individuals, such as *Cryptococcus*, *Histoplasma*, *Coccidioides*, and *Bacillus*. Among them, *Cryptococcus* is the most common causative agent of intracranial fungal infections, which accounts for 40–60% of intracranial fungal infections, and both groups of people are susceptible to infection.

The complexity and diversity of pathological changes in intracranial fungal infections lead to a diversity of imaging manifestations, and some imaging manifestations in immunocompromised patients are not significantly specific, and the different immune status of patients leads to different regression of intracranial fungal infections, so the application of imaging techniques for diagnosis and differential diagnosis, assessment of prognosis, and efficacy should be closely integrated with clinical data and laboratory tests.

Cryptococcus neoformans infections mainly present with changes such as enlarged V-R gaps, gelatinous pseudocysts, abnormal meningeal enhancement, cryptococcal granulomas, and cerebral atrophy, with the basal ganglia and meninges being the most common sites of involvement. Gelatinous pseudocysts, cryptococcal granulomas, or abnormal meningeal enhancement are relatively uncommon in immunocompromised individuals. The early manifestation of *Aspergillus* infection in the brain parenchyma alone involves cerebral infarction or hemorrhage in the basal ganglia region, thalamus, and corpus callosum, followed by rapid spread of *Aspergillus* within the infarcted brain parenchyma and the formation of multiple abscesses. Enhanced T_2-FLAIR sequence scans in addition to conventional MR examinations for CNS *Candida albicans* infections can help in the early diagnosis of the disease. It is useful to distinguish fungal from pyogenic or tuberculous infections by some of the imaging features of fungal infections, such as T_2WI low signal in the wall of fungal abscesses and the tendency of *Aspergillus* infection to cause bleeding [3].

3.3.3 Application of New Imaging Techniques in Craniospinal Fungal Infections

The DWI sequence of cryptococcal infection presents a high signal with restricted diffusion within the lesion, similar to the presentation of brain abscess, and the DWI sequence is more sensitive to show some of the microscopic lesions than the enhanced scan. The center of the cryptococcal lesion on the PWI sequence is hypoperfused, suggesting a lack of blood supply. The ^{1}H-MRS of cryptococcosis showed a decrease in NAA, Cr, Cho, and inositol (mI) peaks and an increase in Lip peaks in the lesion. Together with other imaging techniques, including PWI and MRS, DWI can facilitate the differentiation of abscesses from other similar lesions such as cystic metastases and distinguish fungal or septic lesions.

3.3.4 Comparison of the Diagnostic Value of Imaging Techniques

MRI is more reliable than CT in visualizing fungal infections, especially in demonstrating microabscesses and hemorrhagic infarcts, and it often detects more lesions than CT. However, it is not as good as CT in showing granulomatous calcifications, and since there are similar MRI manifestations in other types of infections, it is not easy to distinguish them by MRI alone, and cytological examination is required.

3.4 Parasitic Infections

3.4.1 Significance of Imaging in Parasitic Infections of the Brain and Spinal Cord

Brain parasitic diseases have not only more species and complex clinical manifestations but also develop slowly. Patients often present nonspecific symptoms such as dizziness and weakness at an early stage, and some patients only present with neurological conditions such as headache, convulsions, and epilepsy, which may easily lead to misdiagnosis and mismanagement. Although etiologic diagnosis is the main criterion for confirming the diagnosis of parasitic diseases, such opportunities are often less available in patients with brain parasitosis, making imaging examination very important. Corresponding imaging manifestations help to detect suspected patients with parasitic diseases in a timely manner and are needed to assist in the diagnosis through auxiliary tests such as immunology and molecular biology.

3.4.2 Conventional Imaging Techniques in Craniospinal Parasitic Infections

There are many parasites that can cause intracranial infections; the common ones include schistosomes, toxoplasma, and cysticercus. The parasitic infection may lead to lesions such as meningitis, encephalitis, and sarcoidosis. As an important part of the diagnosis of brain parasitic infection, imaging examination can reveal the location and number of parasites in the central nervous system, the characteristics of the parasite species, and the degree of damage to the central nervous system, which is of great importance for clear diagnosis and guiding treatment.

Some parasitic infections manifest in CT and MRI with certain characteristics; therefore, imaging examination has a more important significance for the diagnosis of parasitic diseases. For instance, CT presentation of cerebral cysticercosis shows ovoid cystic hypodense lesions which have CT values similar to cerebrospinal fluid, and small dot-like high-density foci can be seen in the cyst, which are cerebral cysticercosis head segments; MRI of cystic ovoid lesions shows low signal in T_1WI and high signal in T_2WI, and eccentric head segments can be seen on the cyst wall, which has an important suggestive role for the diagnosis of cerebral cysticercosis.

MRI can display hemorrhage, inflammatory lesions, edema, and characteristic tunnel-like changes in the brain parenchyma caused by pulmonary schistosome brain migration, which is important for the diagnosis of pulmonary schistosomiasis in the active stage. In the case of encephalocysticercosis (multicysticercosis), MRI can show different signals between the mother and the daughter cysts, and in the case of endocyst separation, the endocyst can collapse and detach, and the detached endocyst membranes can be folded and curled and suspended in the cyst fluid, which can be manifested as the "floating belt sign" and "water snake sign." These features are helpful for the diagnosis of encystment [4].

3.4.3 Application of New Imaging Techniques in Craniospinal Parasitic Infections

^{1}H-MRS showed elevated Cho, lactate, succinate, alanine, lipids, and acetate and decreased Cr and NAA in cerebral cysticercosis cyst fluid. Similar manifestations are found in brain abscesses and their infected lesions, but the typical presentation of septic brain abscesses on DWI is markedly high signal with reduced ADC values. Cerebral cysticercosis shows equal to slightly high signal on DWI relative to cerebrospinal fluid, and its ADC values are close to those of cerebrospinal fluid, indicating unrestricted diffusion of cerebral cysticercosis and contributing to the differential diagnosis of cerebral cysticercosis.

3.4.4 Comparison of the Diagnostic Value of Imaging Techniques

The main diagnostic advantages of MRI for brain parasitic diseases are:

1. High sensitivity to detect parasitic bodies on the top brain surface or in the ventricles of the brain.

2. High specificity: MRI can have characteristic performance for lesions with atypical CT findings.
3. MRI is superior to CT for the display of secondary changes caused by parasites such as cerebral infarction and inflammation.
4. More imaging sequences: DWI, MRS, and PWI have great significance for the localization, characterization, staging, and differential diagnosis of cerebral parasitic diseases.

References

1. Mukherji S. Clinical review articles central nervous system infections. Beijing: People's Army Medical Press; 2015. Wu Yuankui, Liu Xian, Lu Guoshi, trans.
2. Mahan M, Karl M, Gordon S. Neuroimaging of viral infections of the central nervous system. Handb Clin Neurol. 2014;123:149–73.
3. Mathur M, Johnson CE, Sze G, et al. Fungal infections of the central nervous system. Neuroimaging Clin N Am. 2012;22(4):609–32.
4. Stojkovic M, Junghanss T. Cystic and alveolar echinococcosis. Handb Clin Neurol. 2013;114(114):327–34.

4 Application of Imaging Techniques in Craniospinal Autoimmune Diseases

Chunhui Jiang, Hui Xing, Xuening Zhang, and Longlin Yin

4.1 Overview

Autoimmune disease is a disease caused by the immune response of the body to its own antigens, resulting in damage to its own tissues. Autoimmune diseases affect a wide range of populations, mostly women, with complex and diverse clinical manifestations, most of which have unknown etiology. It usually occurs in people with high titers of autoantibodies or sensitized lymphocytes against their own tissue cells. The disease presents with pathological changes associated with an immune response and manifests as a chronic inflammation dominated by lymphocytic and plasma cell infiltration. Generally, the disease course is long, mostly chronic, and prolonged. The progression and remission of the disease alternate repeatedly during the course of the disease. Steroid and immunosuppressive therapy can be effective.

Autoimmune diseases can involve multiple systems throughout the body. Among them, autoimmune disease of CNS includes autoimmune encephalitis, acute disseminated encephalomyelitis (ADEM), neuromyelitis optica spectrum disorder (NMOSD), primary angiitis of the central nervous system (PACNS), Rasmussen's encephalitis (Rasmussen), etc. Autoimmune diseases that can involve the CNS include systemic lupus erythematosus (SLE), Sjögren syndrome (SS), antiphospholipid antibody syndrome (APLS), and multiple sclerosis (MS) [1]. Traditional imaging examinations such as cranial X-ray is not helpful for the diagnosis of the disease. CT and MRI may reveal the location and extent of the lesion better and allow localization and quantitative analysis, while MRI is superior to CT, but the qualitative diagnosis of the disease needs to be combined with clinical manifestations. The sensitivity of angiography is not satisfactory for the diagnosis of PACNS, and a positive result can be used as evidence for the suspected diagnosis of PACNS.

4.2 Conventional Imaging Manifestations of Autoimmune Diseases of the Brain and Spinal Cord

The typical imaging feature of CNS involvement in autoimmune disease is limbic system involvement, which is often unremarkable on early-stage CT scans and may appear as limited or multiple white matter lesions on CT scan of late stage. MRI can reveal abnormal signals in the limbic system. The FLAIR sequences are most sensitive and mainly shows nonspecific multiple focals or fused white matter lesions with poorly defined borders, which manifest as slightly hypointense or isointense on T_1WI and hyperintense on T_2WI and FLAIR (T_2) sequences. The lesions are mostly located in the cerebral hemispheres, but can also occur in the brainstem, cerebellum, and can be combined with brain atrophy. Imaging is dominated by ischemic lesions, demyelinating lesions, vasogenic edema, and cerebral atrophy, and a high degree of suspicion of autoimmune disease is required in patients with these imaging presentations. For example, MRI of autoimmune encephalitis shows predominantly parenchymal brain lesions, accounting for about 80.0% of the involvement, which can involve the occipital lobe, bilateral hippocampus, temporal lobe, frontal lobe, parietal lobe, cerebellum, insula, thalamus, caudate nucleus, etc. Apart from diffuse lesions in the hippocampus, the rest are patchy or "gyrus-like" lesions with hypointense on T_1WI and hyperintense on T_2WI and FLAIR and no abnormal enhancement on enhanced T_1WI [2]. MRI studies in patients with neuromyelitis optica show nonspecific cerebral white matter lesions involving the deep white matter or subcortex of the

C. Jiang · H. Xing
The First Affiliated Hospital of Xinjiang Medical University, Urumqi, China

X. Zhang (✉)
Department of Radiology, The Second Hospital of Tianjin Medical University, Tianjin, China

L. Yin
Sichuan Provincial People's Hospital, Chengdu, China

H. Li et al. (eds.), *Radiology of Infectious and Inflammatory Diseases - Volume 1*,
https://doi.org/10.1007/978-981-99-0039-8_4

cerebral hemispheres, usually <3 mm in diameter, with punctate and speckled hyperintense on T_2WI, similar to microvascular lesions, which increase and accumulate as the disease evolves, forming radiolucent or ink-spattered changes along the white matter fiber bundles [3]. The presence of large fusion lesions in the white matter of the brain often indicates deterioration and a poor prognosis, especially in pediatric patients, and the mechanism of their production may be associated with vasogenic edema. Enhancement of brain lesions in optic neuromyelitis optica is commonly seen in the acute phase, while lesions in remission do not have abnormal enhancement. Cloud-like, pencil-core-like, and abnormal soft meningeal enhancement are characteristic signs of intracerebral enhancement in optic neuromyelitis optica [4]. Multiple sclerosis (MS) is mainly manifested as hypointense on T_1WI and hyperintense on T_2WI. Intracranial lesions are mainly distributed in the lateral paraventricular space, corpus callosum, centrum semiovale, midbrain, cerebellum, etc. They appear as circular or fused patchy shadow, and in severe cases, brain tissue degeneration and atrophy can be seen, the long axis of which is perpendicular to the tangent line of the ventricular wall, and spinal cord lesions are mostly in the form of heterogeneous cords. The enhancement of the lesion can be seen on MRI-enhanced scan, indicating an active lesion with local blood-brain barrier disruption [5]. Therefore, patients with negative imaging cannot be excluded from this disease. Some patients showed no abnormalities in cranial MRI plain and enhanced scan, no abnormalities in routine biochemistry of cerebrospinal fluid, and no abnormalities in autoimmune disease-related antibody tests, and their symptoms have been significantly relieved by antiviral therapy, followed by high-dose hormone shock and immunoglobulin treatment. For this reason, patients with negative imaging and autoimmune-related antibody tests who are not responding to antiviral therapy should also be considered as likely to have autoimmune disease.

4.3 New Imaging Techniques in Craniospinal Autoimmune Diseases

The new MRI technique is able to detect occult injuries that cannot be detected by conventional MRI examinations and is especially important in people with autoimmune diseases that are normal on conventional MRI examinations. New MRI techniques include magnetization transfer imaging (MTI), diffusion-weighted imaging (DWI), diffusion tensor imaging (DTI), spectral imaging (MRS), and functional brain magnetic resonance imaging.

MTI is a selective tissue signal suppression technique. Water molecules in human tissues coexist in two different states, namely, free water molecules and bound water molecules. Free water molecules move freely without restriction, while the combined movement of bound water molecules and macromolecular proteins is restricted. The magnetization transfer ratio (MTR) can be calculated using the corresponding method. MTR is a measure of the magnetization transfer effect and is very sensitive to evaluate the structural integrity of the tissue and is a quantifiable indicator. In CNS demyelinating disorders, MTR reflects the integrity of myelin sheaths, with a decrease in MTR suggesting demyelination and axonal loss and an increase in MTR suggesting myelin regeneration. Ropele et al. [6] studied nine cases of cerebral white matter in patients diagnosed with relapsing-remitting MS and found that MTR was reduced in different types of MS white matter lesions and in cerebral white matter that showed normal on conventional MRI, compared to healthy individuals, and the degree of MTR reduction varied between different types of MS lesions (punctate, patchy, and white matter with no significant abnormalities), which probably indicates different pathological changes. This suggests that MTR can reflect insidious demyelination and the severity of the lesion.

Diffusion is a microscopic, random thermal motion of molecules, also known as Brownian motion. In living organisms, diffusion movement is influenced by cell composition, temperature, etc. The denser the cell composition and the lower the temperature, the more restricted the diffusion movement. Magnetic resonance diffusion imaging labels water molecules through the magnetization of hydrogen protons without interfering with their diffusion process and can give a more realistic picture of the diffusion of water molecules in the examined tissue. Diffusion imaging consists of DWI and DTI, where DTI is developed from DWI to provide a better assessment of the direction of diffusion movement and to show the anisotropy of the tissue. The most commonly used parameters to evaluate the diffusion characteristics of tissues are ADC, mean diffusivity (MD), and partial fractional anisotropy (FA), with larger FA values indicating greater diffusion anisotropy. The DTI technique is widely applied in the histomorphological and pathological study of the central nervous system, as it can display the information of nerve fiber bundle alignment, direction, arrangement, and myelin sheath in a noninvasive and accurate manner. Rocca et al. [7] studied the brain tissue of patients with neuromyelitis optica by DTI technique and found that the MD of gray matter was increased, while the MD of white matter was not altered statistically, suggesting that there may be occult damage to the gray matter in patients with neuromyelitis optica. The presence of whole brain diffusion abnormalities in patients with MS, including white matter lesions and normally behaving white matter, suggests that DTI can be used for MS diagnosis and evaluation of the degree of the damage. Yang Yang et al. [8] conducted tracing of cerebral white matter tracts in patients with MS and found that the ADC of demyelinated plaques in the MS group was lower than that in healthy normal subjects, and the FA value was higher than that in healthy normal subjects, while both the number of tracer fibers and fiber density were negatively correlated with the extended brain disability status score.

4.4 Application of Other Imaging Techniques in Craniospinal Autoimmune Diseases

PET has been shown to have a beneficial effect on the diagnosis of limbic lobe encephalitis, and some patients with negative MRI findings of limbic lobe encephalitis show hypermetabolism in the medial temporal lobe in PET. It has been found [9] that patients with anti-NMDAR encephalitis have increased metabolism in the frontal and temporal lobes with decreased metabolism in the occipital lobe, and the degree of alteration of this metabolic gradient was found to be positively correlated with disease severity, and cortical metabolism returned to normal in these patients after clinical cure.

The application of MRI has greatly improved the accuracy of autoimmune disease diagnosis, which has certain characteristics in MRI manifestation, and the application of MRI can better comprehend the disease characteristics and disease progression of autoimmune diseases. In recent years, more and more new MRI techniques have been applied to clinical practice, allowing physicians to gain a deeper understanding of the disease characteristics of autoimmune diseases, and with the in-depth study of these techniques, new MRI techniques will be more widely used in the study of autoimmune diseases.

References

1. Sweeney M. Autoimmune neurologic diseases in children. Semin Neurol. 2018;38(3):355–70.
2. Kim HJ, Paul F, Lanapeixoto MA, et al. MRI characteristics of neuromyelitis optica spectrum disorder an international update. Neurology. 2015;84(11):1165–73.
3. Stamile C, Kocevar G, Cotton F, et al. A sensitive and automatic white matter fiber tracts model for longitudinal analysis of diffusion tensor images in multiple sclerosis. PLoS One. 2016;11(5):e0156405.
4. Cao D, Zhang L, Guo X, et al. Analysis of clinical manifestations and MRI features of autoimmune encephalitis. Chin J Neuropsychiatr Dis. 2017;43(6):341–5.
5. Qiu X, Zhuangzhi S, Yao L, et al. MRI features of ophthalmoneuromyelitis. Chin Med Imaging Technol. 2017;33(6):944–8.
6. Ropele S, Strasserfuchs S, Augustin M, et al. A comparison of magnetization transfer ratio, magnetization transfer rate, and the native relaxation time of water protons related to relapsing-remitting multiple sclerosis. Am J Neuroradiol. 2000;21(10):1885.
7. Rocca MA, Agosta F, Mezzapesa DM, et al. A functional MRI study of movement-associated cortical changes in patients with Devic's neuromyelitis optica. Neuroimage. 2004;21(3):1061–8.
8. Yang Y, Zhuang K, Yan Z, et al. Quantitative 3D simulation of MRI diffusion tensor imaging brain white matter bundle tracing in patients with multiple sclerosis. Chin J Neurol. 2011;10(10):1048–52.
9. Leypoldt F, Buchert R, Kleiter I, et al. Fluorodeoxyglucose positron emission tomography in anti-N-methyl-D-aspartate receptor encephalitis: distinct pattern of disease. J Neurol Neurosurg Psychiatry. 2012;83(7):681.

Laboratory Diagnostic Techniques and Methods for Infectious and Inflammatory Diseases of the Central Nervous System

5

Mingquan Chen, Yanran Li, and Yunjin Song

5.1 Diagnosis of Pathogens

Mingquan Chen, Yanran Li, and Yunjin Song

5.1.1 Overview

Infections of the central nervous system (CNS) can be easily confused with other diseases due to the lack of specificity of the initial symptoms and signs. It is also difficult to decide the infections caused by different pathogens based merely on clinical manifestations. Therefore, pathogenic diagnosis in laboratory tests has an irreplaceable role in the diagnosis and treatment of CNS infections. Laboratory pathogenic diagnostic methods for CNS infections mainly include cerebrospinal fluid (CSF) smear, CSF cell count and biochemical examination, CSF pathogen culture, and brain tissue biopsy.

5.1.2 CSF Smear

CSF smear is commonly used for the examination of bacteria and fungi infections, which is simple to perform and has a confirmatory value once the result is positive. However, its positive rate is low, while a positive Gram stain of CSF is highly suggestive of bacterial meningitis. In patients without antibiotics, the sensitivity of Gram stain for the diagnosis of bacterial meningitis ranges from 60% to 80%, whereas the sensitivity of Gram stain for the diagnosis of bacterial meningitis is only 40–60% in patients treated with antibiotics [1]. In addition, the sensitivity of Gram stain of CSF smear varies depending on the type of pathogen. The sensitivity of CSF Gram stain for *Haemophilus influenzae* infection ranges from 25% to 65%; the positive rate of CSF Gram stain for *Streptococcus pneumoniae* infection is 69–93%; and the sensitivity of CSF Gram stain for *Neisseria meningitidis* infection is 73–89%. Gram staining has a low detection rate for *Listeria monocytogenes* with a sensitivity of 23–36% [1].

Since different species of fungi have their own typical colony morphology and varying morphology of spores and mycelium, morphological examination by smear is an essential tool for fungal detection. The most readily diagnosed of the various fungal meningitis types by CSF smear is cryptococcal meningitis. The sensitivity of ink staining of CSF smears for the diagnosis of cryptococcal meningitis can be up to 70% [2].

5.1.3 CSF Cell Count and Biochemical Tests

Bacterial (except *Mycobacterium tuberculosis*), *Mycobacterium tuberculosis*, viral, and fungal infections can be broadly distinguished by changes in cell count, glucose, and protein content in the CSF. Bacterial infections: The CSF cell count, predominantly neutrophils, significantly increases to nearly 2000 × 10^6/L. CSF glucose is less than 0.34 g/L, with the ratio of CSF glucose to blood glucose at less than 0.23, and CSF protein exceeds 2.2 g/L. *Mycobacterium tuberculosis* infections: The CSF cell count, mainly lymphocytes, is elevated to nearly 500 × 10^6/L, with the CSF glucose being usually at 0.2–0.4 g/L and protein content >0.5 g/L. Viral infections: The CSF cell count, mainly lymphocytes, is slightly elevated to (10–200) × 10^6/L, and the CSF glucose content is normal and the protein content is basically normal. Fungal infections: The CSF cell count, predominantly lymphocytes, is elevated to nearly 200 × 10^6/L, with a marked decrease in the glucose content

M. Chen (✉)
Huashan Hospital, Fudan University, Shanghai, China
e-mail: mingquanchen@fudan.edu.cn

Y. Li
The First Affiliated Hospital of Xinjiang Medical University, Urumqi, China

Y. Song
School of Medicine, Shanghai University, Shanghai, China

H. Li et al. (eds.), *Radiology of Infectious and Inflammatory Diseases - Volume 1*,
https://doi.org/10.1007/978-981-99-0039-8_5

(most <0.3 g/L) and an increase in the protein content, generally exceeding 1 g/L. CSF cell counts and biochemical tests are more rudimentary in differentiating pathogens, and the cell counts, glucose, and protein cutoff values mentioned above cannot be generalized. Thus, a comprehensive judgment also requires CSF smear and pathogen culture results.

5.1.4 Culture of CSF Pathogens

The results of CSF pathogen cultures are generally used as the gold standard for diagnosis [3]. While viral, bacterial (including *Mycobacterium tuberculosis*), and fungal infections can be identified by this method, the positive rate of CSF cultures for all of these pathogens is low. In addition, CSF bacterial cultures generally require at least 72 h to make a determination, while the sensitivity of *Mycobacterium tuberculosis* cultures is only 22% [3]. Fungal meningitis CSF cultures are similarly time-consuming and have a low positive rate. For viral infections, the experimental conditions for CSF virus culture are demanding, whereas the sensitivity is unsatisfactory. Therefore, although a positive culture of CSF pathogens plays a decisive role in the diagnosis of the disease, it is often detrimental to the early diagnosis and treatment of patients because of its lagging nature and low sensitivity.

5.1.5 Brain Tissue Biopsy

In cases where the diagnosis cannot be confirmed by conventional examination, brain tissue biopsy can be used to examine brain tissue specimens by light microscopy or electron microscopy, both to understand the characteristics of brain tissue lesions and to directly observe the infecting pathogens, such as characteristic viral inclusion bodies that can be observed under light microscopy and viral particles under electron microscopy. However, this method is invasive and not easily accepted by patients.

5.2 Immunological Diagnosis

Mingquan Chen, Yanran Li, and Yunjin Song

5.2.1 Overview

The blood-brain barrier (BBB) of the normal CNS prevents components of the immune system from entering the CNS and is therefore considered "immune-privileged sites." However, when the CNS is invaded by pathogens, the BBB is violated, and thus lymphocytes and associated immune molecules from the blood enter the CSF. On the other hand, in noninfectious inflammatory diseases of the CNS, such as autoimmune encephalitis, patients have increased expression of anti-neuronal antibodies in the serum and CSF. Thus, immunological methods also have an important role in the diagnosis of infectious and noninfectious inflammatory diseases of the CNS.

5.2.2 Rapid Antigen Detection

Cryptococcal antigen testing is widely used in antigen testing for fungal infections of the CNS. This method relies on latex agglutination test to detect the presence of cryptococcus capsular polysaccharide antigen in CSF with a sensitivity and specificity of 80% and 93%, respectively [2]. Cryptococcal latex agglutination test is significantly superior to the conventional culture and microscopy methods for the early and rapid diagnosis of cryptococcal meningitis, but false positives and false negatives are inevitable. Junctional disease and systemic lupus erythematosus are cross-antigens with *Cryptococcus neoformans* podocyte polysaccharide antigen, thus causing false positives. In contrast, the hook effect caused by high concentrations of cryptococcal antigens and the masking effect of unknown nonspecific proteins on cryptococcal antigens in vivo can cause false negatives.

Detection of galactomannan (GM) and 1, 3-beta-D-glucan antigens in CSF is useful in the diagnosis of other invasive fungal infections of the CNS, such as *Aspergillus*. Some studies have reported a decrease in 1, 3-beta-D-glucan antigen concentrations in the CSF of patients receiving antifungal therapy [4]; therefore, detection of 1, 3-beta-D-glucan antigen concentrations in the CSF can be used to monitor the response to treatment of fungal meningitis. For the diagnosis of bacterial meningitis, it is also possible to detect bacterial podocyte polysaccharide antigens in the patient's CSF using the latex agglutination test.

It has been reported that the sensitivity of CSF bacterial podocyte polysaccharide antigen testing is about 78% in patients with *Haemophilus influenzae* type B infection, 59% in patients with *Streptococcus pneumoniae* infection, and 30–89% in patients with meningococcal infection [5]. However, most studies have shown that the positive rate of CSF bacterial podocyte polysaccharide antigen testing is only 7–10% [6]. The clinical use and popularity of the bacterial podocyte polysaccharide antigen test remains limited due to the extremely high false-positive rate.

5.2.3 Antibody Testing

The pathogen causing the infection can be inferred indirectly by detecting specific antibodies in the blood and CSF. The specific antibody test has little significance for early diagnosis because it takes time for antibodies to be produced. The IgM antibody, which emphasizes the comparison of the results of the acute and recovery periods, is of more diagnostic value than the IgG antibody. Nevertheless, the antibodies produced by different pathogens may have cross-reactivity and affect the accuracy of the results, which should be noted clinically. These tests are more widely used, such as coagulation test, sedimentation test, complement binding test, enzyme-linked immunosorbent assay, and immunoblot test for parasitic infections; venereal disease research laboratory (VDRL) or rapid plasma reagin (RPR) (screening test), fluorescent treponemal antibody absorption (FTA-ABS), or micro-hemagglutination assay (MHA-TP) (confirmatory test) for syphilis spirochete infections; and neutralization test, complement binding test, hemagglutination inhibition test, etc., for viral infections.

Autoantibody testing is also important in the diagnosis of noninfectious inflammatory diseases of the CNS, such as Rasmussen's encephalitis, where GluR3 antibodies are detected in serum and CSF, and autoimmune encephalitis, where autoantibodies against neuronal surface antigens are positive.

5.2.4 γ-Interferon Release Test

The technique has shown some advantages in clinical application for the diagnosis of tuberculous meningitis. The long-term presence of antigen-specific memory T cells in the body after *Mycobacterium tuberculosis* infection allows them to rapidly activate and proliferate upon re-stimulation with antigen, releasing γ-interferon. The main principle of this technique is using *Mycobacterium tuberculosis*-specific antigen early secretory targeting antigen 6 (ESAT-6) and culture filtration protein 10 (CFP-10) as stimulators to stimulate the activation and proliferation of Mycobacterium tuberculosis-specific memory T cells in peripheral blood or CSF, thereby detecting gamma-interferon releasing T lymphocytes.

A blank control, a positive control, and two wells with ESAT-6 and CFP-10 peptide libraries as stimulants are provided. The test will be considered valid if the number of spots in the blank control wells is smaller than 10 and the number of spots in the positive control wells is larger than 20. When the number of spots in the blank control wells is smaller than 6 and if the number of spots in any of the test wells is ≥6 after subtracting that of the blank control, the result is interpreted as positive; when the number of spots in the blank control wells is greater than 6 and if the number of spots in any of the test wells is greater than twice that of the blank control, the result is interpreted as positive [7].

5.3 Genetic Diagnosis

Mingquan Chen, Yanran Li, and Yunjin Song

5.3.1 Overview

With the rapid development of molecular biology techniques, the identification of pathogenic microorganisms is no longer limited to general tests such as external morphological structure and physiological properties but goes further to the study of biological macromolecules at the molecular biology level, especially at the nucleic acid level. The understanding of microorganisms has gradually shifted from external phenotypes to internal genetic structure characteristics, and the detection of microorganisms has also shifted from biochemical and immunological methods to genetic-level detection. There are certain advantages to genetic testing for the diagnosis of CNS infections, since normally the CSF, spinal cord, and brain tissue are sterile sites and any evidence showing the presence of microorganisms may represent an infection, and if an infection is present, it is usually monomicrobial. In addition, common inhibitors of nucleic acid amplification methods (such as polymerase chain reaction [PCR]) that can lead to false-negative results, such as heme, nucleic acid endonucleases, and nucleic acid exonucleases, are usually not present in CSF. Therefore, direct detection of nucleic acids in CNS samples may be less likely to produce false-positive results (e.g., contamination or presence of nonpathogenic colonization) or false-negative results (e.g., suppression) than in other parts of the body for a number of common reasons.

Genetic testing provides precise results for identifying the pathogens of CNS infections, which helps to quickly and accurately identify the pathogens and activate antimicrobial drug therapy in a timely manner.

5.3.2 Nucleic Acid Amplification Techniques

5.3.2.1 Conventional PCR and Real-Time Fluorescence PCR Assay Techniques

The conventional PCR assay consists of three steps: sample extraction, target nucleic acid amplification, and amplicon detection. The application of PCR for detection of viral nucleic acid sequences in CNS herpes simplex virus infections is faster and more sensitive than viral isolation and culture and maintains the same specificity [8]. Subsequently, the real-time fluorescent PCR assay was introduced by Applied Biosystems in 1996 and has been internationally recognized as the most effective means of laboratory confirmation of pathogenic microorganisms associated with infectious diseases for its accuracy, rapidity, and sensitivity. The chemistry of fluorescent PCR can be divided into three basic types: DNA-binding dye method, probe method, and quencher dye primer method. The former two methods could detect primer dimers and other nonspecific reaction products with low specificity; therefore, they have been rarely used in the clinical diagnosis of infectious diseases. Probe method is generally recommended for the molecular diagnosis of infectious diseases of the CNS. The probe method, which relies on fluorescence resonance energy migration, including TaqMan probes, molecular beacons, scorpion probes, composite probes, etc., detects only specific amplification products and is therefore highly specific. The most widely used is the TaqMan probe technology.

5.3.2.2 Isothermal Amplification of Nucleic Acid

It is a rapidly developing in vitro nucleic acid amplification technology in recent years. Unlike PCR technology, its amplification reaction is always carried out at a single temperature without the need for temperature-controlled precision experimental instruments and complex experimental procedures, and its easy operation, rapid reaction, and high detection sensitivity have shown good prospects for clinical and field rapid diagnosis. Presently available isothermal amplification techniques consist of loop-mediated isothermal amplification (LAMP), nucleic acid sequence-based amplification (NASBA), chain-substitution isothermal amplification, loop-rolling isothermal amplification, loop-dependent isothermal amplification, single-primer isothermal amplification, and rapid isothermal amplification of nucleic acids. In the detection of infectious disease pathogens, there are more applications of LAMP, NASBA, etc. LAMP has been successfully applied to the detection of EV71, *Mycobacterium tuberculosis*, dengue virus, yellow fever virus, etc., and NASBA has been applied to the detection of various pathogenic microorganisms such as bacteria and viruses. LAMP uses four primers to identify six loci with high specificity, but the primer design is demanding, and the amplification products cannot be used for clone sequencing, which can easily form aerosols and cause false positives, thus affecting the detection results. The NASBA reaction components are more complex, and the use of three enzymes increases the cost of the reaction and is not suitable for DNA-type pathogen detection.

5.3.2.3 GeneXpert Rapid Detection System

It integrates and automates the sample preparation and quantitative PCR processes in a single closed kit, automating sample preparation, nucleic acid purification and concentration, quantitative PCR amplification detection, and analytical output in tens of minutes. Compared with conventional PCR and real-time fluorescence quantitative PCR, GeneXpert rapid detection system has three distinct advantages. (1) More accurate: The unique quantitative PCR reaction design, fully automated operation, and internal reference design ensure accurate and reliable results. (2) Quick and easy: The entire process from sample processing, nucleic acid purification, to quantitative PCR assay is completed automatically. (3) Highly safe: The entire test is performed fully automatically in a closed kit, without the need for complex protection.

It is noticeable that the GeneXpert rapid test has shown its strengths in diagnosing tuberculous meningitis in *Mycobacterium tuberculosis* infections. The Xpert MTB/RIF *Mycobacterium tuberculosis* test kit can detect the presence of *Mycobacterium tuberculosis* and its resistance to rifampicin directly from patient specimens within 2 h. The World Health Organization (WHO) even recommends the Xpert MTB/RIF *Mycobacterium tuberculosis* test kit test as a first-line pathogen test for tuberculosis. In a study from South Africa, a high-HIV-prevalence region, the overall sensitivity and specificity of the Xpert MTB/RIF *Mycobacterium tuberculosis* test kit using 1 mL of non-centrifuged and 3 mL of centrifuged CSF was 62% and 95%, respectively, which was better than the 12% sensitivity of smear staining, and the sensitivity of centrifuged specimens was 82%, which was higher than that of non-centrifuged specimens at 47%. This indicates that the Xpert MTB/RIF *Mycobacterium tuberculosis* test can be a promising method for the diagnosis of tuberculous meningitis in HIV-infected patients, especially when centrifuged CSF is available [9]. However, the high cost of the test largely limits its use. Besides, the Xpert MTB/RIF system cannot distinguish between live and dead *Mycobacterium tuberculosis* and cannot be used to monitor treatment success, failure, or relapse.

5.3.3 Nucleic Acid Molecular Hybridization Techniques

Nucleic acid molecular hybridization is the process of forming heterogeneous duplexes of two single strands of nucleic acid with certain homology under certain conditions according to the principle of base complementary pairing based on the nature of nucleic acid denaturation and complexation. According to the source and nature of probes, nucleic acid probes are divided into four categories: genomic DNA probes, cDNA probes, RNA probes, and oligonucleotide probes, which have their own characteristics and scope of application, and their markers are radionuclides and non-radionuclides, the latter including biotin, digoxin, fluorescein, enzymes, and chemiluminescent markers. Nucleic acid molecular hybridization can be divided into two main categories: solid-phase hybridization and liquid-phase hybridization. Common types of solid-phase hybridization include Southern blot hybridization, Northern blot hybridization, spot or slit hybridization, and colony hybridization. The technique is a specific, sensitive, simple, and rapid detection method that can directly detect pathogenic bacteria in the clinic without the influence of nonpathogenic bacteria. It is of special significance especially to the detection of bacteria that cannot yet be isolated and cultured or are very difficult to culture.

5.3.4 Next-Generation Sequencing (NGS) Technologies

NGS is a novel sequencing method compared to the first-generation DNA sequencing technology. Gene sequencing was made possible by Frederick Sanger's invention of the double deoxygenated chain termination method in 1977. With the innovation of technology, in addition to the standard Sanger sequencing method, new methods such as automated sequencers, fluorescent labeled ends, capillary sequencing, etc., have emerged, but they are essentially based on the technique of Sanger sequencing, which is consequently called the first-generation sequencing technology. NGS is also known as "high-throughput sequencing" or "deep sequencing," which includes second- and third-generation sequencing. The general processes of the second-generation sequencing include (1) sample collection and DNA extraction; (2) generation of template strands to build DNA libraries by bridge PCR or emulsion PCR; (3) sequencing while synthesizing by pyrophosphate sequencing, reversible terminator method, ligation sequencing, etc.; and (4) analysis of the sequencing results and splicing into the required DNA information. The main difference between third-generation sequencing and second-generation sequencing is that single-molecule sequencing is used instead of sequencing after building a DNA library to reduce sequencing errors introduced during the PCR process. The most significant advantage of NGS over first-generation sequencing is that millions or even hundreds of millions of DNA or RNA sequences can be measured simultaneously, greatly accelerating the speed of whole-genome sequencing.

NGS has significant advantages in the detection of pathogens in patients with unexplained encephalitis [10]. NGS can identify novel pathogens infecting the CNS and is dominated by new strains of known viruses. With the ability to assemble genomes from scratch, the unbiased nature of NGS technology allows the discovery of completely novel microorganisms that are undetectable by traditional pathogenic assays or the unearthing of unknown pathogenic capabilities of a known microorganism.

However, as a new genetic diagnostic technique, there is no uniform standard for the analysis and interpretation of CSF NGS results. Unlike serology, PCR, and other tests that target a specific pathogen, CSF NGS usually obtains multiple suspected pathogen gene sequences, which are matched and analyzed against the pathogen genome to obtain diagnostic information. Contamination and mixing of microbial genetic sequences in specimen collection and laboratory testing is inevitable, and contaminated sequencing as background "noise" may significantly affect the judgment of results. Theoretically, the higher the coverage and depth corresponding to a particular pathogen, the more likely it is to suggest the presence of that pathogen in the specimen. Additional confirmatory tests are necessary for highly suspected pathogens detected by NGS screening, including PCR assays, specific serological tests, immunocytochemistry, and in situ hybridization.

References

1. He T, Kaplan S, Kamboj M, et al. Laboratory diagnosis of central nervous system infection. Curr Infect Dis Rep. 2016;18(11):35.
2. Dunbar SA, Eason RA, Musher DM, et al. Microscopic examination and broth culture of cerebrospinal fluid in diagnosis of meningitis. J Ciln Microbiol. 1998;36(6):1617–20.
3. Ubukata K. Rapid identification of meningitis due to bacterial pathogens. Clin Neurol. 2013;53(11):1184–6.
4. Meyer T, Franke G, Polywka SK, et al. Improved detection of bacterial central nervous system infections by use of a broad-range PCR assay. J Ciln Microbiol. 2014;52(5):1751–3.
5. Acosta J, Catalan M, Del PA, et al. Prospective study in critically ill non-neutropenic patients: diagnostic potential of (1, 3)-beta-D-glucan assay and circulating galactomannan for the diagnosis of invasive fungal disease. Eur J Clin Microbiol Infect Dis. 2012;31(5):721–31.
6. Lyons JL, Thakur KT, Lee R, et al. Utility of measuring (1, 3) -beta-d-glucan in cerebrospinal fluid for diagnosis of fungal central nervous system infection. J Ciln Microbiol. 2015;53(1):319–22.
7. Bahr NC, Marais S, Caws M, et al. GeneXpert MTB/Rif to diagnose tuberculous meningitis: perhaps the first test but not the last. Clin Infect Dis. 2016;62(9):1133–5.
8. Tyler KL. Herpes simplex virus infections of the central nervous system: encephalitis and meningitis, including Mollaret's. Herpes. 2004;11(Suppl 2):57A–64A.
9. Ohkusu K. Molecular approaches for the diagnosis of central nervous system infections. Brain Nerve. 2015;67(7):799–811.
10. Wilson MR, Naccache SN, Samayoa E, et al. Actionable diagnosis of neuroleptospirosis by next-generation sequencing. N Engl J Med. 2014;370(25):2408–17.

Part II

Special Contagious Diseases Related to the Central Nervous System

6 Respiratory Infectious Disease-Related Intracranial Infections

Li Li, Yinglin Guo, Dan Zhang, Jun Liu, Wenxiao Jia, Longlin Yin, Meiji Ren, Nuerbiyemu Abulikemu, and Xuening Zhang

6.1 Measles

Li Li and Yinglin Guo

Measles is an acute respiratory infection caused by the measles virus (MV), which is a category B infectious disease among the notifiable diseases in China. Encephalitis associated with measles includes acute measles encephalitis, immunosuppressive measles encephalitis, and subacute sclerosing panencephalitis, mostly thought to be caused by direct invasion of brain tissue by measles virus.

6.1.1 Acute Measles Encephalitis

6.1.1.1 Overview

Measles encephalitis (ME) is a central nervous system complication of the measles course, resulting from direct invasion of the central nervous system by the measles virus or from an immune response to infection. Acute measles encephalitis can occur at any age but is more common in children aged 6 months to 6 years, consistent with the age of onset of measles. Encephalitis occurs mostly on days 2–6 after the rash, and its occurrence is not related to the severity of measles but is mainly due to the direct invasion of brain tissue by the measles virus.

The clinical manifestations of acute measles encephalitis are similar to those of other viral encephalitis, such as fever, headache, vomiting, convulsions, drowsiness or even coma, or personality changes and behavioral abnormalities. Meningeal irritation sign and pathological reflexes are positive. Cerebrospinal fluid examination demonstrates increased lymphocytes and mildly increased protein, but the cerebrospinal fluid is clear and bright in color. About half of the patients with measles have transient electroencephalograph (EEG) abnormalities in the late stages. Mild encephalitis can recover in a few days; some patients are left with sequelae such as mental retardation, epilepsy, and paralysis; a few have fulminant progression and die rapidly; measles virus-specific antibody measurements in serum or cerebrospinal fluid can suggest a diagnosis.

6.1.1.2 Pathological Manifestations

Brain tissue congestion and edema, scattered foci of hemorrhage, perivascular hemorrhage, lymphocytic infiltration, and demyelinating changes.

6.1.1.3 Imaging

1. CT: There is no abnormality in the early stages, while extensive mild atrophy of the cerebral cortex can be seen after a few weeks. The frontoparietal lobe is the most predominant, and limited hypothalamic atrophy is rare.
2. MRI: The manifestation of MRI is mostly normal in the early stage. Mild atrophy of the cerebral cortex, cerebral edema, and demyelination can be seen after a few weeks. The lesions are mostly found in the periventricular white matter, basal ganglia, hippocampus, subcortex (occipital lobe), and cerebellar white matter. It appears as a punctate or lamellar T_1-hypointense and T_2-hyperintense on patho-

L. Li · M. Ren
Beijing You'an Hospital, Capital Medical University, Beijing, China

Y. Guo
Harbin Daowai District Taiping People's Hospital, Harbin, China

D. Zhang · W. Jia (✉) · N. Abulikemu
The First Affiliated Hospital of Xinjiang Medical University, Urumqi, China

J. Liu
The Second Xiangya Hospital of Central South University, Changsha, China
e-mail: junliu123@csu.edu.cn

L. Yin
Sichuan Provincial People's Hospital, Chengdu, China

X. Zhang
Department of Radiology, The Second Hospital of Tianjin Medical University, Tianjin, China

H. Li et al. (eds.), *Radiology of Infectious and Inflammatory Diseases - Volume 1*,
https://doi.org/10.1007/978-981-99-0039-8_6

logical regions, with high signal intensity on T_2-weighted fluid-attenuated inversion recovery (FLAIR). Liu Lumin [1] reported one case of adult measles encephalitis with partial memory loss after discharge from the hospital, considered to be related to hippocampal damage. Mi Changrui et al. [2] reported a case of measles encephalitis complicated by central pontine myelinolysis, which apparents hypointense on T_1-weighted imaging and hyperintense on T_2-weighted imaging at the median edge of the pontine on MRI, with hyperintense in both FLAIR and DWI. The myelinolysis of the central pontine was considered to be related to cerebral edema, hypokalemia, hypocalcemia, and hypomagnesemia after measles encephalitis.

6.1.1.4 Diagnostic Key Points

1. In patients with measles, clinical symptoms such as high fever, headache, convulsions, drowsiness, and even coma are seen.
2. On MR images, multiple T_1-hypointense and T_2-hyperintense lesions can be seen in basal ganglia, hippocampus, and white matter, with restricted diffusion on diffusion-weighted imaging (DWI).
3. Cerebrospinal fluid is positive for measles IgM antibody.

6.1.1.5 Differential Diagnosis

The imaging manifestations of acute measles encephalitis overlap with other viral encephalitis. Confirmation of the diagnosis requires a combination of clinical manifestations and cerebrospinal fluid examination.

6.1.2 Immunosuppressive Measles Encephalitis

6.1.2.1 Overview

Immunosuppressive measles encephalitis, also known as delayed measles encephalitis, most often occurs in immunocompromised measles patients. In the early stage of measles, the symptoms are mostly mild and atypical. When the measles subsides and after an asymptomatic period of 2–5 months, neurological symptoms appear, such as mental abnormalities, drowsiness, coma, convulsions, and hemiparesis. The disease has an acute or subacute onset and a short duration, with death occurring within a few weeks to a few months after the onset of the disease. The laboratory tests can detect measles IgM antibodies in the cerebrospinal fluid or blood.

6.1.2.2 Pathological Manifestations

Diffuse changes are seen in the brain and spinal cord, and inclusion bodies are seen in the cytoplasm and nuclei of neuronal cells and astrocytes. There is extensive neuroblast degeneration, and microglia and astrocytes are all proliferating. Severe hypoxic changes are present in the hippocampal pyramidal layer with normal white matter. Occasional mononuclear cell infiltration can be found in the meninges and around blood vessels.

6.1.2.3 Imaging

1. CT: Multiple patchy hypodense foci at the junction of the basal ganglia and gray-white matter, mostly without enhancement or with mild enhancement on enhanced imaging; late cortical atrophy is evident or total brain atrophy.
2. MRI: T_2WI and FLAIR show multiple lamellar high signal intensity with poorly defined borders. The lesions may involve the thalamus and basal ganglia, bilateral hemianopia centers, gray-white matter junction, cerebellum, and brainstem. After administration of contrast material, few lesions are enhanced, and bilateral lesions are mostly asymmetric.

6.1.2.4 Diagnostic Key Points

1. Neurological symptoms in immunocompromised measles patients.
2. CT shows multiple patchy hypodense foci at the junction of basal ganglia and gray-white matter. In terms of MRI, hyperintense signal intensity can be seen on T_2WI and FLAIR and mostly without enhancement or with mild enhancement on postcontrast imaging.
3. Antibodies to measles IgM can be found in cerebrospinal fluid or blood.

6.1.2.5 Differential Diagnosis

1. Progressive multifocal leukoencephalopathy lesions predominantly located in the parietal, occipital lobe, frontal lobe, and subcortical white matter are more distant from the lateral ventricles, whereas the lesions of measles encephalitis involve the thalamus and basal ganglia, bilateral centrum semiovale, gray-white matter junction, cerebellum, and brainstem, with different sites of predilection. Besides, progressive multifocal leukoencephalopathy is often asymmetric, with progressive enlargement and fusion. MRI shows multiple subcortical demyelinating spots, T_1WI with low signal intensity, T_2WI with high signal intensity, and no occupancy effect. The outer edges of demyelinated spots are sharp, scalloped, or oval.
2. MRI of herpes simplex virus encephalitis shows a round-like or mass-like hypointense T1W signal intensity and hyperintense T_2W signal intensity in the temporal lobe, insula, and frontal lobe, which may show mild enhancement on postcontrast imaging, often with significant occupancy effects and punctate hemorrhage within the lesion.

3. Disseminated encephalitis lesions are mainly located in the periventricular area and less frequently involve the gray matter, showing multiple and diffuse irregular T_1-hypointense and T_2-hyperintense.

6.1.3 Subacute Sclerosing Panencephalitis

6.1.3.1 Overview

Subacute sclerosing panencephalitis (SSPE) is a chronic progressive degenerative lethal disease of the central nervous system caused by persistent infection with defective measles virus, a distant complication of measles, and a chronic or subacute progressive encephalitis.

This disease was first reported by Dawson in 1933 and officially defined as SSPE in 1969 after Greenfield isolated the measles virus from the brain tissue of patients. SSPE is rare, with an incidence of (1–4)/1 million, and often develops 2–17 years (mean 7 years) after the primary measles. It also with poor prognosis and extremely high rate of death. Its mechanism is mainly related to the gene mutation of measles virus, in which the body fails to produce antibodies against matrix proteins, resulting in prolonged latency of the virus in brain cells. The patient gradually develops mental retardation, personality changes, motor incoordination, speech and visual-auditory impairment, and seizures and finally dies from coma and tonic paralysis.

Confirmed diagnosis of SSPE depends on the fluctuating changes of virus antibody ratios in the cerebrospinal fluid and serum measles. SSPE patients have elevated titers of measles virus antibodies in the cerebrospinal fluid. Typical cases contain measles virus IgM and IgG antibodies in both serum and cerebrospinal fluid with consistently high titers and elevated gamma globulin levels and a paralytic colloidal gold curve. The characteristic EEG changes of SSPE manifest as periodic synchronous discharges (PSD), especially extensive periodic compound slow waves, i.e., periodic high amplitude slow and sharp slow waves in low amplitude activity present roughly symmetrical bilaterally and mostly pronounced in the parieto-occipital region.

6.1.3.2 Pathological Manifestations

SSPE: The early histopathological changes are predominantly inflammatory lesions, seen as meningitis and encephalitis. The lesions first involve the occipital, parietal, and posterior temporal lobes and gradually spread from posterior to anterior to the frontal region as the disease progresses. Because the lesions can involve the cerebral cortex, subcortical white matter, basal ganglia, brainstem, and upper cervical medulla, it is called "holoprosencephalitis." There is extensive involvement of the gray and white matter of the brain, with perivascular lymphocytic and plasma cell cuff-like infiltration, glial cell hyperplasia, and nodule formation, hence the term "sclerotic." Intranuclear inclusion bodies are one of the characteristic changes of SSPE [3, 4].

6.1.3.3 Imaging

1. CT: Multiple patchy hypodensity can be seen in the paraventricular and cortical areas and white matter with no enhancement after administration of contrast material. Total brain atrophy may occur at advanced stages.
2. MRI: The lesion is located in the cerebral cortex, subcortical and periventricular white matter, corpus callosum, basal ganglia, thalamus, and brainstem. Cortical, subcortical, and periventricular white matter is commonly involved, which may extend to the corpus callosum, especially the splenium of corpus callosum.

The damage degree of brain parenchymal was significantly correlated with the duration of the disease [5]. The distribution of lesion sites at MRI is time-specific. In the early stage of SSPE, CT and MRI may be without positive findings. At MRI, multiple patches of asymmetry T_1-hypointense and T_2-hyperintense are demonstrated in the cortical and subcortical white matter. The lesions are obvious in the posterior part of the cerebral hemisphere, and about 20–35% involved the basal ganglia. The midline may be displaced due to brain tissue edema, with tumor-like occupying effects and enhancement. With the progress of the disease, T_2WI high-signal-intensity areas may enlarge and extend to the paraventricular and corpus callosum. At the end stage, almost all white matter may loss, the corpus callosum may become thinner, the brainstem demonstrates foci with hyperintense on T_2WI and diffuse brain atrophy may occur, and some cases may be accompanied by cerebellar atrophy. Slowly progressing SSPE just manifests brain atrophy.

6.1.3.4 Diagnostic Key Points

1. Typical clinical course of measles or history of previous measles virus infection.
2. At MRI, diffusion lesions are involved in both gray and white matter, especially the cerebral cortex, subcortical, and periventricular white matter. The lesions may extend to the corpus callosum, especially the splenium of the corpus callosum. Brain atrophy can be seen in advanced stages.
3. Characteristic EEG changes, manifested by periodic synchronous discharges, especially extensive periodic compound slow waves, i.e., periodic high amplitude slow waves and sharp slow waves in the midst of low amplitude activity.
4. The most diagnostic significance is the fluctuating changes in the ratio of cerebrospinal fluid and serum measles virus antibodies, with elevated titers of measles virus antibodies in the cerebrospinal fluid. Typical cases

contain consistently increasing titers of measles virus IgM and IgG antibodies in both serum and cerebrospinal fluid, with elevated gamma globulin levels and a paralytic colloidal gold curve.

5. Brain tissue biopsy or pathological examination revealed pathological changes in holoprosencephalitis. Measles-like virus can be isolated or measles virus antigen can be found in the brain tissue.

6.1.3.5 Differential Diagnosis

1. Progressive multifocal leukoencephalopathy is a multifocal disease that occurs in the subcortical white matter of the parieto-occipital lobe, mostly far from the periventricular area, and can gradually fuse and expand, with cerebral U-shaped fiber involvement as the characteristic manifestation. While SSPE is more common in the cerebral cortex with subcortical white matter and periventricular white matter involvement, the white matter involvement can extend to the corpus callosum, especially the corpus callosum pressure.
   The characteristic EEG changes of SSPE are periodic synchronous discharges, especially extensive periodic compound slow waves, i.e., periodic high-amplitude slow waves and sharp slow waves in the midst of low-amplitude activity.
2. On noncontrast MRI, herpes simplex virus encephalitis demonstrates unilaterally T_1-hypointense and T_2-hyperintense which confined to the temporal lobe and insula. At postcontrast imaging, linear enhancement around the lateral fissure and gyral enhancement in the lesion area are often noted; occupancy effects and intralesion punctate hemorrhage can be seen. However, the lesions on contralateral are milder.
3. Sporadic encephalitis demonstrates irregular T_1-hypointense and T_2-hyperintense lesions primarily located in the white matter with multiple distributions. The lesions are mainly located around the ventricles and the cortex can be less involved.

6.1.3.6 Status and Progress of Research

1. ^{1}H-MRS: In the early stage of SSPE, biomarkers from MRS significantly changed. A decrease of *N*-acetyl aspartate (NAA) and an increase of choline (Cho) and lactate (Lac) suggest demyelination, inflammatory, and increased metabolism of brain tissue, respectively. In the advanced stage, the ratio of NAA to creatinine (NAA/Cre) decreases, and the ratio of choline, inositol, and creatinine increases, which may reflect gliosis, neurogenic fiber tangles, and brain atrophy [5]. ^{1}H-MRS is considered an early diagnostic robust technique of SSPE.
2. **DWI**: Mild diffusion restriction can be seen on DWI.

6.2 Intracranial Tuberculosis

Dan Zhang, Jun Liu, Wenxiao Jia and Longlin Yin

6.2.1 Overview

Intracranial tuberculosis is a rare form of tuberculosis of the central nervous system caused by hematogenous dissemination of *Mycobacterium tuberculosis* [6]. Intracranial tuberculosis can develop at any age and is more common in children and young adults. It may clinically present with symptoms of tuberculosis toxicity such as fever, night sweats, lack of appetite, general lethargy and weakness, and mental depression, as well as symptoms of focal central nervous system damage (e.g., limb paralysis, epilepsy, etc.).

Based on the location of intracranial tuberculosis, imaging often classifies it into three basic types, namely, meningeal tuberculosis, parenchymal tuberculosis, and mixed intracranial tuberculosis [7–10]. Meningeal tuberculosis refers to the simple involvement of the meninges by tuberculosis lesions, which can be divided into three subtypes according to their pathological changes: tuberculous meningitis, meningeal tuberculoma, and subdural (extradural) tuberculous abscess. Secondary changes such as cerebral infarction, cerebral atrophy, and hydrocephalus are often seen in meningeal tuberculosis [11]. Tuberculosis of the brain parenchyma refers to the simple involvement of the brain parenchyma by tuberculosis lesions, which can be classified into five subtypes according to their pathological changes: diffuse miliary tuberculosis, tuberculous nodules, tuberculoma, tuberculous encephalitis, and tuberculous brain abscess. Mixed intracranial tuberculosis is the presence of both meningeal and parenchymal tuberculosis in the same case. Imaging of intracranial tuberculosis varies because of the complex and diverse pathological changes and regression of intracranial tuberculosis.

6.2.2 Pathological Manifestations

Tuberculous inflammation often manifests pathologically as inflammatory exudation, hyperplasia, and degeneration, and these three pathological changes often coexist or are dominated by one or the other, and all three can be interconverted, depending primarily on the number of infected *Mycobacterium tuberculosis*, the size of the virulence, and the immunity and allergic status of the organism. The predominantly exudative lesions appear mainly in the early stages of tuberculosis inflammation or when the lesions worsen and recur, showing localized neutrophil infiltration followed by replacement by macrophages and lymphocytes. The predominantly hyperplasia lesions often occur when the body is more resistant or during the recovery phase of the lesion and manifest as typical tuberculous nodules composed of lymphocytes, epithelioid cells, Langhans giant cells, and fibroblasts. When the virulence of *Mycobacterium tuberculosis* is strong, the amount of infected bacteria is high, and the resistance of the body is low, a yellowish caseous necrosis may appear in the middle of the tuberculosis nodule. Meningeal tuberculosis tends to be predominantly exudative, whereas parenchymal tuberculosis tends to present as hyperplasia and caseous necrosis.

1. Meningeal Tuberculosis

   Massive tuberculous exudate spreads in the subarachnoid space to basal and lateral fissure cistern. Light microscopy reveals a tuberculous exudate consisting of polymorphonuclear leukocytes, macrophages, lymphocytes, and erythrocytes with varying numbers of bacteria in a fibrin network. As the disease progresses, there is a gradual increase in lymphocytes and connective tissue.
2. Tuberculosis of the brain parenchyma. Multiple or solitary small nodules with predominantly caseous necrosis surrounded by granulomas. Intracranial tuberculoma varies in size with clear borders. Pathologically, the tuberculoma has a yellowish caseous necrotic or granulomatous tissue in the center of the section, and microscopic examination shows epithelioid cells, Langhans giant cells, lymphocytes, plasma cells, and neutrophils. Carbolic acid magenta staining can find acid-fast bacilli. In a small number of cases, tuberculomas may be combined with purulent bacterial infections or form tuberculous brain abscesses.

6.2.3 Imaging

1. X-ray examination: Tuberculous meningitis on X-rays is often unremarkable, but sometimes hyperdense calcium spots are seen around the cisterna ambiens and suprasellar cistern near the superior sella in the advanced stages of the disease. The characteristic X-ray of patients with cerebral tuberculoma is calcification, which occurs close to the inner plate of the skull, so the extent of calcification on X-ray does not represent the actual size of the tuberculoma, and the incidence of calcification is not high. X-rays of tuberculous abscesses are similar to those of pyogenic abscesses, except that in tuberculous abscesses there is no gas in the lesion.
2. Angiography: The main manifestation of tuberculous meningitis on angiography is homogeneous or irregular narrowing of the lumen of the arterial trunk at the base of the skull and extensive thinning of the cerebral veins. Most tuberculomas have no vascular supply within them, and the contrast changes are identical to those of other avascular occupying lesions. A small number of tuberculomas may have envelope vascularization and may appear similar to chronic brain abscesses and are located in the cerebral cortex or superficial subcortical layers, often in multiple cases. Focal tuberculous encephalitis angiography may have no abnormal findings, and tuberculous brain abscesses may have occupying effects and abscess wall visualization similar to chronic brain abscesses.
3. CT
   (a) Meningeal tuberculosis
      - Tuberculous meningitis: Commonly found at the base of the brain. It is caused by hematogenous dissemination of *Mycobacterium tuberculosis* into the subarachnoid space and is one of the most serious manifestations of tuberculosis infectious disease and one of the leading causes of death from tuberculosis [12]. Early CT scan reveals increased density in the subarachnoid space, thickened meninges, and hyperdense flocculent deposits in the basal cistern and lateral fissure cistern of the brain, with localized punctate calcification in later stages and linear enhancement of the thickened meninges on enhanced scan (Fig. 6.1).
      - Meningeal tuberculoma: Tuberculomas consist of granulomas and exudative, liquefied centers of caseous necrosis. The granulomas are round or irregular in shape and often fuse with thickened meninges, mostly in the basal pool arachnoid,

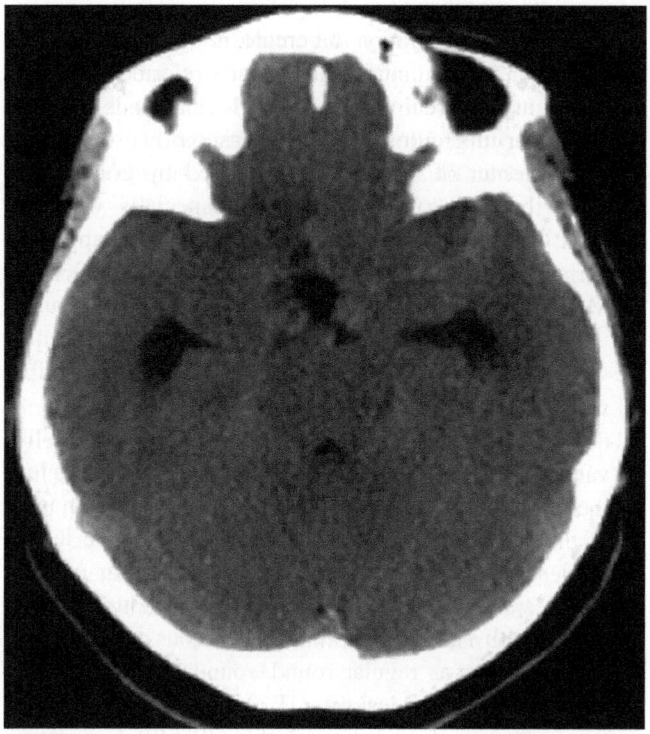

Fig. 6.1 Tuberculous meningitis. CT scan shows increased arachnoid linear and nodular density in the basal and bilateral lateral fissure pools

ventricular canal, and soft meninges, often in clusters. CT scan shows a nodular lesion with higher density than cerebrospinal fluid and similar density to the brain parenchyma, and enhanced scan shows a significantly enhanced granulomatous ring and non-enhancing caseous or liquefied necrotic centers [13]. In tuberculoma with larger diameters, the caseous necrotic center of the lesion manifests as hypodense, and the surrounding granuloma ring manifests as isodense. The lesions manifest ring-like enhancement on enhanced scans.

(b) Parenchymal tuberculosis of the brain
- Tuberculous encephalitis: The pathological basis of tuberculous encephalitis is inflammatory reactive edema and demyelinating changes in the white matter of the brain. CT scan shows a patchy hypodense area visible in the brain and no abnormal enhancement of the lesion on enhanced scan.
- Tuberculous brain abscess: The lesion is often seen on CT as a round or circular hypodense area with an isodense or slightly hyperdense ring around the lesion, and the lesion often shows nodular or irregular ring-like enhancement on enhanced scan. The CT findings of tuberculous brain abscesses are similar to those of larger diameter tuberculomas, and sometimes it is difficult to distinguish those two diseases.
- Diffuse miliary tuberculosis: Nodular lesions <3 mm in diameter are usually referred to as miliary tuberculosis. The pathological basis of nodular tuberculosis lesions is caseous necrosis in the center of the lesion surrounded by granulomas, but due to size limitations, especially when the diameter is <3 mm, most of the lesions appear as solid nodular foci on both CT and MRI. When combined with calcification, a diffuse distribution of hyperdense foci of calcification can be seen on CT scan. Enhanced scan shows diffuse distribution of nodular enhancement (Fig. 6.2).
- Tuberculosis nodules: It refers to nodule-like lesions with a diameter of 3–5 mm. Tuberculous nodules are usually multiple, and their imaging presentation varies due to the size of the lesion. Smaller diameter lesions tend to appear as solid nodules, while larger diameter lesions or those with a greater proportion of caseous necrosis often appear as regular round, round-like, or irregular ring-shaped lesions. CT plain scan may show no abnormal findings or only slightly hyperdense lesions, with ring-like enhancement on enhanced scan (Fig. 6.3).

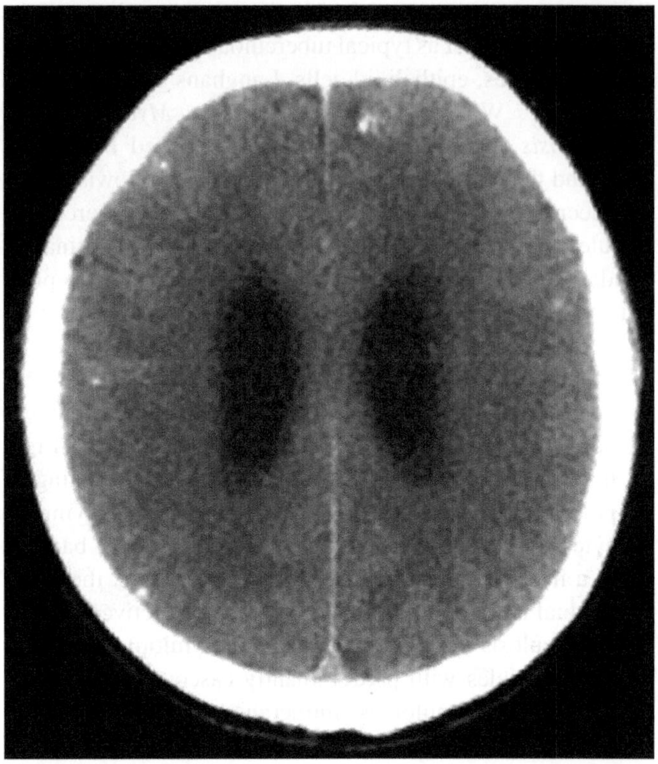

Fig. 6.2 Diffuse miliary tuberculosis of the brain parenchyma. CT scan shows multiple nodular hyperdense calcifications <3 mm in diameter in the brain parenchyma

- Tuberculoma: A nodular lesion >5 mm in diameter, either solitary or multiple, often as a fusion of multiple nodules, preferably in the subcortical or subcortical areas of the cerebral hemispheres and cerebellum. CT plain scan shows an isodense granulomatous ring of the lesion with a slightly hypodense caseous necrotic in the center of the lesion, a more pronounced ring of enhancement on enhanced scan, and a slightly hyperdense lesion with calcification (Fig. 6.4).

(c) Subdural or epidural tuberculous abscesses: The CT presentation of subdural tuberculous abscesses is a crescentic lesion under the intracranial plate, while epidural tuberculous abscesses appear as biconvex lenticular lesions under the intracranial plate with hypodensity and ring-like enhancement on enhanced scans.

4. MRI

(a) Meningeal tuberculosis
- Tuberculous meningitis: MRI (Fig. 6.5) usually shows isointense or slightly hyperintense on T_1WI and isodense or slightly hypodense on T_2WI. The meninges show obvious thickening, more pronounced at the base of the skull. Also due to the accumulation of exudate, MRI plain scan shows

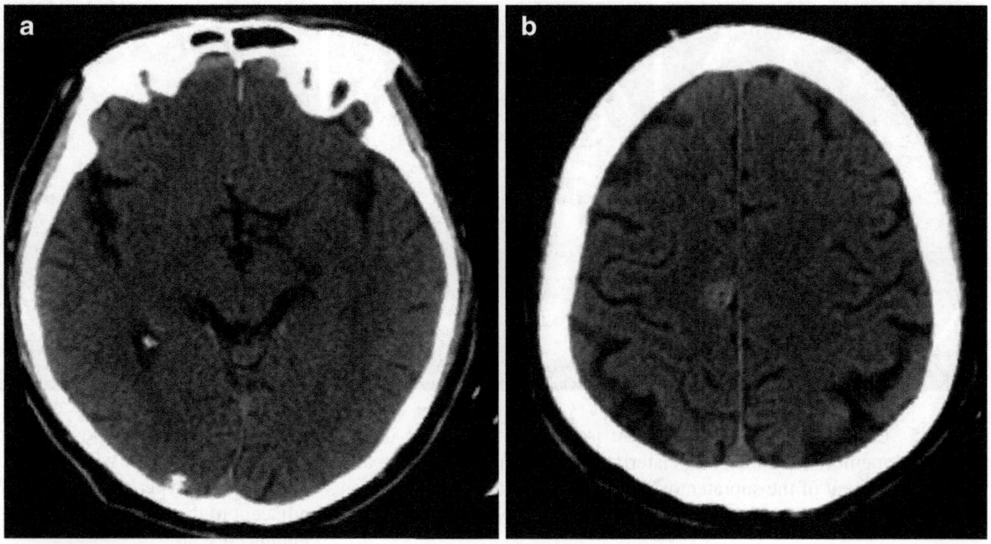

Fig. 6.3 Tuberculous nodules of the brain parenchyma. CT scan shows hyperdense and slightly hyperdense nodular lesions in the right occipital lobe (**a**) and frontal lobe (**b**), respectively, with clear boundaries

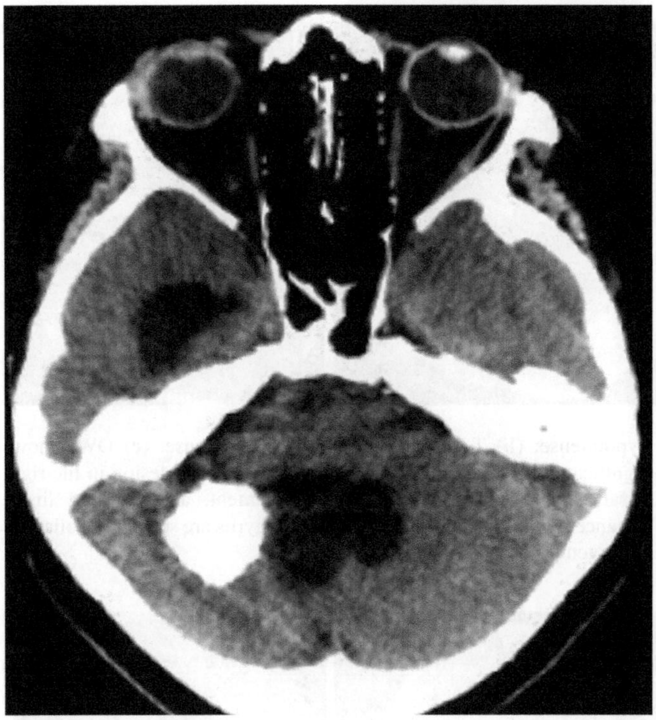

Fig. 6.4 Tuberculoma with calcification in the right cerebellar hemisphere. CT plain scan shows a round-like hyperdense lesion in the right cerebellar hemisphere

narrowing and occlusion of the basal and lateral fissure pools of the brain. The meninges may be significantly thickened and abnormally enhanced on enhanced scans, with each pool at the base of the skull showing more distinctly, mainly as striated, clustered, nodular, and ring-like enhancement of the basal pools and lateral fissure pools (Fig. 6.5). Calcification of the meninges may occur in the later stages of the lesion, when the lesion is slightly hypointense on both T_1WI and T_2WI but not as clearly as on CT. In addition, common changes secondary to tuberculous meningitis include traffic hydrocephalus and cerebral infarction (Fig. 6.6). When cerebral infarction occurs, speckled or patchy lesions, which manifest as slightly hypointense on T_1WI and slightly hyperintense on T_2WI, are seen in the brain parenchyma with no significant abnormal enhancement or abnormal gyrus-like enhancement seen on enhanced scans. These lesions mainly are infarction caused by invasion of *Mycobacterium tuberculosis* into cerebral vessels and mainly are found in basal ganglia and internal capsule. Lesions in the basal cistern arachnoid can cause impaired cerebrospinal fluid circulation and cause secondary hydrocephalus.

- Meningeal tuberculoma: It is often indistinguishable from irregularly thickened meninges on T_1WI and manifests as isointense or slightly hyperintense on T_2WI. The caseous necrotic center of the lesion shows hypointense on T_1WI and various signals on T_2WI, with hyperintense if the lesion is completely liquefied, hypointense if the lesion is not liquefied, and mixed hyper- and hypointense if the lesion is partially liquefied. The granulomatous ring of the lesion is significantly enhanced on enhanced scan, while the caseous necrotic center of the lesion is not enhanced. Whether the focal caseous necrotic center is unliquefied or completely liquefied, it shows hypointense on the DWI sequence (Fig. 6.7).

(b) Parenchymal tuberculosis of the brain

- Tuberculous encephalitis: On MRI, lamellar abnormal signals, which manifest as hypointense on T_1WI and hyperintense on T_2WI, are seen in

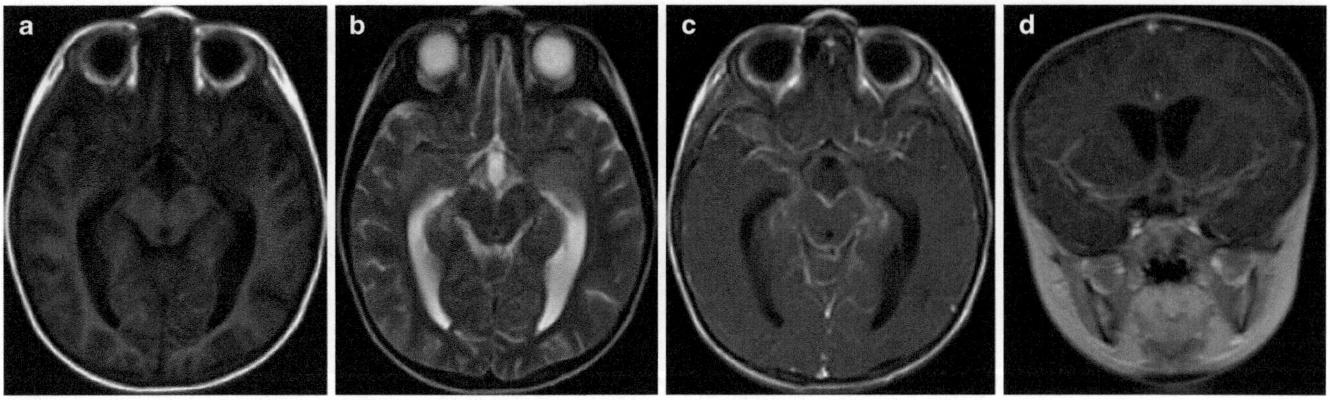

Fig. 6.5 Tuberculous meningitis. There is marked thickening of the arachnoid membrane in the basal cistern and lateral fissure cistern, and mild enlargement of the supratentorial ventricular system. (**a**) MR scan shows isointense on T_1WI; (**b**) T_2WI shows slightly hyperintense; (**c, d**) thickened meninges show multiple linear enhancement on enhanced scan. Edema signal, which manifests as slightly hypointense on T_1WI and slightly hyperintense on T_2WI, is seen in the brain parenchyma adjacent to the thickened meninges, with no abnormal enhancement on enhanced scan

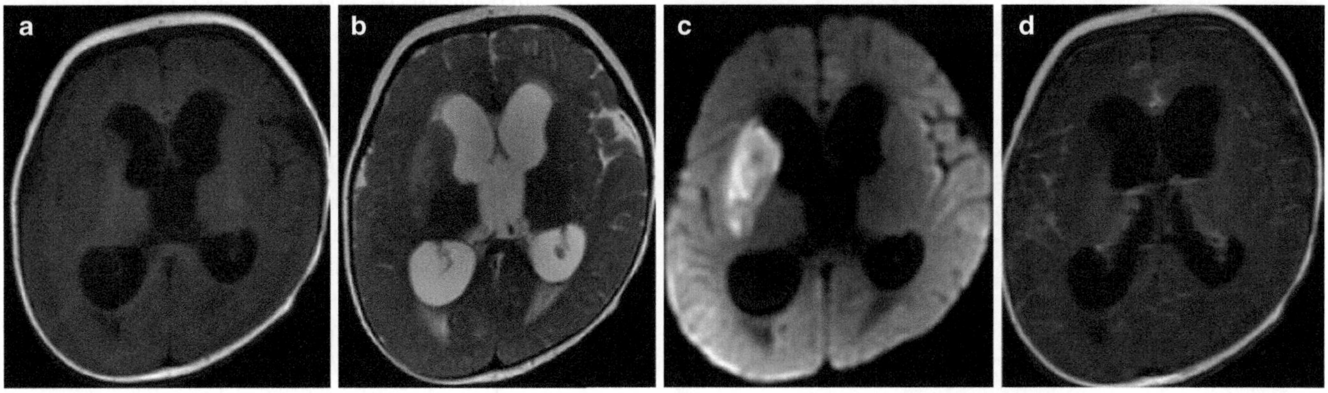

Fig. 6.6 Meningeal tuberculosis secondary hydrocephalus and cerebral infarction in the right basal ganglia region. Enlarged effusion in the third ventricle and bilateral lateral ventricles, with patchy lesions visible in the right basal ganglia region. (**a**) MRI T_1WI scan shows slightly hypointense; (**b**) T_2WI shows slightly hyperintense; (**c**) DWI shows significantly hyperintense; (**d**) enhanced scan of the lesion in the right basal ganglia region shows no enhancement, and multiple linear enhancements distributed along the sulcal gyrus are seen in the bilateral frontotemporal meninges

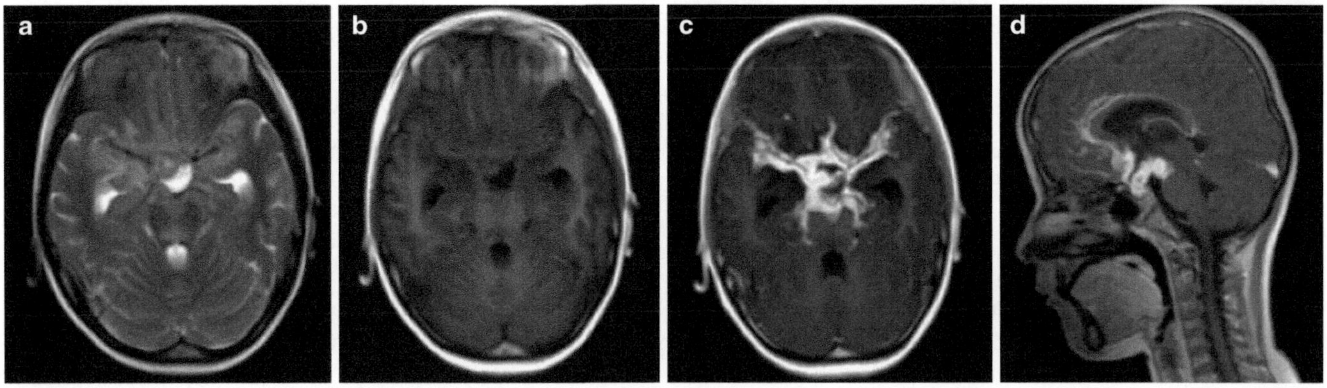

Fig. 6.7 Tuberculoma of meninges. There is marked thickening of the arachnoid membrane in the basal cistern and lateral fissure cistern. (**a, b**) MRI shows nodular granuloma fused with thickened meninges with isointensity on T_1WI and slightly hyperintensity on T_2WI; (**c, d**) enhanced scan shows strip, bead-like, and circular abnormal enhancement

the brain parenchyma, with an occupying effect, and most of the lesions do not have abnormal enhancement on enhanced scans, but sometimes gyrus-like or lamellar enhancement is seen, with non-enhancement nodules or tuberculomas within them.

- Tuberculous brain abscess: The central part of the lesions manifests as hypointense on T_1WI, and the marginal abscess wall manifests as isointense or slightly hyperintense. The abscess wall manifests as isointense or slightly hyperintense on T_2WI with linear hypointense around the lesion edges, and large sheets of edema are seen around the lesion. DWI sequence shows slightly hyperintense with decreased ADC value of the abscess cavity. The lesion shows obvious ring-like enhancement on enhanced scan (Fig. 6.8).
- Diffuse miliary tuberculosis: MRI T_1WI often shows diffusely distributed punctate isointense or slightly hypointense lesions on bilateral cerebral hemisphere, and the lesions manifest as hypo- or slightly hyperintense on T_2WI, and varying degrees of hyperintense edema can be seen around some of the lesions. Lesions manifest as punctate isointense or slightly hyperintense on DWI sequences. The lesions present homogeneous nodular enhancement on enhanced scans (Fig. 6.9).
- Tuberculosis nodules: Tuberculous granuloma or granuloma ring shows isointense or slightly hyperintense on T_1WI and isointense or slightly hyperintense on T_2WI. It may show hypointense when there is increased collagen fiber content, increased free radical content, or calcification in

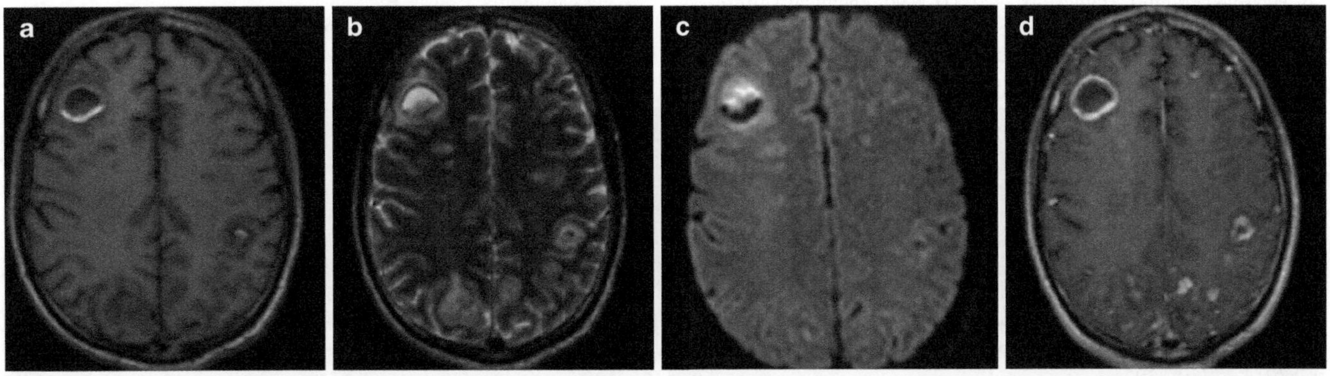

Fig. 6.8 Tuberculous brain abscess. A round-like lesion is seen in the right frontal lobe. (**a**) MRI T_1WI scan shows hypointense in the central region of the lesion, with a ring-shaped slightly hyperintense envelope in the periphery; (**b**) T_2WI shows a hyperintense in the central region of the lesion with a hypointense in the periphery; (**c**) DWI sequence shows hyperintense in the center of the lesion; (**d**) enhanced scan shows ring-shaped enhancement

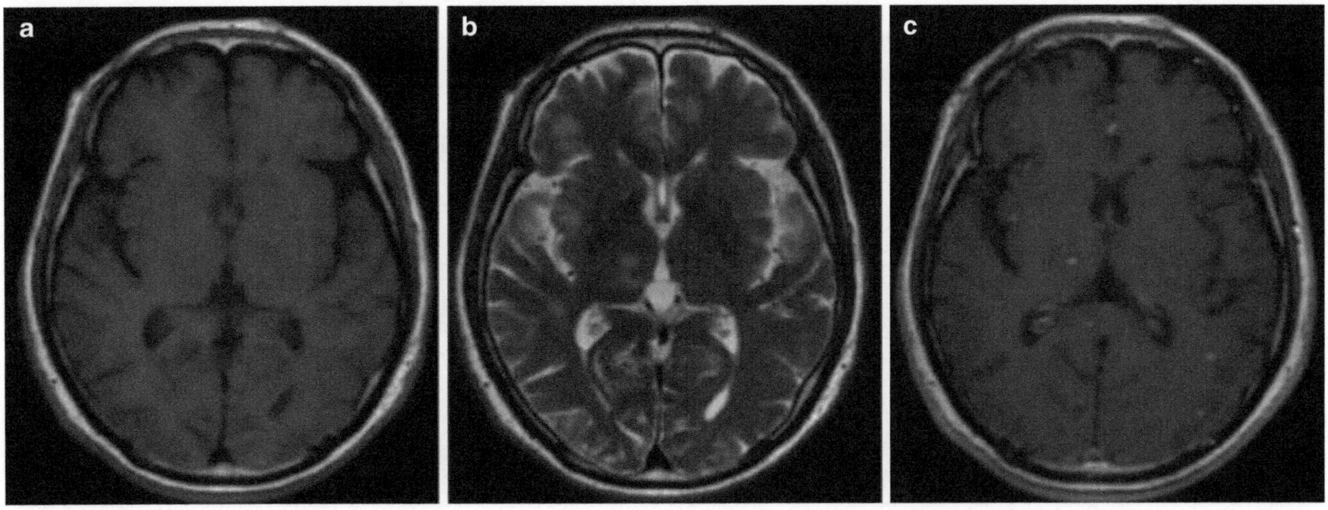

Fig. 6.9 Diffuse miliary tuberculosis of the brain parenchyma. Multiple small nodular lesions <3 mm in diameter are seen in the brain parenchyma. (**a**) MRI T_1WI shows isointense or slightly hypointense; (**b**) T_2WI shows slightly hyperintense; (**c**) nodular-like abnormal enhancement can be seen on enhanced scan

the lesion. Internal liquefaction necrosis manifests as hypointense on T_1WI and hyperintense on T_2WI, while the coagulation necrosis mostly shows hyperintense on T_1WI and hypointense on T_2WI.

- Tuberculoma: Nodules larger than 5 mm have a diverse presentation on MRI (Figs. 6.10 and 6.11), mainly depending on the pathological changes and regression of the lesion. When the lesion is mainly inflammatory exudate, the inflammatory cell content of the lesion is more, and the collagen fiber content is less, so the lesion manifests as isointense or hypointense on T_1WI and hyperintense on T_2WI; surrounding edema shadow can be seen, but it is not clearly demarcated from the lesion. The lesions show homogeneous nodular enhancement on enhanced scan and are clearly demarcated from the surrounding edema. When the lesion is predominantly hyperplastic, T_1WI shows hypointense or isointense, and the T_2WI shows hypointense, with non-enhancement on enhanced scan. When different degrees of liquefied necrosis occur in the central caseous part, T_1WI shows hypointense in the center of the lesion and isointense at the edge of the lesion. T_2WI shows hyperintense in the center of the lesion, surrounded by hypointense at the edge, forming a typical "ring target sign." Lesion shows obvious ring-like enhancement on the enhanced scan with uneven lesion wall. Old tuberculoma lesions may have calcification in the center and are mostly hypointense on T_1WI and T_2WI, with non-enhancing edematous areas surrounding the lesion.

(c) Subdural or epidural tuberculous abscesses: The pus in the abscess cavity of subdural or epidural tuberculous abscess (Fig. 6.12) manifests as hypointense on T_1WI and hyperintense on T_2WI; the abscess wall

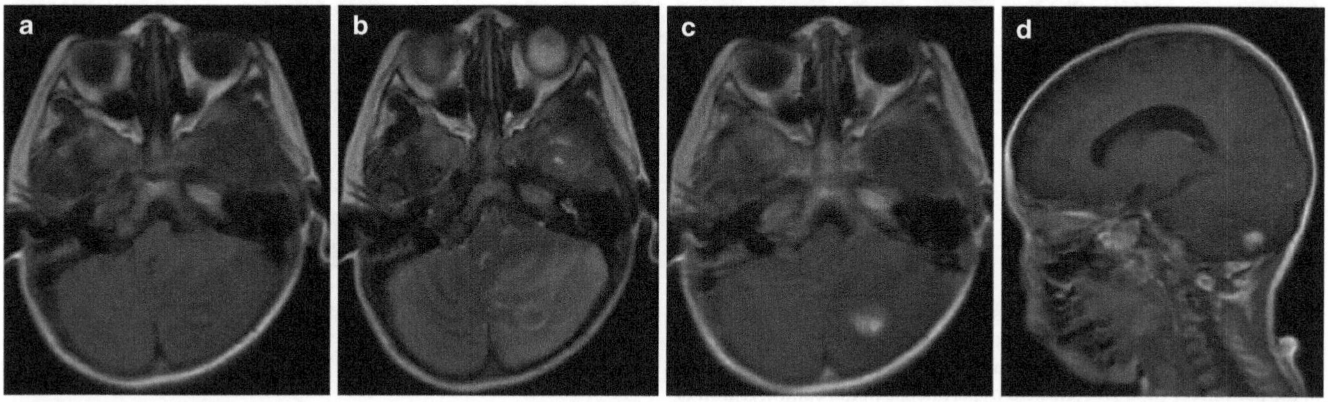

Fig. 6.10 Tuberculoma of the brain parenchyma. A round-like lesion in the left cerebellar hemisphere. (**a**) MRI T_1WI scan shows hyperintense in the central region of the lesion and slightly hypointense in the periphery; (**b**) T_2WI shows hypointense in the central region of the lesion; (**c**) slightly hyperintense is seen at the periphery of the lesion. (**d**) The lesion shows significant heterogeneous abnormal enhancement on the enhanced scan

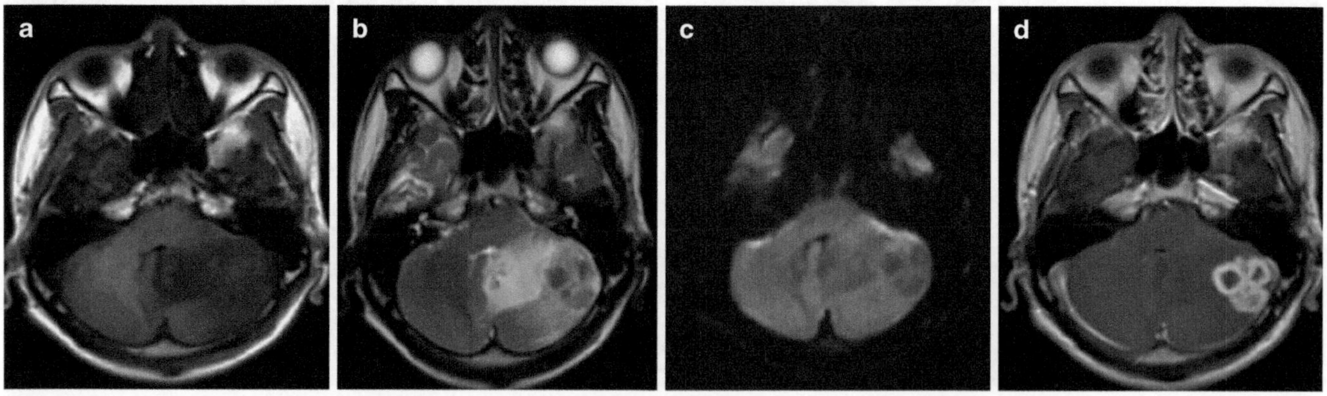

Fig. 6.11 Tuberculoma of the brain parenchyma. Irregularly shaped lesion in the left cerebellar hemisphere. (**a**) Lesion mainly shows isointense on T_1WI; (**b**) lesion mainly shows hypointense on T_2WI with slightly hyperintense in the peripheral edema region; (**c**) lesion shows hypointense on DWI sequence; (**d**) ring-like enhancement can be seen on enhanced scan

shows isointense or slightly hyperintense on T_1WI and T_2WI. The wall of the abscess shows significant ring-like enhancement on enhanced scan, and there is no enhancement of the pus in the abscess cavity.

The pus in the abscess cavity is a viscous macromolecular substance, so its diffusion is restricted and manifests as hyperintense on DWI sequence (Fig. 6.12).

(d) Mixed intracranial tuberculosis: Meningeal tuberculosis and parenchymal tuberculosis occur in the same patient. Sometimes there may be a predominance of meningeal lesions or parenchymal lesions (Fig. 6.13).

6.2.4 Diagnostic Key Points

1. The patient usually has a history of tuberculosis infection in other parts of the body, such as the lungs, and has symptoms of tuberculosis toxicity and meningeal irritation during the course of the disease.
2. It is more common in children and adolescents and occurs more often below the curtain than above it.
3. Radiographic manifestations
   (a) Meningeal tuberculosis: Narrowing and occlusion of the basal cistern and lateral fissure cistern can be seen, and enhancement scans show irregular strips, nodules, rings, and clusters of significant enhancement; secondary changes such as traffic hydrocephalus and cerebral infarction may be present.
   (b) Brain parenchymal tuberculosis: Tuberculosis nodules and tuberculomas appear variously on plain CT and MRI, with calcifications showing hyperdense on CT plain scan and internal caseous necrosis showing hypointense on T_2WI, with nodular and ring-like enhancement on enhanced scans.
   (c) Mixed intracranial tuberculosis: Coexistence of meningeal and parenchymal brain tuberculosis.
4. Cerebrospinal fluid smear and culture: Positive acid-fast stain smear of cerebrospinal fluid and culture of cerebrospinal fluid for *Mycobacterium tuberculosis* can clarify

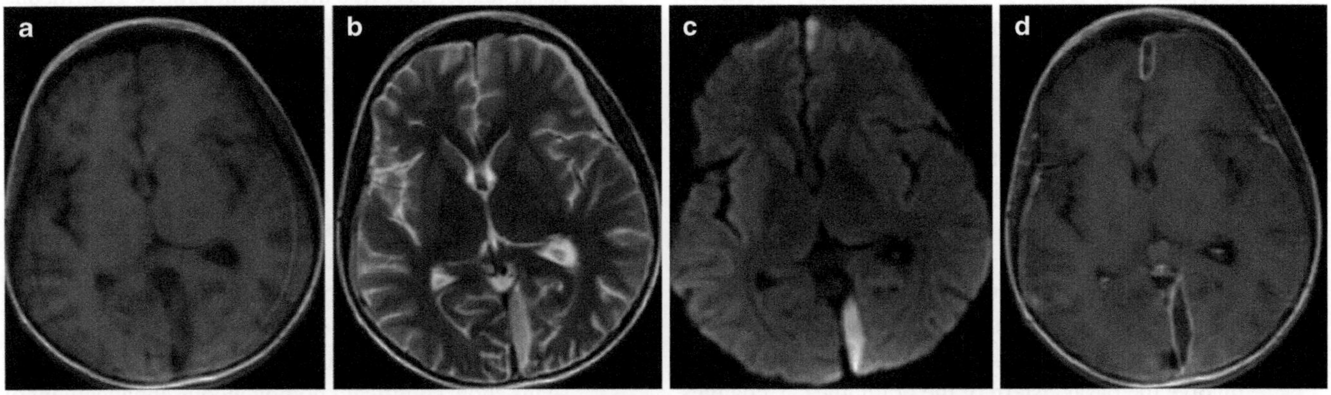

Fig. 6.12 Subdural tuberculous abscess. Posterior longitudinal fissure and anterior longitudinal fissure spindle lesions. (**a**) T_1WI shows hypointense in the central pus and isointense in the peripheral abscess wall; (**b**) T_2WI shows hyperintense in the central pus and isointense in the peripheral abscess wall; (**c**) abscess shows significant hyperintense on DWI; (**d**) ring-like enhancement is seen on enhanced scan

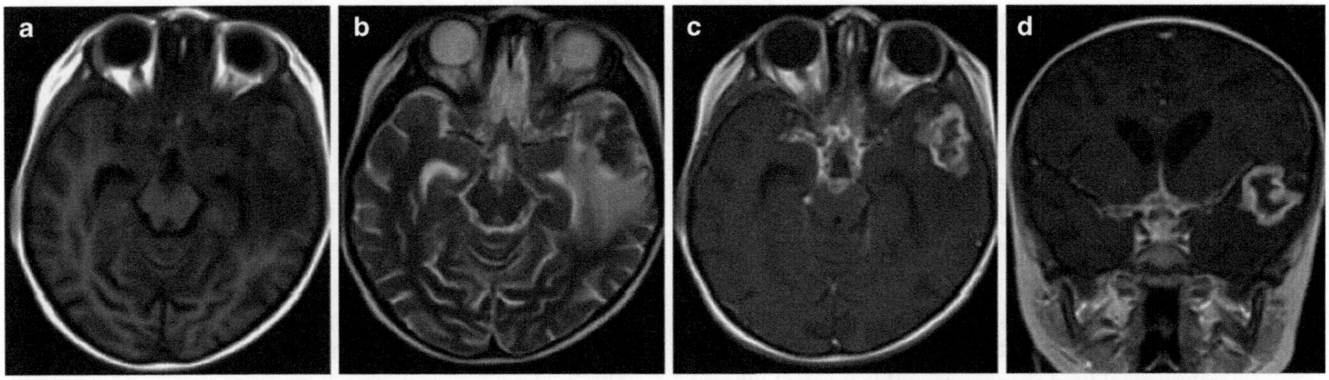

Fig. 6.13 Mixed intracranial tuberculosis. Irregularly shaped tuberculoma lesions are seen in the left temporal lobe. (**a, b**) Lesion shows isointensity on T_1WI and hypointensity on T_2WI; (**c, d**) ring-like enhancement of lesion is seen in the left temporal lobe and thickening of the basal cistern and lateral fissure cistern with significant abnormal enhancement of the meninges

the diagnosis. Cerebrospinal fluid examination: Glucose and chloride levels are reduced, the cerebrospinal fluid glucose-to-blood glucose ratio is usually less than 0.5, and chloride is reduced more markedly than in other properties of meningitis.

6.2.5 Differential Diagnosis

Early diagnosis of intracranial tuberculosis is the key to a good prognosis, but the rapid progression of intracranial tuberculosis and the high rates of disability and death require multiple, multimodal investigations to avoid misdiagnosis or missed diagnosis. The disease should be differentiated from diseases that occur in the meninges, brain parenchyma, subdural or epidural and with similar imaging manifestation of tuberculosis.

1. Tuberculosis occurring in the meninges needs to be differentiated from the following diseases:
    (a) Septic meningitis: Caused by septic bacteria, with acute onset and often with high fever and chills; cerebrospinal fluid leukocyte count is markedly increased, with a predominantly increased proportion of neutrophils and a more pronounced decrease in glucose content than in tuberculous meningitis; growth of pathogenic bacteria is seen on cerebrospinal fluid cytology smears or bacterial cultures. The peripheral blood leukocyte count is significantly increased, and septic foci of infection are seen outside the nervous system, which may cause atypical clinical manifestations after irregular antibiotic treatment and should be differentiated from tuberculous meningitis. In contrast to tuberculous meningitis, which tends to involve the basal cistern of the brain, the CT changes in septic meningitis are predominantly meningeal enhancement on the convex side of the brain, and the basal cistern is often clearer. Tuberculous meningitis is usually distinguished from septic meningitis by a history of close contact with tuberculosis and by signs of tuberculosis on tuberculin testing and chest X-ray.
    (b) *Cryptococcus neoformans* meningitis: It is a fungal meningitis caused by a fungus with a predominant pathology of brain base changes. In contrast to tuberculous meningitis, patients with *Cryptococcus neoformans* meningitis tend not to have an enlarged ventricular system but instead may show a homogeneous narrowing. Cryptococcus meningitis often has a chronic course, and its clinical manifestations and cerebrospinal fluid changes resemble those of tuberculous meningitis, but the systemic inflammatory response to cryptococcal meningitis is less severe, usually without fever or other infectious manifestations, and resolves spontaneously; people with a history of close contact with pigeon droppings and long-term use of broad-spectrum antibiotics or immunosuppressive drugs are susceptible to *Cryptococcus neoformans* meningitis. Cerebrospinal fluid shows positive in ink stain, MGG stain, or Alisin blue stain.
    (c) Viral meningitis: Coxsackievirus, herpes simplex virus, and adenovirus infections are common, with a history of diarrhea or upper respiratory tract infection before onset; with acute onset and often with muscle pain during high fever; manifests as self-limiting course and generally heals in 2–3 weeks. Head CT or MRI examination is mostly normal; cerebrospinal fluid leukocyte count is increased, predominantly with an increased proportion of lymphocytes, and glucose and chloride are slightly below the normal range.
2. Tuberculosis occurring in the brain parenchyma needs to be differentiated from the following diseases:
    (a) Glioma: Tuberculoma needs to be differentiated from glioma with calcification. Glioma is generally irregular in shape; has often diffuse, infiltrative growth; and is poorly demarcated from normal brain tissue, often with cystic necrosis and hemorrhage, and perilesion edema is severe than that of tuberculoma, with obvious occupying effect. It often manifests as irregular enhancement or no significant enhancement on enhanced scan and no more typical "ring target sign."
    (b) Brain metastases: Mostly located in the cortical and medullary junction, the lesions often appear as multiple foci, with small tumors and large edema. Brain metastases have a significant occupying effect because of the presence of severe edema. Enhanced scans show significant homogeneous enhancement of the tumor. A clinical history, primary lesions in extracranial organs, and symptoms can differentiate it from tuberculoma.
3. Tuberculosis occurring subdurally or epidurally needs to be differentiated from purulent brain abscess:
    Purulent brain abscess cavities vary in size, some with subfoci, and their walls are thinner and more uniform. Planes of gas and fluid or bubbles are visible in the pus cavity if anaerobic infection is present, and scattered skull base calcifications are less common. The CT and MRI presentation of purulent brain abscess is very similar to that of tuberculous brain abscess, making it more difficult to diagnose. However, purulent brain abscesses have their own more unique characteristics. First, purulent brain abscesses are more frequent than tuberculous brain abscesses and often have an acute onset, often with extracerebral purulent lesions. Second, purulent brain abscesses tend to progress rapidly, with rapid increases in intracranial pressure, and symptoms of headache and

optic disc edema are more common and pronounced than in tuberculous brain abscesses. Laboratory tests show an increase in total white blood cells and neutrophils in the peripheral blood.

6.2.6 Status and Progress of Research

In recent years, with the development of new magnetic resonance technology and its gradual popularization in clinical practice, the clinical application value of MRI in the diagnosis, differential diagnosis, and posttreatment follow-up of intracranial tuberculosis has been greatly improved. Magnetic resonance perfusion imaging provides information of hemodynamics in intracranial nodules. Magnetic resonance spectroscopy provides information of metabolism in intracranial nodules. Magnetic resonance diffusion imaging can provide information such as the diffusion of water molecules within intracranial nodules. Functional magnetic resonance imaging can provide information of invasion of functional brain areas by intracranial nodules.

1. Hydrogen proton spectroscopy imaging (^{1}H-MRS): It can reflect the physiological metabolism of the lesioned tissue as a noninvasive diagnosis method and can provide metabolic information for the diagnosis of intracranial tuberculosis lesions, and its wave spectrum has certain characteristics, which is useful to improve the diagnostic accuracy on the basis of conventional MRI examination, and is a useful supplement to conventional examination. Santy et al. [14] applied ^{1}H-MRS to the diagnosis of four children with brain tuberculoma and found that the Lip peaks of the brain tuberculoma lesions were significantly elevated in all four children, and no waves of other metabolites were detected. After active antituberculosis treatment in these four children, ^{1}H-MRS was performed again and found that the tuberculoma lesions had shrunk by more than 50% compared with the previous lesion. The Lip peak, although at a rather low level, was still present, and therefore the Lip peak is considered to be a characteristic ^{1}H-MRS manifestation of brain tuberculoma. Pretell et al. [15] found that ^{1}H-MRS in the parenchyma of cerebral tuberculoma showed elevated Lip and Cho peaks with decreased N-acetylaspartate (NAA) and creatine (Cr) peaks, which can be used to differentiate between cerebral tuberculoma and cerebral cysticercosis. Peng Juan et al. [16] found that Cho/Cr and Cho/NAA values in brain tuberculoma were lower than those in high-grade gliomas and brain metastases and therefore suggested that the combination of conventional MRI and ^{1}H-MRS could help distinguish brain TB tumors from high-grade gliomas and brain metastases.

   In summary, an occupying brain lesion that is difficult to diagnose with conventional MRI and shows a mild increase in Lip peak with or without mild increase in Cho/Cr and Cho/NAA values and absence of other positive metabolites on ^{1}H-MRS examinations suggests a high probability of brain tuberculoma.
2. Diffusion-weighted imaging (DWI): DWI is presently the only imaging method that can observe the microscopic movement of water molecules in living bodies and can detect early morphological and physiological changes associated with changes in tissue water content. Studies which evaluated intracranial tuberculoma with DWI are relatively few. Thus, there is no agreement on the DWI presentation of brain tuberculoma. Early studies suggested that the central hyperintense of brain tuberculoma lesions on DWI was characteristic and could be used to identify other intracranial ring-like enhancing lesions. Peng Juan et al. [17] found that tuberculoma lesions and perilesion edema manifest as isointense on DWI. The ADC and relative ADC values (rADC, ADC value of the lesion/ADC value of the normal brain parenchyma in the contralateral hemisphere) of tuberculoma tumors and perilesion edema zone were higher than those of high-grade astrocytoma and brain metastases. Therefore, it is considered that combining conventional MRI and DWI, according to the ADC and rADC values of lesion and perilesion edema, it can help to distinguish brain tuberculoma, high-grade astrocytoma, and brain metastasis. Gupta et al. [18] concluded that DWI sequences are useful in differentiating cerebral tuberculoma from granuloma of cysticercus and that the ADC values of active and metaphase dead cysticercus lesion centers are significantly higher than those of tuberculoma and tuberculous brain abscess, whereas there is no significant difference in the ADC values of tuberculous brain abscess and tuberculoma with high-signal center. The mechanism of DWI manifestation of brain tuberculoma is unclear. It has been suggested that the free fatty acid component of the caseous necrotic substance and vasogenic edema lead to an enlarged extracellular space and accelerated diffusion of water molecules, which may be responsible for the unrestricted diffusion of the lesion or even an elevated ADC value.
3. Magnetic resonance perfusion (PWI): Hemodynamic parameters obtained by PWI, such as cerebral blood volume (CBV) and cerebral blood flow (CBF), as well as physiological parameters such as transfer coefficient (K_{trans}) and leakage volume (Ve), have been used to confirm vascular regeneration in gliomas and tuberculomas. Presently, PWI has been widely used in the study of brain tumors, and fewer studies have been reported in brain tuberculoma. PWI is useful as an adjunct to the evaluation of tuberculomas for lesion characterization

and diagnosis. Ring-enhanced lesions and nodular-enhanced lesions show different perfusion characteristics, with elevated rCBV values within nodular-enhanced lesions, similar to gliomas, and decreased rCBV values around ring-enhanced lesions can help differentiate them. Haris et al. [19] compared PWI parameters in patients with brain tuberculoma before and after treatment and found that rCBV correlated with cell volume, while edema volume influenced the transfer coefficient and leakage volume, implying that PWI parameters can evaluate the treatment effect of brain tuberculoma. Gupta et al. [20] found that rCBV could reflect the vascular regeneration status of brain tuberculoma and is helpful in prediction of future treatment response of brain tuberculoma, which is relevant for the detection of tuberculoma treatment efficacy. Chatterjee et al. [21] retrospectively analyzed the DWI and PWI results of 11 patients with pathologically confirmed brain tuberculoma or metastases and found that the mean rCBV value between the tuberculoma lesion and normal brain white matter is <1, while the mean rCBV value between the metastases lesion and normal brain white matter is >5, but the ADC values of two lesions are similar, so it is considered that the rCBV with value of <1 between parenchyma lesion and normal brain white matter can be used as a basis for the differential diagnosis of brain tuberculoma from brain metastases.

4. Magnetic susceptibility-weighted imaging (SWI): Hemorrhage or iron deposition can cause heterogeneous magnetic field distribution in local tissues, and the SWI technique exploits this magnetic susceptibility difference for imaging and is a further development based on the T_2^* imaging sequence [22]. The SWI technique is sensitive to hypoxia, ischemia, hemosiderin deposition, ferritin, and iron deposition. In addition, the SWI technique can combine filtered images and phase images to achieve self-enhancement of blood vessels, providing effective assistance for clinical angiography [23]. Thus, the SWI technique, to a certain extent, can reflect the vascular inflammatory changes due to tuberculous meningitis. The SWI technique reveals the presence of paramagnetic material, while calcification is antimagnetic; it shows hyperintense on the SWI phase diagram, which clearly distinguishes it from hemorrhage [24, 25]. The massive tuberculous exudate of tuberculous meningitis is rich in polymorphonuclear leukocytes, macrophages, etc.; the tuberculous nodule progresses further with varying degrees of caseous liquefaction and necrosis in the center of the lesion. Calcification may occur around advanced tuberculoma lesions. It is therefore inferred that there is some variation in SWI manifestations in different pathological periods of intracranial tuberculosis. Another study found that [26, 27] abscess-like lesions on SWI often showed a complete, smooth, hypointense ring around the edge of the lesion, which is of great value in the diagnosis of intracranial tuberculous abscesses using the SWI technique. In summary, the SWI technique enables staging of intracranial tuberculoma lesions and provides for treatment follow-up.
5. Magnetization transfer (MT) technique is a physical method to increase the contrast of an image or to create a new contrast. In the early stages of some diseases, conventional MRI scans do not yet show changes, and the MT technique can be useful in detecting lesions when there are differences in protein and bound water content between the diseased and normal tissues. Saxena et al. [28] compared the T_1WI of MT with conventional pressurized water sequences for the number and visibility display of brain nodules and found that MT had the number and clarity of lesions detected on T_1WI higher than those on the pressurized water sequence. The commonly used metric magnetization transfer rate (MTR) in the MT technique can indirectly or even semiquantitatively reflect the transformation of macromolecular protein content in tissues. Gupta et al. [29] concluded that enhanced MT better detects intracranial TB disease, while MTR identifies intracranial TB lesions and infectious lesions with similar MRI presentation to TB. Using MT technique, Pui et al. [30] found that the MTR of the unenhanced center area of tuberculoma lesion was significantly higher than that of the corresponding area of high-grade glioma and higher than that of the cystic area of low-grade glioma and abscess, but the difference was not significant, while the difference in MTR between abscess and tumor was not statistically significant.

6.3 Meningococcal Meningitis

Li Li and Yinglin Guo

6.3.1 Overview

Meningococcal meningitis is a purulent meningitis caused by *Neisseria meningitidis*. The main clinical manifestations are sudden onset of high fever, severe headache, frequent vomiting, mucosal petechiae and petechiae on the skin, meningeal irritation signs, and, in severe cases, fulminant attacks with septic shock and brain parenchymal damage, which can often be life-threatening.

The source of infection for influenza is the patient and the carrier. The patient is infectious both at the end of the incubation period and during the onset of the disease, but the infectious period generally does not exceed 10 days. The pathogen is transmitted directly from the respiratory tract mainly by droplets through coughing and sneezing. The population is generally susceptible.

The severity of influenza varies, and it can generally be characterized by four clinical types, namely, mild, common, fulminant, and chronic. The common type accounts for about 90% of all those who develop the disease after *Neisseria meningitidis* infection, and according to the pathogenesis, rheumatic encephalitis is divided into prodromal phase (upper respiratory infection phase), septic phase, meningitis phase, and recovery phase 4. The prodromal phase is often overlooked because of its rapid onset and progression. The rash is mainly seen in the septic phase, which is characterized by petechiae and petechiae on the skin mucosa, and this phase lasts 1–2 days before entering the meningitis phase. In addition to high fever and intoxication, the main manifestations of the meningitis phase are severe headache, frequent vomiting, apathy or lethargy, cervical tonicity, and signs of meningeal irritation. After treatment, the body temperature gradually decreased to normal, the skin petechiae and petechiae disappeared, the neurological examination was normal, and the patient entered the recovery period. The fulminant form is characterized by rapid onset, rapid change of condition, and high mortality rate, which can be life-threatening within 24 h if left untreated. Fulminant forms are subdivided into shock, fulminant meningoencephalitis, and mixed three types.

Cerebrospinal fluid testing is an important method for confirming the diagnosis of rheumatoid brain. In typical meningitis, cerebrospinal fluid examination reveals increased pressure, cloudy appearance, and a significantly higher white blood cell count of 1.0×10^9/L or more, with predominantly multinucleated cells; sugar and chloride are significantly reduced, and protein content is elevated. Serum immunological tests are mainly used for the early diagnosis of the disease, with a positive rate of over 90%.

Diagnosis is confirmed by culture of *Neisseria meningitidis* in cerebrospinal fluid or blood or detection of *Neisseria meningitidis* group-specific polysaccharide antigen, positive test for *Neisseria meningitidis*-specific nucleic acid fragments, or positive anti-*Neisseria meningitidis* antibodies in the patient's serum in the acute or recovery phase.

6.3.2 Pathological Manifestations

Neisseria meningitidis primarily involves the soft meninges and arachnoid, causing septic inflammation. Early manifestations are vascular congestion, hemorrhage, and edema. The late stage shows septic changes with massive neutrophil, fibrin, and plasma exudate in the cerebrospinal fluid. Due to viscous pus at the base of the skull and direct invasion of septic lesions, there can be meningeal adhesions, and septic inflammation can cause cerebral nerve damage. The fulminant meningoencephalitis type of lesion is mainly located in the brain parenchyma, with necrosis, congestion, hemorrhage, and edema in the brain tissue, increased intracranial pressure, and, in severe cases, brain herniation, which can be seen as herniation of the foramen magnum and herniation of the occipital foramen.

6.3.3 Imaging

1. CT: No abnormal reveal in the early stage at CT. With the progress of the disease, the enlargement of ventricles and subdural fluid accumulation are revealed. Focal or diffuse hypodense shadow in the brain parenchyma is noted, and the density of the brain pool is increased. Marked enhancement of the meninges shows on postcontrast imaging.
2. MRI: Subdural effusion or pus and supratentorial hydrocephalus are generally revealed at MRI [31]. Pathological sulci and subarachnoid space are obscured and show a moderately low signal intensity on T_1WI. FLAIR shows that the sulcus in the lesion area is filled with moderately high signal or high signal in the form of lines and strips. In cases of concurrent brain parenchymal inflammation, patces of slightly high signal on T_2WI and FLAIR were seen in the adjacent brain parenchyma, and the diffusion was restricted on DWI [32]. After administration of contrast material, linear enhancement of the meninges and arachnoid is revealed. Besides, the spinal cord may be swelling, and patchy high signal intensity can be seen on T_2WI [33]. Boos et al. [34] reported an atypical chronic rheumatoid braincase, which presents with cerebral infarction but not a meningeal enhancement. Van de Beek et al. [35] reported a case of brainstem infarction in a 25-year-old woman; traffic hydrocephalus found by CT and FLAIR revealed patchy high signal intensity in the right posterior aspect of the medulla oblongata and septic ventricular meningitis. O'Farrell et al. [36] reported a case of transverse myelitis caused by the rheumatoid brain, which showed high signal intensity on T_2-weighted imaging in the lower medulla, upper cervical medulla, and cerebellar tonsils.

6.3.4 Diagnostic Key Points

1. There is an epidemiological history of epidemic meningitis.
2. Clinical presentation and cerebrospinal fluid examination are consistent with manifestations of septic meningitis with skin mucosal petechiae and petechiae.

3. Based on imaging, the enlargement of supratentorial ventricles, subdural effusion or pus, and accompanying meningeal enhancement, epidemic meningitis should be considered.
4. Pathogenic or serologic testing positive for *Neisseria meningitidis*.

6.3.5 Differential Diagnosis

1. Tuberculous meningitis: Most of them have a history of tuberculosis or close contact, with a slow onset and long duration of illness, low fever, night sweats, wasting and other symptoms of tuberculosis toxicity, late appearance of neurological symptoms, and no petechiae or petechiae on the skin mucosa. Epidemic meningitis generally has an associated epidemiologic history, and clinical manifestations and cerebrospinal fluid examination are consistent with the manifestations of septic meningitis with skin mucosal petechiae and petechiae. Tuberculous meningitis often involves the soft meninges of the skull base and the basal cistern system of the brain, with thickened meninges and scattered calcifications. Most epidemic meningitis may present with subdural effusion, supratentorial hydrocephalus, and also subdural pus accumulation. The patient may have a positive acid-fast stain on the cerebrospinal fluid smear, culture of *Neisseria meningitidis* in the cerebrospinal fluid or blood or detection of *Neisseria meningitidis* group-specific polysaccharide antigens, positive *Neisseria meningitidis*-specific nucleic acid fragments, or positive anti-*Neisseria meningitidis* antibodies in the patient's serum during the acute or recovery phase.
2. Epidemic B encephalitis is common in children, with the onset of the disease mostly in July to September. The patient has an acute onset with high fever, impaired consciousness, convulsions, tonic spasms, and signs of meningeal irritation. The skin mucosa is usually free of petechiae. MRI findings show low or mixed T_1WI signal intensity, high T_2WI signal intensity, and high FLAIR signal intensity on the midbrain, thalamus, and basal ganglia.

6.3.6 Status and Progress of Research

Strains of *Neisseria meningitidis* can be classified into at least 12 serogroups based on the characteristics of their podoconjugates. Serogroups A, B, C, W135, and Y are the main pathogenic groups, and with the widespread use of serogroup A, C, Y, and W135 rheumatoid vaccines, serogroup B has become one of the main prevalent groups of meningitis. Two new multicomponent vaccines, Trumenba and Bexsero, were successfully developed by Wyeth and Novartis, respectively, for the prevention of serogroup B influenzae strains in people aged 10–25 years and approved by the US Food and Drug Administration (FDA) in 2014 and 2015 [37].

6.4 Pertussis Encephalopathy

Li Li and Yinglin Guo

6.4.1 Overview

Whooping cough (pertussis) is an acute respiratory infection caused by *Bordetella pertussis*. Clinical features include paroxysmal spasmodic cough, cockle-like inspiratory sounds, and peripheral blood lymphocytosis. The disease has a long course, and untreated cough symptoms can be prolonged for 2–3 months, hence the name "whooping cough."

It occurs most often in children, especially those under 5 years of age.

Pertussis encephalopathy is the most serious complication of whooping cough and occurs mainly during the spasmodic cough phase. The mechanism of occurrence is cerebral vascular spasm caused by severe spasmodic coughing, leading to hypoxia and hemorrhage in brain tissue. Clinical manifestations include convulsions or repeated convulsions, hyperthermia, impaired consciousness, coma, etc. Severe cases are often life-threatening. Patients can be left with sequelae such as epilepsy and mental retardation after encephalopathy [38]. Laboratory tests present elevated blood leukocyte and lymphocyte counts, positive serology for antibodies to pertussis toxin, and positive PCR for *Bordetella pertussis*.

6.4.2 Pathological Manifestations

Brain tissue edema, congestion, punctate hemorrhage and cortical atrophy, neuronal cell degeneration, etc. [39].

6.4.3 Imaging

1. CT: Cerebral edema and hypoxia mostly occurred in the symmetrical basal ganglia region. Scattered and indistinct edges of hypodense lesions can be seen in CT. The margin of gray and white matter is poorly defined, and in some cases, sulci are disappeared. A punctate, patchy, or round-like high-density surrounded with low-density edema in the brain parenchyma is typical of intraparenchymal hemorrhage. In case of subarachnoid hemorrhage, the cerebral sulcus and pools disappear, and the density increases, also known as the "castellated" sign.

2. MRI: Cerebral edema and hypoxia in the symmetrically basal ganglia region manifest multifocal/diffuse lamellar hypointense on T_1-weighted images and hyperintense on T_2-weighted images. On DWI sequence, cytotoxic edema shows diffusion restriction with high signal intensity, and ADC values are significantly decreased; notably, interstitial edema does not show the high signal intensity, and ADC values are moderately increased. Hematomas can have variable T_1W and T_2W signal intensity, depending on the evaluation of the blood products. Subacute and chronic hematomas exhibit high signal intensity in both T_1WI and T_2WI [40].

6.4.4 Diagnostic Key Points

1. Children with whooping cough.
2. Clinical signs of impaired consciousness, hyperthermia, and coma are present.
3. Image finding shows cerebral edema and hypoxia.
4. Laboratory tests: Positive serology for antibodies to pertussis toxin and positive PCR for *Bordetella pertussis*.

6.4.5 Differential Diagnosis

1. Viral encephalitis demonstrated unilaterally or bilaterally hypodense foci in the cerebral hemispheres at CT, with blurred margins, and linear or ring enhancement on post-contrast images. At MRI, it appeared as low T_1 signal intensity and high T_2 signal intensity with occupancy effects. When lesions partially involved the cerebral cortex, gyrus-like hyperintense T_2-weighted signal intensity can be seen.
2. CT findings of carbon monoxide toxic encephalopathy show symmetric hypodense foci in the bilateral basal ganglia.
   At MRI, bilateral basal ganglia symmetrically revealed as low T_1 signal intensity and high T_2 signal intensity, with high signal intensity on FLAIR. The involvement of bilateral nucleus pulposus is specificity. The patient had a clear history of carbon monoxide poisoning.
3. Wilson's disease shows symmetric hypodensity in bilateral basal ganglia on CT. On MRI-based T_1-weighted images, the nucleus pulposus shows low signal intensity, and the pallidum demonstrates iso-signal intensity. In contrast, the nucleus pulposus shows high signal intensity, and the pallidum reveals characteristically low signal intensity on T_2-weighted images. The patient had a specific corneal K-F ring and abnormal laboratory tests regarding copper metabolism.

6.4.6 Status and Progress of Research

1. New epidemiological features of pertussis: "The recurrence of pertussis" with a new epidemiological feature has emerged, namely, a rebound in the incidence of adolescents and adults [41].
2. The new pertussis vaccine has been studied by means of biofilms, with the new discoveries of outer membrane vesicles, new antigens, etc., and the application of new technologies represented by genetic engineering and nanotechnology. It is believed that the new pertussis vaccine is expected to make a breakthrough and will be effective against the recurrence of pertussis epidemics and the rise in its incidence [42].

6.5 Rubella Virus Encephalitis

Li Li and Meiji Ren

6.5.1 Overview

Rubella is an acute respiratory infection caused by rubella virus (RV) infection, with acquired infection manifested by mild upper respiratory tract inflammation, fever, red maculopapular rash, and swollen lymph nodes behind the ear and occiput, and infection in early pregnancy can lead to fetal malformation or stillbirth.

Rubella virus encephalitis is a more serious complication of rubella and is seen mainly in children. The severity of symptoms in school-age children who develop the disease may be related to the high virulence of rubella infection in older children. The onset is often 1–7 days after the rash, with headache, drowsiness, neck stiffness, convulsions, paralysis of limbs, etc. The course of the disease is short, mostly in 3–7 days, a few left with sequelae. The morbidity and mortality rate are about 20%, with death mostly occurring within a few days after symptoms of encephalitis due to coma and respiratory failure [43]. Rubella virus can also persist in brain tissue for long periods of time, often causing progressive rubella panencephalitis (PRP) at 10–30 years of age, with an incubation period of up to 12 years. Laboratory examination of pharyngeal swabs, urine or cerebrospinal fluid specimens may isolate rubella virus or detect rubella virus nucleic acid; serum rubella IgM antibody is positive (no live attenuated rubella vaccine within 1 month); serum rubella IgG antibodies or rubella hemagglutination-inhibiting antibody titers in the recovery phase are fourfold higher than that in the acute phase; negative antibody in the acute phase and positive antibody in the recovery phase can be found.

6.5.2 Pathological Manifestations

Brain tissue edema, perivascular lymphocytic infiltration, neuronal cell degeneration, mild meningeal reaction, and demyelination of white matter in the brain, brainstem, cerebellum, and spinal cord.

6.5.3 Imaging

1. **CT**

   Calcifications can be found in the cerebral cortex and basal ganglia and appeared as nodular, striated, and punctate [44]. Subventricular linear calcification is a typical manifestation of rubella virus encephalitis. The density of the limbic system and deep white matter is reduced, and the cerebellar cortical is atrophied. The cerebral sulci and brain pools are broadening, and the lateral ventricular body, triangle, and the fourth ventricle ventricular dilatation are most pronounced.
2. **MRI**

   The degeneration of deep and subcortical white matter can appear due to cerebrovascular damage and ischemic necrosis, manifested by multiple linear and speckled high signal intensity on T2-weighted images in bilateral white matter, pronounced located in the white matter of frontal and parietal lobes [45, 46]. Periventricular subcortical high T2 signal intensity in infants and children suggests delayed myelin formation. Ventricular dilatation is common.

6.5.4 Diagnostic Key Points

1. Sudden convulsions, coma, headache, and vomiting during rubella epidemic should be considered first as possible encephalitis.
2. Imaging findings reveal changes such as calcification of basal ganglia, subventricular and ventricular dilatation, and cerebral atrophy.
3. Rubella virus may be isolated, or rubella virus nucleic acid may be detected in throat swabs, urine, or cerebrospinal fluid specimens, and serum rubella IgM antibodies are positive.

6.5.5 Differential Diagnosis

1. In congenital toxoplasmic encephalitis, the typical CT manifestations are intracerebral calcification, decreased density of brain parenchyma, and hydrocephalus. Confirmation of the diagnosis is based on the measurement of specific anti-*Toxoplasma* IgM and IgG antibodies.
2. The clinical manifestations of hypoparathyroidism are characterized by twitching of the hands and feet, epilepsy, and convulsions. Based on imaging, calcifications can be found in the basal ganglia, thalamus, and corticomedullary junction, and biochemical examinations show hypocalcemia and hyperphosphorus changes.
3. Congenital cytomegalovirus (CMV) encephalitis: Microcephaly is common in infected children, with clinical manifestations of fever, abnormal sensation, convulsions, visual deficits, lethargy, and coma. In noncontrast CT images, it is depicted as brain atrophy, ventricular dilatation, and calcifications in the brain parenchyma, most commonly in the periventricular. MR images reveal ectopic malformations of neurons, brain softening, and delayed myelin formation. Positive blood and cerebrospinal fluid CMV antigen and anti-CMV IgM help to confirm the diagnosis.

6.5.6 Status and Progress of Research

Wang Xizhen et al. [47] showed that rubella virus IgM antibody positivity can increase the risk of primary hypertension but is not a major influencing factor.

6.6 Influenza A H1N1-Related Brain Changes

Li Li and Meiji Ren

6.6.1 Overview

Influenza A H1N1, referred to as influenza A, is an acute respiratory infection caused by the mutated new influenza A virus H1N1 subtype, mainly through respiratory transmission; most patients have mild clinical manifestations, a small number of cases present severely and progress rapidly. Pediatric patients may develop central nervous system complications, the most common clinical manifestations being convulsions, encephalopathy, and persistent status epilepticus.

Influenza A H1N1 central nervous system complications include convulsions, encephalopathy, or encephalitis within 5 days of the onset of influenza-like symptoms, with laboratory tests confirming the presence of respiratory influenza A H1N1 virus infection and no evidence of other possible etiologies.

Simple convulsions are defined as a rapid return of consciousness after a convulsion. Encephalopathy is defined as altered consciousness (agitation, drowsiness, or coma) for more than 24 h, in which symmetrical bilateral thalamic necrosis occurs, which is called acute necrotizing encephalopathy (ANE). Encephalitis is defined as the presence of more than two or two of the following manifestations underlying the encephalopathy: (1) fever, with a body temperature exceeding 38.5°C; (2) signs of focal neuropathy; (3) elevated cerebrospinal fluid lymphocyte count; (4) EEG suggestive of encephalitis; and (5) neuroimaging suggestive of infection or inflammation.

The first case of central nervous system complications of influenza A H1N1 was reported in the United States, included four cases of 7–17-year-old boys, among whom three cases present with encephalopathy and one case with convulsion. The clinical manifestations were all mild and they all discharged with recovery [48], followed by a reported one case 12 of previously healthy female influenza A H1N1 ANE deaths [49]. Three cases of ANE deaths were reported at Shenzhen Children's Hospital in China. The main clinical manifestations are drowsiness, irritability, convulsions, and coma after 1–4 days of acute fever with or without respiratory symptoms.

ANE is a rare and serious central nervous system complication of viral infection, mostly caused by influenza viruses, and rarely can be caused by parainfluenza virus, herpes simplex virus 6, etc. ANE was first reported by Mizuguchi et al. [50] in 1995, and ANE cases are mostly from Japan and rare in our country.

ANE occurs mostly in children under 5 years of age; most children have prodromal symptoms of fever and acute upper respiratory tract infection and develop central nervous system symptoms after prodromal symptoms 24–48 h. The clinical features are multifocal, symmetric brain damage involving the bilateral thalamus, brainstem periaqueductal, periventricular white matter, and cerebellar medulla. Laboratory tests may present negative results in blood and some cases may present hypokalemia in blood biochemistry test; elevated creatine kinase (CK), aspartate aminotransferase (AST), alanine aminotransferase (ALT), lactate dehydrogenase (LDH) can be also seen in few cases. Influenza A H1N1 virus can be isolated from respiratory specimens, and serum levels of influenza A H1N1 virus-specific antibodies can be increased four times or more in double copies.

6.6.2 Pathological Manifestations

The brain tissue was visible to the naked eye as swollen and off-white, with still clear cortical and medullary demarcation and marked liquefied necrosis in the occipital lobe, cerebellar hemispheres, brainstem, and hippocampus. Microscopically, the brain tissue showed liquefied necrosis and demyelinating changes of myelinated nerve fibers and multiple foci of microglial cell proliferation infiltration, and microglia in the focal area became round due to loss of spines and transformed into phagocytes surrounding the neurons and engulfing dead cell debris, suggesting an activated state of microglia. No neutrophil, lymphocyte, or dendritic cell infiltrate was seen in the brain tissue. No influenza AH1N1 genes were detected in cerebrospinal fluid and brain tissue RT-PCR [51].

6.6.3 Imaging

Kimura et al. [52] classified influenza-associated brain changes into five grades based on cranial CT and MRI imaging findings: grade I showing no abnormalities (i.e., influenza-associated encephalopathy), grade II with cortical involvement, grade III with brainstem edema, grade IV with symmetrical involvement of the thalamus (i.e., ANE), and grade V with postinfectious meningitis.

1. CT: The deepening of the cerebral sulci and the enlargement of the ventricles can be found in the mid- to late stages. The imaging manifestation of brain of recovered patient can change back to normal. Tang Zhengzhen et al. [53] reported two cases with early presentation of cerebral edema and the disease progressed rapidly to soften and liquefy. One case presented with cerebral hemorrhage and two patients both died. This result suggests a poor prognosis for those with early presentation of cerebral edema. Kong D.W. et al. [54] reported one case of bilateral cerebellar hemispheres and cerebral hemispheres with multiple cortical and subcortical patchy hypodense lesions with blurred margins, evident in the parietal lobe. In this case, the lesion changed rapidly, and on review after 2 days, the lesion was less dense than before, and on review after 7 days, the lesion was significantly reduced.
2. MRI: Diffuse demyelination of cerebellar hemispheres, brainstem, and white matter of the brain. Enhanced scan showed patchy, cerebral gyrus enhancement of variable size in the brain parenchyma of the bilateral cerebellar hemispheres, brainstem, and cerebral hemispheres. Haktanir reported [55] one case of meningoencephalitis, mainly presenting with bilateral frontoparietal junctional area. Hyperintense in T_2WI can be seen in the thalamus. T1WI enhanced scan shows significant enhancement of the right frontoparietal junctional area and bilateral cerebral hemispheric meninges. Magnetic sensitivity imaging (SWI) based on gradient echo sequence shows pronounced high signal intensity in the right frontoparietal junctional area, without cerebral edema.

Symmetrical multifocal brain damage is a characteristic manifestation of ANE. The lesions were mainly located in

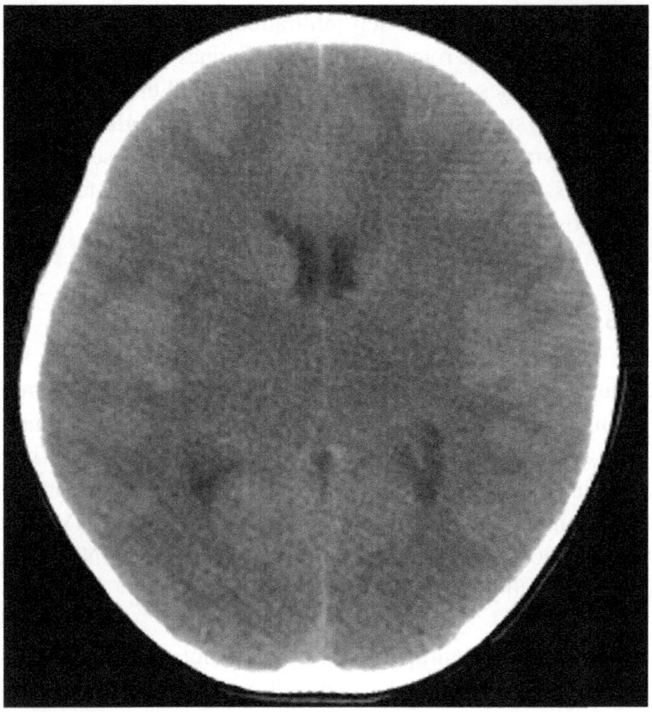

Fig. 6.14 Influenza A H1N1 complicated by encephalitis. Cranial CT shows the density of bilateral cerebral white matter, basal ganglia, and symmetrical thalamus decreased and shallowing of the cerebral sulcus. (Image courtesy of Li Ping, the Second Hospital of Harbin Medical University)

the thalamus, the periaqueductal cover of the brainstem, the white matter around the lateral ventricles, and the cerebellar medulla. CT shows symmetrical hypodensity in the white matter of the brain in the bilateral thalamus, posterior limb of the internal capsule, brainstem, and bilateral fronto-parieto-occipital lobes (Fig. 6.14), as well as diffuse cerebral edema with loss of the sulcus and fourth ventricle, brainstem edema, and bilateral basal ganglia infarction. MRI shows symmetrical low T_1 signal intensity and high T_2 signal intensity in bilateral thalamus, basal ganglia, brainstem, corpus callosum pressure, bilateral centrum semiovale, and paraventricular white matter. FLAIR shows high signal intensity. Enhanced scan shows linear and circumferential enhancement of the semi-oval center and thalamus, without enhancement of the meninges. DWI shows hyperintense in the bilateral thalamus or hypointense in the center with ring-like hyperintense at the edge, and hyperintense in the rest of the lesion area. ADC map shows a slightly hyperintense in the center surrounded by a ring-like slightly hypointensity (low ADC values). Cerebellar involvement may manifest as slightly low T_1 signal intensity and high T_2 signal intensity, slightly high signal intensity on FLAIR, and high signal intensity on DWI in the medulla of the cerebellar hemispheres bilaterally and in the middle peduncle of the right cerebellum. Marked enhancement of the cerebellar meninges can be seen after contrast administration. Low signal in the central area of the bilateral thalamic lesion on DWI is pathologically based on necrosis. In contrast, high signal intensity on DWI is mainly due to cytotoxic edema. The ADC values decreased in the center of the thalamus and increased in the periphery, and ADC values are elevated due to vascular edema of origin.

Zeng Hongwu et al. [56] found the main MRI manifestations of patients with influenza A H1N1 central nervous system complications are as follows: (1) thickening, swelling, and deformation of the brainstem with visible hemorrhage, edema, and necrotic signals; (2) cerebellar tonsillar hernia; and (3) diffuse involvement of the gray and white matter of the bilaterally cerebral and cerebellar. Presumably, the MRI manifestation reflects further exacerbation of cerebral edema, hemorrhage, and neuronal and glial cell necrosis at the time of ANE deterioration compared to the previous condition.

Zeng Hongwu et al. [57] reported one case of influenza A H1N1 complicated by intracranial *Trichophyton* infection, with a slightly low T_1-weighted signal intensity and slightly high T_2-weighted signal intensity in the brain parenchyma with marginal linear enhancement, with marked enhancement of the meninges. MRI follow-up showed cerebral bridge involvement, suggesting further aggravation of the lesion. The child eventually died of multiple organ failure syndrome and intracranial fungal infection.

6.6.4 Diagnostic Key Points

1. A child with influenza presents with multifocal, symmetrical brain damage, characterized by bilateral thalamic involvement, which may involve bilateral basal ganglia, brainstem periaqueductal, periventricular white matter, and cerebellar white matter, with hypointense CT and MRI with long T_1 and long T_2 signal.
2. Positive nucleic acid test for influenza A H1N1 virus, isolation of influenza A H1N1 virus, or double serum influenza A H1N1 virus-specific antibody level elevated four times or more.

6.6.5 Differential Diagnosis

1. Wernicke encephalopathy is caused by vitamin B_1 deficiency from various causes. It mainly involves the brain parenchyma around the third and fourth ventricles and bilateral thalamus can be symmetrically involved. The signal changes are similar to ANE, but no hemorrhagic can be seen. It commonly occurs in chronic alcoholism and severe vomiting during the pregnancy.

2. Epidemic B encephalitis: It is common in summer and is more common in children under 10 years of age. It is characterized clinically by high fever, convulsions, impaired consciousness, and signs of meningeal irritation. The thalamus and midbrain substantia nigra can be involved, either bilaterally or asymmetrically and less frequently in the brainstem. Severe cases may present with hemorrhage, and the diagnosis is confirmed by serum and cerebrospinal fluid IgM antibodies.
3. Reye's syndrome: It is common to develop acute cranial symptoms of encephalopathy such as increased intracranial pressure, impaired consciousness, convulsions, etc., with liver abnormal liver function, hyperammonemia, hypoglycemia, and lactic acidemia. Imaging is mainly diffuse or limited with signs of cerebral edema, and parenchymal brain damage is rare. The disease is fierce and can kill within 24 h; survivors mostly improve in 2–3 days.
4. EV71 central nervous system complications of hand, foot, and mouth disease lesions. It is variable in location, asymmetrical, with a susceptibility to brainstem involvement, and easier to identify when combined with the clinical presence of herpes in the hand, foot, and mouth area.
5. Autosomal dominant acute necrotizing encephalopathy occurs mainly in children and presents as a sudden onset of encephalopathy symptoms 2–3 days after febrile illness. Lesions are mainly symmetrically distributed in the thalamus and brainstem, similar to ANE. The disease has a tendency to recur, and recurrence damage is severe.

6.6.6 Status and Progress of Research

Wong et al. [58] proposed the MRI scoring system, which was approved by many experts. This system has a score of 0–4 points: Scores of 1 or 0 are assigned according to the occurrence of hemorrhage, cyst formation, brainstem damage, and white matter (cerebral, cerebellar, or both) damage, respectively; the higher the score, the worse the prognosis. It has been empirically demonstrated that it correlates well with clinical prognosis.

6.7 COVID-19-Related Encephalopathy

Ablikemu Nurbiyemu, Xuening Zhang, and Wenxiao Jia

6.7.1 Overview

Corona virus disease (COVID-19) outbreak in late 2019 poses a significant global public health threat [59]. By the end of 2020, the number of COVID-19 infections is increasing worldwide, and research on COVID-19 is constantly progressing. This section focuses on the central nervous system alterations associated with COVID-19 based on the present phase of literature.

On Nov 11, 2020, the World Health Organization officially named the corona virus-infected pneumonia as "COVID-19," and the International Committee on Taxonomy of Viruses named the virus as "SARS-CoV-2" (severe acute respiratory syndrome coronavirus-2). The virus is the seventh virus found in the coronavirus family that can infect humans. The main mechanism of infection is the binding of the S protein on the surface of the virus to the corresponding receptor on the target cell and the production of a series of corresponding changes [60]. The human-to-human transmission route of SARS-CoV-2 is similar to that of severe acute respiratory syndrome coronavirus (SARS-nCoV) and Middle East respiratory syndrome coronavirus (MERS-nCoV), and mainly transmitted through respiratory, close contact and aerosol.

Patients infected with SARS-CoV-2 mostly showed clinical symptoms such as fever, dry cough, dyspnea, muscle pain, etc. Their chest CT showed bilateral ground glass-like changes, which are similar to SARS-nCoV and MERS-nCoV. However, patients with SARS-CoV-2 infection rarely present with significant upper respiratory signs and symptoms (e.g., runny nose, sneezing, sore throat, etc.), suggesting that the target cells may be located in the lower respiratory tract. In addition, patients with SARS-CoV-2 infection also rarely present with GI signs and symptoms (e.g., diarrhea, nausea, vomiting, etc.), which are unlike those with SARS-nCoV and MERS-nCoV infections [59]. In addition to the respiratory system, SARS-CoV-2 can involve multiple organs throughout the body, and it is primarily caused by cytokine storms [59]. Some patients with SARS-CoV-2 infection develop neurological symptoms such as impaired consciousness, abnormal skeletal muscle function, and dysosmia and can be combined with diseases such as acute necrotizing encephalopathy (ANE), acute cerebrovascular disease, acute disseminated encephalomyelitis, Guillain-Barre syndrome, and many other neurological disorders [61, 62]. Most neurological manifestations appear in the early stages of the disease and may be caused by SARS-CoV-2 invasion of the CNS via hematogenous or retrograde neuronal pathways [61]. Studies have shown that patients with more severe infections are more likely to have neurological symptoms and are often accompanied by elevated D-dimers and intravascular thrombosis, which may explain why patients with severe infections are more likely to have cerebrovascular symptoms [61]. Laboratory tests reveal blood features of viral infection (i.e., lymphopenia, leukopenia, or normal), and SARS-CoV-2-related nucleic acids can be detected in nasopharyngeal swabs and cerebrospinal fluid.

6.7.2 Pathological Manifestations

Hematoxylin- and eosin-stained sections of brain tissue from SARS-CoV-2-infected patients showed marked tissue edema and neuronal degeneration, and virus particles were detectable under electron microscopy, and ultrastructural analysis of the tissue revealed the presence of 80–110 nm virus-like particles and characteristic rod-like protrusions with two different spike-like protein structures, which are typical characteristics of β-corona viruses. In addition, SARS-CoV-2 viral particles can also be found in the vascular endothelial cells of the central nervous system. This phenomenon may explain the pathway by which the virus enters the central nervous system: In the blood transmission route, the virus enters the central nervous system by infecting the endothelial cells of the blood-brain barrier and the epithelial cells of the blood-brain barrier in the choroid plexus, which in turn invades a large number of neurons, while eventually causing extensive neuroglial cell proliferation, inflammatory cell infiltration, neuronal degeneration, edema, and necrosis through immune-mediation [63, 64].

6.7.3 Imaging

SARS-CoV-2 involves the central nervous system with manifestations similar to SARS-nCoV, which may include acute necrotizing encephalopathy, acute brain injury, acute disseminated encephalomyelitis, ischemic stroke, and cerebral hemorrhage, among which acute hemorrhagic necrotizing encephalopathy is the main manifestation. Most lesions may show no significant abnormalities on CT, but MRI is helpful in the diagnosis of CNS-related disorders.

1. CT findings: When SARS-CoV-2 affects the central nervous system, early CT may not be abnormal in cases where ANE is the predominant presentation. In the middle and late stages, patchy, symmetrical hypodense foci may appear in the bilateral basal ganglia and thalamus, and hyperdense foci may be seen in the foci with hemorrhage [65]. When encephalitis occurs, there is no significant cerebral edema or acute changes in CT, and there may be microvascular ischemic changes [66–68]; in the case of cerebral infarction, multiple hypodense foci of infarction may be seen in the brain parenchyma, occasionally a single foci, and hyperdense thrombi may be seen in the blood vessels which supply the infarcted area; in the case of cerebral hemorrhage, punctate or lamellar hyperdense shadow of the brain parenchyma can be seen, which may be combined with hydrocephalus and occupying effect [69, 70]; central nervous system vasculitis may also occur (see Chap. 19, Sect. 19.1).
2. MRI findings: Some cases of SARS-CoV-2-infected patients present with an imaging syndrome of ANE, which is characterized by symmetric multifocal brain damage, with lesions mainly distributed in the thalamus, deep white matter of the brain, brainstem tegmentum, and cerebellar medulla. The existing reported SARS-CoV-2-infected patient presented with ANE as a characteristic symmetrically distributed bilateral thalamic lesion with T_1WI showing hypointense and T_2WI and DWI showing hyperintense. When hemorrhage occurs, SWI sequences can sensitively detect the hypointense of the hemorrhagic component. On the enhanced scan, lesion shows linear and ring-like enhancement [65].
When complicated with encephalitis, lesion tissues may swell, and T_2WI shows hyperintense in the temporal lobe, hippocampus, and cerebellar peduncle area, and enhanced scan may show no enhancement or gyrus-like enhancement and hyperintense distributed along the lateral ventricular wall that can be seen on DWI sequence [66–68]; when complicated with cerebral infarction, the infarct foci manifest as hypointense on T_1WI and hyperintense on T_2WI, mainly multifocal, with acute or subacute infarcts that manifest as significant hyperintense on DWI and hemorrhagic infarcts or microhemorrhages that manifest as significant hypointense on SWI sequence, which helps in the diagnosis [69, 70]; when complicated with acute disseminated encephalomyelitis, lesions in brain parenchyma may involve basal ganglia, thalamus, etc., and periventricular fusion white matter lesions can be seen. The lesions manifest as hyperintense on T_2WI and DWI with corresponding changes in apparent diffusion coefficient [69]; when complicated with Guillain-Barre syndrome, there may be demyelinating changes in the brain parenchyma and significant abnormal enhancement of the affected nerves on enhanced scans [69]. In addition, studies have reported that majority of patients who have SARS-CoV-2 involvement of the central nervous system show decreased perfusion in different regions of the brain, mostly in the bilateral frontal and temporal lobes, on PWI [71].
3. Cerebral angiography: When central nervous system lesions are predominantly ischemic, hemorrhagic cerebral infarction or cerebral hemorrhage, cerebral angiography reveals rupture of the involved artery, arterial stenosis or intra-arterial thrombosis.

6.7.4 Diagnostic Key Points

1. History of SARS-CoV-2 infection.
2. There may be corresponding imaging manifestations of acute brain damage, acute disseminated encephalomyelitis, ischemic stroke, cerebral hemorrhage, and central nervous system vasculitis.
3. When SARS-CoV-2 infection involves the central nervous system manifesting as ANE, imaging shows characteristic symmetric multifocal brain damage with lesions mostly located in bilateral thalamic and basal ganglia regions. The

necrotic area of brain parenchyma appears as a patchy hypodense lesion on CT and hypointense on T_1WI and hyperintense on T_2WI, with mixed signal on DWI and significant linear and ring-like enhancement on enhanced scan. When complicated with hemorrhage, relative changes can be found, and SWI sequence can be sensitive to detect small hemorrhagic foci. PWI sequence can show hypoperfusion at different sites in frontotemporal brain parenchyma.

4. SARS-CoV-2 is detected in cerebrospinal fluid or brain tissue, or there is evidence of SARS-CoV-2-specific intrathecal antibodies, and no other explainable pathogen or cause is found [69].

6.7.5 Differential Diagnosis

1. Epidemic encephalitis B: Imaging features are similar to ANE, and CT may have no positive features. MRI shows varying degrees of hyperintense on T_2WI in bilateral thalamic regions, with significant hyperintense on DWI and hypointense on ADC. As malacia occurs in the lesion, signal on T_2WI and DWI gradually decreased. Differentiation of ANE led by encephalitis B and SARS-CoV-2 relies mainly on laboratory tests [72].
2. Percheron arterial infarction. It is a rare, normal variant of disease in which arteries become infarcted. DWI shows hyperintense in bilateral thalamus with hypointense on ADC, which is similar to ANE caused by SARS-CoV-2; However, Percheron artery infarction has an anatomical arterial variant basis, whereas ANE caused by SARS-CoV-2 has a normal anatomical structure. Therefore, cerebral angiography can be used as a method of differentiation between those two diseases [73].
3. Deep cerebral vein thrombosis: It can lead to bilateral thalamic swelling and venous infarction. MRI shows bilateral thalamic hypointense on T_1WI and hyperintense on T_2WI and DWI. A region of deep venous hypointense beside thalamus can be seen on SWI, suggesting deep venous thrombosis. In contrast, ANE caused by SARS-CoV-2 does not involve the deep veins of the thalamus, so the manifestations of two diseases are different and can be distinguished [74].

6.7.6 Status and Progress of Research

Few CNS involvements due to SARS-CoV-2 infection have been reported so far, with most patients only undergoing conventional MRI examinations and treatment for brain complications. According to the available reports, it can be found that examination techniques such as DWI, SWI, and PWI are helpful in the diagnosis of SARS-CoV-2 neurological complications.

1. Magnetic resonance diffusion-weighted imaging (DWI): It has a high specificity in the diagnosis of acute cerebral infarction. The diffusion of various CNS lesions caused by SARS-CoV-2 infection is restricted, and most of them manifest as hyperintense on DWI, especially cerebral infarction. In addition to helping to diagnose neurological lesions caused by SARS-CoV-2 infection, DWI has a significant role in the differential diagnosis of this disease, and the DWI sequence is recommended for routine use in patients with SARS-CoV-2 infection who have central nervous system symptoms.
2. Magnetic susceptibility-weighted imaging (SWI): It has a high sensitivity and specificity in the diagnosis of microvascular hemorrhage and thrombosis, which are more common in central nervous system involvement due to SARS-CoV-2 infection. Among the diagnoses of acute hemorrhagic necrotizing encephalopathy, which is specific in CNS involvement, the SWI sequence shows symmetrical scattered hypointense within the necrotic foci, suggesting microhemorrhage in the lesion area and contributing to the diagnosis of acute hemorrhagic necrotizing encephalopathy. In addition, because of the elevated D-dimer in patients with SARS-CoV-2 infection, it is prone to thrombus formation in cerebral vessels, leading to ischemic cerebral infarction, and the intravascular thrombus appears as intravascular hypointense foci on SWI and also contributes to the diagnosis of cerebral involvement caused by SARS-CoV-2 infection.
3. Perfusion-weighted imaging (PWI): The study reported that reduced perfusion of frontotemporal brain parenchyma is common in CNS lesions caused by SARSCoV-2 infection, and PWI can sensitively detect blood perfusion in various regions of the brain. It is recommended that patients with SARS-CoV-2 infection and CNS symptoms actively use PWI scanning to improve the diagnostic efficiency.

References

1. Liu L. Adult measles encephalitis 1 cases. J Mod Integr Med. 2010;19(3):353–4.
2. Mi C, Wang J, Zhang A, et al. Pontocerebral central myelinolysis due to measles encephalitis 1 example. Chin J Pract Pediatr. 2009;24(7):566–7.
3. Liu H, Xiao E, Tan L, et al. Fulminant subacute sclerosing holoprosencephalitis in young children MRI diagnostic. J Clin Radiol. 2012;31(9):60–2.
4. Xiong F, Deng SY, Wan ZM, et al. Current status and progress of research on subacute sclerosing holoprosencephalitis. J Clin Radiol. 2012;31(9):1193–5.
5. Oguz KK, Celebi A, Anlar B. MR imaging, diffusion weighted imaging and MR spectroscopy findings in acute rapidly progressive subacute sclerosing panencephalitis. Brain Dev. 2007;29(5):306–11.
6. Gupta RK, Kumar S. Central nervous system tuberculosis. Neuroimaging Clin N Am. 2011;21(4):795–814.
7. Tang S, Gao W. Clinical tuberculosis. Beijing: People's Medical Publishing House; 2011.

8. Guo L, Lv Y, Zhou X. MRI features of intracranial tuberculosis and dynamic score of anti-tuberculosis treatment. J Clin Radiol. 2012;31(9):202–6.
9. Bernaerts A, Vanhoenacker FM, Parizel PM, et al. Tuberculosis of the central nervous system: overview of neuroradiological findings. Eur Radiol. 2003;13(8):1876–90.
10. Bartzatt R. Tuberculosis infections of the central nervous system. Cent Nerv Syst Agents Med Chem. 2011;11(1):321–7.
11. Gao Y, Cai Y, Cai Z. Diagnostic magnetic resonance imaging. Beijing: People's Medical Publishing House; 1997.
12. Feng Y, Liu Z, Zhang S, et al. Clinical and pathological aspects of tuberculous meningitis 129 cases. Chin J Tuberc Respir. 1997;20(3):161–3.
13. Dui H, Hou DL, Zhang X, et al. Exploration of the advantages of multilayer spiral CT delayed scanning for the display of intracranial tuberculosis lesions. J Clin Radiol. 2012;31(9):1207–11.
14. Santy K, Nan P, Chantana Y, et al. The diagnosis of brain tuberculoma by (1)H-magnetic resonance spectroscopy. Eur J Pediatr. 2011;170(3):379–87.
15. Pretell EJ, Martinot CJ, Garcia HH, et al. Differential diagnosis between cerebral tuberculosis and neurocysticercosis by magnetic resonance spectroscopy. J Comput Assist Tomogr. 2005;29(1):112–4.
16. Peng J, Luo T, Luo F, et al. Differential diagnostic value of hydrogen proton MR spectroscopy for brain tuberculoma, glioma and brain metastases. J Third Mil Med Univ. 2009;31(12):1213–6.
17. Peng J, Luo T, Luo F, et al. The value of MRI diffusion-weighted imaging to identify brain tuberculoma and high-grade astrocytoma and brain metastases. Chin J Radiol. 2007;41(9):926–30.
18. Gupta RK, Prakash M, Mishra AM, et al. Role of diffusion weighted imaging in differentiation of intracranial tuberculoma and tuberculous abscess from cysticercus granulomas—a report of more than 100 lesions. Eur J Radiol. 2005;55(3):384–92.
19. Haris M, Gupta RK, Husain M, et al. Assessment of therapeutic response in brain tuberculomas using serial dynamic contrast-enhanced MRI. Clin Radiol. 2008;63(5):562–74.
20. Gupta RK, Haris M, Husain N, et al. Relative cerebral blood volume is a measure of angiogenesis in brain tuberculoma. J Comput Assist Tomogr. 2007;31(3):335–41.
21. Chatterjee S, Saini J, Kesavadas C, et al. Differentiation of tubercular infection and metastasis presenting as ring enhancing lesion by diffusion and perfusion magnetic resonance imaging. J Neuroradiol. 2010;37(3):167–71.
22. Haacke EM, Mittal S, Wu Z, et al. Susceptibility-weighted imaging: technical aspects and clinical applications. Part I. Am J Neuroradiol. 2009;30(1):19–30.
23. Barnes SRS, Haacke EM. Susceptibility-weighted imaging: clinical angiographic applications. Magn Reson Imaging Clin N Am. 2009;17(1):47–61.
24. Wu Z, Mittal S, Kish K, et al. Identification of calcification with magnetic resonance imaging using susceptibility-weighted imaging: a case study. J Magn Reson Imaging. 2009;29(1):177–82.
25. Mittal S, Wu Z, Neelavall J, et al. Susceptibility-weighted imaging: technical aspects and clinical applications. Part 2. Am J Neuroradiol. 2009;30:232–50.
26. Toh CH, Wei KC, Chang CN, et al. Differentiation of pyogenic brain abscesses from necrotic glioblastomas with use of susceptibility-weighted imaging. Am J Neuroradiol. 2012;33(8):1534–8.
27. Rangarajan K, Das CJ, Kumar A, et al. MRI in central nervous system infections: a simplified pattern approach. World J Radiol. 2014;28(9):716–25.
28. Saxena S, Prakash M, Kumar S, et al. Comparative evaluation of magnetization transfer contrast and fluid attenuated inversion recovery sequences in brain tuberculoma. Clin Radiol. 2005;60(7):787–93.
29. Gupta RK, Kathuria MK, Pradhan S. Magnetization transfer MR imaging in CNS tuberculosis. Am J Neuroradiol. 1999;20(5):867–75.
30. Pui MH, Ahmad MN. Magnetization transfer imaging diagnosis of intracranial tuberculomas. Neuroradiology. 2002;44(3):210–5.
31. Yip K, Gosling R, Jones V, et al. An unusual case of meningococcal meningitis complicated with subdural empyema in a 3 month old infant: a case report. Cases J. 2009;2(1):6335.
32. Izzo I, Pileri P, Merello M, et al. A typical clinical presentation of meningococcal meningitis: a case report. Infez Med. 2016;24(3):234–6.
33. Kastenbauer S, Winkler F, Fesl G, et al. Acute severe spinal cord dysfunction in bacterial meningitis in adults. MRI findings suggest extensive myelitis. Arch Neurol. 2001;58(5):806–10.
34. Boos C, Daneshvar C, Hinton A, et al. An unusual case of chronic meningitis. BMC Fam Pract. 2004;5(1):21.
35. van de Beek D, Patel R, Wijdicks EF. Meningococcal meningitis with brainstem infarction. Arch Neurol. 2007;64(9):1350–1.
36. O'Farrell R, Thornton J, Brennan P, et al. Spinal cord infarction and tetraplegia-rare complications of meningococcal meningitis. Br J Anaesth. 2000;84(4):514–7.
37. Liu JD, Zhang JF, Zheng HF. Research progress of epidemic encephalomyelitis vaccine of group B. Chin J Biol Prod. 2019;32(4):472–5.
38. Zhang L, Zhou X. Modern epidemiology. 2nd ed. Beijing: People's Medical Publishing House; 2010.
39. Li L, Ren H. Epidemiology. 3rd ed. Beijing: People's Medical Publishing House; 2010.
40. Aydin H, Ozgul E, Agildere AM. Acute necrotizing encephalopathy secondary to diphtheria, tetanus toxoid and whole-cell pertussis vaccination: diffusion-weighted imaging and proton MR spectroscopy findings. Pediatr Radiol. 2010;40(7):1281–4.
41. Zhang T, Chen Z, He Q. Progress in the study of mechanisms related to immune protection against pertussis and evaluation indicators. Adv Microbiol Immunol. 2019;47(2):47–51.
42. Luo P, Ma X. Advances in research on novel pertussis vaccines. Adv Microbiol Immunol. 2018;46(5):91–5.
43. Zhang L, Zhou X. Modern epidemiology. 2rd ed. Beijing: People's Medical Publishing House; 2010.
44. Numazaki K, Fujikawa T. Intracranial calcification with congenital rubella syndrome in a mother with serologic immunity. J Child Neurol. 2003;18(4):296–7.
45. Takano T, Morimoto M, Bamba N, et al. Frontal-dominant white matter lesions following congenital rubella and cytomegalovirus infection. J Perinat Med. 2006;34(3):254–5.
46. Lane B, Sullivan EV, Lim KO, et al. White matter MR hyperintensities in adult patients with congenital rubella. Am J Neuroradiol. 1996;17(1):99–103.
47. Wang X, Wang Y, Liu X, et al. Association of rubella virus IgM antibodies with essential hypertension joint study. Chin Foreign Med Res. 2017;15(35):1–3.
48. Centers for Disease Control and Prevention (CDC). Neurologic complications associated with novel influenza A (H1N1) virus infection in children-Dallas, Texas, May 2009. Morb Mortal Wkly Rep. 2009;58(28):773–8.
49. Lyon JB, Remigio C, Milligan T, et al. Acute necrotizing encephalopathy in a child with H1N1 influenza infection. Pediatr Radiol. 2010;40(2):200–5.
50. Mizuguchi M, Abe J, Mikkaichi K, et al. Acute necrotising encephalopathy of childhood: a new syndrome presenting with multifocal, symmetric brain lesions. J Neurol Neurosurg Psychiatry. 1995;58(5):555–61.
51. Cao J, Li C, Wen F, et al. 2009 Year A H1N1 influenza virus-associated acute necrotizing encephalopathy 3 histopathologi-

cal observation of brain cases. Chin J Pract Pediatr. 2012;27: 595–8.
52. Kimura S, Ohtuki N, Nezu A, et al. Clinical and radiological variability of influenza-related encephalopathy or encephalitis. Acta Paediatr Jpn. 1998;40(3):264–70.
53. Tang Z, He Y, Zheng Y, et al. Children 2009 A H1N1 Influenza-related nerves systemic complications reported. Chin J Pract Pediatr. 2010;25(2):129–31.
54. Kong D, Wu W. A case of brain damage due to influenza A H1N1. J Clin Radiol. 2010;29(7):876.
55. Haktanir A. MR imaging in novel influenza A(H1N1)-associated meningoencephalitis. Am J Neuroradiol. 2010;31(3):394–5.
56. Zeng H, Gan Y, Huang Document, et al. Clinical and imaging analysis of acute necrotizing encephalopathy in children. J Clin Radiol. 2012;31(9):1209–11.
57. Zeng H, Huang Document, Gan Y, et al. Imaging manifestations of central nervous system complications of critical childhood A H1N1 influenza. Radiol Pract. 2010;25(9):947–50.
58. Wong AM, Simon EM, Zimmerman RA, et al. Acute necrotizing encephalopathy of childhood correlation of MR finding and clinical outcome. Am J Neuroradiol. 2006;27(9):1919–23.
59. Huang CL, Wang YM, Li XW, et al. Clinical features of patients infected with 2019 novel coronavirus in Wuhan, China. Lancet. 2020;395:497–506.
60. Su S, Li XC, Artemisia, et al. Advances in the study of novel coronaviruses. J Xi'an Jiaotong Univ (Med Ed). 2020;41(4):479–82, 496.
61. Mao L, Jin H, Wang M, et al. Neurologic manifestations of hospitalized patients with coronavirus disease 2019 in Wuhan, China. JAMA Neurol. 2020;77(6):1–9.
62. Wang L, Shen Y, Li M, et al. Clinical manifestations and evidence of neurological involvement in 2019 novel coronavirus SARS-CoV-2: a systematic review and meta-analysis. J Neurol. 2020;267(10):2777–89.
63. Paniz-Mondolfi A, Bryce C, Grimes Z, et al. Central nervous system involvement by severe acute respiratory syndrome coronavirus-2 (SARS-CoV-2). J Med Virol. 2020;92(7):699–702.
64. Neurologist Branch, Shenzhen Physicians Association, Central Nervous System Infection and Immunology Group, Neurology Branch, Shenzhen Physicians Association. Treatment plan for central nervous system infections and immune-related diseases during the novel coronavirus pneumonia outbreak (trial version 1). GDMS. 2020;41(6):549–54.
65. Poyiadji N, Shahin G, Noujaim D, et al. COVID-19-associated acute hemorrhagic necrotizing encephalopathy: imaging features. Radiology. 2020;296(2):119–20.
66. Moriguchi T, Harii N, Goto J, et al. A first case of meningitis/encephalitis associated with SARS-coronavirus-2. Int J Infect Dis. 2020;94:55–8.
67. Sohal S, Mossammat M. COVID-19 presenting with seizures. IDCases. 2020;20:00782.
68. Wong PF, Craik S, Newman P, et al. Lessons of the month 1: a case of rhombencephalitis as a rare complication of acute COVID-19 infection. Clin Med (Lond). 2020;20(3):293–4.
69. Ellul MA, Benjamin L, Singh B, et al. Neurological associations of COVID-19. Lancet Neurol. 2020;19(9):767–83.
70. Beyrouti R, Adams ME, Benjamin L, et al. Characteristics of ischaemic stroke associated with COVID-19. J Neurol Neurosurg Psychiatry. 2020;91(8):889–91.
71. Helms J, Kremer S, Merdji H, et al. Neurologic features in severe SARS-CoV-2 infection. N Engl JMed. 2020;382(23):2268–70.
72. Arahata Y, Fujii K, Nishimura T, et al. Longitudinal magnetic resonance imaging changes in Japanese encephalitis. Brain Dev. 2019;41(8):731–4.
73. Khanni JL, Casale JA, Koek AY, et al. Artery of Percheron infarct: an acute diagnostic challenge with a spectrum of clinical presentations. Cureus. 2018;10:e3276.
74. Taniguchi D, Nakajima S, Hayashida A, et al. Deep cerebral venous thrombosis mimicking influenza-associated acute necrotizing encephalopathy: a case report. J Med Case Rep. 2017;11(1):281.

7 Gastrointestinal Infectious Disease-Related Central Nervous System Infections (Poliomyelitis)

Xiaodan Du, Junle Yang, Jin Li, and Jian Wang

7.1 Overview

Poliomyelitis is an acute infectious disease caused by infections of poliovirus, with humans as the only natural host, and mostly occurs in children. The incidence gradually increases over 6 months of age, decreases after 5 years of age, and is rare in adults. Poliomyelitis is a contact infectious disease that is highly contagious and is transmitted mainly through fecal-oral infection from patients in the acute phase and asymptomatic poliovirus carriers, with an incubation period of 3–35 days, mostly 5–14 days [1]. After poliovirus infection, most people are asymptomatic or have nonspecific symptoms, including mild fever, malaise, headache, sore throat, and gastrointestinal discomfort. Of patients with nonspecific disease symptoms, 1–2% may develop paralytic disease. Paralysis progresses rapidly with fever, often resulting in asymmetric muscle atrophy, but there is no impairment of sensation and bladder or rectal function. Poliomyelitis is also known as "poliomyelitis" or "infantile paralysis" because of the clinical manifestations of decreased muscle tone and asymmetric flaccid paralysis [2]. Patients with poliomyelitis are more commonly seen with occult infection and non-paralytic cases, most of which can be cured, with a few patients left with paralytic sequelae. With the extent of vaccination and improved immunity in the population, the incidence has decreased significantly, and the disease is almost exclusively seen in vaccine-associated cases, namely, vaccine-associated paralytic poliomyelitis (VAPP). WHO defines VAPP as acute flaccid paralysis occurring in 4–40 days after oral administration of live-attenuated polio vaccine, in which vaccine-like poliovirus is isolated from fecal samples of patients and the virus is identified as the cause. In addition, polio-associated neurological sequelae must occur at least 60 days after the onset of paralysis [3]. The incidence of VAPP neonates in the country is 1–2.4/1 million [4].

After entering the body orally, poliovirus mainly invades the nasopharynx and intestinal lymphoid tissues and proliferates and excretes the virus. Depending on whether the virus enters the bloodstream and invades the nervous system, the clinical manifestations can be divided into four types:

1. Occult infection (asymptomatic poliomyelitis), which accounts for 90–95% of all infections. The virus does not enter the bloodstream or central nervous system after infection, and there are usually no clinical symptoms or only mild discomfort.
2. Abortive poliomyelitis (mild), which accounts for 4–8% of infected patients, causes mild viremia when the virus enters the bloodstream and does not invade the central nervous system but only has prodromal symptoms such as respiratory and gastrointestinal tracts.
3. Non-paralytic poliomyelitis. The virus proliferates in the lymphoid tissues of the body and enters the bloodstream in large numbers and invades the central nervous system and presents not only abortive symptoms but also neurological symptoms; however, no paralysis occurs. It mainly involves the motor cells of the anterior horn of the spinal cord, in which the virus proliferates and causes cell necrosis. During this course, changes of nerve and muscle function have not appear and are difficult to distinguish with other aseptic meningitis; virological or serological examination is required.

X. Du
Zhuhai Hospital of Integrated Traditional Chinese and Western Medicine, Zhuhai, China

J. Yang
Journal of Practical Radiology, Xi'an, China

J. Li
The First Affiliated Hospital of Xinjiang Medical University, Urumqi, China

J. Wang (✉)
Medical Imaging Center, First Affiliated Hospital of Xinjiang Medical University, Urumqi, China

Shanghai Universal Medical Imaging Diagnostic Center, Shanghai University, Shanghai, China

H. Li et al. (eds.), *Radiology of Infectious and Inflammatory Diseases - Volume 1*,
https://doi.org/10.1007/978-981-99-0039-8_7

4. Paralytic poliomyelitis, which accounts for 1–2% of infected patients and is characterized by paralysis on the basis of clinical manifestations of the non-paralytic type, plus involvement of the gray matter of the anterior horn of the spinal cord, brain, and cerebral neuropathy. This type is divided into five phases according to clinical manifestations: prodromal phase; pre-paralytic phase; paralytic phase (this phase can be divided into the following types according to the site of the lesion: the spinal cord type [the lesions mostly occur in the cervical and lumbar spinal cord, mostly presenting as asymmetric unilateral flaccid limb paralysis, usually with lower limb paralysis. Symptoms appear earlier in the proximal muscle groups and are more severe than in the distal muscle groups, with the paralysis involving different muscle groups, and thus the corresponding symptoms occur]; the brainstem type, most of which occurs simultaneously with spinal cord type and has viral invasion of the medulla oblongata and pons; the encephalitis type [symptoms of brain damage occur in this type and manifest as diffuse or focal encephalitis]; and mixed type, where two or more types occur at the site of lesion occurrence, with spinal and brainstem types occurring together more often); recovery phase; and posterior phase [1]. Laboratory tests may isolate wild-type poliovirus from feces, pharynx, cerebrospinal fluid, and brain or spinal cord tissue; in cases with no oral polio vaccine (OPV) or exposure to the vaccine virus within 6 weeks before and after the onset, anti-polio virus IgM antibodies can be detected in cerebrospinal fluid or blood within 1 month after paralysis, or specific IgG antibody titers 4 times higher than that of in the acute phase in serum during recovery.

7.2 Pathological Manifestations

Poliovirus can involve any structure of the nervous system, but the virus tends to affect larger neurons, especially those in the anterior horn of the spinal cord and medullary motoneuron [5], mostly in the cervical and lumbar spinal cord, but also in the brainstem and other areas, less frequently in the cerebral cortex. It is a neurotropic virus. Pathological changes include (1) nerve cell damage, chromosomal lysis that occurs in nerve cells, loss of niosomes in the cytoplasm, and visible eosinophilic inclusion bodies and (2) inflammatory response, secondary to nerve cell damage, with surrounding tissue congestion and edema and perivascular inflammatory cell infiltration. When swollen tissue compresses adjacent brain nerves, patients may experience temporary corresponding loss of function; early mild lesions are reversible, and generally after 3–4 weeks of onset, the corresponding damaged nerve cell function may gradually recover due to gradual disappearance and decompensation of lesion edema and inflammation. In more severe cases, the nuclei of damaged cells become concentrated, necrotic, and eventually cleared by phagocytes; in severe cases, the damaged cells develop irreversible lesions and scar formation, leading to permanent paralysis [2].

7.3 Imaging

1. CT shows poorly for lesions in the spinal cord but can show associated complications due to polio sequelae.
2. MRI. Poliomyelitis lesions are most often seen in the cervical lumbar spinal cord, with motor nerve damage most pronounced in the anterior horn of the spinal cord, with involvement of the brainstem and other sites (mostly in the substantia nigra, dorsal aspect of the medulla oblongata), and less frequently in the cerebral cortex [6]. Only 10–15% of cases have no medulla oblongata involvement; most cases present as mixed medulla oblongata plus spinal cord involvement, with VII, IX, and X pairs of cerebral nerves most commonly involved [7]. Abnormal hyperintensity is seen in the central anterior gray matter horn of the spinal cord on axial T_2WI in the acute and subacute stages of poliomyelitis, and sagittal T_2WI shows continuous strip-like hyperintensity in the anterior part of the spinal cord, which may be due to inflammatory changes, neurophilic effects, gliosis, and cell destruction in the anterior horn of the spinal cord caused by poliovirus, with or without abnormal enhancement on the enhanced scan. Patients with advanced poliomyelitis are seen to have abnormal hyperintensityl in the spinal cord at T_2WI, and most are seen to have spinal cord atrophy [8], which may be due to atrophy or absence of motor neurons, reactive gliosis, and inflammatory changes in the perivascular and parenchymal areas [9]. Late stages of paralytic polio patients may be combined with spinal cord cavitation.

7.4 Diagnostic Key Points

1. The patient has a history of contact with a confirmed polio victim or a history of residence in a polio-endemic area.
2. Clinical manifestations are mostly fever, nausea and vomiting, muscle aches and pains, decreased muscle tone, and asymmetric flaccid paralysis.
3. Lesions are mostly located in the cervical and lumbar spinal cord, with the most significant damage to the motor nerves in the anterior horn of the spinal cord, and the brainstem and other areas can also be involved; cerebral cortex involvement is rare.

4. MRI plain scan: In acute and subacute phase, T_1WI shows hypointensity, and axial T_2WI shows abnormal hypointensity in the anterior horn of the spinal cord with sagittal T_2WI showing continuous strip-like hyperintensity in the anterior part of the spinal cord. In late phase, T_2WI shows abnormally hypointensity in the spinal cord, which may appear as atrophy, with or without abnormal enhancement on enhanced scan.
5. Poliovirus can be isolated from the patient's feces, pharynx, cerebrospinal fluid, and brain or spinal cord tissue.
6. In the cases with no inactivated polio vaccine or oral live-attenuated polio vaccine within 6 weeks before or after onset of illness and no exposure to vaccine virus, the anti-poliovirus IgM antibodies can be detected in the body within 1 month after paralysis, or serum-neutralizing antibodies or specific IgG antibodies during the recovery period. A titer more than four times higher than in the acute phase may help confirm the diagnosis.

7.5 Differential Diagnosis

Patients with poliomyelitis do not show characteristic early manifestations, and CT and MRI plain scans often show no early abnormalities and lack specificity. They can often be distinguished from other types of encephalitis, acute flaccid paralysis (AFP) by their clinical history (patients with poliomyelitis may show excessive sweating, irritability, drowsiness, and marked headache due to central nervous system stimulation) and laboratory tests [10]. Acute disseminated encephalomyelitis (ADEM) is rarely associated with oral administration of live-attenuated polio vaccine and usually has a monophasic clinical course with varying degrees of encephalopathy and focal neurological signs, and most patients respond well to glucocorticoid therapy and can recover completely without neurological sequelae.

7.6 Status and Progress of Research

Systematic studies about the polio MRI are scarce, with only a few case reports. Typical presentation is a marked increase in signal intensity in the central gray matter anterior horn of the spinal cord in T_2WI, generally without occupancy effects and enhancement. A combination of clinical signs and isolation of poliovirus is required to make the diagnosis.

References

1. National Health and Family Planning Commission of the People's Republic of China. Polio diagnostic criteria. Beijing: China Standard Press; 2016. WS 294-2016.
2. Li H. Practical infectious disease imaging. Beijing: People's Health Press; 2014.
3. Ferraz-Filho JRL, dos Santos TU, de Oliveira EP, et al. MRI findings in an infant with vaccine-associated paralytic poliomyelitis. Pediatr Radiol. 2010;40(1):S138–40.
4. Wu W, Wang H, Li K, et al. Recipient vaccine-associated paralytic poliomyelitis in China, 2010-2015. Vaccine. 2018;36(9):1209–13.
5. Malzberg MS, Rogg JM, Tate CA, et al. Poliomyelitis: hyperintensity of the anterior horn cells on MR images of the spinal cord. Am J Roentgenol. 1993;161(4):863–5.
6. Choudhary A, Sharma S, Sankhyan N, et al. Midbrain and spinal cord magnetic resonance imaging (MRI) changes in poliomyelitis. J Child Neurol. 2010;25(4):497–9.
7. Maloney JA, Mirsky DM, Messacar K, et al. MRI findings in children with acute flaccid paralysis and cranial nerve dysfunction occurring during the 2014 enterovirus D68 outbreak. Am J Neuroradiol. 2015;36(2):245–50.
8. França MCJ, Schmutzler KM, Garibaldi SG, et al. Bilateral substantia nigra involvement in vaccine-associated poliomyelitis. Neurology. 2006;66(10):1597–8.
9. Ziller MG, Stommel EW. Spinal magnetic resonance imaging in chronic poliomyelitis. J Clin Neuromuscul Dis. 2014;16(1):24.
10. Nelson GR, Bonkowsky JL, Doll E, et al. Recognition and management of acute flaccid myelitis in children. Pediatr Neurol. 2016;55:17–21.

Entomophila Infection-Related Intracranial Infections

8

Xiaodan Du, Shuang Ding, Jian Wang, Chunhui Jiang, Jun Liu, Ling Wu, Hanqiu Liu, Weiwei Wang, Dan Zhang, and Jun Lu

8.1 Epidemic B Encephalitis

Xiaodan Du, Shuang Ding, and Jian Wang

8.1.1 Overview

Epidemic encephalitis B is an acute infectious disease of the central nervous system caused by the encephalitis B virus, which is neurotropic in nature, with inflammation of the brain parenchyma as the main change. The disease is also called Japanese encephalitis because it was the first successful isolation of B encephalitis virus in Japan. The virus is transmitted between animal and human hosts through mosquito vectors and is prevalent in summer and autumn, mostly affecting children. The virus multiplies in the mononuclear phagocyte system after being bitten by a virulent mosquito and then enters the bloodstream to form viremia. The onset and severity of the disease depends mainly on the number of viruses, their virulence, and the immunity of the infected individuals. In people with competent immunity, the infection is mostly latent, while in people with weak immunity, the encephalitis B virus destructs the blood-brain barrier and invades the central nervous system, causing encephalitis, which has a high mortality rate and is prone to sequelae. Most infected individuals do not develop the disease and are latent infected. Epidemic encephalitis B mainly affects children under the age of 10. It is more frequent in the population aged 2–6 and more often in male than in female. Epidemic encephalitis B can also occur in adults in non-endemic areas. Clinical symptoms such as acute fever, convulsions, impaired consciousness, meningeal irritation, and respiratory failure with sequelae may occur in severe cases [1].

According to the clinical stages of development, the disease can be divided into four stages. (1) Early period: On days 1–3 of the course of the disease, the patient develops acute fever, which may be accompanied by headache, vomiting, convulsions, and impaired consciousness, representing the viremia phase. (2) Extreme period: On the 4th to 10th day of the disease, patients develop symptoms of systemic viremia and brain damage, such as high fever, hyperspasmia, convulsions, impaired consciousness, meningeal irritation signs, and even lethargy and coma, and the deeper and longer the coma, the more serious the disease. In severe cases, parenchymal brain lesions can lead to central respiratory failure. (3) Recovery period: The body temperature drops to normal or near normal after the acute period, and most patients gradually recover to normal, and some patients with slow recovery tend to revert to normal within 6 months after active treatment. (4) Sequelae period: The sequelae period is defined as when the recovery period symptoms are still present after 6 months [1, 2].

The disease can be classified into four types according to the severity of clinical manifestations. (1) Mild type: Body temperature is 38–39 °C, headache and vomiting may occur, patients are mostly conscious or drowsy and usually free of convulsions, some children may have convulsions, and they will recover within 1 week without sequelae. (2) Normal type: The temperature reaches about 40 °C and usually lasts

X. Du
Zhuhai Hospital of Integrated Traditional Chinese and Western Medicine, Zhuhai, China

S. Ding · C. Jiang · L. Wu · D. Zhang · J. Lu
Medical Imaging Center, First Affiliated Hospital of Xinjiang Medical University, Urumqi, China

J. Wang (✉)
Medical Imaging Center, First Affiliated Hospital of Xinjiang Medical University, Urumqi, China

Shanghai Universal Medical Imaging Diagnostic Center, Shanghai University, Shanghai, China

J. Liu
The Second Xiangya Hospital of Central South University, Changsha, China
e-mail: junliu123@csu.edu.cn

H. Liu · W. Wang
Huashan Hospital, Fudan University, Shanghai, China

H. Li et al. (eds.), *Radiology of Infectious and Inflammatory Diseases - Volume 1*,
https://doi.org/10.1007/978-981-99-0039-8_8

4–5 days. Patients experience headache, vomiting, semiconsciousness or transient coma, occasional convulsions, partial loss of superficial reflexes, hyperactive deep reflexes, and meningeal stimulation signs. It usually recovers in 7–9 days without sequelae in general. (3) Severe type: Patients with persistent temperature of 40–41 °C, vomiting, irritability or coma, recurrent convulsions, loss of deep and superficial reflexes, and obvious signs of meningeal irritation mostly enter the recovery period after 10 days and rarely have sequelae. (4) Fulminant type: The patient's body temperature rises sharply, with pyrexia or hyperthermia and recurrent strong convulsions, and patients may develop deep coma in 1–2 days, with central respiratory failure, brain herniation, and death due to respiratory failure in severe cases, while survivors are left with sequelae [1, 2]. Laboratory examinations of the blood total leukocyte count is mostly (10–20) × 10^9/L, and neutrophils can reach 80% or more; cerebrospinal fluid pressure is increased, with a clear appearance and an elevated leukocyte count, mostly at (50–500) × 10^6/L, with mildly increased total protein. Serological tests suggest that blood or cerebrospinal fluid of unvaccinated individuals within 1 month is positive for encephalitis B virus IgM antibodies; encephalitis B virus can be isolated, or encephalitis B virus-specific nucleic acids can be detected in the cerebrospinal fluid or serum of early infected individuals.

8.1.2 Pathological Manifestations

Epidemic encephalitis B lesions can involve the gray matter of the brain with severity of cortical, thalamic, midbrain substantia nigra, basal ganglia >pons, cerebellum, and medulla oblongata >spinal cord [3]. Visual observation shows soft pia mater congestion, edema, and hemorrhage. Microscopic examination may show:

1. Vascular changes and inflammatory response, with dilatation and congestion of the vessels, widening of their surrounding gaps, and edema of the brain tissue. The inflammatory response is dominated by lymphocyte, plasma cell, and monocyte infiltration, mostly centered on necrotic and degenerated neurons, or by the formation of vascular sleeves in the perivascular spaces.
2. Degeneration, necrosis, and swelling of neurons; solidification, dissolution, and disappearance of neuronal nuclei; disappearance of nisus vesicles; vacuolation; nuclei deviation; etc. Proliferating oligodendrocytes can be seen around the necrotic degenerated nerve cells (satellite phenomenon); microglia are also seen surrounding the necrotic degenerated neurons and engulfing the necrotic degenerated neurons (neuronophagia phenomenon).
3. The formation of malacic foci, with sieve-like malacic foci, caused by necrosis and liquefaction of focal nerve cell and with certain characteristics.
4. Glial cell proliferation and microglia proliferate to form microglial nodules [1, 2].

8.1.3 Imaging

1. **CT**: Epidemic encephalitis B lesions can involve the gray matter of the brain, but their predominant predilection is in the thalamus, followed by the basal ganglia, frontal lobes, and temporal lobes. Early CT scan mainly shows patchy slightly hypodense foci with blurred margins and may show different degrees of brain tissue edema and hydrocephalus, while some patients may not show significant abnormalities on CT. In the extreme period, multiple or single lamellar hypodense foci with clear or indistinct borders are seen in the brain parenchyma, with no significant enhancement on enhanced scans, which may be accompanied by occupying effects, cerebral edema, hydrocephalus, and other changes. In cases with hemorrhage, CT shows hyperdensity in strips of brain parenchyma. In a few cases, no significant abnormalities can be seen in the extreme period of CT, and some malacic foci can be seen in the recovery and sequelae period, which may be accompanied by different degrees of hydrocephalus and brain atrophy. Some patients with complete recovery may not show significant abnormalities in their CT findings.
2. MRI: The main manifestation is multiple patchy abnormal signals in the brain parenchyma, mostly located in the thalamus, basal ganglia region, midbrain, cerebral cortex, cerebellum, pons, and anterior horn of the spinal cord. In the acute phase, the lesion shows slightly hypointense on T_1WI, slightly hyperintense on T_2WI, and slightly hyperintense on FLAIR sequence (Figs. 8.1 and 8.2), and no significant abnormal enhancement is seen on the enhanced scan; in the recovery phase, the lesion shows equal or slightly hypointense on T_1WI, slightly hyperintense on T_2WI, and slightly hyperintense on DWI and FLAIR sequence. The signal on MRI in the presence of hemorrhage is variable at different stages. It has been reported that the characteristic imaging pattern of epidemic encephalitis B is speckled to homogeneous with hyperintensity on DWI and FLAIR images [4].
3. SPECT: The SPECT findings suggest hyperperfusion of the epidemic encephalitis B lesion in the acute period and hypoperfusion in the subacute or chronic period. These changes are of little diagnostic value but help in understanding the sequelae, especially movement disorders [1].

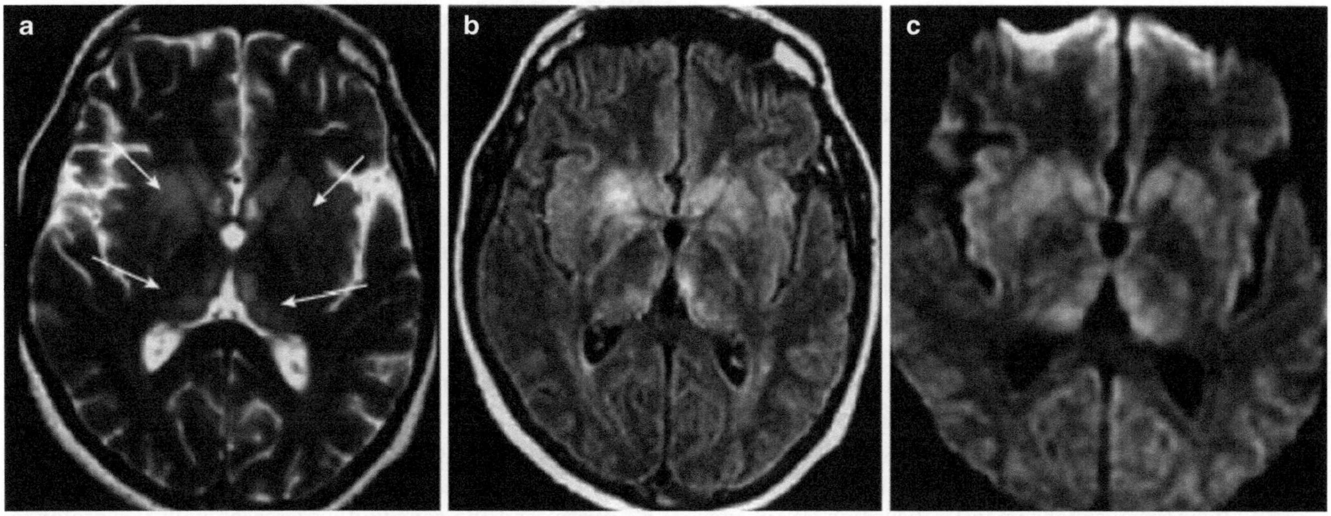

Fig. 8.1 Epidemic encephalitis B (1). Multiple patchy lesions can be seen in the bilateral dorsal thalamus and basal ganglia regions. (**a**) T_2WI with slightly hyperintense; (**b**) FLAIR sequence with slightly hyperintense; (**c**) DWI sequence with slightly hyperintense (b = 1000 mm^2/s). (Courtesy for the case and images from Sawlani V. Diffusion-weighted imaging and apparent diffusion coefficient evaluation of herpes simplex encephalitis and Japanese encephalitis. J Neurol Sci, 2009, 287(1–2): 221–226)

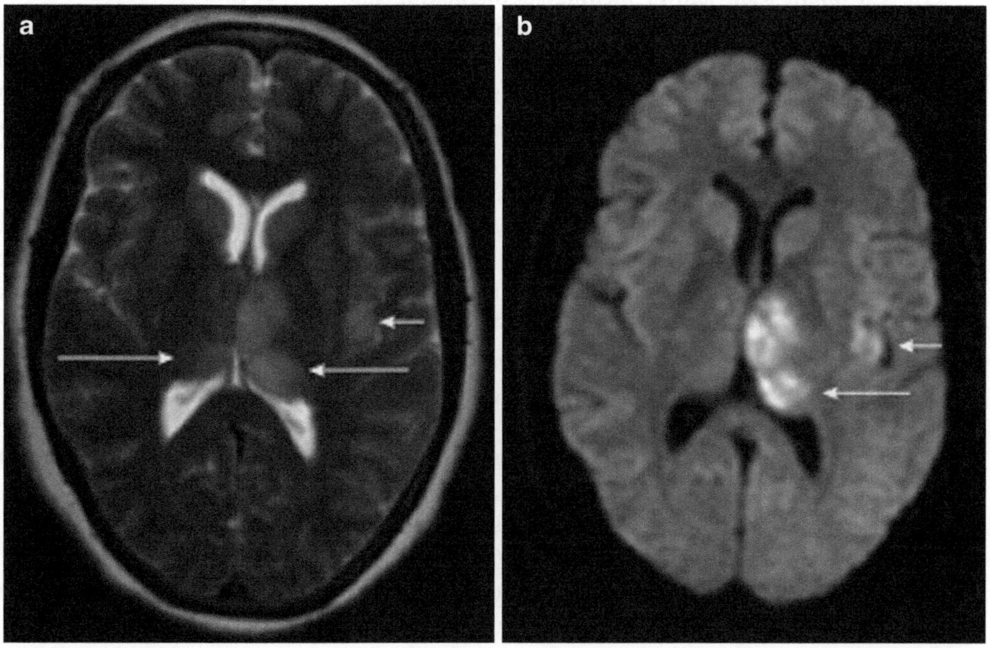

Fig. 8.2 Epidemic encephalitis B (2). Patchy lesions are seen in the bilateral dorsolateral thalamus and left insula. (**a**) T_2WI shows slightly hyperintense with blurred border (white arrow); (**b**) DWI shows restricted diffusion in the left dorsal thalamus and insula (white arrow). (Image courtesy of Professor Xia Shuang, Tianjin First Central Hospital)

8.1.4 Diagnostic Key Points

1. History of residency in endemic areas of epidemic encephalitis B, with a tendency to occur in children.
2. The clinical manifestations in the acute period are mostly fever, headache, projectile vomiting, and positive meningeal irritation signs.
3. CT scan in the extreme phase: Multiple lamellar hypodense foci in the thalamus, basal ganglia, and cerebral hemispheres. MRI scan in the extreme phase: The lesion shows slightly hypointense on T_1WI, slightly hyperintense on T_2WI, and slightly hyperintense in FLAIR sequence. Lesions in acute and subacute phase manifest as slightly hyperintense at DWI and in recovery phase DWI shows isointense.
4. Laboratory tests: The diagnosis can be confirmed by mildly increased intracranial pressure, positive epidemic encephalitis B antigen test results, positive specific IgM antibody test, and isolation of epidemic encephalitis B virus from brain tissue.

8.1.5 Differential Diagnosis

1. **Bacterial meningitis**. It is mostly characterized by inflammatory exudate covering the meninges of the brain surface, with extensive lesions. CT scan shows blurring between the gyri and increased density in the sulci and pools, and enhanced scan shows meningeal linear-like or gyral-like abnormal enhancement. In addition to meningeal manifestations, bacterial meningitis may be accompanied by signs of encephalitis, brain abscess, and subdural pus accumulation. Epidemic encephalitis B mainly shows patchy abnormal density and signal in multiple sites such as thalamus, basal ganglia area, midbrain, cerebral cortex, cerebellum, and pons. Early atypical cases are not easily distinguished from epidemic encephalitis B and require a combination of clinical symptoms and laboratory tests.
2. **Tuberculous meningitis**: Tuberculous meningitis often involves the leptomeninges at the base of the skull, the basal cistern, the ambient cistern, and the sylvian cistern. CT plain scan shows meningeal thickening and scattered calcifications, and enhanced scan shows varying degrees of meningeal thickening and abnormal linear or nodular enhancement in the basal cistern system. The incidence of tuberculous meningitis is generally seasonless, with a slow onset and long course and a history of other sites of tuberculosis. The smear or culture may find *Mycobacterium tuberculosis*. The basal cistern violation in epidemic encephalitis B is less common than that in tuberculous meningitis.
3. **Metabolic encephalopathies such as Wilson's disease, Creutzfeldt-Jakob disease, and Wernicke encephalopathy**: Wilson's disease is mainly located in the bilateral nucleus accumbens, the gray matter around the cerebral aqueduct, the cerebral peduncle, and the basal ganglia; Creutzfeldt-Jakob disease is mainly characterized by symmetric hyperintensity in the bilateral caudate nucleus and the nucleus accumbens on T_2WI; Wernicke encephalopathy is characterized by symmetric hyperintensity around the third ventricle and the aqueduct on T_2WI. Epidemic encephalitis B mainly manifests as abnormal signals in bilateral thalamus, cerebral peduncle, and basal ganglia areas, and its clinical manifestations help to differentiate it. The acute phase of epidemic encephalitis B presents with high fever and increased blood leukocyte count, which combined with laboratory tests help to differentiate it.
4. **Other types of viral encephalitis**: (1) Herpes simplex viral encephalitis: The lesion mostly involves the temporal lobe unilaterally or bilaterally first, but the border of the nucleus accumbens is clear and the lesion easily fuses into large patches; (2) EV71 infection with hand-foot-mouth disease encephalitis: The lesion mostly involves the midbrain, the posterior medulla, the dentate nucleus, the nucleus accumbens, and the deep white matter of the lateral paraventricular area. In contrast, when the temporal lobe of the cerebral brain is involved in epidemic encephalitis B, it is mostly accompanied by thalamic involvement and involves the substantia nigra of the midbrain, which can be differentiated by clinical history and laboratory tests.

8.1.6 Status and Progress of Research

1. **Magnetic resonance diffusion-weighted imaging (DWI)**: DWI is more sensitive to lesions in the acute phase, and the sensitivity decreases with the prolongation of the disease. Neurological symptoms appear early, and lesions can be detected within a few hours, but T_2WI and FLAIR are more sensitive than DWI within 48 h of onset, which may be attributed to the early cytotoxic edema of brain tissue damage caused by epidemic encephalitis B virus, followed by the emergence of viral pathological stages that transform into vasogenic edema [5]. However, the changes in the DWI and ADC maps are more apparent in the recovery and sequela periods than in conventional MRI.
2. **Hydrogen proton magnetic resonance spectroscopy imaging (^{1}H-MRS)**: It can quantitatively evaluate the alterations of common metabolites in the brain of patients with epidemic encephalitis B. Epidemic encephalitis B in ^{1}H-MRS most often shows varying degrees of decrease in NAA peaks and little change in Cho and Cr peaks, while most of the patients exhibit elevated Lac peaks, and a few patients exhibit MI peaks. There are reports of patients found to have significantly decreased NAA peaks with possible sequelae, while patients with mildly decreased NAA peaks have a good prognosis, and those with low Lac peak concentrations have a better prognosis than those with high concentrations [6].

8.2 Echinococcosis

Chunhui Jiang, Jun Liu, Ling Wu, and Jian Wang

Hydatid disease (echinococcosis) is a parasitic disease caused by human infection with the larvae of the *Echinococcus* species and is a global zoonosis. It is prevalent in areas with developed animal husbandry all over the world, and in China it is mainly concentrated in the northern or northwestern part of the country. Echinococcosis is an endemic and common disease in nomadic areas such as Xinjiang, Qinghai, Tibet, Ningxia, and Inner Mongolia. With the increasing number of dogs kept in cities in recent years, the incidence of the disease among urban residents who are not susceptible to echinococcosis is also on the rise. In areas where echinococcosis is endemic, the susceptibility of the population is about 1%, the prevalence of echinococcosis in *Canis familiaris*, herding, and wild dogs is 20–70%, and the prevalence of echinococcosis in livestock such as sheep and cattle is 30–90% [7]. There are many types of *Echinococcus* species, which can lead to different types of echinococcosis, and presently the common types in China are cystic echinococcosis and alveolar echinococcosis. The former is caused by the infection of *Echinococcus granulosus* and mainly appears as a cyst after the patient is infected with *Echinococcus* eggs, while the latter is caused by the infection of alveolar *Echinococcus* and can form a local mass at the site of the disease, which resembles a malignant tumor, or a metastasis of a malignant tumor when it occurs more frequently. In the past, alveolar echinococcosis was regarded as a "malignant tumor" and called "insect carcinoma." The morphology, pathological changes, and clinical manifestations of the worms are different between the two types.

The liver is the most common site of infection, followed by the lung and brain, while other sites of infection, such as the lung and brain, are mostly due to blood circulation. The incidence of cerebral echinococcosis accounts for 1–4% of the incidence of systemic echinococcosis, and the incidence of cystic echinococcosis accounts for 80% of the total incidence, with a significantly higher incidence in children than in adults. The incidence of cerebral alveolar echinococcosis is low, accounting for only 1–3% of systemic metastatic lesions in alveolar echinococcosis [8]. The clinical diagnosis of cerebral alveolar echinococcosis is very difficult, so the imaging diagnosis is crucial. In recent years, with social progress and continuous improvement of sanitary conditions, various variants of echinococcosis have emerged, and imaging manifestations tend to be complicated. Laboratory tests reveal eosinophilia in more than half of the patients with both types of echinococcosis and positive immunologic tests for echinococcosis-specific antibodies such as cephalomere antibodies and cystic fluid antibodies. Most patients with primary cerebral cystic echinococcosis have mostly negative serum immunologic tests, and the rate of positive serum immunologic tests for cerebral alveolar echinococcosis is high.

8.2.1 Cerebral Cyst Echinococcosis

8.2.1.1 Overview

Cerebral cyst echinococcosis (CCE), also known as hydatid cyst, is a parasitic infection of the brain caused by human infection with larva of the *Echinococcus granulosus*. *Echinococcus granulosus* can be parasitized in any part of the brain, with the middle cerebral artery supply area being the most common and the parietal and frontal lobes being the most frequent.

Primary infection is more common in cerebral cystic echinococcosis, and the most important source of infection is the dog, which is the end host of *Echinococcus*. Adult *Echinococcus granulosus* parasites are found in the upper part of the small intestine of dogs, and their eggs are excreted with the feces, contaminating soil, food, or water. Humans and even-toed ungulates such as sheep are the intermediate hosts. When people live in places contaminated with eggs, the eggs enter the body by hand, food, or water through the mouth and hatch out of the hexacanth embrasure by the action of digestive juices in the gastrointestinal tract. The hexacanth embrasure then escapes and burrows into the intestinal wall vein and invades the liver through the portal vein blood flow, which is the first and most frequently involved part of human cystic echinococcosis. A small number of hexacanth embrasure reenter the circulation through the hepatic sinusoids and enter the brain via the internal carotid artery, where they grow and develop to form hydatid cyst. WHO classifies cerebral cystic echinococcosis into five types according to the activity of cysticercus: type I and type II have the ability to reproduce; type III is the transitional stage; type IV and type V are metaphase, inactive, and have no ability to reproduce. On the other hand, it can be divided into mono-, multi-, and subcapsular, calcified, ruptured, and infected types according to the imaging presentation.

There are no obvious symptoms and signs in the early stage of cerebral cystic echinococcosis, but when the cysts are large, they produce compression symptoms such as headache, nausea, vomiting, optic disc edema, etc., or focal symptoms such as hemiplegia, aphasia, hemianesthesia, seizures, etc.

8.2.1.2 Pathological Manifestations

1. Macroscopic observation: The simple hydatid cysts are milky white and translucent, with smooth and shiny surface and uniform wall thickness of 1–3 mm in diameter. In addition to a large parent cyst, multiple sub-cysts of varying sizes are also visible inside the parent cysts. The sub-cysts are similar in structure to the parent cysts and are milky white or translucent vesicles.
2. Light microscopic observation: The cyst wall of an encapsulated cyst is divided into two parts: the outer and the inner capsule. The outer capsule is a fibrous capsule wall formed by the immune response to host infection with echinococcosis and is a fibrous connective tissue envelope composed of new fibroblasts surrounded by plasma cells and multinucleated macrophage infiltration. The inner capsule, the hydatid itself, is divided into two layers: the outer layer is the stratum corneum and the inner layer is the germ layer. The stratum corneum is formed by the secretions of the cells of the hair growth layer and does not contain cellular structures. The germ layer is composed mainly of germ cells and is the base for the

proliferation of embryonic larvae. On the inner surface of the germ layer grow many tiny granular brood sacs and chick sacs. The brood sac has a very thin envelope containing multiple protoscolex. The protoscolex is ovoid, white, and granular, with four suction cups and rostellum, with two circles of head hooks on the rostellum, which are ovoid when the rostellum is protruding into the body and duck-pear shaped when the rostellum is protruding from the body. Inclusion of hydatid cysts is filled with aqueous cyst fluid, which is a derivative of host blood and contains a variety of components such as proteins, carbohydrates, metabolites of the inclusion worm, and host body fluids. Cystic echinococcosis lesion is surrounded by an intact parasitic cystic membrane (inner capsule) and a reactive layer of compressed host tissue (outer capsule). The cystic membrane produces cystic fluid that expands the lesion distensively in the periphery, and the subcapsules give the cysts a multi-compartmental character; cystic fluid thickening and wall/capsule content calcification occur when the cysts degenerate; various signs of cystic membrane detachment can occur when the inner capsule is detached from the outer capsule [9].

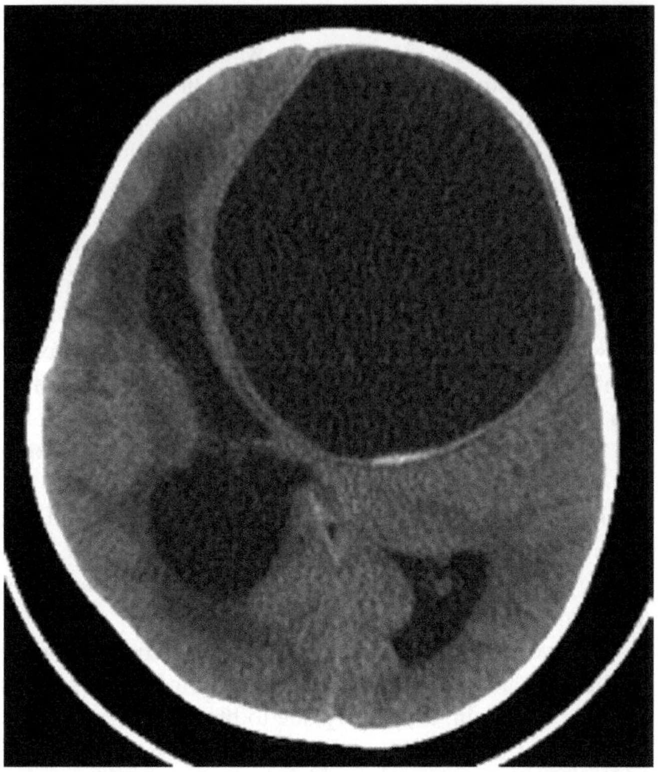

Fig. 8.3 Left frontal lobe cerebral cystic echinococcosis: simple cystic type. CT scan shows a watery hypodensity inside the lesion, with a uniform isodense envelope and a small amount of calcification

8.2.1.3 Imaging

1. **X-rays**: X-rays are usually unremarkable, even when cystic echinococcosis is combined with calcification. When cystic echinococcosis involves the skull, single or multiple cystic swelling bone destruction may occur, easily penetrating the bone plate to form intracranial and extracranial soft tissue masses. Those confined to the skull base lack the characteristics of single or multiple sacs and show osteosclerosis, usually without periosteal reaction. Cystic echinococcosis in the brain parenchyma can produce signs of increased intracranial pressure when they are large and can manifest as bone resorption in the posterior clinoid process, enlargement of the sellar, and displacement of calcium spots in pineal gland. Pediatric patients may present with skull finger indentation, thin skull, and even skull defects.
2. **Angiography**: Cystic echinococcosis is not specifically demonstrated on cerebral angiography. When the hydatid cyst of cystic echinococcosis is large, the surrounding veins may be displaced in an arc. Generally, the cysts show a nonvascular area, and the blood vessels around the cysts are arcuately compressed and displaced, surrounding the nonvascular area in a "hand holding the ball" sign, and the cerebral blood vessels are drawn and thinned, with the same diameter, resembling a "spider foot."
3. CT findings
   (a) Simple cystic cerebral cystic echinococcosis: Solitary is common; occasionally multiple lesions may occur. CT scan shows a round or ovoid cystic mass with smooth and sharp edges, generally no edema around the lesion, homogenous internal density, close to the cerebrospinal fluid density, and a homogenous isodense envelope around the periphery. When the cyst is large, it may compress adjacent brain tissue, ventricles, and midline structures causing a dominant effect. In the case of hydatid cyst degeneration, the cyst wall may be combined with calcification, which is a characteristic manifestation of hydatid cysts. The cyst is usually not abnormally enhanced on enhanced scans, but the cyst wall may be mildly enhanced when the hydatid cyst is coinfected [10] (Fig. 8.3).
   (b) Multicystic cerebral cystic echinococcosis: The presence of a variable number of daughter cysts within the hydatid cyst is a characteristic sign of a "cyst within a cyst (daughter cyst)" or separation within the cyst, with the density of the daughter cysts being slightly lower than that of the parent cyst (Fig. 8.4).
   (c) Calcified cystic echinococcosis (degeneration type): Curved, shelled, or ring-shaped hyperdense calcification can be seen in the walls of the hydatid cyst, and density of the cyst contents increased. Calcification of the detached endocapsular membrane, cysts, and ceph-

alomere can occur, to the extent that the whole hydatid is calcified, but the calcification is mostly uneven.

(d) Multiple cystic echinococcosis (disseminated type): It can be hematogenous or medically disseminated, most often with a history of hydatid removal surgery or combined with other sites of hydatid cysts. Features include multiple foci, mostly unilocular, which may be distributed in clusters. This type can be seen anywhere in the brain parenchyma (including the ventricular system).

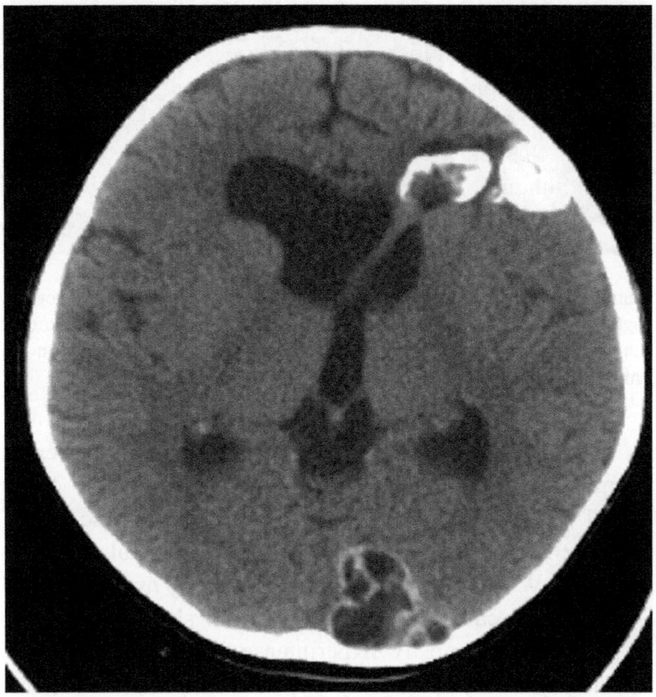

Fig. 8.4 Left frontal lobe cerebral cystic echinococcosis: multicystic cystic type. CT scan shows hypodense cystic fluid within the lesion, with multiple separations and multiple small daughter cysts nested within the parent cyst

4. MRI: The simple cyst type presents as a single or multiple cystic occupying foci, with approximately 85% of cysts >4.5 cm in diameter. The internal cystic fluid shows hypointense on T_1WI and hyperintense on T_2WI, surrounded by a continuous and uniformly thick cystic wall, which is characterized by hypointense on T_2WI. The vesicular fluid is suppressed to hypointense as is cerebrospinal fluid at FLAIR sequence. The cyst wall is generally not enhanced on enhanced scans and may be mildly enhanced in the presence of coinfection (Fig. 8.5).

   The multicystic type is characterized by multiple daughter cysts of different sizes within the parent cyst, and the daughter cysts are mostly arranged along the periphery of the parent cyst, showing the "rose petal sign" or "wheel sign," and both the parent cyst and the daughter cyst fluid present hypointense on T_1WI, but the signal of the daughter cyst fluid is lower than that of the parent cyst, and the wall of the daughter cyst is usually poorly visualized, and both the parent cyst and the daughter cyst fluid present hyperintense on T_2WI, and the wall of the parent cyst and the daughter cyst both present slightly hypointense. Both cysts showed no obvious enhancement on the enhanced scans and may be ring like enhanced in the presence of coinfection (Fig. 8.6). When the combined internal cysts rupture, the internal cysts float in the cyst fluid, forming the "floating band sign" (Fig. 8.7).

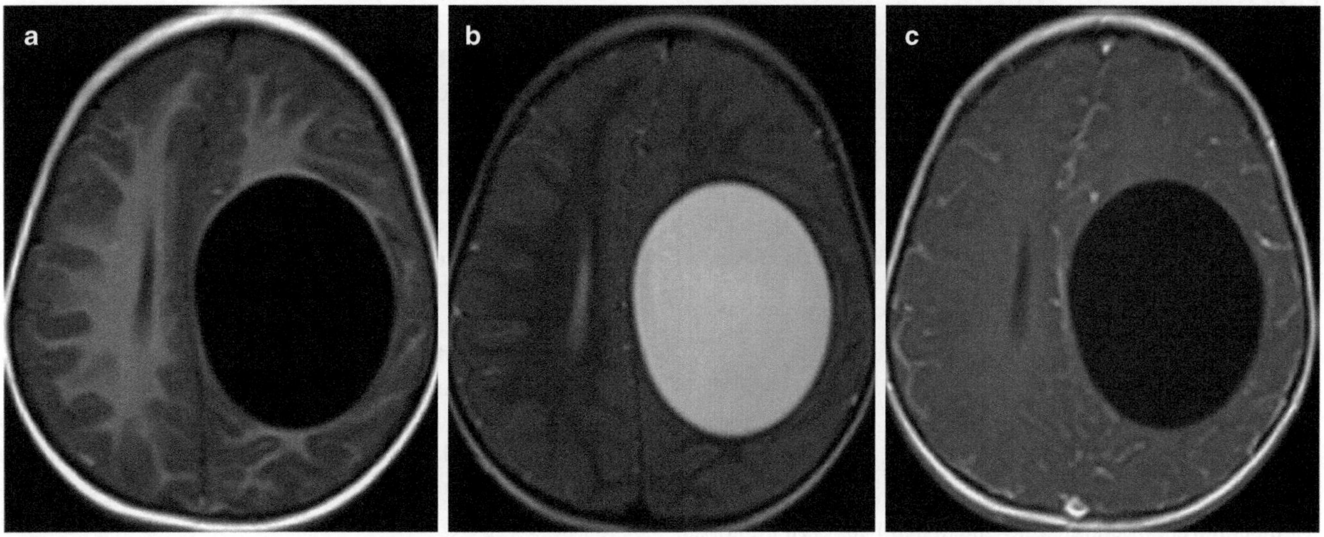

Fig. 8.5 Cerebral cystic echinococcosis (simple cystic type) in the left frontal parietal junctional area. (**a**) T_1WI shows a hypointense cystic fluid and a uniformly thick and thin isointense cystic wall around the lesion; (**b**) T_2WI shows a hyperintense cystic fluid and a slightly hypointense cystic wall around the lesion, with enhanced scans; (**c**) neither the cystic contents nor the cystic wall is enhanced

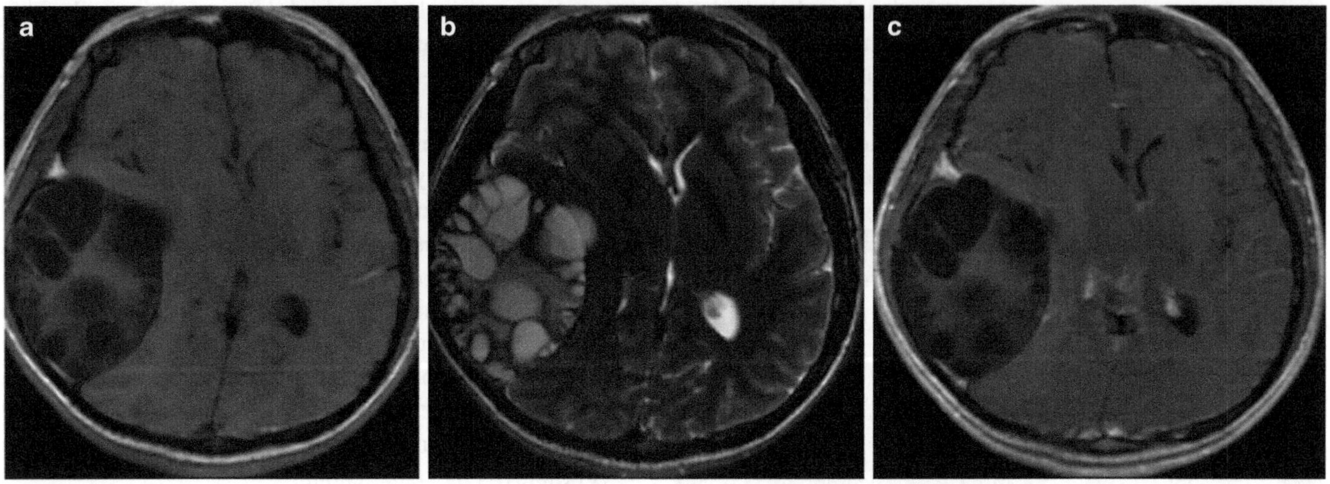

Fig. 8.6 Right temporal cerebral cystic echinococcosis. (**a**) T_1WI shows a hypo- and isointense mixed signal, and multiple daughter cysts of different sizes can be seen within the parent cyst, and the signal of the daughter cyst is lower than that of the parent cyst; (**b**) T_2WI shows a mixed signal with mainly hyperintense inside the lesion, and the signal of the daughter cyst is higher than that of the parent cyst, and part of the wall of the daughter cyst manifests as hypointense; (**c**) no significant enhancement is seen on the enhanced scan

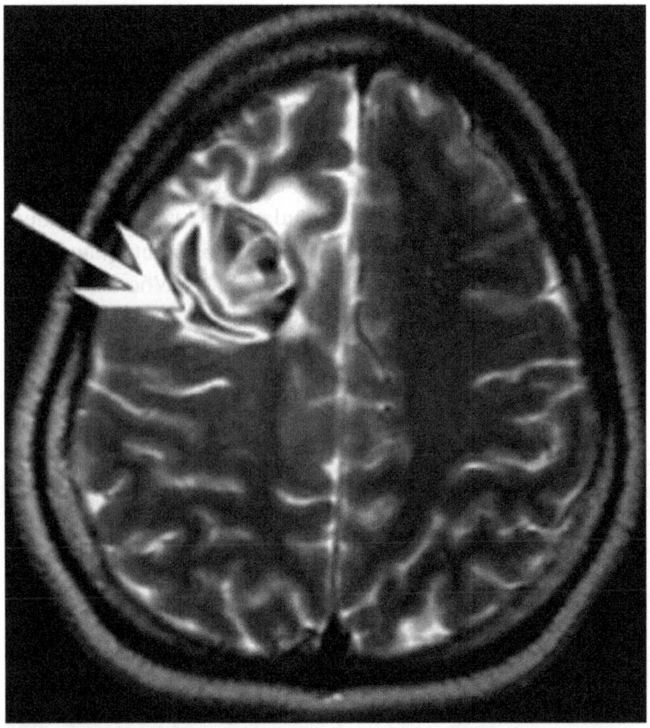

Fig. 8.7 Right frontal cerebral cystic echinococcosis (ruptured internal cyst type). T_2WI sequence shows rupture of the inner cyst of hydatid cyst, with the "floating band sign" visible inside

8.2.1.4 Diagnostic Key Points

1. History of residence in endemic areas or contact with infectious agents and susceptible animals; high incidence in children, preferably in the frontal or parietal lobes, with inapparent occupying effects.
2. Single or multiple cystic lesions with uniform wall thickness and "floating band sign" when the inner capsule ruptures; "rose petal sign" and "wheel sign" can be seen in multiple cysts.
3. CT scan shows uniform hypodensity in the cystic cavity, and the cystic wall may be combined with calcification; MR T_1WI sequence shows predominantly hypointense in the cystic cavity, and the cystic wall shows isointense; T_2WI shows mostly hyperintense in the cystic cavity. The cyst wall is slightly hypointense; enhanced scans are mostly without abnormal enhancement, and abnormal enhancement of the cyst wall is seen in cases of coinfection.
4. Immunologic tests can assist in the diagnosis of this disease, and the hydatid-specific antibody test has a high diagnostic value for this disease.

8.2.1.5 Differential Diagnosis

Cerebral echinococcosis is a rare type of echinococcosis, but its imaging manifestations are characteristic, and the identification is not difficult when combined with the history of residence in endemic areas, the source of infection, or the contact history of susceptible animals. This disease needs to be differentiated from arachnoid cysts, epidermoid cysts, and brain abscesses.

1. **Arachnoid cysts**: It is the most common intracranial cystic lesion, while hydatid cyst is also an intracerebral cystic lesion, so the two need to be differentiated. Arachnoid cyst is usually located in the subarachnoid space, outside the brain parenchyma, and has an irregular shape. In contrast, hydatid is a more regular, round-like mass, mostly located within the brain parenchyma, and arachnoid lesion is rare. The hydatid cyst has a distinct wall due to the presence of an internal and external cyst, whereas

arachnoid cyst tends to show poorly due to a thin wall. It is not difficult to distinguish them when combined with the history of living in the area where the disease is endemic or the history of contact with infectious sources or susceptible animals.

2. **Epidermoid cyst**: It is also known as cholesteatoma, which is a more common intracranial cystic occupying lesion. They are mostly found in the cerebellopontine angle or within the subarachnoid cistern system and occur in less than 10% of the brain parenchyma, whereas hydatid cyst occurs mostly in the brain parenchyma. Epidermoid cyst is soft, burrows when it occurs, and generally grows along the cerebral sulcus and cerebral pool cast. In contrast, cerebral cystic echinococcosis usually occurs in the brain parenchyma, and the characteristic "rose petal sign" or "floating ribbon sign" is seen internally. Epidermoid cysts and hydatid cysts have similar CT findings and are predominantly hypodense, but CT values for epidermoid cysts are closer to fat density, whereas hydatid cysts are closer to water density. Epidermoid cysts are characteristically hyperintense on DWI, and hydatid cysts are hypointense on DWI. Epidermoid cysts show no enhancement on the enhanced scans. Generally, cerebral cystic echinococcosis show no enhancement, but in the presence of infection, mild enhancement can be seen in the cyst wall. The two present differently and are easily identified.
3. **Brain abscesses**: The onset of the disease is generally more rapid with a clear history of bacterial infection, whereas cystic echinococcosis generally has a slow onset with a history of residence in an endemic area or contact with infectious agents or susceptible animals. Although both brain abscesses and hydatid cysts have a distinct cyst wall, the cyst wall of hydatid cysts generally has no abnormal enhancement, whereas the cyst wall of brain abscesses may show distinct ring-like enhancement with a smooth inner wall. Brain abscesses are characterized by significant hyperintense on DWI images due to restricted diffusion of their contents, whereas cystic echinococcosis generally manifests as hypointense on DWI. Brain abscesses are distinguished by elevated amino acid and Lac peaks and elevated acetate and succinate peaks on ^{1}H-MRS, while cerebral cystic echinococcosis appears to be distinguished by decreased NAA, Cr, and Cho peaks; elevated Lac and Ala peaks; and elevated acetate, pyruvate, and succinate peaks.

8.2.1.6 Status and Progress of Research

1. **Diffusion-weighted imaging (DWI)**: Similar to most water-rich cystic lesions, the diffusive movement of water molecules in the cystic fluid within the cystic lumen of cerebral cystic echinococcosis is not restricted and therefore appears as a hypointense on the DWI sequence. DWI helps to presume the cystic versus solid component of the lesion and to differentiate it from cystic lesions with mixed components in the cystic cavity (e.g., abscesses).
2. **Hydrogen proton magnetic resonance spectroscopy imaging (^{1}H-MRS)**: ^{1}H-MRS can be an important complement to conventional MRI and DWI. ^{1}H-MRS of internal cyst fluid from cerebral cystic echinococcosis lesions showed decreased NAA, Cr, and Cho peaks and increased Lac and Ala peaks, as well as increased acetate, pyruvate, and succinate peaks. ^{1}H-MRS can be used to differentiate cerebral cystic echinococcosis from brain abscesses. Bacterial brain abscesses, which result from hypoxia of the lesion, accumulation of lactic acid in the pus cavity, and necrosis of the cell membrane, lead the release of lipids and proteins from the cytosol. The protein is in turn broken down into a variety of amino acids by a large number of protein hydrolases, so lactic acid and amino acids are elevated. The occurrence of Lac and AA peaks (amino acid peaks) within untreated bacterial brain abscesses was close to 100%. The AA peak has not been detected on examination of necrotic or cystic lesions other than bacterial abscesses (including in vivo lesions of cerebral cystic echinococcosis and fungal abscesses), and therefore its sensitivity and specificity for the diagnosis of bacterial brain abscesses is extremely high, and the AA peak is considered a key marker for bacterial brain abscesses and can be used to differentiate them from cerebral cystic echinococcosis.
3. **Magnetic resonance hydrography (MRH) technique**: It is one of the rapidly developing magnetic resonance imaging techniques in recent years. This technique can not only clearly display the tissue structure containing fluid and sensitively show the subtle structures such as cystic hydatid microcysts but also outline the lesion and show the relationship between the hydatid microcysts and the adjacent involved structures such as the ventricles, which has special advantages for the diagnosis of hydatid disease. On the MRH sequence, simple cerebral cystic echinococcosis exhibits a round-like hyperintense with well-defined margins; multicystic cerebral cystic echinococcosis exhibits a grape bunch-like or rose-petal-like hyperintense.

8.2.2 Cerebral Alveolar Echinococcosis

8.2.2.1 Overview

Cerebral alveolar echinococcosis (CAE) is a parasitic infection of the brain caused by the larvae of alveolar *Echinococcus*. Lesions are often multiple. Almost 100% of cerebral alveolar echinococcosis originates from hematogenous metastases of hepatic alveolar echinococcosis, and therefore the lesions are located in the corticomedullary junction area, with abundant blood supply.

The end hosts of alveolar *Echinococcus* are mainly foxes, followed by dogs, and the intermediate hosts are rodents represented by rats, and the dogs are considered to be the main source of infection for alveolar *Echinococcus*. The pathway of human infection with alveolar *Echinococcus* is similar to that of *Echinococcus granulosus*, which is mainly parasitized in the liver, and in the middle and advanced stages, the lesions invade the blood vessels and metastasize systemically, with a few entering the cerebral through the internal carotid artery, mostly in the cortical or subcortical areas [11]. The eggs of the tapeworm are excreted along with the feces of the dog and contaminate the surrounding environment. After ingestion of food contaminated with eggs, the eggs enter the duodenum of the host, and the larvae pass through the intestinal wall, enter the liver via the portal vein, and reach the whole body via the heart and lungs, so the distribution of disease in human organs is related to the sequence of larval passage.

The clinical presentation of cerebral alveolar echinococcosis is similar to that of cerebral cystic echinococcosis.

8.2.2.2 Pathological Manifestations

1. **Macroscopic observation**: The lesions are lumpy or nodular, yellowish or off-white in color, resembling substantial tumors in section, yellowish brown or off-white in color, fine in texture, and sponge-like in shape, and multiple vesicles of varying sizes are visible. The margins of the lesions are irregular, without envelope, and small nodules growing prominently outward are visible.
2. **Light microscopic observation**: Alveolar *Echinococcus* vesicles of different sizes scattered in the brain tissue are its characteristic manifestation [12]. Because humans are not suitable intermediate hosts for alveolar echinococcosis, protoscolex is rarely seen in the vesicles, and generally only the stratum corneum, which is thin, is visible, and occasionally the unicellular germ layer can be seen. The vesicles are mostly round, dendritic, or fissured in shape, surrounded by eosinophilic infiltration, with typical granulation tissue formation and hyperplasia of fibrous tissue. The vesicles are scattered or clustered within fibrous tissue, and coagulative necrosis may also occur in the brain tissue between the vesicles. Alveolar echinococcosis grows in a budding fashion (internal and external budding), mostly as an exogenous budding growth. The wall of the parent cyst of alveolar echinococcosis shows multiple small warty protrusions, which gradually grow and extend outward, while forming multiple small vesicles, which gradually increase in size to form daughter and grandchild cysts and further proliferate outward and infiltrate into adjacent tissues. The peripheral nerve tissue is correspondingly damaged and extruded, and the lesion is indistinctly demarcated from adjacent tissues. Small vesicles continue to proliferate peripherally, and clusters or nests of vesicles and scattered tiny vesicles extend outward to form infiltrative zone. Numerous small vesicles of 1–10 mm in diameter form solid proliferative nodules or masses surrounded by lymphocyte-dominated inflammatory cell infiltrates, with fibroblasts, epithelioid cells, and a few multinucleated giant cells disturbed in the periphery of inflammatory cell infiltration, forming tuberculosis-like granulomas. This "tumor-like" growth pattern is unique to alveolar echinococcosis; hence, it is also called "insect carcinoma" [13].

8.2.2.3 Imaging

1. **CT**: The lesion appears as a soft tissue density mass or nodule with punctate or granular calcifications visible inside, which is the result of degeneration of the vesicle wall and calcium salt deposition within the small vesicles and is a characteristic manifestation of cerebral alveolar echinococcosis. Enhanced scans show distinct irregular ring enhancement mostly, and the lesions are often surrounded by more obvious edema and occupying effects. CT scan cannot clearly identify the characteristic small vesicles of alveolar echinococcosis (Fig. 8.8).

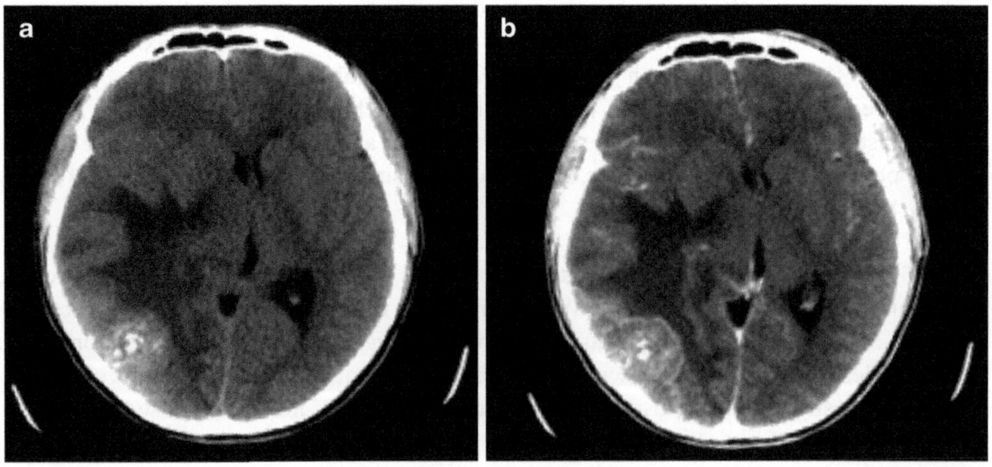

Fig. 8.8 Right parietal occipital junction area cerebral alveolar echinococcosis. A round-like lesion in the junctional area of the right parieto-occipital lobe. (**a**) CT scan shows slightly hyperdense with central speckled calcification; (**b**) CT enhancement image shows ring-like enhancement

2. **MRI**: Cerebral alveolar echinococcosis is found in cortical or subcortical areas with abundant blood supply and shows infiltrative growth in the brain parenchyma, often as a round-like or irregular-shaped mass, mostly with marked occupying effects and perifocal edema. T_1WI shows iso- or slightly hyperintense, and T_2WI shows mixed signal with predominant hypointensity, interspersed with multiple hyperintense vesicles of varying sizes. The unique signal characteristics on T_2WI are the characteristic manifestation of alveolar echinococcosis [14]. Enhanced scans show mostly irregular circular enhancement of cerebral alveolar echinococcosis (Fig. 8.9).
3. ^{18}**F-FDG PET**: In the proliferative infiltrative zone of cerebral alveolar echinococcosis lesions, ^{18}F-FDG is perfused into the microvasculature through blood circulation and participates in cellular metabolism, and the cytokines secreted by the alveolar echinococcosis themselves can promote the growth of microvasculature in the surrounding granulation tissue. The denser the vessels, the higher the uptake of ^{18}F-FDG. In addition, the more inflammatory cells there are, the higher the uptake of ^{18}F-FDG, while there is no clear uptake of ^{18}F-FDG in the central area of calcification and necrosis due to the absence of neovascularization and inflammatory cells. Therefore, ^{18}F-FDG PET in cerebral alveolar echinococcosis showed a circular heterogeneous distribution of radioactive concentrations (Fig. 8.10).

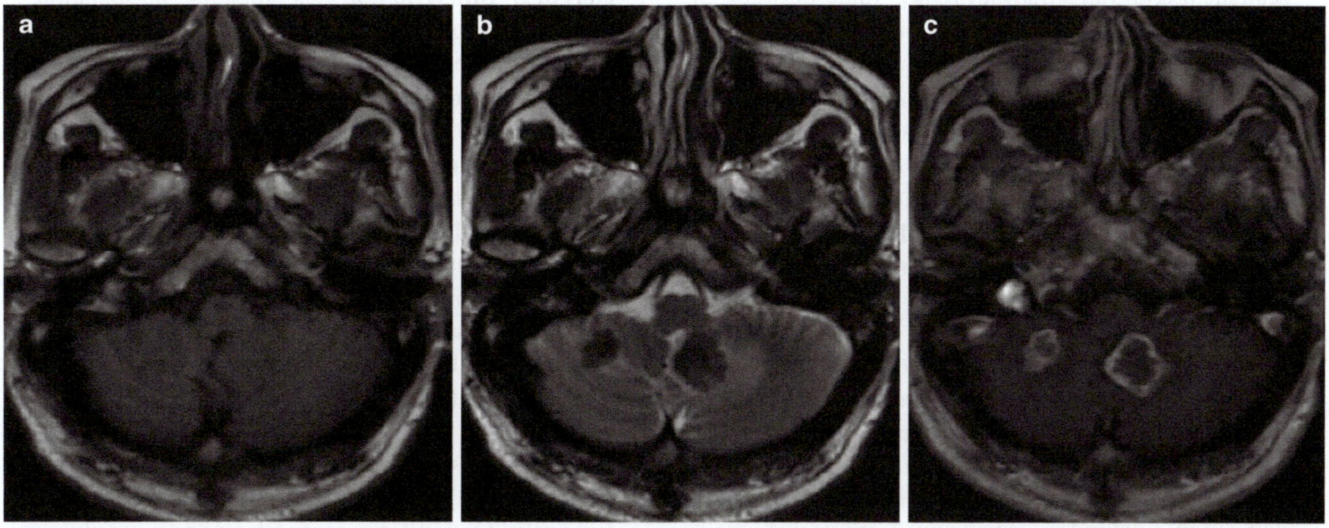

Fig. 8.9 Bilateral cerebellar hemispheres with multiple alveolar echinococcosis. Multiple round-like lesions in the bilateral cerebellar hemispheres. (**a**) T_1WI shows isointense; (**b**) T_2WI shows hypointense, with multiple slightly hyperintense vesicles of different sizes in the center; (**c**) enhanced scan shows ring-like enhancement

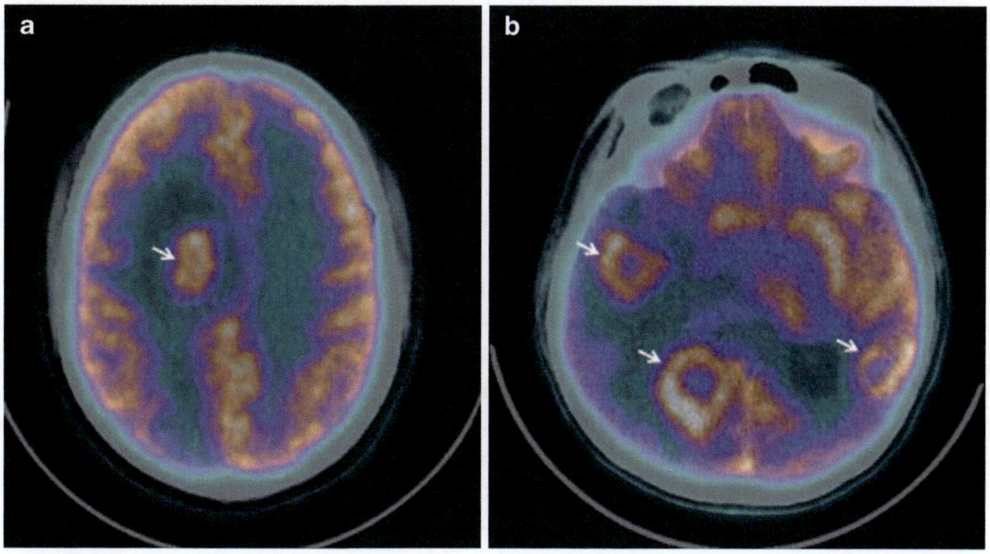

Fig. 8.10 Multiple intracerebral parenchymal alveolar echinococcosis. (**a**) ^{18}F-FDG PET shows well-defined mass-like foci of radiolucent distribution visible in the right parietal lobe; (**b**) ^{18}F-FDG PET shows ring-shaped heterogeneous foci of radiolucent distribution visible in the right temporal lobe and bilateral occipital lobes

8.2.2.4 Diagnostic Key Points

1. History of residence in endemic areas or contact with infectious sources or susceptible animals.
2. Single or multiple foci in the brain parenchyma with infiltrative growth, indistinctly demarcated from surrounding tissues, mostly with occupying effect, preferably in the cortical or subcortical areas.
3. CT scan mostly shows isodensity solid masses, which may be combined with calcification; MR scan T_2WI shows predominantly hypointense with hyperintense vesicles of variable size, which is its characteristic presentation and is better shown on MR water imaging; enhanced scan shows irregular ring enhancement.
4. Immunologic tests can assist in the diagnosis of this disease, and the echinococcosis-specific antibody test has a high diagnostic value for this disease.

8.2.2.5 Differential Diagnosis

Cerebral alveolar echinococcosis is a rare type of echinococcosis, but its imaging manifestations are characteristic, and the identification is not difficult when combined with the history of residence in endemic areas, the source of infection, or the contact history of susceptible animals. This disease needs to be differentiated from brain metastases, brain tuberculoma, and melanoma.

1. **Brain metastases**: They are more common intracerebral tumors, and their sites of predilection are similar to those of cerebral alveolar echinococcosis, both of which are located in the cutaneous medullary junction area. The metastases are also prone to combined hemorrhage and can also show hypointense on T_2WI, which can be easily confused with cerebral alveolar echinococcosis. However, metastases often have a history of extracerebral malignancy, and liquefied necrosis often occurs in the center of the tumor, with marked peripheral edema that is disproportionate to the size of the tumor, usually accompanied by extensive edema when the tumor is very small. Enhanced scans may show abnormal enhancement such as nodular, annular, and "flower lace," and the inner wall may be accompanied by irregular attached nodules. ^{1}H-MRS shows an elevated Cho peak, a significantly lower creatinine peak, and a reduced or absent NAA peak. In PWI sequence, the solid portion of the tumor shows significant hyperperfusion and elevated rCBV values. MRH shows no microvesicles. In contrast, cerebral alveolar echinococcosis often has a clear history of hepatic alveolar echinococcosis and presents as a single or multiple foci in the brain parenchyma with infiltrative growth, poorly demarcated from the surrounding tissue, and with some occupying effect. CT scan shows an isodense solid mass, which may be combined with hyperdense calcification; MR T_2WI scan presents predominantly hypointense with multiple slightly hyperintense vesicles of varying sizes, which is a characteristic manifestation different from metastases, and metastases are prone to combined hemorrhage which is rare in alveolar cerebral alveolar echinococcosis. ^{1}H-MRS reveals varying degrees of decrease in Cho, NAA, and creatinine peaks and obvious Lip peaks with or without Lac peaks. In PWI sequence, the solid internal part of the lesion is hypoperfused, and the peripheral inflammatory reaction zone is relatively hyperperfused. Characteristic small vesicular manifestations are seen in the form of a "honeycomb sign" in MRH. The manifestations of two diseases are different and can be identified.
2. **Cerebral tuberculoma**: The imaging presentation of cerebral tuberculoma is similar to that of cerebral alveolar echinococcosis in that they both appear as multiple nodules of varying sizes with internal calcification and hypointense on T_2WI, with ring-like enhancement on enhanced scans. However, tuberculoma of the brain is usually caused by hematogenous dissemination of tuberculosis from the lungs or other parts of the body and is often accompanied by signs of tuberculous meningitis. In contrast, cerebral alveolar echinococcosis is usually secondary to hepatic alveolar echinococcosis, and the characteristic small vesicle shadow is seen on T_2WI, which is different from that of tuberculoma. In addition to the variously reduced Cho, NAA, and creatinine peaks seen on the ^{1}H-MRS sequence, which is similarity to alveolar echinococcosis, tuberculomas may also show significant Lip peaks. On DWI, the brain tuberculoma mostly manifests as hypointense and may display hyperintense when combined with abscess formation. However, the solid portion of the cerebral alveolar echinococcosis manifests as hypointense, and the surrounding inflammatory reaction zone displays hyperintense on DWI. In MRH, tuberculoma of the brain shows no signs of the characteristic vesicles of cerebral alveolar echinococcosis. These two diseases are easily identified.
3. **Melanoma**: Both of them show hypointense on T_2WI, but the T_2WI of cerebral alveolar echinococcosis can show multiple small vesicle-like "honeycomb-like" changes, and melanoma is less likely to have calcification, and it is not difficult to make a diagnosis when combined with the immunologic test and clinical history of echinococcosis.

8.2.2.6 Status and Progress of Research

1. **DWI**: It can provide important information for the diagnosis and differential diagnosis of cerebral alveolar echinococcosis. Cerebral alveolar echinococcosis lesion with

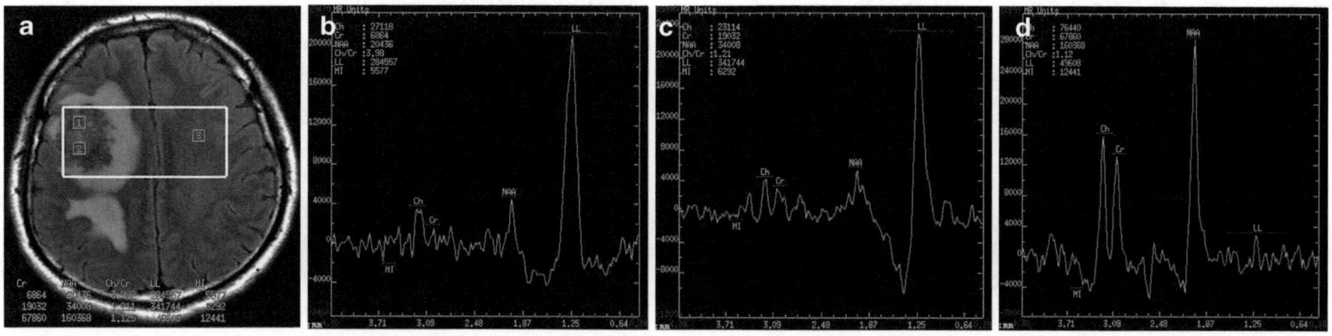

Fig. 8.11 Right temporal cerebral alveolar echinococcosis. (**a**) ^{1}H-MRS localization phase; (**b**) single-peaked proliferative lesion (region 1 in (**a**)). The NAA peak, Cho peak, and creatinine peak are reduced, and a high sharp Lip peak is visible; (**c**) bimodal proliferative lesions (region 2 in (**a**)). The NAA and Cho peaks are reduced, and a moderately upright Lip peak with an inverted Lac peak can be seen; (**d**) the normal spectrum in the control region (region 3 in (**a**))

numerous dense vesicles and clusters of vesicles in the main body of the lesion, resulting in restricted diffusive movement of water molecules, manifests as slightly hyperintense on DWI images [15]. On ADC images, the ADC values are increased, and the eADC values are decreased in the focal area of cerebral alveolar echinococcosis compared to normal brain tissue. In addition, relative ADC (rADC) values can be applied to differentiate cerebral schistosomiasis from high-grade gliomas and brain metastases. rADC values are significantly lower in cerebral schistosomiasis than in brain metastases, and rADC values are significantly higher in proximal perifocal edema in cerebral schistosomiasis than in high-grade gliomas.

2. **Hydrogen proton spectroscopy imaging (^{1}H-MRS)**: It can be an important complementary imaging method to conventional MRI and DWI. The characteristic features of the ^{1}H-MRS of cerebral alveolar echinococcosis are Cho and NAA peaks with varying degrees of reduction and a distinct Lip peak with or without Lac peak, which is a representative spectral feature of proliferative lesions (Fig. 8.11) and a point of differentiation between cerebral alveolar echinococcosis, metastases, and gliomas [16–18].
3. **Magnetic resonance perfusion imaging (PWI)**: It reflects the blood supply characteristics of CAE, with hypoperfusion within the lesion and relative hyperperfusion in the peripheral inflammatory zone. The findings of a MRI perfusion study of cerebral alveolar echinococcosis showed reduced rCBV within the lesion and increased perfusion in the inflammatory zone around the lesion. In another study, the rCBV values of different regions of the cerebral alveolar echinococcosis were found to be marginal > control > edema > parenchymal, indicating that the marginal region had the highest perfusion and the most abundant blood supply, while the parenchymal region had the lowest perfusion and lacked in blood supply. Some of the studies showed that rCBV, rCBF, and MTT values in the parenchymal area of cerebral alveolar echinococcosis were lower than those in the control area. The main reason may be that there are numerous dense vesicles and clusters of vesicles inside the lesion, which require high energy and relatively lack in blood supply, thus causing necrosis and liquefaction, resulting in hypoperfusion in the lesion parenchyma area, while the hyperperfusion in the marginal zone may be due to vascular proliferation around the lesion and the presence of a granulation tissue reaction zone at the edge of the parenchyma of the lesion.

   The parenchymal areas of other tumors, represented by metastases, tend to be hyperperfused, while the marginal areas become hypoperfused.
4. **Magnetic resonance hydrography (MRH)**: It has particular advantages for the diagnosis of echinococcosis, as it not only clearly shows fluid-containing tissue structures but also outlines the lesion. Compared with conventional MRI, MRH can show the small vesicles of cerebral alveolar echinococcosis and its relationship with adjacent structures such as the ventricles and can improve the detection rate of cerebral alveolar echinococcosis when combined with conventional MRI. Compared with conventional MRI, MRH is not only able to show the extent of cerebral alveolar echinococcosis but also has important value for the diagnosis and differential diagnosis of cerebral alveolar echinococcosis. The many small vesicles and clusters of vesicles are the basic features of cerebral alveolar echinococcosis and the main point of differentiation from tuberculomas, metastases, and other diseases with hypointensity on T_2WI.

8.3 Cerebral Schistosomiasis

Hanqiu Liu, Weiwei Wang, and Dan Zhang

8.3.1 Overview

Blood flukes are also known as schistosoma, and the three species of schistosomes that cause disease in humans are *Schistosoma egypti*, *Schistosoma mansoni*, and *Schistosoma japonicum*. *Schistosoma japonicum* is endemic in China and is found in the Yangtze River basin and in rural areas of 13 southern provinces and cities [19]. The eggs of schistosomes in feces contaminate the water source and hatch into cercaria in the intermediate host, the *Oncomelania*. After contact with infected water, the larvae invade the human body through the skin or mucous membrane and develop into adult worms in the portal vein system, with symptoms appearing within a few months, or may be delayed for 1–2 years. *Schistosoma japonicum* often involves the portal system but causes little damage outside the portal system, which is called ectopic schistosomiasis, of which ectopic damage is common in the brain, accounting for 2–4% of schistosomiasis, called cerebral schistosomiasis (CSM) [20]. Present studies suggest the following possible routes of schistosome entry into the CNS [21]: (1) adult worms parasitizing the portal venous system oviposit to form emboli that are transmitted via the pulmonary vasculature from the left ventricle into the brain or through the venous system with anastomosing branches of the Batson's vertebral veins against the flow; (2) adults located in the cerebral veins (mainly females) are deposited mainly by direct oviposition.

Laboratory tests: In acute cerebral schistosomiasis, peripheral blood eosinophil levels are increased, serum globulins are elevated, and eggs can be found on fecal examination (often repeated several times). Blood and cerebrospinal fluid specimens from patients with schistosomal immunoassay, i.e., indirect hemagglutination assay (IHA) and enzyme-linked immunosorbent assay (ELISA), are positive, and the detection of schistosome eggs or trichuriasis in the stool and cerebrospinal fluid is the gold standard for laboratory diagnosis.

8.3.2 Pathological Manifestations

Schistosoma eggs are deposited in brain tissue via the circulation, commonly in the brain; mostly in the parietal, occipital, and frontal lobes; and less frequently in the cerebellum, brainstem, soft cerebrum, and choroid plexus [22]. The reactions elicited can be classified as both atopic and nonspecific. Atopic lesions refer to characteristic schistosomal granulomas, i.e., including calcification of schistosome egg nodules or egg remnants surrounded by a large eosinophilic, lymphocytic infiltrate and associated fibrous tissue hyperplastic granulomas. The eggs cause nonspecific changes as inflammatory edema and focal softening of perifocal brain tissue. One to several mature eggs are visible in the center of the nodule. The nonspecific reactions are glial cell reaction, brain softening, and brain edema. Inflammatory changes in the blood vessels are more prominent in cerebral schistosomiasis, and the lesions often involve small- and medium-sized vessels, causing total arteritis, phlebitis, and capillary hyperplasia, which can lead to secondary cerebral infarction.

8.3.3 Imaging

1. CT: The scan shows hypodense lesions with multiple small nodules (1–3 mm) and large nodules (5–45 mm) that may fuse into clusters, and the morphology and size of the lesions are characteristic; perifocal edema is obvious, and most of the lesions are surrounded by obvious hypodense edema, which is "Buddha's hand" or "finger sleeve" edema (Fig. 8.12a). The majority of cases show punctiform (1–3 mm) enhancement, "clusters" of large nodules (5–45 mm), or mass-like enhancement on enhanced scans (Fig. 8.12b). Dynamic enhanced scans demonstrate gradual enhancement with time, which is a "slow-in, slow-out" phenomenon.
2. MRI: The scan shows isointense or slightly hypointense in T_1WI and hyperintense or slightly hyperintense in T_2WI. Most of the lesions are located in the cortical or subcortical white matter areas, predominantly supratentorial, but can also occur in the subcortex, surrounded by large "finger-like" edema extending into the cortex. The edema also varies depending on the course of the disease and the effectiveness of clinical treatment. Enhanced scans may show various forms of enhancement, including punctate, nodular, patchy, and fusion of multiple small nodular lesions in "clusters" or masses, with some cases showing multiple clusters of clustered punctate nodules with central linear enhancement, which has been referred to as the characteristic "dendritic sign" [23] (Fig. 8.13).

8.3.4 Diagnostic Key Points

1. The patient is from an area where schistosomiasis is endemic or has a history of exposure to infected water.
2. CT- and MRI-enhanced scans show typical "dotted enhancement, clustered aggregation sign" or "dendritic sign" enhancement features.
3. Combined with a positive serum immunologic test result and a positive cerebrospinal fluid schistosome antibody test (ELISA method), the diagnosis is essentially clear.

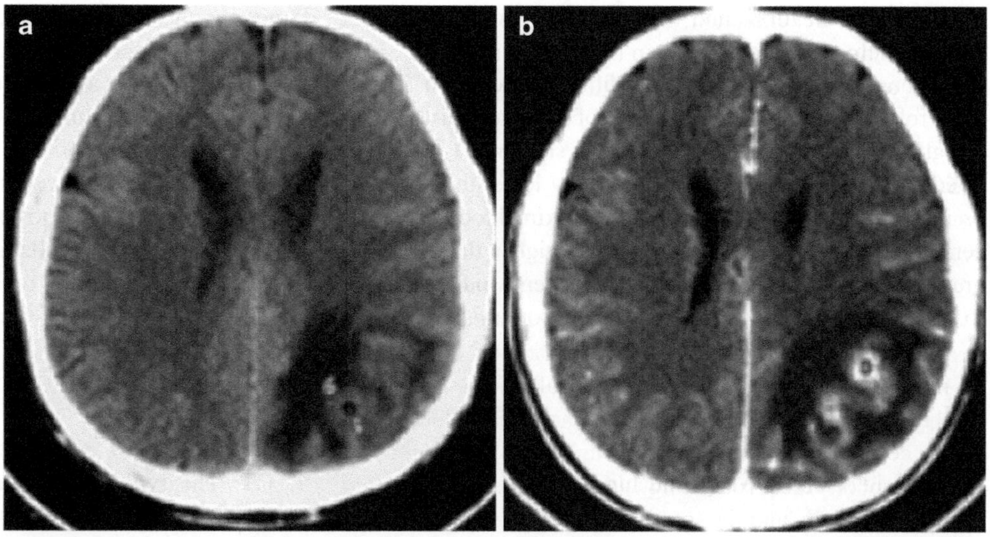

Fig. 8.12 Schistosomal granuloma of the left parietal brain. (**a**) CT scan shows a lesion with isodense cerebral gray matter and marked “finger-like” edema around the lesion; (**b**) enhanced scan shows several clustered clusters of punctate enhancing nodules

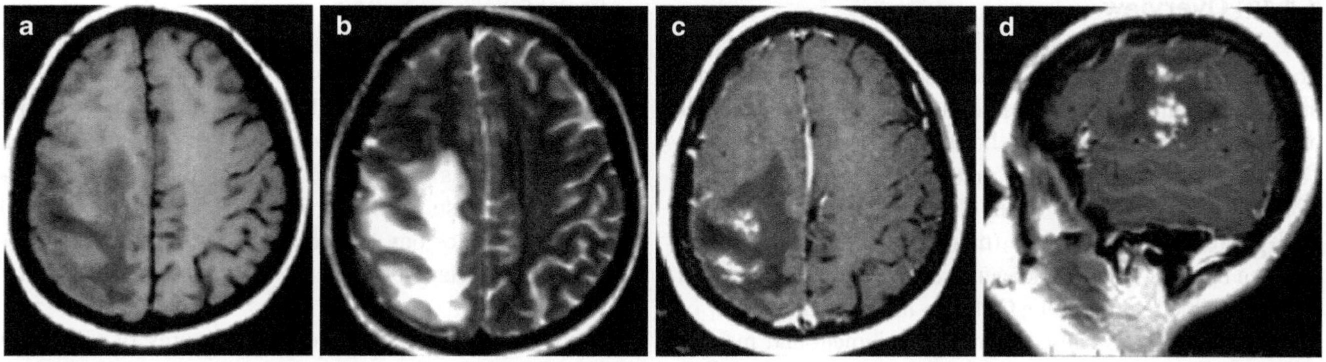

Fig. 8.13 Multiple cerebral schistosomal granulomas in the right parietal lobe. Multiple patchy lesions in the right parietal lobe. (**a**) T_1WI shows that the lesion is isointense as the gray matter of the brain; (**b**) T_2WI shows that the lesion is surrounded by a distinct “finger sleeve”; (**c, d**) T_1WI-enhanced scan shows multiple clustered clusters of nodular enhancement nodules in the right frontal lobe with central linear enhancement, i.e., “dendritic sign” (axial, sagittal)

The gold standard of laboratory tests is the detection of schistosome eggs or trichuriasis in the stool and cerebrospinal fluid.

8.3.5 Differential Diagnosis

1. Brain cysticercosis also often occurs in the cortex and subcortex, but brain cysticercosis commonly involves small cysts with eccentric, dense cephalic nodules visible within the cysts, the “target sign.”
2. Cerebral tuberculoma often has a history of primary tuberculosis, and the lesion can be located anywhere in the brain, with isointense or hypointense in the center of the lesion on T_2WI scan, with circumferential enhancement after enhancement, and the “target sign” can be seen.
3. Malignant glioma in the brain is mostly located in the deep white matter area, with wreath-like enhancement after enhancement and hyperintense on DWI in the area of enhancement, which highly supports the diagnosis of glioma if the lesion invades the corpus callosum.
4. Brain metastases: Patients often have a history of a primary malignancy; they are usually multiple foci in the brain, mostly located in the subcortical region, with significant perifocal edema and no signs of clustered aggregation of lesions.
5. Cerebral infarction: Patients are generally older and have a history of sudden-onset disease, and recent infarct foci can be seen on DWI, whereas patients with schistosome cerebral infarction are generally younger and have a history of schistosome infection.

8.3.6 Status and Progress of Research

The diagnosis of cerebral schistosomiasis relies on MRI and laboratory tests, especially MRI-enhanced scans. X-rays can show indirect signs such as calcification of cerebral schistosomiasis but are of limited value for the diagnosis of specific intracranial lesions. MRI has high soft tissue resolution, and its multi-sequence, multimodal examination can provide a wealth of information for the localization, characterization, and even quantitative diagnosis of cerebral schistosomiasis.

Among them, the DWI apparent diffusion coefficient (ADC) has a role in the differential diagnosis of cerebral schistosomiasis, gliomas, and metastases. It has been shown that [24] ADC in cerebral schistosomiasis is significantly lower than ADC in brain metastases, and ADC in areas of proximal focal edema in cerebral schistosomiasis is significantly higher than in high-grade gliomas. ADC and proximal focal edema may contribute to an accurate diagnosis of cerebral schistosomiasis.

8.4 Cerebral Malaria

Hanqiu Liu, Weiwei Wang, and Jun Lu

8.4.1 Overview

Malaria is a common tropical and subtropical insect-borne disease that causes about 100 million deaths per year [25], half of which occur in patients with cerebral malaria (CM). The CM is an aggressive form of malaria that occurs mostly in falciparum malaria, mainly in African children and Asian adults, with the vast majority (more than 90%) occurring in children aged 5 years or younger in sub-Saharan Africa, who are susceptible to developing CM after infection due to low or no immunity. CM is caused by malaria pigment and malaria parasites infecting the red blood cells in the microvasculature of the cerebral cortex. The infected red blood cells increase in size and adhesion, forming emboli, causing microcirculatory disorders and disseminated intravascular coagulation (DIC), resulting in brain tissue hypoxia, congestion, edema, inflammation, and focal necrosis. The pathogenesis of CM involves several processes, including microvascular obstruction due to *Plasmodium falciparum*-parasitized red blood cells, excessive pro-inflammatory cytokine production, microvascular thrombosis, loss of endothelial barrier function, and endothelial cell dysregulation. The main clinical manifestations are sudden chills, high fever, headache, impaired consciousness, and convulsions, with some patients having atypical symptoms or even no fever [26, 27]. Thick and thin blood film smears are used clinically to detect *Plasmodium vivax* as the gold standard for malaria diagnosis. Immunologic tests are commonly used for screening of transfusion recipients, epidemiological studies of malaria, and clinical adjuncts.

8.4.2 Pathological Manifestations

The classical pathology of brain tissue in patients who died due to CM appears as follows: the cerebral vasculature is extensively filled with infected red blood cells, which adheres to the vascular endothelium, resulting in the production of large amounts of lactic acid, as the infected red blood cells block the microcirculation and cause hypoxia in the brain tissue. It is often associated with circumferential hemorrhage, perivascular inflammatory cell infiltration, platelet activation, and thrombin deposition, and immunohistochemical studies reveal activation of endothelial cells. Autopsy pathology of patients who died of CM revealed the presence of infected red blood cells adhering to the microcirculation of brain tissue in 96% of patients, compared to 13% of patients who died of non-CM [27, 28].

8.4.3 Imaging

1. CT: The typical presentation on cranial CT is diffuse brain swelling (Fig. 8.14), while localized intracranial lesions are less common and may also appear as normal cranial CT.
2. MR: The MRI shows brain swelling more clearly than CT, showing focal or diffuse signal changes in brain tissue, hyperintense in T_2WI or FLAIR sequences, and cerebral gyrus-like enhancement of the lesion on enhanced scans (Fig. 8.15). Patients may develop irreversible necrosis of the perivascular myelin sheath and hemorrhagic lesions if effective treatment is not introduced at this stage of CM.

In conclusion, although the MRI features of CM have been reported to be diverse, the diagnosis of cerebral malaria should be strongly considered when patients with a history of residence in endemic areas present with systemic symptoms and acute hemorrhagic cerebral infarction.

8.4.4 Diagnostic Key Points

1. Most of them have a history of staying in malaria-endemic areas.
2. Accompanied by systemic symptoms such as chills, fever, unconsciousness, or anemia and thrombocytopenia.
3. CT shows diffuse brain tissue swelling.
4. MRI shows diffuse brain swelling and multiple hemorrhagic cerebral infarcts.
5. Laboratory tests: Thick and thin blood film smear stained for detection of *Plasmodium* can confirm the diagnosis.

8.4.5 Differential Diagnosis

1. **Epidemic B encephalitis**: It occurs in mosquito-prone areas in summer. In a typical patient, abnormal high signal on T_2WI and FLAIR sequences is seen on MR, involving the deep gray matter nuclei of the brain, including the bilateral thalamus and basal ganglia.

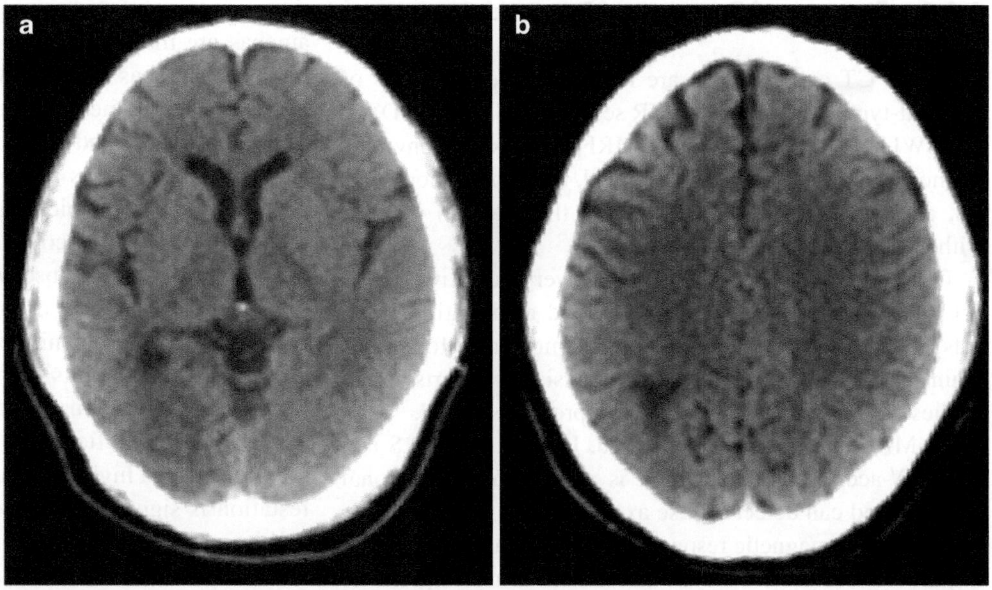

Fig. 8.14 Cerebral malaria (1). (**a**, **b**) CT scan shows swollen brain parenchyma with narrowing of the cerebral sulcus and cerebral fissure. (Image courtesy of Dr. Wang Haochu of Zhejiang Provincial People's Hospital)

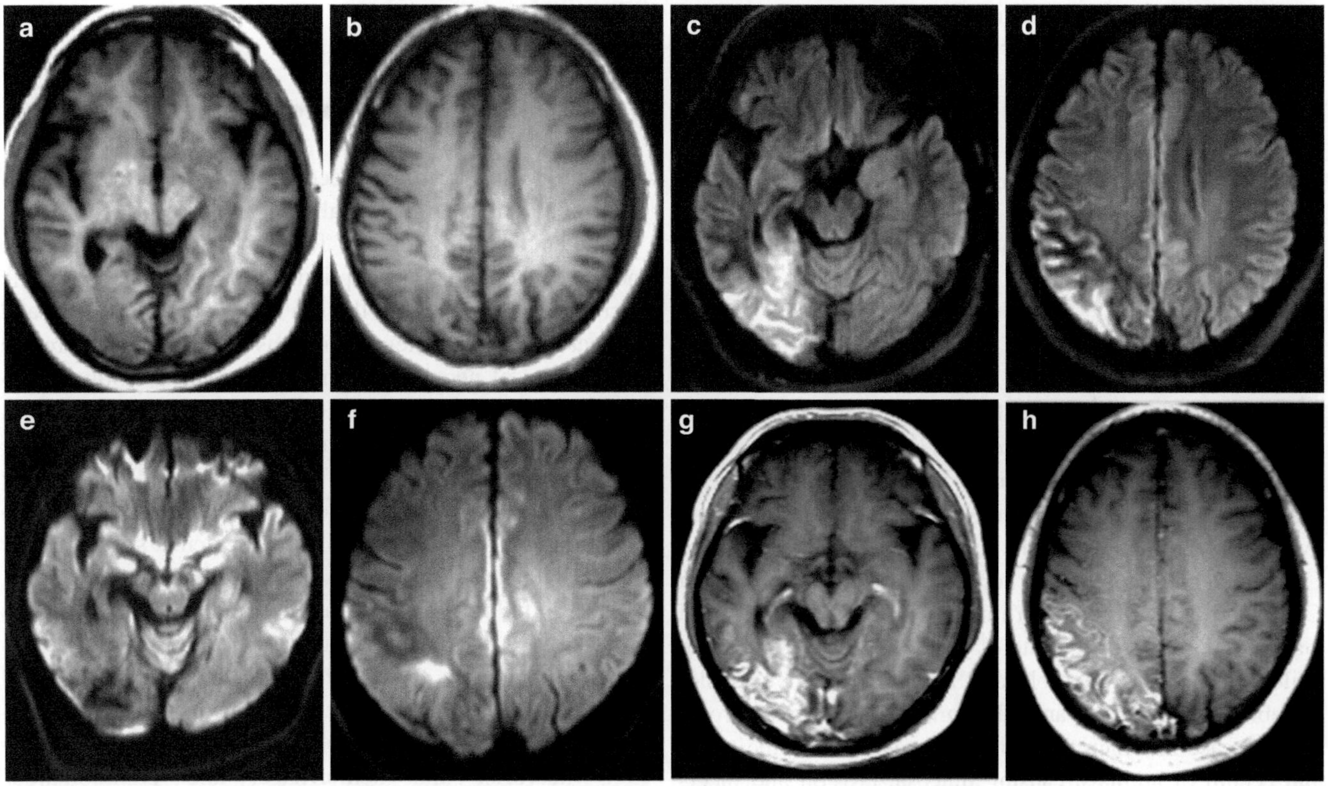

Fig. 8.15 Cerebral malaria (2). Swelling of the brain parenchyma in the right temporo-occipital lobe. (**a**, **b**) T_1WI shows hypointense; (**c**, **d**) FLAIR sequence shows hyperintense; (**e**, **f**) DWI shows lesion with uneven signal. (**g**, **h**) T_1WI-enhanced scan of the lesion showed cerebral gyrus-like enhancement. (Image courtesy of Dr. Wang Haochu, Zhejiang Provincial People's Hospital)

2. **Bacterial meningoencephalitis**: There is a clear history of purulent bacterial infection, and the subarachnoid space is indistinct and hypodense on CT scan. The T_1WI and T_2WI may appear normal, and the DWI sequence of the cerebral sulcus shows significant hyperintense, and the enhanced scan shows linear enhancement of the soft meninges. Cerebrospinal fluid examination shows a significant increase in white blood cells, increased protein, and decreased glucose; associated pathogens can be detected in the cerebrospinal fluid.
3. **Cerebral infarction**: The patient has a clear history of sudden onset, mostly in the elderly. It is easy to distinguish it from CM with a clear history of sudden onset, mostly in elderly patients with hypertension, and the occupying effect will diminish after follow-up review.

8.4.6 Status and Progress of Research

MRI and CT examinations are helpful in the diagnosis of cerebral-type malaria, where MR sequence of FLAIR, DWI, and SWI has certain advantages. MRI provides a noninvasive method to assess the basic anatomical, metabolic, biochemical, and functional characteristics of the brain in patients with CM.

DWI, GRE imaging and SWI are very sensitive to the detection of cytotoxic edema and blood degradation products, and can show acute infarcts and hemorrhagic foci in the brain [28, 29]. However, there are inconsistent reports across studies as to whether the lesions are spread restricted.

^{1}H-MRS can measure lactic acid. In addition, MRS can detect *N*-acetylaspartate, which is an indicator of axonal integrity and can detect diffuse axonal injury.

Functional magnetic resonance imaging has the potential to provide information about the distribution of regions of neural activity during coma and recovery, helping to determine whether severe neurological deficits in CM originate in specific regions of the brain or whether the process is diffuse throughout the brain.

8.5 Cerebral Amebiasis

Hanqiu Liu, Weiwei Wang, and Dan Zhang

8.5.1 Overview

Amebiasis is a disease caused by *Entamoeba histolytica* of Endamoebidae and *Entamoeba* [30–33], which mainly occurs in tropical and subtropical regions, with a high prevalence in eastern South America, Southeast Asia, and Mexico and an average infection rate of more than 20% in the population. In China, it is more common in northwest, southwest, and north China and more serious in Yunnan, Guizhou, Xinjiang, and Gansu, with an infection rate of more than 2%, common in children under 14 years old and adults over 40 years old. Amebiasis is a human-animal commensal intestinal protozoan disease in which the pathogen is parasitic in the colon and cecum of animals, causing mucosal erosion and ulceration of the large intestine. It has a slow onset and is characterized clinically by intractable diarrhea but can also cause secondary amebiasis by hematogenous transit or occasionally by direct invasion. According to the WHO-recommended clinical staging, it can be divided into asymptomatic carrier infections (which account for more than 90% of infections, the majority of which are noninvasive species of the complex) and symptomatic invasive infections.

Amebic infections of the central nervous system are rare and are mainly divided into amebic infections of lysosomes and free-living amebic infections. Lysogenic amebic infections cause secondary amebic brain abscesses; free-living amebas are the Fowler's naive amebas, spiny amebas, and mandelic amebas that are widely found in nature. Among them, Fowler's ameba causes primary amebic meningoencephalitis (PAM) and echinococcosis, and mandelic ameba causes granulomatous amebic encephalitis (GAE). Patients with secondary amebic brain abscess have both primary abscess lesions in the colon and metastatic abscesses in the liver and lungs. Most abscesses in their brain are secondary to abscesses in the liver or lungs.

Primary amebic meningoencephalitis is most often seen in healthy young adults with a history of swimming, freshwater exposure, or dust inhalation prior to the onset of the disease. Patients often have an acute onset and rapid progression, with a high mortality rate. The main clinical manifestation is signs of meningeal irritation, and symptoms of brain parenchymal damage may appear in the late course of the disease. A high titer of amebic antibodies, if detected in the serum, can be strong evidence for the diagnosis of this disease.

8.5.2 Pathological Manifestations

The pathological features of secondary amebic brain abscesses are similar to those of bacterial brain abscesses [34].

The main pathological features of primary amebic meningoencephalitis are septic meningitis and hemorrhagic necrotizing encephalitis; the pia maters are congested and edematous, and purulent secretions can be seen; there are diffuse foci of necrosis and hemorrhage in the brain, cerebellum, and brainstem, and the foci can sometimes fuse. The microscope often presents with perivasculitis in the superficial and basal layers of the cortex. Distinctive amebic vascular sheaths, i.e., clustered distribution of amebic trophozoites densely arranged in the perivascular spaces and/or vessel walls, are seen in areas of hemorrhage and necrosis.

The pathology of granulomatous amebic encephalitis is characterized by scattered localized necrotic cystic lesions containing amebic trophozoites, which are mostly found around blood vessels and have a tendency to erode them, surrounded by a granulomatous reaction with visible inflammation, necrosis, and hemorrhage, and granulomatous encephalitis can progress to necrotizing arteritis or even the formation of aneurysms.

8.5.3 Imaging

There is no characteristic appearance. CT shows multiple foci of low density with fuzzy borders in the cerebral cortex or subcortex, with moderate occupancy effect, and no significant enhancement in and around the lesion after enhancement (Fig. 8.16). MRI demonstrates multiple morphologically

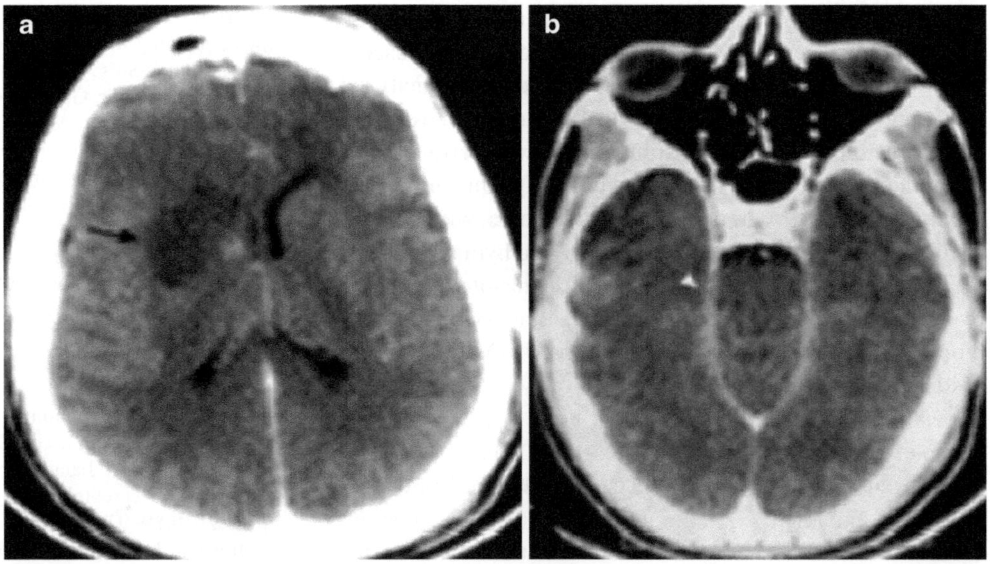

Fig. 8.16 Cerebral amebiasis (1). (**a**) CT scan shows a round-like hypodense shadow in the right basal ganglia; (**b**) linear enhancement is seen in the periaqueductal brain pool after enhancement. (Image courtesy of Professor Li Hongjun of Beijing Youan Hospital, Capital Medical University)

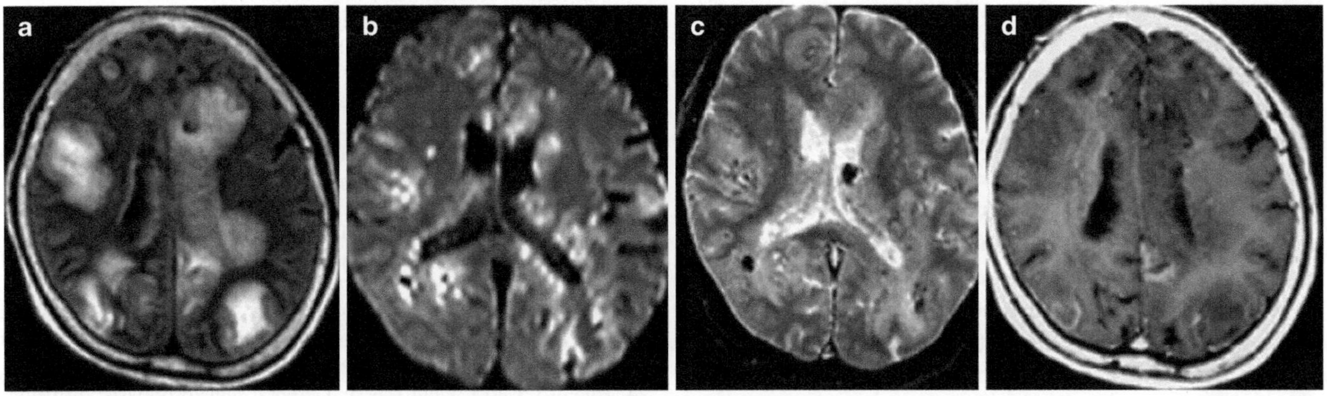

Fig. 8.17 Cerebral amebiasis (2). Multiple round-like abnormal signals are seen in the bilateral basal ganglia region, bilateral occipital lobes, and posterior horn of the lateral ventricles. (**a**) FLAIR sequence with hyperintense; (**b**) DWI with slightly hyperintense; (**c**) T_2WI with hypointense in the center of the lesion and hyperintense at the periphery; (**d**) enhanced lesion with circular enhancement. (Image courtesy of Prof. Li Hongjun, Beijing Youan Hospital, Capital Medical University)

irregular abnormal signals in the brain with hypo- or isointense in T_1WI and iso- or hyperintense in T_2WI, often with significant edema, and may be accompanied by occupational effects. Enhanced scan shows heterogeneous, circumferential, or linear enhancement (Fig. 8.17).

8.5.4 Diagnostic Key Points

1. Secondary amebic brain abscess with colonic primary foci and liver and lung metastases.
2. Primary amebic meningoencephalitis develops rapidly, mostly in young adults who are fit and have a history of swimming, freshwater exposure, or dust inhalation prior to the onset of the disease.
3. Granulomatous amebic encephalitis develops slowly; is often associated with chronic wasting disease, immunosuppressive use, or acquired immunodeficiency syndrome; and develops without a history of swimming or freshwater exposure.
4. The imaging presentation is non-characteristic and may resemble encephalitis and fungal brain abscess, bacterial brain abscess, and/or tuberculous brain abscess presentations.
5. Pathological examination: Culture or identify trophozoites and encapsulation of amebae from the lesioned tissue. Serum tests: Positive amebic antibodies, or the presence of high titers of amebic antibodies, are also strong evidence for the diagnosis of the disease.

8.5.5 Differential Diagnosis

1. The T_2WI signals of both nodular granulomas are similar, and intracerebral nodular calcifications are common, and the presence of a distinct lipid peak in the wave spectrum also contributes to the diagnosis of cerebral nodules.

2. Bacterial brain abscess is seen as continuous circumferential enhancement with thin and homogeneous abscess wall after enhancement, and it also needs to be analyzed in combination with clinical history and the results of routine blood and cerebrospinal fluid examination.
3. Intracerebral malignant glioma: Malignant glioma is mostly located in the deep white matter area, with wreath-like enhancement after enhancement and hyperintense on DWI in the area of enhancement. If the lesion invades the corpus callosum, the diagnosis of glioma is highly supported; magnetic resonance spectroscopy (MRS) helps to differentiate the two.

8.5.6 Status and Progress of Research

MRI and CT can be useful for the examination of intracranial amebic infections. MRI features high soft tissue resolution, and its multi-sequence and multimodal examination can provide extensive information for the localization, characterization, and even quantitative diagnosis of intracranial amebic infection and is the preferred recommended examination method. Techniques such as DWI and MRS may have some value in differentiating intracranial ameba from other intracranial occupying lesions. CT can be widely used in the screening of intracranial lesions because of its fast-scanning speed and low cost. CT is superior to MRI in showing microcalcifications and cortical bone destruction. However, the soft tissue resolution of CT is relatively low, and the diagnostic accuracy is not as good as that of MRI.

References

1. Misra UK, Kalita J. Overview: Japanese encephalitis. Prog Neurobiol. 2010;91(2):108–20.
2. Li H. Practical infectious disease imaging. Beijing: People's Medical Publishing House; 2016.
3. Basumatary LJ, Raja D, Bhuyan D, et al. Clinical and radiological spectrum of Japanese encephalitis. J Neurol Sci. 2013;325(1/2):15–21.
4. Arahata Y, Fujii K, Nishimura T, et al. Longitudinal magnetic resonance imaging changes in Japanese encephalitis. Brain Dev. 2019;41(8):731–4.
5. Sawlani V. Diffusion-weighted imaging and apparent diffusion coefficient evaluation of herpes simplex encephalitis and Japanese encephalitis. J Neurol Sci. 2009;287(1/2):221–6.
6. Bai G, Ye X, Yan Z, et al. Magnetic resonance spectral characteristics and follow-up study of pediatric epidemic encephalitis B. Radiol Pract. 2010;25(10):1094–6.
7. Zhang W, Li J, Mcmanus DP. Concepts in immunology and diagnosis of hydatid disease. Clin Microbiol Rev. 2003;16(1):18–36.
8. Stojkovic M, Junghanss T. Cystic and alveolar echinococcosis. Handb Clin Neurol. 2013;114(114):327–34.
9. Zhang YF, Xie ZR, Ni YQ, et al. Curative effect of radiotherapy at various doses on subcutaneous alveolar echinococcosis in rats. Chin Med J. 2011;124(18):2845–8.
10. Wani NA, Kousar TL, Gojwari T, et al. Computed tomography findings in cerebral hydatid disease. Turk Neurosurg. 2011;21(3):347–51.
11. Okuri A. Magnetic resonance spectroscopy and magnetic resonance imaging findings of the intracerebral alveolar echinococcosis. Craniofac Surg. 2014;25(4):1352–3.
12. Pu P, Liu L, Wang G, et al. CT and MRI manifestations of cerebral alveolar echinococcosis in relation to pathology. J Clin Radiol. 2012;31(9):1238–42.
13. Karçaalincaba M, Sirlin CB. CT and MRI of diffuse lobar involvement pattern in liver pathology. Diagn Interv Radiol. 2010;17(4):334–42.
14. Zhang JX, Ren YL, Wang L, et al. CT and MRI manifestations and diagnosis of cerebral alveolar hydatid. Chin J Radiol. 2011;44:1148.
15. Becce F, Pomoni A, Uldry E, et al. Alveolar echinococcosis of the liver: diffusion-weighted MRI findings and potential role in lesion characterisation. Eur J Radiol. 2014;83(4):625–31.
16. Wang J, Yao WH, Yi BN, et al. Proton magnetic resonance spectroscopy in the evaluation of infiltration zone of cerebral alveolar echinococcosis. Chin Med J. 2012;125(13):2260.
17. Wang J, Ibanu A, Jiang C, et al. Characterization of MR proton spectrum of cerebral alveolar echinococcosis. J Clin Radiol. 2012;31(9):89–92.
18. Yang GC, Zhang QX, Tang GB, et al. Role of magnetic resonance spectroscopy and susceptibility weighted imaging in cerebral alveolar echinococcosis. Iran J Parasitol. 2015;10(1):122–7.
19. Wong KH. Important strategies for parasitic disease control—health promotion. Chin J Parasitol Parasitic Dis. 2003;21(3):129, 130.
20. Roberts M, Cross J, Pohl U, et al. Cerebral schistosomiasis. Lancet Infect Dis. 2006;6(12):820.
21. Ching HT, Clark AE, Hendrix VJ, et al. MR imaging appearance of intracerebral schistosomiasis. Am J Roentgenol. 1994;162(3):693, 694.
22. Wang C, Yang Y, Gao Z. Diagnosis and staging of MR of cerebral schistosomiasis (with analysis of 10 cases). Chin J Clin Med Imaging. 2002;13(6):437, 443.
23. Liu H, Lim CC, Feng X, et al. MRI in cerebral schistosomiasis: characteristic nodular enhancement in 33 patients. Am J Roentgenol. 2008;191(2):582–8.
24. Huang J, Luo J, Peng J, et al. Cerebral schistosomiasis: diffusion-weighted imaging helps to differentiate from brain glioma and metastasis. Acta Radiol. 2017;58(11):1371–7.
25. Shikani HJ, Freeman BD, Lisanti MP, et al. Cerebral malaria: we have come a long way. Am J Pathol. 2012;181(5):1484–92.
26. Hora R, Kapoor P, Thind KK, et al. Cerebral malaria-clinical manifestations and pathogenesis. Metab Brain Dis. 2016;31(2):225–37.
27. Idro R, Jenkins NE, Newton CR. Pathogenesis, clinical features, and neurological outcome of cerebral malaria. Lancet Neurol. 2005;4(12):827–40.
28. Mohanty S, Taylor TE, Kampondeni S, et al. Magnetic resonance imaging during life: the key to unlock cerebral malaria pathogenesis. Malar J. 2014;13:276.
29. Nickerson JP, Tong KA, Raghavan R. Imaging cerebral malaria with a susceptibility-weighted MR sequence. Am J Neuroradiol. 2009;30(6):e85–6.
30. Zhu Y, Xu Y, Feng L, et al. A case of granulomatous amoebic encephalitis. J Clin Radiol. 2012;31(9):335, 336.
31. Itoh K, Yagita K, Nozaki T, et al. An autopsy case of Balamuthia mandrillaris amoebic encephalitis, a rare emerging infectious disease, with a brief review of the cases reported in Japan. Neuropathology. 2015;35(1):64–9.
32. Takei K, Toyoshima M, Nakamura M, et al. An acute case of granulomatous amoebic encephalitis-Balamuthia mandrillaris infection. Intern Med. 2018;57(9):1313–6.
33. Linam WM, Ahmed M, Cope JR, et al. Successful treatment of an adolescent with Naegleria fowleri primary amebic meningoencephalitis. Pediatrics. 2015;135(3):e744–8.
34. Lu D, Luo L, Xu Q. A clinicopathological study of granulomatous amebic encephalitis. J Clin Radiol. 2012;31(9):169.

Contagious Disease-Related Intracranial Infections

9

Li Li, Meiji Ren, Rui Huang, Yan Wang, Jian Wang, and Yupeng Liu

9.1 Rabies Encephalitis

Li Li and Meiji Ren

9.1.1 Overview

Rabies is an acute zoonotic disease caused by rabies virus (rabies virus) that mainly attacks the central nervous system and is usually transmitted to humans by the bite of a sick animal through saliva. Clinical manifestations include manic and paralytic types. The manic type, also known as the classic or encephalitic type, has symptoms of characteristic hydrophobia, fear of sound, fear of wind, fear of restlessness, pharyngeal muscle spasms, and progressive paralysis, and it's also known as hydrophobia because of the more prominent symptoms of hydrophobia. There is no specific treatment for this disease and the mortality rate is 100%.

Rabies virus has a strong affinity for nerve tissue, and after invading the body from a break in the skin or mucous membrane, it spreads retrograde and centripetal to the center through the nerves. The pathogenic process is divided into three phases: a small multiplication of the virus in the tissues, the invasion of the central nervous system from the peripheral nerves, and the spread of the virus from the central nervous system to the organs.

Manic rabies is divided into three phases according to clinical manifestations. (1) In the prodromal phase, patients present with nonspecific symptoms similar to a cold, such as malaise, lack of appetite, fever, and headache, followed by sensitivity to stimuli such as sound, wind, and light and a feeling of tightness in the throat. An early symptom of diagnostic significance is an unusual sensation such as itching, pain, numbness, or ankylosis in the healing wound and its innervated area. (2) During the excitement phase, the patient presents with high fever, high excitement, fear of restlessness, fear of water, fear of light, fear of wind, etc. Fear of water is its typical symptom, but not in every case. Patients may be accompanied by high fever and sympathetic hyperactivity, and are more likely to be lucid, but may also experience psychosis, hallucinations, and hallucinations. (3) In the paralytic phase (coma or death phase), the patient's spastic convulsions cease, followed by general flaccid paralysis, gradual coma, and eventually death due to respiratory, circulatory, and systemic failure. Laboratory tests are positive for rabies virus antigen in saliva and cerebrospinal fluid, and rabies virus can be isolated in saliva and cerebrospinal fluid; confirmation of diagnosis depends on examination for viral antigen, positive viral nucleic acid test for rabies virus nucleic acid, or detection of endogenous vesicles in autopsy brain tissue.

9.1.2 Pathological Manifestations

The main pathological change of the disease is acute diffuse encephalomyelitis with mostly normal meninges. Lesions were most evident in the basal hippocampal parahippocampal gyrus, brainstem sites (midbrain, pons, and medulla), and cerebellum, manifesting as congestion, edema, and microhemorrhages in the brain parenchyma and spinal cord. Microscopy showed nonspecific neuroblastic degeneration

L. Li · M. Ren
Beijing You'an Hospital, Capital Medical University, Beijing, China

R. Huang
Department of Radiology, Xijing Hospital, Air Force Military Medical University, Xi'an, China

Y. Wang
The Second Affiliated Hospital of Xiamen Medical School, Xiamen, China

J. Wang (✉)
Medical Imaging Center, First Affiliated Hospital of Xinjiang Medical University, Urumqi, China

Shanghai Universal Medical Imaging Diagnostic Center, Shanghai University, Shanghai, China

Y. Liu
First Hospital of Qinhuangdao, Qinghuangdao, China

H. Li et al. (eds.), *Radiology of Infectious and Inflammatory Diseases - Volume 1*,
https://doi.org/10.1007/978-981-99-0039-8_9

with inflammatory cell infiltration in the brain parenchyma. The characteristic lesions are eosinophilic inclusion bodies in neuronal cells, i.e., endosomal vesicles, round or ovoid, 3–10 μm in diameter, stained cherry red. Endosomes are colonies of rabies virus, commonly found in hippocampal and cerebellar Purkinje cells, with one or two endosomes in each cell, but about 20% of patients are negative [1].

9.1.3 Imaging

1. At **CT**, multiple hypodense lesions in the basal ganglia, periventricular white matter, hippocampus, and brainstem are revealed, without enhancement of the lesion on postcontrast images [2].
2. **MRI** examination shows important diagnostic value in rabies virus encephalitis. The changes in MRI signal intensity correlate with the stage of disease and are available for clinical diagnostic evaluation. MRI shows gray matter involvement, including basal ganglia, thalamus, hippocampus, midbrain, etc. The lesions show hypointense on T_1-weighted images and hyperintense on T_2-weighted images and FLAIR. The borders are poorly defined and mostly symmetrically distributed [3]. On diffusion-weighted images, high signal intensity with diffusion restriction appeared, without enhancement on contrast enhancement images. Necrotizing encephalitis has been demonstrated in the brainstem and hippocampus of patients with rabies.

9.1.4 Diagnostic Key Points

1. History of bites from rabid dogs or diseased animals.
2. The clinical diagnosis can be made by the presence of typical symptoms such as fear of water, fear of wind, laryngeal spasm, or abnormal sensations such as photophobia, vocalophobia, excessive sweating, salivation and numbness, itching, and pain at the site of the bite.
3. Based on imaging findings, symmetric hypodense lesions are seen in the basal ganglia, hippocampus, and brainstem on CT, with low T_1 signal intensity and high T_2 signal intensity on MRI. Most are without enhancement on postcontrast images.
4. Definitive diagnosis relies on examination for viral antigens, viral nucleic acids, or autopsy of endogenous vesicles in brain tissue.

9.1.5 Differential Diagnosis

1. **Viral encephalitis**. The changes in mental status are obvious, without anemophobia, hydrophobia, phengophobia, and salivation but also mainly presents basal ganglia and brainstem changes, while there are slight changes in the cortex and white matter, prone to diffuse intracranial hemorrhage, while rabies virus encephalitis hemorrhage is extremely rare.
2. **Poliomyelitis**. The involvement of motor cells in the anterior horn of the spinal cord is the most significant, and the general symptoms are mild, and myalgia is obvious. When limb paralysis occurs, most of the other symptoms have subsided and there is no hydrophobia. The presence of scattered lamellar high-T_2 signal intensity at the spinal cord on is also MRI T_2WI. Heterogeneous ring enhancement was revealed on postcontrast images.

9.1.6 Status and Progress of Research

Functional magnetic resonance imaging (fMRI) contributes to the diagnosis of the disease. In an event of neuronal cell swelling or cytotoxic edema, the cell gap narrows, leading to diffusion restriction of the water molecule. DWI shows a high signal intensity and the ADC values decreases. Diffusion tensor imaging (DTI) can be used to assess the integrity of white matter tracts. FA values can decrease during demyelination, and quantification of FA values in diseased compared with normal conditions can help in the early detection of demyelination. Besides, when neurons are damaged or with inflammatory changes and gliosis, MRS shows a decrease in NAA peak, which indicates injury of neural cells; and the cell membrane rupture leads to an increase in Cho peak. Huang et al. [4] reported good immune persistence after rabies exposure using the "2-1-1" procedure for human rabies vaccination, with a good immune response after two doses of booster immunization within 3 years.

9.2 Neurobrucellosis

Rui Huang, Yan Wang, and Jian Wang

9.2.1 Overview

Brucellosis is a common zoonotic disease of natural origin with varying degrees of prevalence in many parts of the world, including East Asia, Central Asia, and Mediterranean countries. The main endemic areas in China include Inner Mongolia, Xinjiang, Heilongjiang, and Jilin. The disease is caused by *Brucella* spp., and humans were infected with the disease through direct contact with infected animals, exposure to pathogenic bacteria from cuts and abrasion wounds or inhalation of infected aerosols, or ingestion of unpasteurized milk or milk products. The disease often occurs in young adults, and the clinical manifestations varied, with continuous or intermittent irregular fever (also known as wave fever) being the most common symptom, followed by sweating and bone, joint involvement, as well as hepatomegaly, splenomegaly, and genitourinary complications (epididymitis, glomerulonephritis). When *Brucella* invades the central nervous system, direct infection and the specific immune inflammatory response triggered by its released endotoxin can lead to central nervous system damage, known as neurobrucellosis. Clinical symptoms may include neurological symptoms such as headache, malaise, chills, impaired sensory awareness, convulsions, hypoacusis, hypoplasia, and abducens nerve paralysis. The modes of initiation of neurobrucellosis include encephalitis, meningoencephalitis, inflammatory demyelination, and peripheral neuropathy. Laboratory tests include elevated cerebrospinal fluid protein levels, normal or low blood glucose levels, elevated white blood cells predominantly lymphocytes, and a positive serum or cerebrospinal fluid *Brucella* agglutination test; serum or cerebrospinal fluid cultures are less likely to be positive for *Brucella*.

9.2.2 Pathological Manifestations

Brucella primarily invades the cells of the human reticuloendothelial system and multiplies within macrophages, lymphocytes, and other cells. Its production of virulence factors increases the likelihood that these organisms will use unique mechanisms to evade host defenses. Smooth lipopolysaccharides regulate the intracellular environment by penetrating host cells and altering intracellular traffic to avoid lysosomal degradation and killing, enabling long-term intracellular survival and recirculation of *Brucella* [5]. The cells of the reticuloendothelial system show diffuse proliferation in the acute phase and granulomatous lesions consisting of epithelioid cells, giant cells, plasma cells, and lymphocytes in the chronic phase, which are characteristic of allergic diseases. Similar lesions can occur in the liver, spleen, lymph nodes, and bone marrow. In sheep and pig brucellosis, especially in pig brucellosis, there is often septic granuloma formation.

9.2.3 Imaging

Imaging manifestations of neurobrucellosis are often encephalitis and meningitis, restrictive or diffuse demyelinating changes, and vascular lesions [6] (Fig. 9.1).

1. **Encephalitis and meningitis** are the most common imaging presentations of neurobrucellosis. MRI enhanced scan shows abnormal enhancement of the cerebellar curtain, meninges, basal nuclei, and nerve roots, which can be reduced in extent or disappear with treatment.
2. **Limited or diffuse demyelination**. MRI plain scan shows multiple abnormal signals in the bilateral subcortical white matter, lateral paraventricular white matter, brainstem, corpus callosum, and cerebellum. T_1WI shows hypointense and T_2WI shows hyperintense with FLAIR sequence shows hyperintense. Patchy abnormal enhancement is seen on enhanced scan [7].
3. **Vascular lesions**. They may present as lacunar cerebral infarction, cerebral hemorrhage, venous embolism, or cerebral small vessel lesions. Cranial CTA, MRA, DSA can show corresponding changes in cerebral vessels [8].

9.2.4 Diagnostic Key Points

1. Prevalent in young adults with a history of exposure to susceptible animals or a history of ingestion of unpasteurized dairy products, etc.
2. Persistent or intermittent irregular fever (wavy fever), and neurological symptoms such as headache, malaise, chills, impaired consciousness, convulsions, hypoacusis, hypopsia, and abducens nerve paralysis.

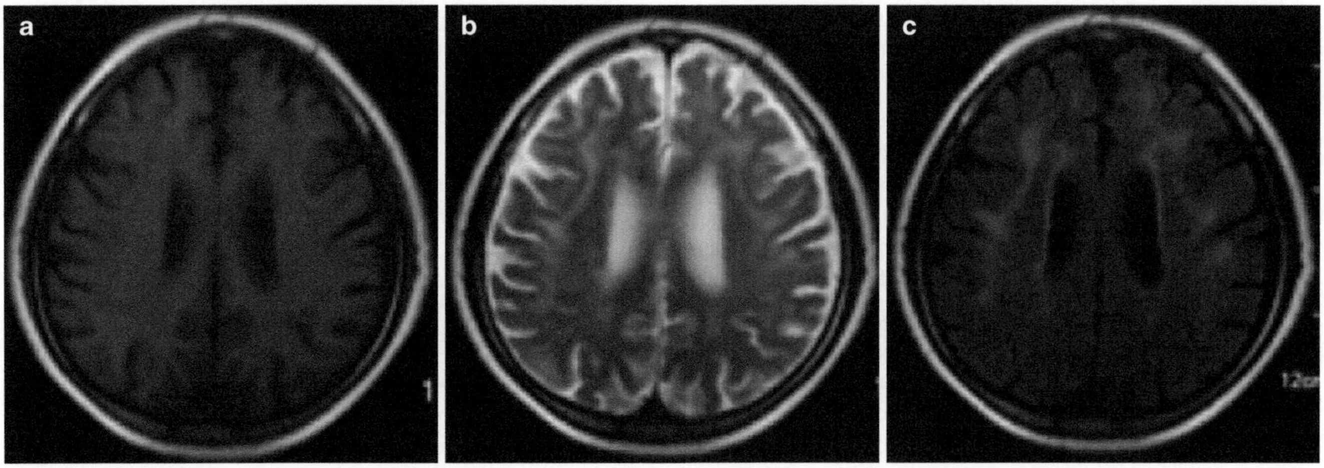

Fig. 9.1 Neurobrucellosis. (**a**) Irregularly shaped lesion in the subcortical white matter area of bilateral cerebral hemispheres, T_1WI with slightly hypointense; (**b**) T_2WI with slightly hyperintense; (**c**) FLAIR sequence with slightly hyperintense. (Image courtesy of Dr. Wang Yan, Sixth People's Hospital of Xinjiang Uygur Autonomous Region)

3. Imaging manifestations include encephalitis and meningitis, limited or diffuse demyelinating changes, lacunar cerebral infarction, cerebral hemorrhage, venous embolism, and cerebral small vessel lesions.
4. Serum or cerebrospinal fluid isolation of Brucella or positive serum or cerebrospinal fluid Brucella agglutination test.

9.2.5 Differential Diagnosis

1. **Multiple sclerosis** (MS). It is more common in young women and has no obvious inducement before onset, characterized by a multitemporal course and recurrent episodes, whereas brucellosis is more common in young adults, most of whom have a history of direct contact with infected animals or ingestion of unpasteurized milk or milk products before onset. MS lesions are often occurs multiply and the most common site is bilateral paraventricular, the long axis of the lesion is "perpendicular" to the ventricle; T_1WI shows hypo or slightly hypointense, T_2WI shows a "core + halo" sign. Around fresh lesions, circumferential/semi-circular enhancement or speckle/patchy enhancement can be seen on enhanced scan; old and new lesions may co-exist. While demyelinating changes in neurobrucellosis show multiple abnormal signals in the subcortical white matter, lateral paraventricular white matter, brainstem, corpus callosum, and cerebellum bilaterally. T_1WI shows hypointense, T_2WI shows hyperintense, FLAIR sequence shows hyperintense, and enhanced scan shows partial enhancement.
2. **Tuberculous meningoencephalitis** (TM) is most commonly seen in adolescents and the elderly, with clinical manifestations often including afternoon hypothermia, night sweats, headache, and signs of meningeal irritation, whereas brucellosis is more common in young adults, with a history of exposure to susceptible animals or ingestion of unsterilized dairy products before onset, and the most common clinical manifestation is undulating fever, which can be differentiated from tuberculous meningoencephalitis. MRI of tuberculous meningoencephalitis shows occlusion of the basal pool of the brain, with the suprasellar pool being the most common, followed by the circumferential and lateral fissure pools. T_1WI shows slightly hyperintense and T_2WI shows hyperintense with FLAIR sequence showing hyperintense. Enhanced scan shows marked thickening of the meninges of the basal pool of the brain and the subarachnoid space may also be involved. When accompanied by intracerebral tuberculoma formation, nodular or ring-like enhancement may be seen. Neurobrucellosis with encephalitis and meningitis changes on enhanced scan showed enhancement of the cerebellar curtain, meninges, basal nuclei, and nerve roots, which can shrink or disappear with treatment.
3. **Acute disseminated encephalomyelitis** (ADEM). This is prevalent in children under 10 years of age, and most patients have a history of infection or vaccination in the weeks before onset; ADEM of cranial MRI shows extensive abnormal signal in the subcortical white matter on both sides of the brain. T_1WI shows slightly hypointense and T_2WI shows slightly hyperintense, with the white matter around the lateral ventricles being more common, with visible peripheral edema and narrowing of the ventricular system due to parenchymal edema compression; the imaging presentation is similar to neurobrucellosis and lack of specificity and can be based on serologic cultures, serum agglutination tests, etc. for differentiation.

9.2.6 Status and Progress of Research

With the widespread use of imaging technology in clinical practice, a variety of imaging techniques have significantly improved the diagnostic efficiency of brucellosis. Brain DSA can detect cerebrovascular lesions in patients with brucellosis; CT can show cerebral edema, cerebral abscess, and cerebrovascular injury in patients with brucellosis; MRI is more valuable for the diagnosis of the disease. In addition to the conventional plain and enhanced scans, MRI new technology offers additional advantages for the diagnosis of brucellosis. MR diffusion-related techniques, including DWI and DTI, can better show the diffusion motility of water molecules within the lesion and the overall picture of diffusion resistance and cerebral white matter fiber bundle alignment. Susceptibility weighted imaging (SWI) can show hemorrhage, calcification, iron deposits, etc. in the lesion. DTI is able to show the alignment and spatial structure of nerve fiber bundles in biopsies, clearly show various pathological changes in nerve fiber bundles, and more accurately show early fine structural changes and quantify them with apparent diffusion coefficients (ADC) and anisotropy scores (FA). ADC value reflects the diffusion of water molecules; the higher the value of ADC, the better the diffusion ability of water molecules and vice versa. FA value reflects the degree of myelination and restriction of water molecules by nerve fibers and can reflect the anisotropy of water molecules. The higher the value of FA, the stronger the anisotropy and vice versa [9].

9.3 Neurosyphilis

Li Li and Yupeng Liu

9.3.1 Overview

Syphilis is a chronic infectious disease caused by the syphilis spirochete (TP), which is a chronic infectious disease mainly transmitted through through sexual contact. In the early stage, it mainly affects the skin and mucous membranes, but in the late stage it can affect the vascular and central nervous system and organs of the body. When the central nervous system is invaded, it is called neurosyphilis (NS). Neurosyphilis can occur at any stage from a few weeks to several years after the initial syphilis infection, and its clinical manifestations are so varied that it is called the "great imitator."

According to the clinical manifestations and pathological changes, neurosyphilis can be divided into five types, namely, asymptomatic type, meningeal type, meningeal vascular type, parenchymal type, and syphilitic dendritic type, with the meningeal vascular type being more common. (1) In asymptomatic type, patients may not have any neurological signs and symptoms; cerebrospinal fluid examination may show only mild abnormalities and positive syphilis serology tests. This type can progress to symptomatic neurosyphilis if not treated systematically. (2) For the meningeal type, one of the early neurosyphilis manifests itself mainly as symptoms of meningitis, such as headache, vomiting, neck stiffness, and even impaired consciousness, convulsive seizures, and cerebral nerve palsy. In subacute or chronic disease, meningeal involvement at the base of the skull is most common, with lesions mainly involving pairs II–VI and VIII cerebral nerves [10], and intracranial hypertension may also occur if cerebrospinal fluid circulation is affected. (3) In the meningeal vascular type, headache and neurological dysfunction associated with vascular lesions are most common. Neurological symptoms appear slowly or suddenly, with signs related to the occluded blood vessels, and may include hemiparesis, hemianesthesia, hemianopsia, and aphasia; they are often accompanied by abnormal changes in the cerebrospinal fluid. (4) For the brain parenchymal type, this is paralytic dementia, the result of diffuse and extensive damage to the brain parenchyma, with symptoms dominated by progressive dementia with signs of neurological damage to the brain [11], or paralysis, hemianesthesia, hemianopia, and aphasia if accompanied by vascular lesions. (5) Finally, for the syphilitic dendritic type, occupational lesions of the nervous system, characterized by the presence of neoplastic, brain abscesses and tuberculoma-like symptoms, are more difficult to diagnose. A positive serological syphilis test and a positive blood and cerebrospinal fluid VDRL test confirm the diagnosis.

9.3.2 Pathological Manifestations

The meningeal vascular type is syphilitic endarteritis of the meninges and intracerebral parenchymal vessels as TP invading the endothelial cells of the vessels, causing necrosis of the intima and epithelium, leading to thrombosis, local ischemia, and infarction [12].

Dendrites are well-defined granulomatous masses formed by the intense inflammatory reaction of the meninges in the early stages of syphilis, and brain dendrites often originate from the brain parenchyma around the connective tissue and blood vessels of the meninges, overlying the convex surface of the brain, and are closely related to the brain parenchyma and meninges, often solitary or multiple. Caseous necrosis is seen inside the dendritic swelling; TP is rare.

9.3.3 Imaging

The involvement sites vary with different pathological types of neurosyphilis and their imaging manifestations are diverse and nonspecific. However, imaging findings can help to observe the extent and location of neurosyphilis involvement.

1. **Asymptomatic type**. No significant abnormalities in brain parenchyma.
2. **Meningeal type**. Meningeal lesions at the base of the brain are more serious, often involving the upper cervical spinal cord and cerebral nerves, with no abnormal findings in early CT. At MRI, it shows extensive meninges thickening and marked cerebral gyrus-like enhancement. Cerebral (spinal) membrane is extensively thickened, and the signal intensity of cerebrospinal fluid in the basal pool on T_2WI is higher than that in the ventricles suggesting possible obstruction [13]. If the lateral and median foramina of the fourth ventricle are closed due to fibrous connective tissue, obstructive hydrocephalus may develop, leading to enlargement of the ventricles. The pathological changes are mainly inflammation of the meninges caused by small vasculitis.

   Cerebral nerve involvement is a characteristic feature of acute meningeal neurosyphilis, and the susceptible nerves are, in order, the vestibulocochlear nerve, facial nerve, optic nerve, and ophthalmic nerve. Kou Cheng et al. [14] found that regarding brain nerve involvement, a single group of cerebral nerve involvement is common. However, Zhao X. et al. [15] and Cao J. et al. [16] reported cases of neurosyphilis in which multiple groups of brain nerves were involved simultaneously, suggesting that neurosyphilis can also cause multiple groups of brain nerve involvement. Li Lin et al. [17] studied 12 patients with syphilitic optic neuritis and found that orbital MRI revealed morphological and signal abnormalities in 83.33% of patients.
3. **Meningeal vascular type**. Single or multiple foci of cerebral infarction are often seen in the anterior and posterior circulation, with variable, wandering lesions of variable size, located mainly in the subcortical and deep cerebral white matter, including the corpus callosum and internal capsule. CT shows heterogeneous or homogeneous hypodense lesions. Visible low signal intensity on T1WI and high signal intensity on T2WI on MR images (Fig. 9.2). Contrast enhancement shows patchy or cortical gyrus-like enhancement after gadopentetate glucosamine

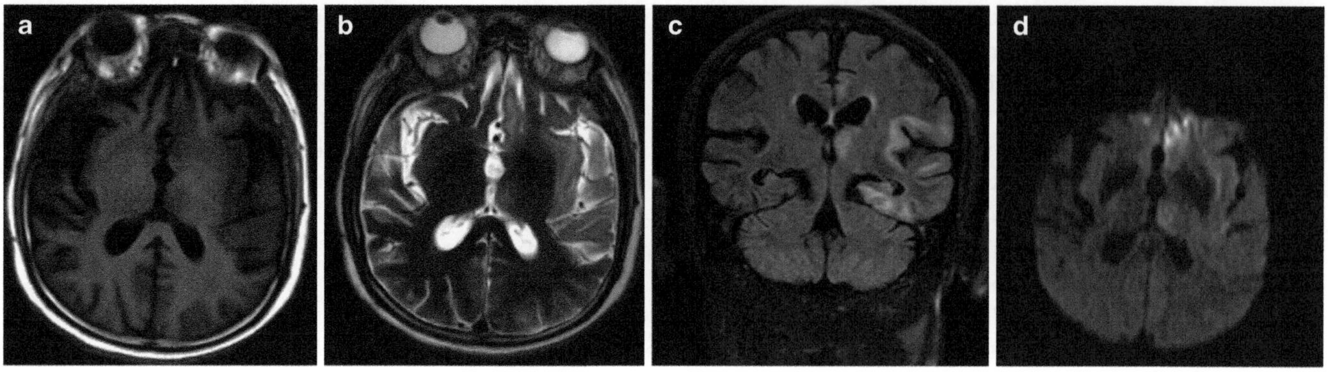

Fig. 9.2 Neurosyphilis (1). Axial brain MRI, relatively low signal intensity on T_1-weighted image (**a**) and relatively high signal intensity on T_2-weighted image (**b**) with wedge-shaped, involving left temporal lobe cortical, subcortical white matter, and insula. Bilateral hemispheres moderate atrophy. FLAIR (**c**) and DWI (**d**) show high signal intensity. (Image courtesy of Tang Yonghua, Ruijin Hospital, Shanghai Jiao Tong University School of Medicine)

(Gd-DTPA) injection, with the same signal as cerebrospinal fluid after encephalomalacia [18]. Liu Renwei et al. [19] reported that T_2-FLAIR could clearly show the protein-containing high-signal nodular shadow in the subarachnoid space and soft meningeal surface in patients with meningeal vascular type; therefore, it was concluded that T_2-FLAIR can effectively improve the sensitivity of MRI to meningeal inflammation in patients with meningeal vascular type. The predilection sites of syphilitic vasculitis are mostly the middle cerebral artery, the anterior cerebral artery, the posterior inferior cerebellar artery, and the anterior spinal artery supply area [20].

4. **Brain parenchymal type**. Early CT shows widespread hypodense changes with edema and late diffuse cortical atrophy with dilated lateral ventricles. MRI shows cortical atrophy and subcortical gliosis, especially in the anterior region [21] (Fig. 9.3). Some studies have shown that frontotemporal lobe atrophy due to paralytic dementia predicts a poor prognosis, and it is believed that MRI has a corresponding value in determining the prognosis of neurosyphilis [22].
5. **Syphilitic dendritic type**. It presents with single or multiple foci, hypo- or isointense lesions, with circumferential enhancement of the lesion on enhanced scan. On MRI T_1WI sequence, the lesion appears to be circular in shape, with a diameter of 2.0–2.5 cm, and is located in the cerebral cortex and subcortex. The caseous necrosis in the center of the lesion presents with hypo- to isointensity and low mixed signal foci, surrounded by a large area of low signal edema, and the occupancy effect is visible. The caseous necrosis shows high signal or isosignal with mixed high and low signal intensity on T_2WI, and the surrounding edema zone is usually high signal. The lesion shows irregular circumferential enhancement on enhanced scan, which is due to immature blood-brain barrier of neovascularization of inflammatory granulation tissue around the necrotic area. Adjacent meningeal enhancement represents meningeal involvement.

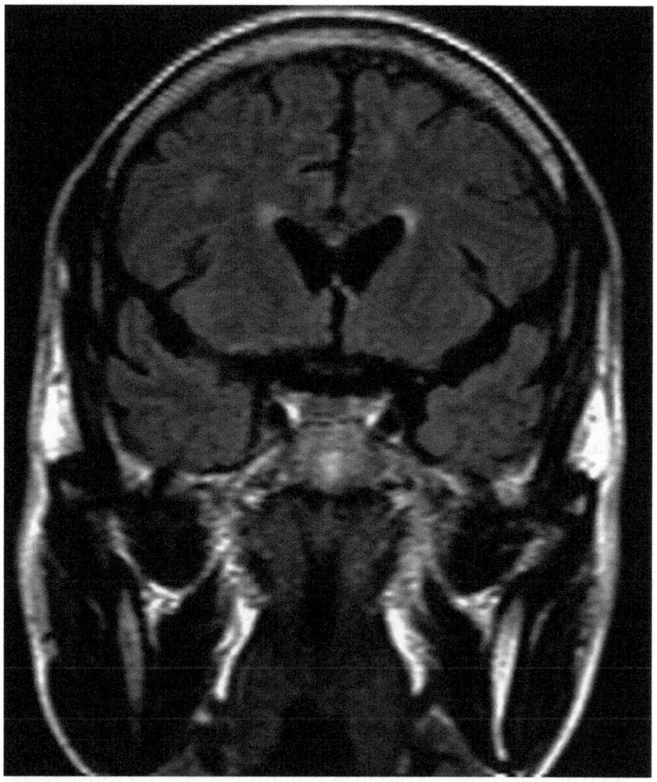

Fig. 9.3 Neurosyphilis (2). Coronal T2-FLAIR image of the brain, multiple demyelinating can be seen in the bilateral frontal lobes. (Image courtesy of Tang Yonghua, Ruijin Hospital, Shanghai Jiaotong University School of Medicine)

9.3.4 Diagnostic Key Points

1. There is a history of transmission by sexual contact.
2. The clinical manifestations are varied, mainly invading the skin and mucous membranes in the early stage, but in the late stage, it may invade the blood vessels, central nervous system, and all organs of the body.
3. Different types of image performance. The parenchymal type shows single or multiple foci of cerebral infarction;

the parenchymal type shows cerebral atrophy with dilated lateral ventricles, more often in the frontotemporal lobe, with edema; the syphilitic dendritic type shows single or multiple round-like foci in the brain, surrounded by edema, with an occupying effect, and the foci are circumferentially enhanced on enhanced scans.

4. A positive serological syphilis test and a positive blood and cerebrospinal fluid VDRL test confirm the diagnosis.

9.3.5 Differential Diagnosis

1. **Atherosclerotic cerebral infarction**. Patients with simple cerebral infarction have a rapid-onset, negative blood and cerebrospinal fluid syphilis tests, and the infarct area is consistent with the extent of innervation of large blood-supplying arteries, mostly with high risk factors for cerebrovascular disease such as hypertension, hyperlipidemia, and diabetes mellitus, while the meningeal vascular type has a slow-onset, positive blood and cerebrospinal fluid syphilis tests, with poorly defined lesion borders and a more limited extent, or a wide but scattered extent, due to syphilis causing occlusion of small arteries.
2. **Herpes simplex virus encephalitis (HSE)**. The onset of disease is rapid. It often progresses from a single side to bilateral involvement and usually located in the medial temporal lobe, where gradually extends to the frontal and limbic systems. Extensive edema and hemorrhagic spots were present in the cortex and subcortex, mostly with occupancy effects, and the lesions showed linear or gyral-like enhancement on enhanced scans. Hobbs et al. [23] suggest that its characteristic presentation, i.e., a lesion with a clear boundary to the outer edge of the nucleus pulposus, convex to the outside, and with a knife-like margin, is related to the fact that the virus does not invade the nucleus pulposus. HSE brain atrophy due to HSE occurs mostly in the advanced stages of the disease as secondary progressive brain atrophy, and extensive brain softening may also occur. Neurosyphilis has a slower onset than HSE and often presents with mild temporal lobe atrophy. The brain parenchymal type of neurosyphilis has an abnormal high signal intensity in the medial temporal lobe on T_2WI, which is one of its characteristic manifestations. A combination of laboratory tests and imaging findings can help in the differential diagnosis of the two.
3. **Intracranial gliomas, tuberculomas, metastases**. The gliomas are more commonly seen at the gray-white matter junction and are highly invasive, which have a heavier occupying effect than the syphilitic dendritic type, whereas the solitary intracranial syphilitic dendritic neurosyphilis is usually located in the cerebral convexity of the gray matter and has a lighter occupying effect. Tuberculoma is multiple, with nodular enhancement on enhanced scans, characterized by the "target sign"; syphiloma shows massive or nodular hypodensity on CT with mild surrounding edema, and a few lesions may show nodular or circumferential enhancement, while MRI is similar to tuberculoma, with nodular enhancement on enhanced scans. It is difficult to distinguish between the two based on imaging alone, but the combination of clinical history of infection can provide an important basis for differentiation. Multiple intracranial syphilitic dendritic neurosyphilis is mostly associated with thickening and intensification of adjacent meninges, mostly originating from the meninges and closely related to the meninges, and the margins of the lesions often intersect the surrounding meninges at an obtuse angle, whereas tuberculomas are mostly located in the brain parenchyma and do not appear to intersect the meninges at an obtuse angle, which can also be a point of differentiation; metastases show multiple necrosis, located at the gray-white matter junction and appear to have extensive meningeal enhancement and nodules are rarely seen, which is not difficult to differentiate when combined with the primary history.
4. **Degenerative brain atrophy (Parkinson's disease, Alzheimer's disease)**. Degenerative brain atrophy has a relatively older age of onset and is generally symmetrical brain atrophy; neurosyphilitic brain atrophy is diffuse and is atrophy of some specific structures, especially the medial temporal lobe, and is thought to be characteristic of paralytic dementia. Paralytic dementia clinically presents with cognitive decline and memory loss, while MRI shows significant temporal lobe atrophy. Dementia caused by syphilis needs to be differentiated from dementia caused by Parkinson's disease and Alzheimer's disease.
5. Tuberculous meningitis. It occurs more frequently at the base of the skull and is often an early lesion. Mycobacterium tuberculosis invades the skull through the blood circulation and deposits first on the soft meninges and ventricular meninges at the base of the skull, causing an inflammatory reaction in the meninges through an immune response, with edema and massive exudate appearing at an early stage, with the exudate mainly accumulating in the suprasellar pool. The CT and MRI manifestations of syphilitic meningitis are similar to those of other meningitis; the MRI manifestations of different clinical phenotypes of neurosyphilis have some overlap and lack specificity; their basic manifestations mainly include brain atrophy, encephalitis, meningitis, cerebral infarction, multiple ischemic foci, and other changes; and multiple lesions can coexist. Neurosyphilis presents with symmetric or asymmetric high signal in the temporal lobe bilaterally, and cranial MRI in patients with syphilitic meningitis shows enlarged ventricles, with linear enhancement of the meninges seen on early enhanced scans. Magnetic resonance angiography (MRA) exhibits

varying degrees of vascular changes, from local stenosis to occlusion. Combined with the clinical history, positive syphilis can be identified when found with the above imaging findings. Tuberculous meningitis, in which the meningeal reinforcement accumulates mainly in the suprasellar pool, is not characterized by syphilitic meningitis and can be differentiated by a history of tuberculosis or syphilis infection.

9.3.6 Status and Progress of Research

1. MRS is less useful in the diagnosis of neurosyphilis. The region of interest (ROI) mainly shows a decrease in both NAA peak and Cho peak compared with normal sites; Cho/NAA is about 1.18, suggesting neuronal damage and loss, but not specific.
2. Magnetic resonance arterial spin labeling (ASL) is a method for obtaining relatively clear images of cerebral vascular perfusion without contrast injection and can obtain whole brain CBF values. Li J. et al. [24] demonstrated that the CBF values of frontal, parietal, and temporal lobes were higher in patients with neurosyphilis than in the control group, with the most lesions occurring in the frontal and temporal lobes, and the involved sites were mainly located in the distribution of blood supply to the anterior cerebral artery and middle cerebral artery, significantly more than in the distribution of vertebral-basilar artery, considering that it may be related to the vertebral-basilar artery system which only accounts for 1/5 of the whole brain blood supply. In addition, spontaneous brain activity in neurosyphilis patients at rest is also significantly different from normal [25], indirectly suggesting that TP invades the central nervous system and affects the whole brain.

The damage of syphilis to the brain is a dynamic process; by reviewing the patient's routine cranial MRI and ASL, it was found that the CBF value was increased, and the CBF value decreased after treatment, suggesting that the encephalitis caused by the TP infection disappeared and showed a trend of improvement, corresponding to the patient. The CBF value decreased, and the CBF value did not change after treatment, suggesting ischemic infarction in this area and finally brain atrophy; the CBF value increased, and the CBF value continued to increase and then decreased after treatment. This suggests that the inflammatory response in the brain did not decrease and tended to worsen, and finally the inflammation in the brain disappeared and tended to improve. Therefore, comparing the change in CBF values before and after treatment can be used as a reference to evaluate the treatment effect.

The CBF value of ASL also enables earlier detection of cerebral perfusion alterations than MRI, providing an important basis for early diagnosis and treatment of neurosyphilis.

9.4 Hand, Foot, and Mouth Disease Complicating Brainstem Encephalitis

Li Li and Yupeng Liu

9.4.1 Overview

Hand-foot-mouth disease (HFMD) is an acute infectious disease caused by enteroviruses, with coxsackievirus A group 16 (Cox A16) and enterovirus 71 (EV71) infections the most common. The clinical manifestations are typically rashes, herpes, or ulcers on the skin and mucous membranes of the hands, feet, and mouth, with most symptoms being mild and self-limited. Some EV71 infections can cause central nervous system complications such as aseptic meningitis, encephalomyelitis, and even brainstem encephalitis.

EV71 is a highly neurotropic virus that is most likely to infect the brainstem, causing brainstem encephalitis and neurogenic pulmonary edema, leading to rapid progression and deterioration of the child's condition and death in severe cases. Huang et al. [26] classify brainstem encephalitis into three classes according to the severity of neurological clinical symptoms. Grade I presents with myocardial tremor and ataxia, leaving permanent neurological sequelae in 5% of children; Grade II presents with myocardial tremor and cerebral nerve involvement, leaving sequelae in 20% of children; Grade III presents with rapid cardiopulmonary failure, killing 80% of children and leaving severe sequelae in survivors. Studies have shown that vomiting, tachycardia, hypertension, and dysphagia are important signs of abnormal brainstem function. Laboratory test results exhibit increase in peripheral blood leukocyte count and blood glucose, early hypersensitivity of C-reactive protein, and increased cell count and elevated protein in cerebrospinal fluid examination. EV71 or Cox A16 viruses and other enteroviruses causing HFMD can be isolated from cerebrospinal fluid; specific nucleic acid tests are positive, and serum-neutralizing antibodies can increase fourfold or more in the recovery phase than in the acute phase.

9.4.2 Pathological Manifestations

The pathogenesis of HFMD complicated by encephalitis is an acute demyelinating lesion induced by direct viral infection and post-viral infection, which manifests early as limited or diffuse edema of brain tissue, degenerative necrosis of neuronal cells, glial cell proliferation, inflammatory cell infiltration, and later formation of softening foci reflecting irreversible destruction of brain tissue [27].

Experimental animal studies have shown that EV71 can spread along damaged or degenerated synapses along brain nerves or peripheral nerves [28]. After invading the central nervous system, EV71 mainly invades the gray matter of the spinal cord, the dorsal vagal nucleus of the medulla oblongata, the nucleus of the isolated fasciculus and the reticular system, as well as the hypothalamus and the dentate nucleus of the cerebellum [28].

9.4.3 Imaging

Brainstem encephalitis caused by EV71 has its specific site of predilection, mainly pontine and medulla oblongata. MRI is the examination of choice to visualize the site, extent, and degree of lesions and to monitor their progression and regression. In addition, MRI manifestations are closely associated with HFMD complicating the pathological development of encephalitis. In the early stage of the lesion, it shows neuronal degeneration and inflammatory cell infiltration, which is not obvious in T_1WI, and slightly high signal in T_2WI (Fig. 9.4), or normal in flat scan with mild enhancement. Most lesions are reversible at this time. Neuronal necrosis may appear in the progressive stage of the lesion, with low signal in T_1WI, significant high signal intensity in T_2WI with clear borders, high signal intensity in both FLAIR and DWI, and indistinct occupancy effect. In some cases, the brainstem atrophies and thinning in the later stages and the central brainstem cavity formation are observed. For the diagnosis of patients with suspected HFMD complicating encephalitis, a thin layer sagittal scan should be performed after the enhanced MRI scan to improve the detection rate.

Huang et al. [26] ranked 17 cases of brainstem encephalitis exhibiting T_2WI brainstem high signal in order of susceptibility to involvement, in the order of the pontine tegmentum (72%), medulla oblongata (55%), midbrain (44%), and dentate nucleus (22%); the more severe the symptoms, the more extensive the involvement, which is called rhombencephalitis because of the absence of abnormal signal and enhancement of the supratentorial brain tissue. Chen F et al. [29] classified brainstem encephalitis into two types based on the imaging findings as follows: type I, limited lesion involving predominantly gray matter nuclei, mostly symmetrically distributed, with or without anterior horn damage of the spinal cord; type II, which presents with a vague patch of slightly low T_1W and slightly high T_2W signal intensity in the posterior part of the brainstem and is more widespread. The follow-up study found that children with type II exhibiting focal long T_1 and long T_2 relaxation time lesions with vague patches in the brainstem had a better prognosis than children with posterior brainstem. The prognosis of type I children with unilateral or bilateral limited punctate hypointense T_1 and hyperintense T_2 signal intensity was better than that of type II children with unilateral or bilateral punctate. It is speculated that this may be related to the less severe damage.

HFMD with simple encephalitis is less common, and brainstem encephalitis with concomitant thalamic and cerebellar dentate nucleus involvement is more common. Bu Chunqing et al. [30] reported that lesions located in the brainstem are mostly bilateral, symmetrical, and patchy, thalamic lesions are speckled or small, basal ganglia lesions are mostly speckled abnormal signal, and lesions in the white matter area of the brain are mostly multiple punctate abnormal signals, which may be considered to be related to the

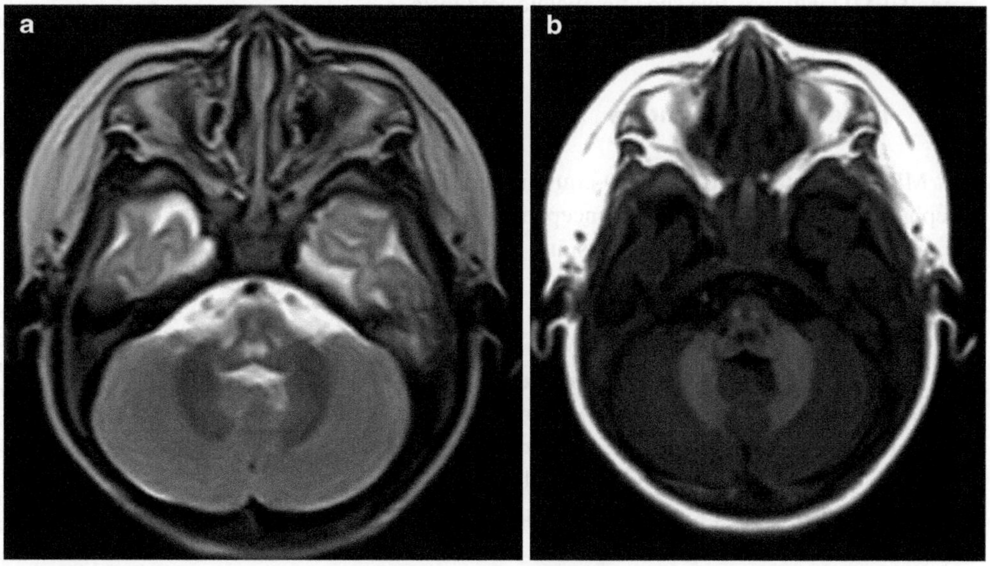

Fig. 9.4 Hand, foot, and mouth disease complicating brainstem encephalitis. Axial brain MR images shows low signal intensity on T1WI (**b**) and high signal intensity on T2WI (**a**) in brainstem (请把病灶位置标号出来) with clear borders; DWI shows slightly high signal intensity and mildly decreased ADC values. (Image courtesy of Laoqun of Hangzhou Children's Hospital)

route of viral invasion, the intensity of virulence, and the different responses to viral invasion in different sites.

HFMD with brainstem encephalitis is often accompanied by myelitis, MRI mainly shows a low T_1WI and high T_2WI signal intensity involving multiple vertebral segments with blurred borders and no obvious occupancy effect. Zeng et al. [31] reported brainstem encephalitis with cervical medullary transverse myelitis as a critical sign, MRI showed diffuse swelling of the cervical medulla with a slightly low T_1WI and high T_2WI signal intensity with simultaneous gray and white matter involvement, poorly demarcated, and contiguous with abnormal medullary signal.

9.4.4 Diagnostic Key Points

1. The main clinical manifestation is the appearance of maculopapular rash and herpes on the hands, feet, and mouth.
2. Complications such as aseptic meningitis, encephalomyelitis, and even brainstem encephalitis occur as a result of involvement of the central nervous system. Unilateral or bilateral cerebral nerve involvement manifested as ophthalmoplegia, dysphagia, ataxia, myoclonus, and limb movement or sensory disorders, and in severe cases, there is a rapid onset of respiratory failure.
3. HFMD-complicated encephalitis occurs in the brainstem (midbrain, pons, or medulla oblongata) and is commonly associated with involvement of the thalamus and dentate nucleus of the cerebellum. Brainstem lesions tend to be bilaterally symmetrical patchy, thalamic lesions are speckled or small, basal ganglia lesions tend to be speckled with abnormal signal, and lesions in the white matter areas of the brain tend to be multiple punctate with abnormal signal.
4. Laboratory tests. Cerebrospinal fluid can be isolated from EV71 or Cox A16 viruses and other enteroviruses causing HFMD with positive specific nucleic acid tests.

9.4.5 Differential Diagnosis

The MRI presentation of HFMD-complicated brainstem encephalitis is similar to other viral encephalitis, but the clinical manifestations and the site of lesions are different and therefore need to be differentiated.

1. **Epidemic B encephalitis**. The lesions are mostly located in the basal ganglia and thalamus and develop symmetrically to both sides; there are seasonal, regional, and epidemiological features such as seasonal, regional, cyclical, and childhood prevalence, and the incubation period can be followed by the epidemiological features of the disease which include seasonal, regional, cyclical, and childhood epidemics.
2. **Measles virus encephalitis and mumps virus encephalitis**. The lesions are mostly located in the basal ganglia and thalamus and symmetrical to both sides. Patients usually have the history of corresponding measles and mumps.
3. **Herpes simplex virus encephalitis and herpes zoster virus encephalitis**. Along the olfactory and trigeminal nerves, herpes simplex virus causes bilateral anterior middle temporal lobe lesions; herpes zoster virus invades the skull along the facial nerve and causes bilateral temporal lobe lesions. Herpes simplex virus encephalitis and herpes zoster virus encephalitis present with recurrent, more painful herpes rashes around the mouth, face, and ears, respectively, followed by neurologic symptoms.

9.4.6 Status and Progress of Research

Chen F et al. [32] concluded that staging the imaging manifestations of HFMD complicated by encephalitis can help determine the prognosis. The prognosis was significantly better in the fuzzy lesion border type than in the clearer type. In addition, the prognosis of patients with single-site lesions in brainstem encephalitis due to EV71 infection is better than that of patients with multiple lesions or combined AFP [33]. DWI is more sensitive than conventional magnetic resonance imaging sequences in detecting EV71 encephalitis in the acute phase, and when cytotoxic brain edema occurs, DWI shows high signal intensity and significantly lower ADC values.

References

1. Zhang L, Zhou X. Modern epidemiology. Page 2 version. Beijing: The People's Army Medical Press; 2010.
2. Awasthi M, Parmar H, Patankar T, et al. Imaging findings in rabies encephalitis. Am J Neuroradiol. 2001;4(22):677–80.
3. Desai RV, Jain V, Singh P, et al. Radiculomyelitic rabies: can MR imaging help? Am J Neuroradiol. 2002;4(23):632–4.
4. Huang C, Su J-L, Cheng H-C, et al. Observation of the persistence of immunity after rabies exposure using the "2-1-1" procedure for human rabies vaccination (Vero cells) 3 years and the effect of 2 doses of booster immunization. Chin J Dis Control. 2019;23(5):607–12.
5. Franco MP, Mulder M, Smits HL, et al. Human brucellosis. Lancet Infect Dis. 2007;7(12):775–86.
6. Ozkavukcu E, Tuncay Z, Selçuk F, et al. An unusual case of neurobrucellosis presenting with unilateral abducens nerve palsy: clinical and MRI findings. Diagn Interv Radiol. 2009;15:236–8.
7. Liu T, Xie S. Neurobrucellosis imaging presentation 1 example. Med Imaging Technol China. 2018;34(9):1439. 1440
8. Cao Y, Fan S, Yao M, et al. Analysis of seven cases of neurological brucellosis with cerebrovascular disease as the main manifestation. Chin J Neurol. 2019;52(4):298–303.

9. Wu P, Zhang Y, Guo H, et al. Diagnostic value of diffusion tensor imaging for spinal neurotypical brucellosis spondylitis. Chin J Endem Dis. 2019;38(3):193–8.
10. Wang N, Zhang XY, Zhang WQ, et al. New advances in the diagnosis and treatment of neurosyphilis. Chin J Mod Neurol Dis. 2016;16(7):397–403.
11. Das S, Kalyan A, Garg K, et al. A case of very early neurosyphilis presented as schizophrenia-like psychosis. Asian J Psychiatr. 2018;31(92):93.
12. Nagappa M, Sinha S, Taly AB, et al. Neurosyphilis: MRI features and their phenotypic correlation in a cohort of 35 patients from a tertiary care university hospital. Neuroradiology. 2013;4(55):379–88.
13. Good CD, Jager HR. Contrast enhancement of the cerebrospinal fluid on MRI in two cases of spirochaetal meningitis. Neuroradiology. 2000;42(6):448–50.
14. Kou C, Xu D, Gao J, et al. Clinical analysis of 20 cases of neurosyphilis patients with cranial nerve involvement as the main manifestation. Chin J Exp Clin Infect Dis. 2019;13(2):172–6.
15. Zhao X, Hou X. Neurosyphilis with multiple cranial nerve damage as the first symptom 1 case report. J Neurol Neurorehabilit. 2004;1(3):157–61.
16. Cao J, Li J, Xiao X, et al. Neurosyphilis with multiple groups of cranial nerve damage as the first symptom 1 case report. J Stroke Neurol Disord. 2018;35(2):176, 177.
17. Li L, Wang J. Syphilitic optic neuritis 12 clinical analysis of cases. Chin J Mod Neurol Dis. 2016;16(7):416–23.
18. Schmidley JW. 10 questions on central nervous system vasculitis. Neurologist. 2008;14(2):138, 139.
19. Liu RW, Fang JZ, Zhang YZ. Analysis of MRI manifestations of meningeal vascular type neurosyphilis. Electron J Emerg Infect Dis. 2018;3(1):25–9.
20. Escobar-Valdivia E, Medina-Piñón I, García-Sarreon A. Concomitant neurosyphilis and herpes simplex encephalitis in an immunocompetent patient: a case report. Neurol Sci. 2018;39(1):185–7.
21. Kodana K, Okada S, Komatsu N, et al. Relationship between MRI findings and prognosis for patients with general paresis. J Neuropsychiatry Clin Neurosci. 2000;12(2):246–9.
22. Serrano-Cardenas KM, Sánchez-Rodriguez A, Pozueta A, et al. Mesial encephalitis: an uncommon presentation of neurosyphilis: a case report and review of the literature. Neurol Sci. 2018;39(1):173–6.
23. Hobbs E, Vera JH, Marks M, et al. Neurosyphilis in patients with HIV. Pract Neurol. 2018;18(3):211–8.
24. Li J, Ye J, Zhang H. Neurosyphilis MRI manifestations and perfusion studies. Chin J Med Imaging. 2019;27(1):25–8.
25. Bi J, Wang H, Yu Y. Resting state fMRI evaluation of functional changes in neurosyphilic brain. Med Imaging Technol China. 2015;32(4):523–6.
26. Huang CC, Liu CC, Chang YC, et al. Neurologic complications in children with enterovirus 71 infection. N Engl J Med. 1999;341(13):936–42.
27. Lim CC, Lee KE, Lee WL, et al. Nipah virus encephalitis: serial MR study of an emerging disease. Radiology. 2002;222(11):219–26.
28. Wong KT, Munisamy B, Ong KC, et al. The distribution of inflammation and virus in human enterovirus 71 encephalomyelitis suggests possible viral spread by neural pathways. J Neuropathol Exp Neurol. 2008;67(2):162–9.
29. Chen F, Li J, Liu T, et al. Enterovirus type 71 infection of hand, foot and mouth disease combined with brainstem encephalitis MRI characteristics and mechanism discussion. J Chongqing Med Univ. 2011;36(9):1097–100.
30. Bu C, Di Y, Wang J, et al. MRI manifestations and features of enterovirus 71 infection of hand, foot and mouth disease combined with encephalitis. J Med Imaging. 2012;22(8):1234–6.
31. Zeng H, Wen F, Gan Y, et al. MRI and associated clinical characteristics of EV71-induced brainstem encephalitis in children with hand-foot- mouth disease. Neuroradiology. 2012;54(6):623–30.
32. Chen F, Li J, Liu T, et al. Enterovirus type 71 infection of hand, foot and mouth disease combined with neurological system uniform impairment of MRI manifestation. Chin J Radiol. 2010;44(9):946–9.
33. Chen F, Liu T, Li J, et al. MRI characteristics and follow-up findings in patients with neurological complications of enterovirus 71-related hand, foot, and mouth disease. Int J Clin Exp Med. 2014;7(9):2696–704.

10 AIDS-Related Intracranial Infections (Blood-Borne Infection-Associated Intracranial Infections)

Yongxiao You, Lulu Liu, Shui Wang, Jian Wang, Xingbo Liu, Yanling Zhou, Kang Li, Qiang Liu, Xiaodan Du, Yibanu, Min Luo, Jinying Wang, Yuxin Yang, Aniwar Ulam, and Xin Gao

AIDS, or acquired immunodeficiency syndrome, is caused by the human immunodeficiency virus (HIV), which was first reported in the United States in 1981. HIV infection has spread almost globally and has become a worldwide problem that poses a serious threat to human health.

Approximately 73–80% of patients with AIDS have central nervous system involvement, which can present with neurological symptoms involving the brain, spinal cord, and peripheral nerves and muscles, the vast majority of which are caused by infection, including direct invasion of the central nervous system by HIV (a neurotropic virus), or by immunodeficiency opportunistic infections. The latter includes a wide range of bacterial, viral, fungal, and parasitic infections secondary to AIDS, with the risk of most infections occurring positively correlated with CD4+ T cell counts, including toxoplasma infections, cytomegalovirus infections, progressive multifocal leukoencephalopathy (JC viral infections), *Mycobacterium tuberculosis* infections, cryptococcal infections, syphilis, etc.

HIV-associated encephalitis can occur at any age but is more common in young and middle-aged patients, followed by infants (mother-to-child transmission), and can occur at any stage of infection, but mainly in the late AIDS phase. The most prominent clinical manifestation is progressive dementia, hence named AIDS dementia syndrome. It is characterized by diminished mental capacity; cognitive, motor, and behavioral dysfunction; and in some cases, hemiplegia, paraplegia, or seizures. In addition, it is often accompanied by cerebral nerve palsy, and involvement of the fifth, seventh, or eighth pair of cerebral nerves is common.

AIDS-related neurological infections are more common with intracranial infections and are increasingly receiving high attention from clinicians in neurology and related disciplines because of their high morbidity and mortality. However, diagnosis is extremely challenging due to the wide variety of pathogens. And neuroimaging, as the most important adjunct, plays a large role in the identification process.

10.1 Human Immunodeficiency Virus-Related Encephalitis

Yongxiao You, Lulu Liu, Shui Wang, and Jian Wang

Y. You
Beijing Shunyi Maternal and Child Health Hospital, Beijing, China

L. Liu · J. Wang · Yibanu · X. Gao
Medical Imaging Center, First Affiliated Hospital of Xinjiang Medical University, Urumqi, China

J. Wang (✉)
Medical Imaging Center, First Affiliated Hospital of Xinjiang Medical University, Urumqi, China

Shanghai Universal Medical Imaging Diagnostic Center, Shanghai University, Shanghai, China

S. Wang
Beijing Children's Hospital Xinjiang Hospital, Beijing, China

X. Liu
Xinjiang Bortala Mongolian Autonomous Prefecture People's Hospital, Bole, China

Y. Zhou
Xiaolan People's Hospital, Southern Medical University, Zhongshan, China

K. Li
Chongqing Hospital, University of Chinese Academy of Sciences, Chongqing, China

Q. Liu
Shandong Provincial Hospital, Jinan, China

X. Du
Zhuhai Hospital of Integrated Traditional Chinese and Western Medicine, Zhuhai, China

M. Luo
Zigong Fourth People's Hospital, Zigong, China

Y. Yang
The Sixth People's Hospital of Xinjiang Uygur Autonomous Region, Urumqi, China

A. Ulam
The Eight Affiliated Hospital of Xinjiang Medical University, Urumqi, China

H. Li et al. (eds.), *Radiology of Infectious and Inflammatory Diseases - Volume 1*,
https://doi.org/10.1007/978-981-99-0039-8_10

10.1.1 Overview

Intracranial HIV primary infections refer to diseases that cause brain damage from HIV direct infection of the central nervous system, including HIV-associated encephalitis and AIDS-associated aseptic meningitis. HIV is a neurotropic virus that can be phagocytosed by macrophages and infects the central nervous system directly through the blood-brain barrier, and central nervous system infection is one of the main causes of increased mortality from AIDS. HIV can cause a range of neurological syndromes and peripheral vascular diseases, as well as demyelinating diseases of the central and peripheral nervous systems.

Human immunodeficiency virus encephalitis (HIVE) is a direct infection of the central nervous system by HIV causing brain damage and corresponding psychoneurological symptoms, also known as AIDS encephalopathy. The main clinical manifestation is dementia, hence named AIDS dementia syndrome. A direct consequence of AIDS damage to the central nervous system is HIV-associated encephalitis, which is three times more prevalent than opportunistic infections and ultimately leads to AIDS dementia syndrome. HIV-associated encephalitis is an infection caused by direct invasion of the brain by HIV, which accounts for 34–47% of neurological complications and is not an opportunistic infection.

Recent studies have concluded that the primary mechanism of CNS damage from HIV is widespread immune activation and inflammatory response and that HIV-associated encephalitis occurs primarily in the late AIDS phase. The pathogenesis includes the following: (1) HIV infects the vascular endothelial cells of the nervous system, causing damage to the blood-brain barrier; (2) HIV infects macrophages and microglia, which have toxic effects and indirectly damage nerves; (3) HIV induces autoimmune reactions; (4) and children with AIDS have underdeveloped autoimmune systems and are more vulnerable to HIV infection. The disease may develop acutely but is more common in the late stages of HIV infection and can be divided into two types: acute and chronic, both with headache and signs of meningeal irritation, but meningeal irritation is common in the acute form with cerebral nerve palsy, and nerve involvement is common in pairs V, VII, or VIII. The main clinical symptoms are brain atrophy and progressive dementia. Patients usually present with weakness and loss of libido and later develop incontinence, progressive dementia, and confusion. Some patients may develop hemiplegia, paraplegia, or seizures due to diffuse microglial nodules and glial cell proliferation in the gray matter and white matter of the brain and perivascular demyelination in the white matter. HIV-specific antibody test is positive after 2–6 weeks of infection, and HIV P24 antigen can be detected in the early stage, but only as an auxiliary diagnosis; HIV can be isolated from cerebrospinal fluid; CD4 T lymphocyte count and function are reduced in immune function test; and the ratio of CD4 T lymphocytes to CD8 T lymphocytes is reduced.

10.1.2 Pathological Manifestations

The pathology is characterized by scattered distribution of microglial nodules, multinucleated giant cell infiltrates, large white matter sparseness, demyelination, and cerebral atrophy changes in cerebral white and gray matter.

HIV enters the brain parenchyma via macrophage carriage or directly infects endothelial cells into the brain, and the target organs are mainly macrophages and microglia, less frequently invading neuronal cells [1]. But HIV accumulates in glial cells or perivascular macrophages and produces HIV protein that causes abnormal oxidative stress, impairs cellular activity, disrupts tight junctions in endothelial cells, and leads to neuronal cell damage and apoptosis.

Brain tissue may be normal on gross observation or may be markedly atrophied, especially in the frontal and temporal lobes, with dilated ventricles and reduced total brain parenchyma seen in advanced stages. HIV first invades the white matter of the brain, followed by the basal ganglia, gray matter, brainstem, and cerebellum, and may also show brain atrophy changes, and in severe cases, large patches of brain tissue may develop necrosis. Light microscopy showed HIV-associated encephalitis with predominance of nodular encephalitis and multinucleated giant cell encephalitis. Nodular encephalitis manifests as microglial cell proliferation aggregating to form small nodules, and widely distributed microglial nodular infiltrates are seen within the lesion, which is characteristic of HIV-associated encephalitis. Multinucleated giant cell encephalitis presents as multinucleated giant cell infiltration in brain tissue. The pathological diagnosis of HIV-associated encephalitis is based on microglial cell nodules and multinucleated giant cell infiltrates with scattered focal demyelination and vacuolar degeneration seen in the involved cerebral white matter. Patients with thrombocytopenia may manifest with hemorrhage.

10.1.3 Imaging

10.1.3.1 CT Findings

CT may not show any significant abnormalities. The majority of cases show lamellar hypodensity in the white matter of the brain bilaterally, which may involve multiple lobes and basal ganglia, mostly in the periventricular and cutaneous medullary junction areas, with brain tissue edema in the early stages, mostly without obvious occupying effects, and no abnormal enhancement on enhanced scans [2]. The lesion may have a dominant effect when it is large or combined with other complications. In the middle and late stages, there is mainly a reduction in total brain tissue, with predominantly gray matter involvement, often with diffuse brain atrophy changes (Fig. 10.1). Calcifications in the basal ganglia are seen in about 1/3 of children with neonatal HIV-associated encephalitis.

10.1.3.2 MRI Findings

MR may show no significant abnormalities. In typical cases, MRI shows diffuse or patchy abnormal signal in the deep white matter of the periventricular and centrum ovale areas, which may involve the basal ganglia, brainstem, and cerebellum. The lesion manifests as hypointense on T_1WI and hyperintense on T_2WI with unclear borders, and the early occupying effect is not obvious. The enhanced scan presents no obvious abnormal enhancement, which should be considered as a combined opportunistic infection if abnormal enhancement occurs. The lesions often involve both sides but are mostly asymmetrical and may fuse. There may be limited or diffuse brain atrophy in the mid to late stages. The imaging changes of the lesions located in the periventricular white matter are similar to those of subcortical atherosclerotic encephalopathy, whereas subcortical atherosclerosis is associated with hypertension and older age of onset, and the presence of AIDS can be differentiated from it (Fig. 10.2).

10.1.4 Diagnostic Key Points

1. HIV-associated encephalitis occurs in young and middle-aged people, with the main clinical manifestations being progressive dementia and motor dysfunction.
2. Multiple patchy lesions in the periventricular or deep white matter area, which can be fused, mostly without obvious edema and occupying effects, with hypodense on CT scan, hypointense on MR T_1WI scan, and hyperintense on T_2WI, without significant abnormal enhancement on enhanced scan, which can be accompanied by focal or whole brain atrophy, with predominant gray matter involvement.
3. The imaging presentation can be unremarkable, but most patients show diffuse brain atrophy with multiple patchy lesions in the deep cerebral white matter or around the ventricles as the main feature.
4. HIV can be isolated from cerebrospinal fluid in laboratory tests, and the confirmation of the diagnosis is based on brain biopsy, and the pathological diagnosis is mainly based on the presence of microglia nodules and multinucleated giant cell infiltration in brain tissue.

10.1.5 Differential Diagnosis

HIV-associated encephalitis should be distinguished from cytomegalovirus encephalitis (CE), AIDS-combined progressive multifocal leukoencephalopathy (PML), subacute spongiform encephalopathy (SSE), and subacute sclerosing panencephalitis (SSPE).

10.1.5.1 Cytomegalovirus Encephalitis (CE)

Both cytomegalovirus encephalitis and HIV-associated encephalitis can be caused by congenital in utero infection or acquired infection. The pathology of cytomegalovirus encephalitis is characterized by microglial nodules involving

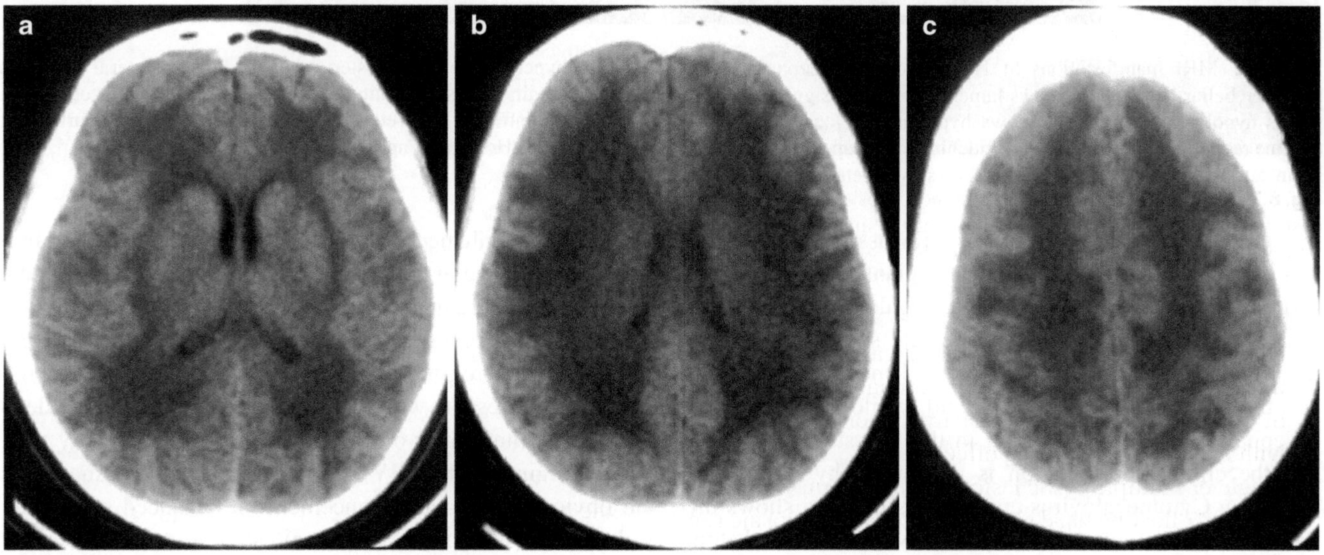

Fig. 10.1 CT findings of HIV-associated encephalitis. (**a–c**) CT plain scan shows symmetrical large patchy hypodensities in the white matter of the brain around the lateral ventricles bilaterally, mostly in the periventricular white matter and cutaneous medullary junction area

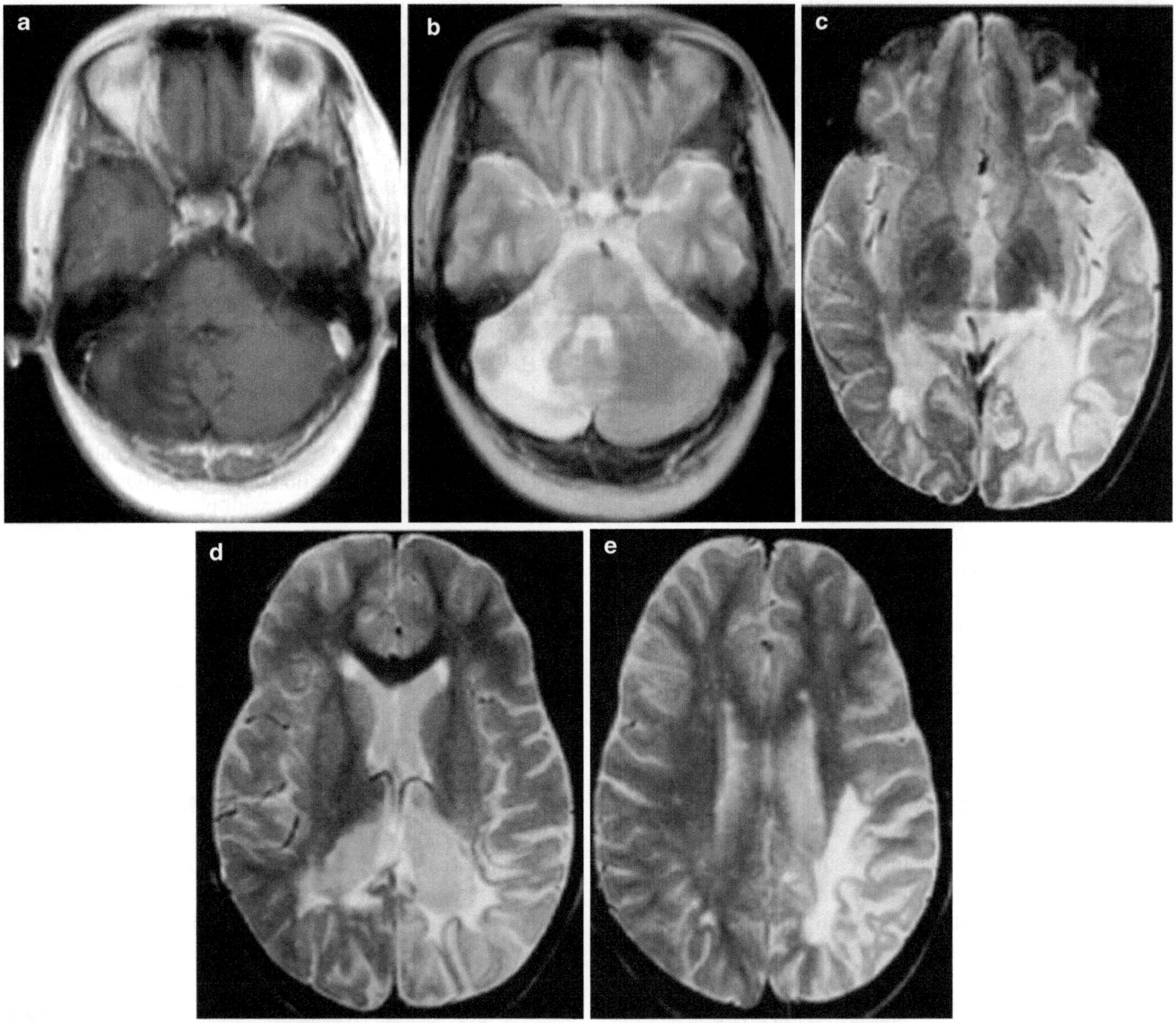

Fig. 10.2 MRI manifestations of HIV-associated encephalitis. The right cerebellar hemisphere shows lamellar abnormal signal. (**a**) T_1WI shows hypointense; (**b**) T_2WI shows hyperintense, local brain tissue volume reduction, and brain sulcus widening and deepening, indicating brain atrophy changes; (**c–e**) T_2WI shows symmetrical cap-like and lamellar hyperintense in the posterior horn of bilateral lateral ventricles and local brain sulcus deepening and widening, and the posterior horn of lateral ventricles is stretched and enlarged. (Image courtesy of Beijing Youan Hospital, Capital Medical University)

the cortex, whereas the pathology of HIV associated encephalitis is characterized by multinucleated giant cell infiltration in addition to microglial nodules. Cytomegalovirus encephalitis is usually characterized by neurological symptoms such as fever, lethargy, coma, convulsions, and motor disturbances, and the onset of the disease is rapid, while HIV-associated encephalitis is most often seen in the late stages of AIDS, and the clinical presentation is dominated by progressive dementia. Cytomegalovirus encephalitis imaging shows diffuse or limited foci in the brain parenchyma distributed along the cerebral vascular pathways, and enhanced scans often show diffuse enhancement of the ventricular canal. Cerebral atrophy, ventricular enlargement, and calcifications in the brain parenchyma are seen in congenitally infected individuals, and intracerebral calcifications are most common in the periventricular region. In contrast, HIV-associated encephalitis mostly presents with multiple patchy lesions in the deep cerebral white matter or around the ventricles, mostly with diffuse brain atrophy. HIV-associated encephalitis usually has no obvious abnormal enhancement on enhanced scans, and calcification is rare. The two manifestations are different and can be distinguished from each other.

10.1.5.2 AIDS Combined with Progressive Multifocal Leukoencephalopathy (PML)

It is more common in adults, while HIV-associated encephalitis develops at a younger age and can also occur in newborns. AIDS combined with PML presents with focal motor sensory deficits, while HIV-associated encephalitis presents mainly with cognitive deficits and dementia, and the clinical presentation of these two diseases is important to confirm the diagnosis. The pathological basis of AIDS combined with PML is demyelination and white matter necrosis, and HIV-associated encephalitis is mainly glial cell nodule formation. The lesions of AIDS combined with PML are mainly distributed in the parieto-occipital and frontal lobes, asymmetrical, progressively enlarged and fused, and located mainly in the subcortical white matter, mostly far from the periventricles, while the lesions of HIV-associated encephalitis are distributed in the deep white matter area, and the periventricular area is also a prone site, but there is little difference between density and signal of the two lesions, and there is no significant abnormal enhancement of the lesions after the enhanced scan. It is difficult to identify the two in the early stage. The confirmed diagnosis depends on pathological biopsy. The pathological changes of AIDS combined with PML are inclusion bodies in oligodendrocytes, lacto-polypoid virus particles can be seen on electron microscopy, and immunohistochemistry can confirm the presence of lacto-polypoid virus antigens, while the pathological changes of HIV-associated encephalitis are mainly microglia nodules and multinucleated giant cell infiltration in brain tissue. The differentiation between the two needs to be combined with the clinical presentation.

10.1.5.3 Subacute Spongiform Encephalopathy (SSE)

It is a rare sporadic central nervous system disease caused by prion infection. The clinical manifestation is characterized by progressive dementia, ataxia, myoclonus, and characteristic periodic EEG changes. The pathology of SSE is characterized by spongy degeneration of the cerebral cortex, basal ganglia, and cerebellum, with decidual necrosis of neuronal cells, heavy proliferation of glial cells, and pore-like vacuole formation, but no inflammatory changes, whereas the pathology of HIV-associated encephalitis is characterized by microglial nodules and multinucleated giant cell infiltration. SSE imaging shows scattered lamellar lesions in the fronto-temporal lobes and basal ganglia bilaterally, which may be associated with progressive brain atrophy and dementia, whereas the main imaging findings in HIV-associated encephalitis are multiple lesions in the periventricular or deep white matter areas, mostly bilateral, with extensive or limited brain atrophy and rare calcifications. However, typical SSE on T_2WI and DWI is characterized by symmetric abnormal hyperintense in the bilateral basal ganglia region, especially the gyrus-like abnormal hyperintense along the cortical gyrus on DWI. It can be distinguished from HIV-associated encephalitis easily.

10.1.5.4 Subacute Sclerosing Panencephalitis (SSPE)

It is a slowly progressive disease caused by persistent central nervous system infection with a variant of measles virus. SSPE is seen after variant measles virus infection, while HIV-associated encephalitis is seen after HIV infection. The imaging findings of the two diseases are similar, with extensive brain parenchymal atrophy and multiple brain white matter lesions, but the SSPE lesions are mostly symmetrically distributed, whereas the HIV-associated encephalitis lesions are mostly asymmetrical. SSPE often has the typical EEG presentation of episodic multiple high waves per second and biphasic waves simultaneously, whereas HIV-associated encephalitis does not have this EEG presentation. Differentiation between the two requires a combination of clinical history and EEG presentation.

10.1.6 Status and Progress of Research

10.1.6.1 Hydrogen Proton Spectroscopy Imaging (^{1}H-MRS)

It is the only technique currently available for noninvasive observation of in vivo tissue metabolism. HIV-associated encephalitis lesions may show decreased NAA and NAA/Cr values, increased Cho and mI values, increased lipid and lactate peaks in the lesion area, and increased Cho/Cr values in the bilateral basal ganglia area. The gradual decrease and increase in NAA/Cr values in some patients after treatment may provide an imaging basis for assessing patient outcomes.

10.1.6.2 Magnetic Resonance Diffusion-Weighted Imaging (DWI)

DWI sequences may show diffuse or patchy fusion hyperintense in the deep white matter around the lateral ventricles bilaterally.

10.1.6.3 Magnetic Resonance Diffusion Tensor Imaging (DTI)

It is the development and deepening of DWI. Nakamoto et al. [3] found that DTI can suggest microstructural changes associated with abnormal glucose metabolism in the caudate nucleus and hippocampus of HIV-infected patients. Filippi et al. [4] concluded the reduction of anisotropy in white matter and increase of the mean water diffusion rate in the splenium and genu of corpus callosum and frontal and parietal subregions along with increasing viral load, whereas conventional MRI was unable to show differences in these regions. Pomara et al. [5] found that FA values in the frontal white matter abnormally decreased in six HIV-infected patients compared to nine controls. In addition, abnormally elevated values of FA in the internal capsule suggest the breakage or absence of some of the crossed fibers. Inflammatory mechanisms affecting white matter fibers are one of the factors by which HIV infection affects the brain, and these studies provide evidence for this hypothesis. In addition, the DTI study has the potential to provide early information on the eventual development of dementia in individual HIV-infected patients.

10.1.6.4 Magnetic Resonance Perfusion Weighted Imaging (PWI)

Bladowska et al. [6] found reduced rCBV values in the bilateral frontal and temporoparietal cortices of patients with HIV-associated encephalitis and areas of hypoperfusion suggestive of central nervous system damage due to HIV infection. Furthermore, HIV-positive patients treated with combination antiretroviral therapy (cART) have more pronounced perfusion changes (decreased perfusion) than untreated patients, which may be caused by neurotoxicity from antiretroviral drugs or by pretreatment brain damage (HIV infection and high viral load).

CT and MRI are the preferred imaging methods for HIV-associated encephalitis; CT is inexpensive, and MRI can improve the detection rate of microscopic lesions but does not show calcifications as well like CT. In recent years, with the development of new MRI technology, MRI has been widely used in the diagnosis and differential diagnosis of AIDS-related conditions. PET/CT also has some significance in the diagnosis of primary intracranial HIV infection, which can understand the glucose metabolism, pathophysiology, and morphology of the lesion and significantly improve the accuracy of the diagnosis. However, its cost is high and its application value is limited.

10.2 Toxoplasmic Encephalitis

Yongxiao You, Xingbo Liu, and Jian Wang

10.2.1 Overview

Toxoplasmic encephalopathy (TE) is a zoonotic disease caused by toxoplasma infection. The pathogen infects the body via food or water, presents as focal or diffuse necrotizing inflammation, and is one of the most common intracranial infections in AIDS patients, with an incidence rate of 10% to 30% and is a common cause of death in patients with AIDS. AIDS-associated toxoplasmic encephalopathy has a subacute onset and lacks specificity in its clinical and imaging manifestations. Patients may have symptoms of diffuse brain damage such as altered mental status, delusional behavior, fever, headache, drowsiness, or even coma and may die within days or weeks. Meningeal involvement may be associated with meningitis, and the "pseudotumor sign" may be followed by symptoms of transient intracranial hypertension, with imaging resembling a tumor or brain abscess or another occupying lesion. Neuropsychiatric symptoms such as hemiparesis, seizures, visual impairment, confusion, unconsciousness, and seizures are signs of focal neurological impairment of the brainstem and spinal cord; fever and signs of meningeal irritation are less common. Laboratory tests for cerebrospinal fluid smears reveal toxoplasma and positive test results for toxoplasma antibodies (IgG and IgM), circulating antigens (CAg), and specific nucleic acids.

10.2.2 Pathological Manifestations

AIDS-associated toxoplasmic encephalopathy may present as focal or diffuse meningoencephalitis with necrosis and microglial cell nodules. Gross visual observation shows that the patient's brain is swollen, often congested on the surface, locally softened, with foci of necrosis visible on the cut surface [2]. AIDS-associated toxoplasmic encephalopathy can develop acute or chronic inflammatory lesions in the brain. Perivasculitis, inflammatory cell infiltration, and glial cell hyperplasia are seen in milder lesions. In more severe cases, foci of necrosis are seen in the gray and white matter, often multiple, small focal necrosis. The foci of infection are coagulative necrosis, with atypical mononuclear cell inflammatory reactions, patches of lymphocyte and plasma cell infiltration, and less frequent eosinophils, which form granuloma-like structures with proliferating glial cells. It may also form toxoplasmic abscess, a necrotic lesion centered on cellular debris and surrounded by edema and inflammatory brain tissue; the necrotic tissue is surrounded by characteristic comma-like tachyzoites (trophozoites) and multiple pseudocapsules of varying sizes. Abnormal vascular manifestations include perivascular and intravascular mononuclear cell and lymphocyte infiltration, endothelial cell swelling, thrombosis, fibrinoid necrosis of the vessel wall, and occlusion by luminal fibrosis.

10.2.3 Imaging

AIDS-associated toxoplasma encephalopathy can be classified into ventricular, parenchymal, and mixed types depending on the locations of AIDS-associated toxoplasma encephalopathy. The lesions are found in the basal ganglia and the cutaneous medullary junction and may involve the cerebellum, brainstem, ventricles, and posterior cranial fossa. The lesions were mostly bilateral and multiple, and a few were single, with a lesion diameter of 0.4–3.0 cm.

10.2.3.1 CT Findings

CT scan shows multiple hypodense or isodense lesions, single lesions are rare, multiple lesions can be fused into patches, with perifocal edema and occupying effect, often cannot clearly distinguish between infected foci and perifocal edema [7]. Enhanced scans show nodular, ring-like, or ring target-shaped distinctly abnormal enhancement, with ring-like enhancement being more common, and the enhancing ring is often thin and smooth, with irregular thick walls seen in larger lesions (Fig. 10.3). If it occurs in the ventricles, the lesion appears as a dense mass shadow with well-defined margins because of the difference between the density of the cerebrospinal fluid and the density of the lesion.

10.2.3.2 MRI Findings

The detection rate of MRI lesions is significantly higher than that of CT. Lesions are usually found in the basal ganglia, cutaneous medullary junction area, thalamus, and cerebellum and appear as multiple lesions or single lesion. The lesions may manifest as isointense or hypointense on T_1WI and slightly hyperintense on T_2WI (Fig. 10.4a), with distinct perilesion edema and occupying effect may be seen, and the signal between the lesions and perilesion edema is not easy to distinguish. Lesions also can manifest as iso- or hypointense on T_2WI with the perilesion edema manifesting as hyperintense; enhanced scans show nodular, annular, or ring target-like enhancement (Fig. 10.4d). The appearance of circular target-like enhancement is called the "target sign" (the

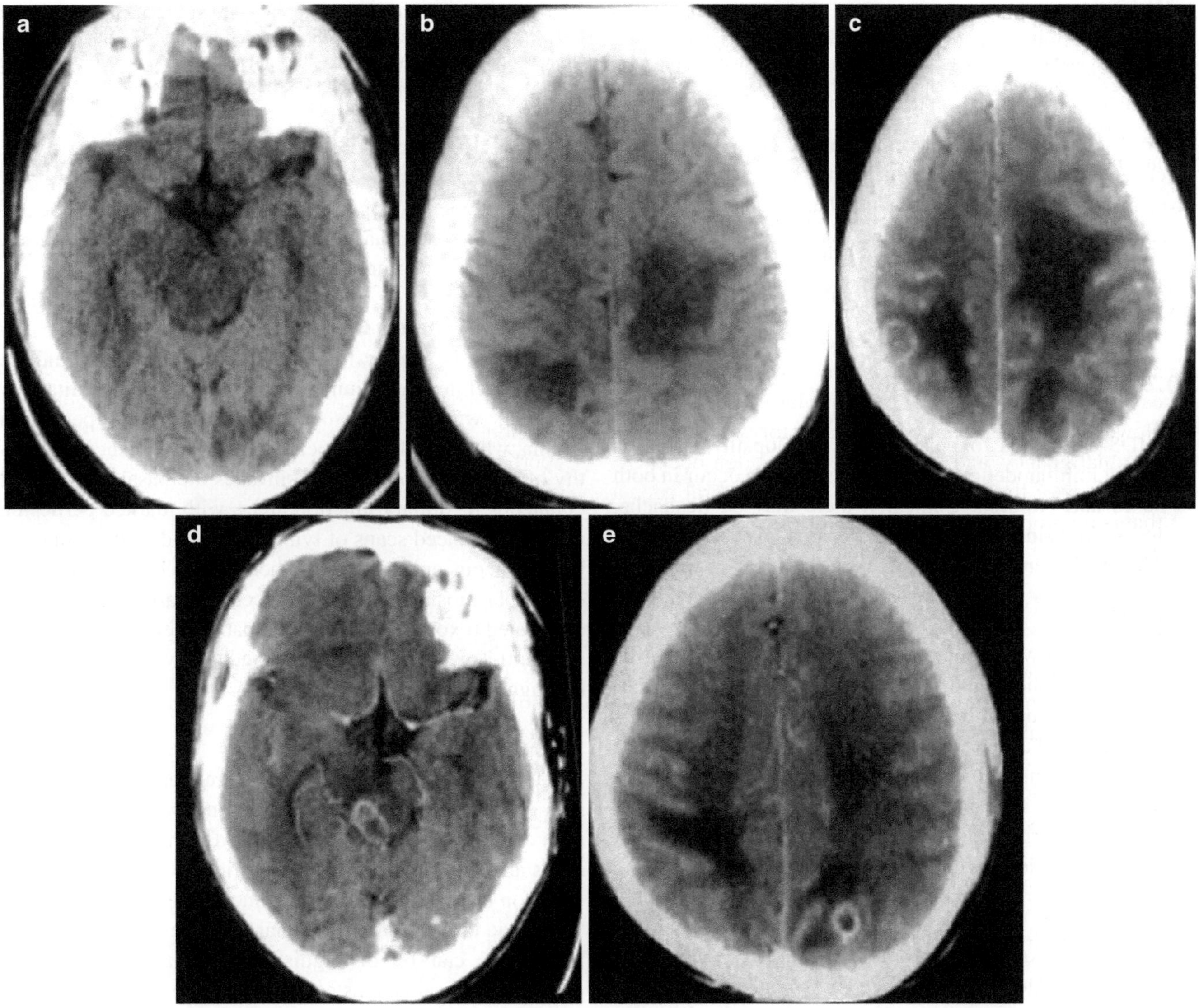

Fig. 10.3 CT presentation of AIDS-associated toxoplasmic encephalopathy. (**a–c**) CT scan shows bilateral parieto-occipital lobe and brainstem patchy hypodense foci with blurred edges; (**d**, **e**) CT enhanced scan shows bilateral occipital lobe and brainstem multiple ring-shaped enhancing foci with surrounding hypodense edema area. (Image courtesy of Professor Li Hongjun of Beijing Youan Hospital, Capital Medical University)

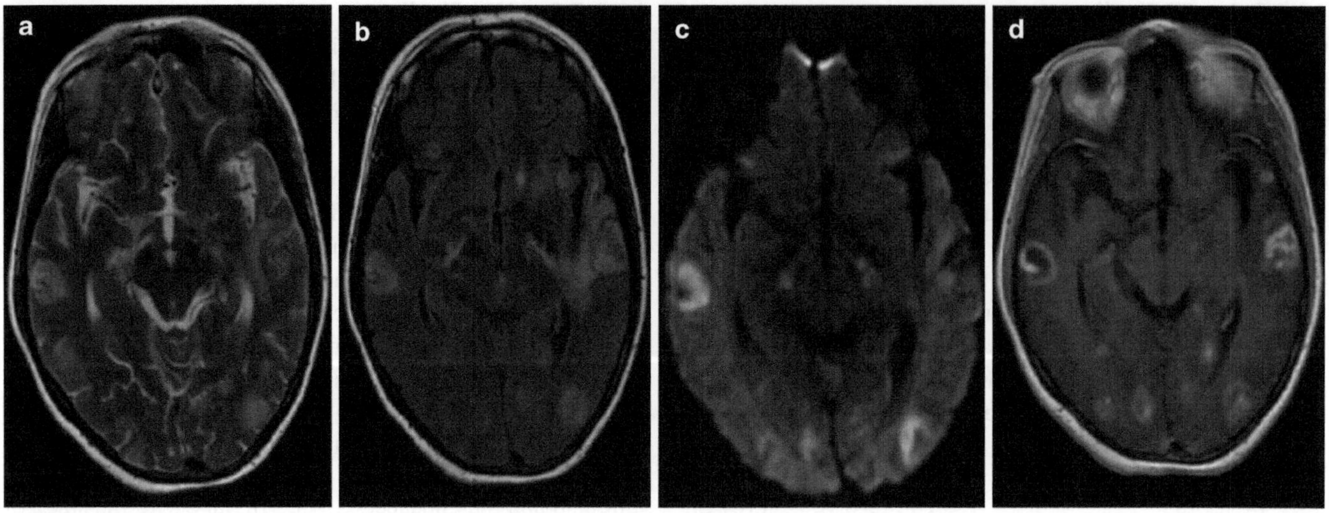

Fig. 10.4 MRI manifestations of AIDS-associated toxoplasmic encephalopathy. (**a**) T_2WI shows multiple round-like slightly hyperintense in the temporal and occipital lobes bilaterally, with punctate hypointense in some lesions and perilesion slightly hyperintense edema; (**b**) FLAIR sequence shows slightly hyperintense, with clearer perilesion edema; (**c**) DWI sequences show significant hyperintense; (**d**) enhanced scans show nodular and circular target-like enhancement (target sign), and the right temporal lobe lesion shows the typical "target sign"

innermost layer is the center of enhancement, the middle layer with hypointense enhancement, and the outermost layer is hyperintense enhancement). The appearance of ring target enhancement is highly suggestive of the disease, which can have both "concentric target sign" and "eccentric target sign," with the latter being more specific [8].

10.2.4 Diagnostic Key Points

1. AIDS-associated toxoplasmic encephalopathy is prevalent in immunodeficient individuals and can occur in both sexes and children. Clinically, there may be headache, fever, drowsiness, and even altered mental status.
2. The lesions are mostly bilateral, multiple, and rarely single. It occurs in the basal ganglia, cutaneous medullary junction area, thalamus, and cerebellum.
3. CT scan shows multiple patchy hypodense lesions, MR T_1WI scan shows mostly isointense or slightly hypointense, T_2WI may show hyper- and hypointense mixed signal, and enhanced scan shows nodular, annular, ring target abnormal enhancement. The presence of ring target enhancement is highly suggestive of the disease, and the "eccentric target sign" is seen in some lesions. Perifocal edema is obvious, with occupying effect.
4. Slightly hyperintense on DWI; decreased NAA, Cr, Cho, and mI peaks on MRS, with increased Cho/Cr and distinct Lip peaks, and also combined with Lac peaks.
5. Toxoplasma gondii found on cerebrospinal fluid smear or free trophozoites or intracellular trophozoites found in tissues or body fluids or in nucleated cells can confirm the diagnosis of the disease.

10.2.5 Differential Diagnosis

AIDS-associated toxoplasmic encephalopathy should be differentiated from primary brain lymphoma, brain metastases, and brain tuberculoma.

10.2.5.1 Primary Cerebral Lymphoma

The disease is usually found in the periventricular midline and gray-white matter junction areas and is often solitary or multiple, with marked occupying effect and perilesion edema, whereas AIDS-associated toxoplasmic encephalopathy often occurs multiple and invades the basal ganglia and cutaneous medullary junction areas, with marked perilesion edema. Enhanced scans of lymphomas tend to show marked homogeneous enhancement, whereas the characteristic sign of toxoplasmosis is usually the "eccentric target sign." AIDS-associated toxoplasmic encephalopathy is effectively treated with anti-Toxoplasma treatment, and the two diseases can be distinguished.

10.2.5.2 Brain Metastases

It is located mostly at the gray-white matter junction, perilesion edema is common, and the lesions are often combined with central necrosis. The density and signal of CT and MR scans are diverse, and nodular and ring-like enhancement is common in the enhanced scan of metastases. In addition, the "eccentric target sign" is the characteristic sign in toxoplasmosis and can be distinguished from metastases. Most patients with brain metastases have a history of extracerebral malignant tumor, and the diagnosis can often be made by combining with the medical history, and the two can be distinguished.

10.2.5.3 Cerebral Tuberculoma

The lesions can be single or multiple, and calcification and necrosis are common. The granuloma portion of tuberculoma manifests as isointense or slightly hyperintense on T_1WI and isointense or hypointense on T_2WI, and the hypointensed tuberculoma on T_2WI is one of its characteristic features; the nodular and circular abnormal enhancement is common on enhanced scan, while the "eccentric target sign" can be seen on enhanced scan of toxoplasmic encephalopathy, and tuberculoma is often combined with tuberculous meningoencephalitis, and tuberculoma has a history of extracerebral tuberculosis in most cases. The two diseases are not difficult to distinguish when combined with laboratory tests.

10.2.6 Status and Progress of Research

10.2.6.1 Magnetic Resonance Diffusion-Weighted Imaging (DWI)

HIV-associated infections and tumor DWI sequences possess different ADC values, which can provide a diagnostic and differential imaging basis for the tumor. One study found that the ADC values (mean) were significantly lower in the solid areas of toxoplasmic encephalopathy lesions compared to control areas, and follow-up studies found that water molecule diffusion was restricted in the early stages of abscess formation in the lesions and DWI shows hyperintense generally. After treatment, as the necrotic tissue liquefied, the water molecule diffusion restriction gradually decreased and the ADC values increased [9]. Diagnosis of *Toxoplasma gondii* encephalitis requires a comprehensive multi-series analysis.

10.2.6.2 Hydrogen Proton Spectroscopy Imaging (^{1}H-MRS)

It is the only noninvasive technique to observe the metabolism of living tissues. AIDS-associated toxoplasmic encephalopathy presents reduced or complete absence of common brain metabolites (e.g., NAA, Cr, Cho, and mI) in the lesion with significantly lower, NAA/Cr and NAA/Cho and lower NAA/Cr in the acute phase compared to the remission phase. Cho/Cr is elevated with a distinct Lip peak is visible, and a Lac peak can be combined. After anti-Toxoplasma treatment, NAA/Cr may return to normal levels completely, and Cho/Cr decreases in some patients or may remain elevated.

10.2.6.3 Magnetic Resonance Perfusion Weighted Imaging (PWI)

It is an important tool for the diagnosis and differential diagnosis of *Toxoplasma gondii* encephalopathy. Ernst et al. [10] reported significant differences in rCBV values for toxoplasmic encephalopathy and lymphoma lesions. It was found that almost all foci of toxoplasmosis presented a lack of blood supply, and the reason for the significantly lower rCBV values may be related to the lack of blood supply in the lesions. Due to the low immune status of AIDS patients, there is a lack of significant inflammatory response around the lesions. One study found that the mean rCBV value and the maximum rCBV value were reduced for toxoplasmic lesions, as well as the rCBV value for perilesion edema. The hypoperfusion manifestation of the lesion and surrounding edema may be related to lack of vascularity within the lesion or increased interstitial pressure in the surrounding edema leading to vasoconstriction. The efficacy of treatment can be assessed using PWI after anti-Toxoplasma treatment, with significant lesion resorption within 2 months and with the resorption of perilesion edema preceding the resorption of the lesion itself.

The clinical and imaging manifestations of AIDS-associated toxoplasmic encephalopathy are complex and varied, and imaging diagnosis is difficult; CT is a low-cost imaging method to screen for the disease, while MRI is the most sensitive and effective imaging method for the disease.

10.3 Cytomegalovirus Encephalitis

Yongxiao You, Yanling Zhou, Jian Wang, and Kang Li

10.3.1 Overview

Cytomegalovirus (CMV) is one of the most common pathogens of viral infections in humans and infects the central nervous system causing cytomegalovirus encephalitis. Humans are the only host of cytomegalovirus, and cytomegalovirus infections are distributed worldwide, with rates varying from country to country and region to region. Cytomegalovirus infections occur in immunocompromised individuals, and most cytomegalovirus infections have no clinical symptoms. Cytomegalovirus can be latent in the body for long periods of time and is activated when cellular immune function is impaired. Cytomegalovirus infection is commonly seen in the late stage of AIDS disease ($CD4^+T$ cell count $<50/mm^3$) and can cause multi-organ infections. In recent years, the incidence of cytomegalovirus infection has been increasing year by year with the increases of immunosuppressed patients with AIDS, radiation injury, organ transplantation, and malignancy. China is a major country of cytomegalovirus infection. Studies have reported cytomegalovirus antibody positivity rates of 59.1–96.1% in healthy populations. Cytomegalovirus infection is the most common opportunistic viral infection in patients with AIDS, with rates of infection reaching up to 40% at the end of

AIDS and often involve the cerebra, cerebellum, spinal cord, and spinal nerve roots.

CNS infections are mostly transmitted through the placenta, resulting in congenital cytomegalovirus infections that can cause fetal malformations, mental retardation, and developmental delays. Cytomegalovirus infections in adults often result in systemic infections, often involving the blood vessels, retina, lungs, and gastrointestinal tract. Clinical presentation is dominated by fever and respiratory, neurological, and hematological symptoms, with temperatures ranging from hypothermia to 40 °C. There may be drowsiness, coma, convulsions, motor disturbances, cerebral palsy, hydrocephalus, mental retardation, and retinal chorioretinitis. Routine biochemical examination of cerebrospinal fluid reveals abnormal lymphocytes, mildly elevated cerebrospinal fluid leukocytes, and elevated cytomegalovirus antibody potency titers; cytomegalovirus can be detected by cerebrospinal fluid PCR.

10.3.2 Pathological Manifestations

Cytomegalovirus infection is a sexually transmitted disease caused by cytomegalovirus that often involves the ventricular canal and occasionally causes extensive destruction of the gray and white matter of the brain. Cytomegalovirus is an DNA virus. Cytomegalovirus infection is characterized by enlarged cells with swollen nuclei containing eosinophilic viral contents and surrounded by a halo, known as the "hawk eye" sign.

10.3.3 Imaging

10.3.3.1 CT Findings

For HIV-associated cytomegalovirus encephalitis, brain atrophy is most common on CT, while hypodense lesions in the white matter of the brain are sometimes seen, mainly in the basal ganglia but also in the paraventricular, pontine, and medulla oblongata. The lesion is a lamellar demyelination-like hypodense lesion on CT with poorly defined borders and no obvious occupying effect (Fig. 10.5) [2].

The diagnosis is further supported by the frequent presence of punctate hyperdense areas, suggesting hemorrhagic necrosis. CT is insensitive to cytomegalovirus encephalitis, and enhanced scans show ring-like or nodular enhancement of the lesion, as well as linear enhancement around the ventricles and in the subependymal.

10.3.3.2 MRI Findings

It mainly involves the basal ganglia, with hypointense on T_1WI and hyperintense on T_2WI, and may have significant edema and occupying effect (Fig. 10.6). T_2WI and FLAIR show multiple punctate and linear hyperintense in the lateral subependymal and other areas of injury. In addition to cerebral atrophy, T_2WI may show patchy hyperintense around the ventricles, and there are often areas of hypointense within larger lesions. Enhanced scans show significant subependymal enhancement, while white matter lesions do not enhance, which is of high diagnostic value. Inflammation can cause adhesions in the middle cerebral aqueduct or lateral foramina, eventually leading to ventricular enlargement and hydrocephalus.

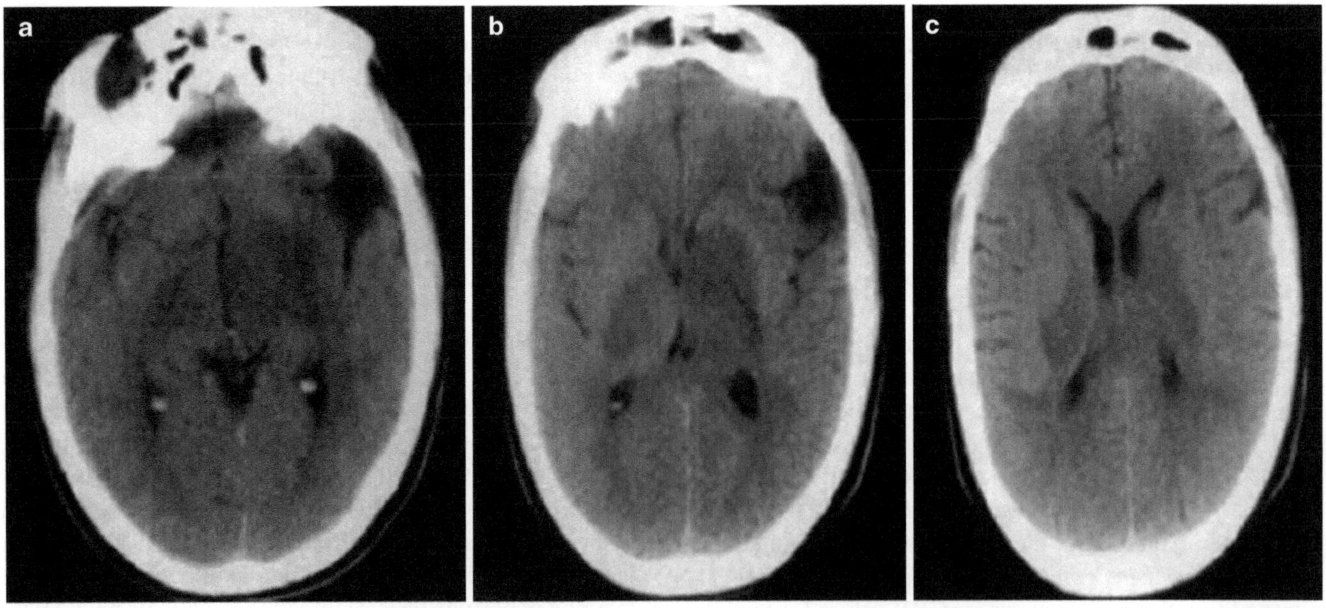

Fig. 10.5 CT findings of AIDS-associated cytomegalovirus encephalitis. (**a**–**c**) CT plain scan shows bilateral symmetrical hypodense areas in the basal ganglia with indistinct borders and insignificant occupancy effects

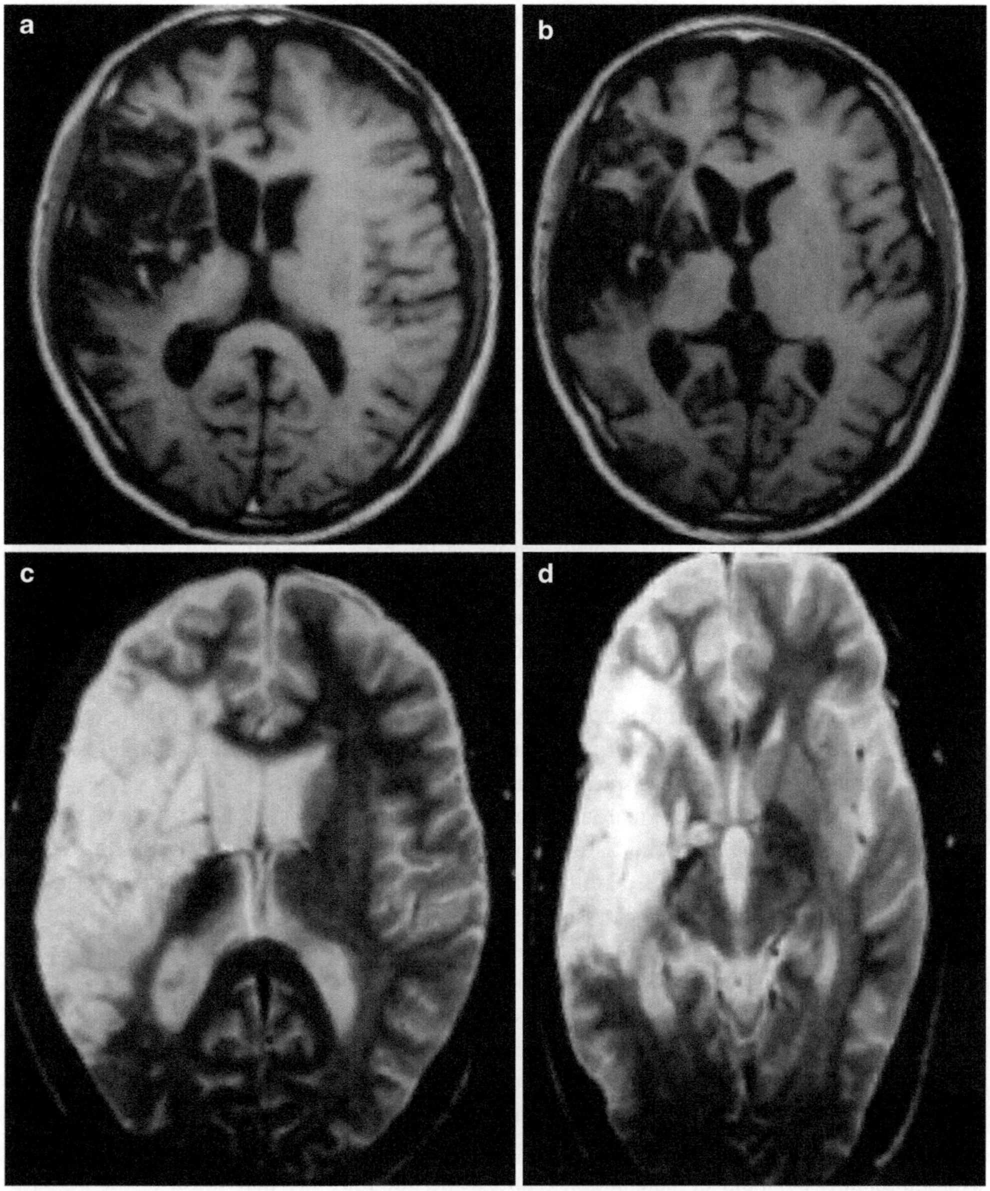

Fig. 10.6 MRI of AIDS-associated cytomegalovirus encephalitis. (**a, b**) T_1WI shows a large lamellar lesion in the right temporal parietal lobe and basal ganglia; (**c, d**) T_2WI shows hyperintense, the occupying effect and brain tissue edema are not obvious, the sulcus is deepened and widened, and the right lateral ventricle is enlarged. (Image courtesy of Li Hongjun of Beijing Youan Hospital, Capital Medical University)

10.3.4 Diagnostic Key Points

1. A history of viral infection with an acute onset and simultaneous cytomegalovirus infection in multiple organs helps in the diagnosis.
2. Clinical manifestations include fever, lethargy, coma, convulsions, and progressively worsening neuropsychiatric symptoms.
3. It is primarily involved in the basal ganglia, but lesions may also be located in the paraventricular space, pons, and medulla. Atrophy of the brain is common, and CT scan shows lamellar demyelination-like hypodense lesions, and the diagnosis is further supported by the frequent presence of punctate hyperdense areas, suggesting hemorrhagic necrosis. MR T_1WI scan shows hypointense and T_2WI shows hyperintense. In enhanced scan, distinct subependymal enhancement can be seen and no abnormal enhancement occurs in periventricular white matter, which provides a high diagnostic value.
4. Mildly elevated cerebrospinal fluid leukocytes, elevated cytomegalovirus antibody potency titers, and cerebrospinal fluid isolation of virus confirm the diagnosis.
5. The diagnosis is confirmed by brain tissue biopsy in which eosinophilic inclusion bodies are seen in neuronal cells or cytomegalovirus particles are found electron microscopically.

10.3.5 Differential Diagnosis

AIDS-associated cytomegalovirus encephalitis should be differentiated from herpes zoster virus encephalitis,

HIV-associated encephalitis, and acute disseminated encephalomyelitis (ADEM).

10.3.5.1 Herpes Zoster Virus Encephalitis

The prognosis is good with mild lesions. The main clinical manifestations are blurred consciousness and ataxia. Most people have a history of cutaneous herpes zoster of the chest and lower back and herpes zoster virus antigens, antibodies and nucleic acids can be detected in serum and cerebrospinal fluid. Cranial CT shows that the lesion mainly involves the cortical part of the cerebral hemisphere, presenting lamellar or mass-like hypodense areas with marked edema and no obvious hemorrhagic necrosis. In contrast, AIDS-associated cytomegalovirus encephalitis often has cerebral atrophy, and hypodense in white matters combined with punctate hyperdense, which suggests hemorrhagic necrosis, can be seen. MRI shows lamellar or mass-like cortical areas of the cerebral hemispheres, with hypointense on T_1WI and hyperintense on T_2WI, with obvious edema and no obvious hemorrhagic necrosis, which support the differentiation.

10.3.5.2 HIV-Associated Encephalitis

Both HIV-associated cytomegalovirus encephalitis and HIV-associated encephalitis manifest similarly in MRI, in which patchy abnormal signals are seen around the ventricles, with slightly hypointense on T_1WI and slightly hyperintense on T_2WI. Both are associated with cerebral atrophy, and HIV-associated cytomegalovirus encephalitis shows no abnormal enhancement on enhanced scans, while HIV-associated cytomegalovirus encephalitis shows significant enhancement in subependymal and no enhancement in white matter lesions, which can be distinguished from each other.

10.3.5.3 Acute Disseminated Encephalomyelitis (ADEM)

There is usually a history of vaccination or infection, and the typical imaging presentation is a multilamellar periventricular demyelinating lesion with patchy enhancement on enhanced scans. In contrast, AIDS-associated cytomegalovirus encephalitis demonstrates no abnormal enhancement in brain parenchyma lesions and distinct enhancement in subependymal lesions. The two diseases manifest differently and can be distinguished easily.

10.3.6 Status and Progress of Research

10.3.6.1 Magnetic Resonance Diffusion-Weighted Imaging (DWI)

The DWI shows multiple punctate hyperintense in the ependyma and periventricular white matter, with reduced ADC values and no significant edema, and fine lines of hyperintense in the subependymal of the lateral ventricles [11]. This prolonged diffusion restriction indicates the presence of ependymitis, which is consistent with the autopsy findings. The histological explanation for the prolonged diffusion restriction is cytotoxic edema caused by cytomegalovirus contents [12].

10.3.6.2 Hydrogen Proton Spectrum Imaging (^{1}H-MRS)

Midya et al. [13] concluded that magnetic resonance spectroscopy showed a decrease in NAA and an increase in the choline peak, as well as the presence of a lactate/lipid bimodal peak.

MRI and CT can be used for the examination of immunodeficiency-associated intracranial infections, with MRI predominating. MRI is characterized by high resolution, and compared with CT, MRI is able to detect more lesions and their surrounding structures without enhancement, which is of great clinical value in reflecting the whole picture of immunodeficiency-associated intracranial infection and improving its sensitivity and specificity. Thus, MRI examination is significantly superior to CT, but the CT presentation of immunodeficiency-associated intracranial infections is also characteristic and indispensable.

10.4 Progressive Multifocal Leukoencephalopathy

Yongxiao You, Qiang Liu, Jian Wang, and Kang Li

10.4.1 Overview

Progressive multifocal leukoencephalopathy (PML) is a demyelinating disease of the central nervous system caused by activation of the JC virus (*Papovaviridae*) with progressive or insidious onset and progressive exacerbation. PML is mainly seen in patients with defective cellular immune responses and has a prevalence of more than 4% in patients with AIDS. As the incidence of AIDS increases, the detection rate of PML in patients with AIDS is also increasing. The development of the lesion is complex, the clinical manifestations varied, and the mortality rate is high. AIDS-associated PML is insidious, has a variety of clinical manifestations, and can occur at any age, but is commonly seen in adult males over the age of 50. Symptoms such as characteristic neurological deficits, progressive mental decline, personality changes, and mental deterioration may occur early in the course of the disease. Depending on the extent of demyelination, patients may experience visual impairment, hemiparesis, quadriplegia, aphasia, and apraxia. Consciousness disturbance and even coma may occur in the late stage. Fever and headache are rare throughout the course of the disease, and about 10% of patients develop headache or epilepsy. The disease progresses rapidly, with death occurring in an average of 3–6 months. In the laboratory, antigen of papovavirus can be detected by immunocytology; JC virus gene can be detected by PCR of cerebrospinal fluid or brain tissue.

10.4.2 Pathological Manifestations

PML is a subacute demyelinating disease of the central nervous system when the organism is immunocompromised. Previous exposure to JC virus and suppressed T cell-associated immune defenses are primary susceptibility factors. The JC virus continues to replicate and spread due to impaired host T lymphocyte immunity against the JC virus, which is unable to inhibit the reactivation of the JC virus. The JC virus of the *Papovaviridae* family has been shown to be the causative agent of PML, and the development of disease in carriers of the virus is associated with the presence or absence of abnormalities in the body's immunity [2]. Immunofluorescence and in situ hybridization studies suggest that PML is caused by papovavirus infection of brain astrocytes and oligodendrocytes in AIDS patients. Pathological autopsy of AIDS-associated PML shows multiple focal demyelinating masses and granular yellow foci of malacia in the white matter of the brain, with diffuse asymmetric distribution and fused lesions up to several centimeters. As oligodendrocytes are selectively destroyed by papovavirus, there is multifocal demyelination in the white matter of the brain, the demyelinating lesions can gradually fuse, the axons remain relatively intact, there is significant local loss of oligodendrocytes and enlargement of surrounding oligodendrocytes, and in most cases vascular changes and inflammatory responses are not evident. The lesions are commonly found in the white matter of the cortical area of the centrum semiovale on both sides of the brain, followed by involvement of the periventricular white matter and even the deep gray matter nuclei, with the cerebral hemispheres being more susceptible than the cerebellum and brainstem.

10.4.3 Imaging

10.4.3.1 CT Findings

CT scan shows heterogenous distributed multiple hypodense foci with poorly defined borders, mostly in the bilateral centrum semiovale. The early lesions are round or oval in shape and then gradually fuse and enlarge; enhanced scans show that most of the lesions present no abnormal enhancement, but very few may demonstrate enhancement. In the late stage of the disease, the ventricles are enlarged, the sulci are deepened and widened, the gyri are narrowed, and other cerebral atrophy changes are observed.

10.4.3.2 MRI Findings

PML is a progressive demyelinating disorder that typically develops in the subcortical white matter and cerebellar peduncles. Supratentorial lesions are often multiple and symmetrically distributed in the cerebral hemispheres, located in the subcortical white matter where blood flow is most abundant; the distribution of multiple foci does not coincide with the cerebrovascular distribution area, and a few are unilateral or isolated, with parieto-occipital involvement being the most common, followed by the temporal and frontal lobe; splenium of corpus callosum involvement is uncommon, and supratentorial lesions are located mainly in the cerebellar peduncles, with unilateral or bilateral onset, and the lesions spread to the midbrain and medulla oblongata [14]. The U-fiber involvement of the brain is the characteristic manifestation, and the involvement of multiple brain gyri resembles a shell shape. The lesion manifests as hypointense on T_1WI and hyperintense on T_2WI and FLAIR, with clear borders and no occupying effect. There is no edema around the lesion (Fig. 10.7), and no abnormal enhancement on enhanced scans, but there may be partial abnormal enhancement when combined with immune reconstitution inflammatory syndrome.

10.4.4 Diagnostic Key Points

1. It occurs in adult males over the age of 50, progresses rapidly, and may present with symptoms of progressive brain damage.
2. The lesions are multifocal, preferably in the subcortical white matter of the parieto-occipital lobe, away from the periventricular area, and can gradually fuse and enlarge, with cerebral U-shaped fiber involvement as the characteristic manifestation.
3. Multiple lamellar hypodense lesions can be seen in the white matter. T_1WI shows slightly hypodense and T_2WI shows iso- or hyperdense with inapparent occupying effect. Enhanced scan shows peripheral enhancement on partial lesions. DWI shows hyperintense with poorly defined borders and hypointense in the center of the lesion, which are typical features of PML.
4. Cerebrospinal fluid examination does not show significant abnormalities and the EEG may show diffuse or focal abnormalities.
5. The histopathological biopsy of the brain is characterized by multifocal cerebral white matter demyelination. JC virus gene could be detected in brain tissue or cerebrospinal fluid by PCR technique.

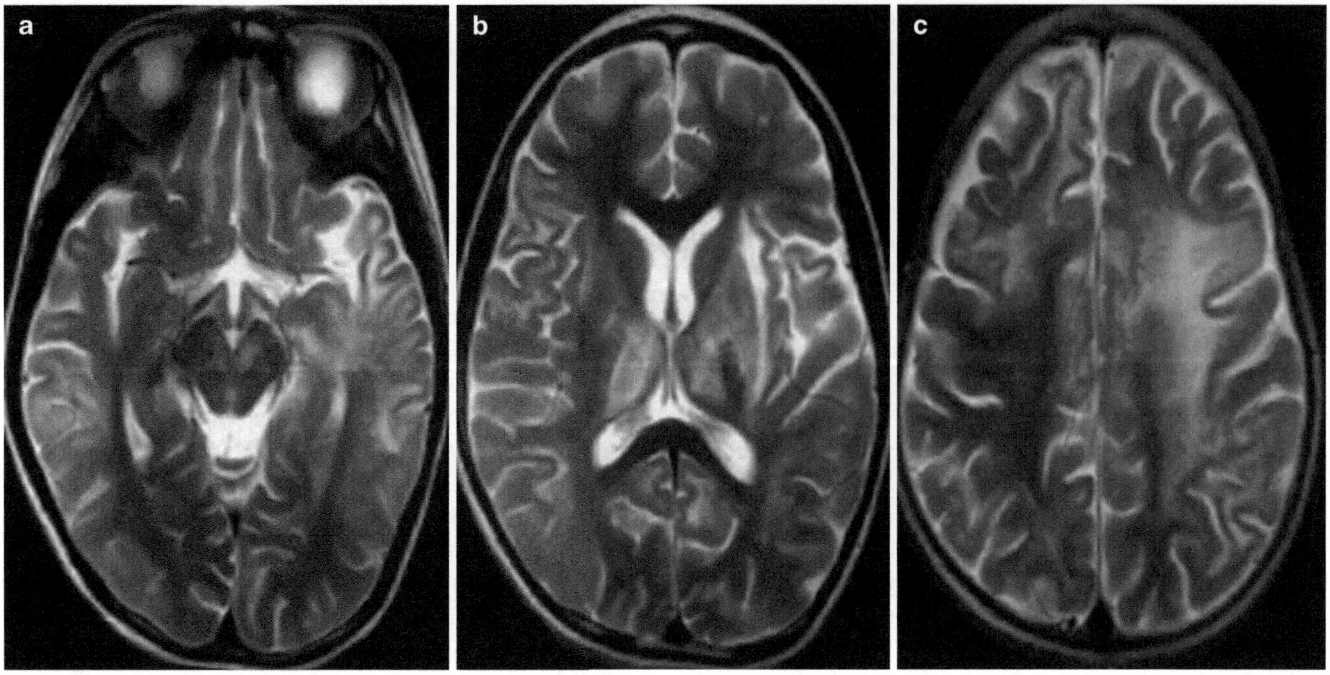

Fig. 10.7 MRI of AIDS-related progressive multifocal leukoencephalopathy. (**a**) T_2WI shows punctiform and lamellar hyperintense in the left temporal lobe and pons, with no obvious edema and occupying effect; (**b**) T_2WI shows bilateral symmetric lamellar hyperintense in the basal ganglia, with still clear borders and no obvious edema and occupying effect; (**c**) T_2WI shows bilateral asymmetric lamellar hyperintense in the center of the centrum semiovale, mainly on the left side. (Image courtesy of Prof. Li Hongjun, Beijing Youan Hospital, Capital Medical University, China)

10.4.5 Differential Diagnosis

With the gradual increase in the incidence of AIDS, the detection rate of PML is increasing among AIDS patients. The lesions are more complex in development and have a variety of clinical presentations with a high mortality rate. Advances in imaging technology have led to an increasing detection rate of PML and an increasingly important role of imaging in the diagnosis of AIDS-associated PML. HIV-associated PML should be differentiated from HIV-associated encephalitis, multiple sclerosis (MS), and cerebrovascular disease.

10.4.5.1 HIV-Associated Encephalitis

It mainly shows glial cell nodule formation. Lesions show iso- or slightly hypointense on T_1WI, mostly diffuse, symmetrical distribution and mostly located around the ventricles, while PML pathological basis is demyelinating changes, and lesions manifest as hypointense on T_1WI and disseminated, asymmetrically distributed, and preferentially located in the subcortical white matter, away from the periventricular area. HIV-associated encephalitis mainly presents with cognitive impairment and dementia, whereas PML mainly presents with focal motor sensory impairment, making the clinical presentation important for confirming the diagnosis.

10.4.5.2 Multiple Sclerosis (MS)

It is the most common of the demyelinating lesions of the central nervous system, of unknown etiology, which is a predominantly white matter inflammatory demyelinating disease that occurs bilaterally around the ventricles, with recurrent worsening and remission and progressive exacerbation. MRI typically shows a periventricular white matter oval-like lesion with a perpendicular ventricular distribution, i.e., Dawson finger sign with ring-like or nodular enhancement in the acute phase and no significant abnormal enhancement of the lesion in the stable phase [15]. PML is dominated by subcortical white matter lesions, which are far from the periventricular area and have no fixed relationship with the ventricles and most of them have no obvious abnormal enhancement. It is not difficult to distinguish the two diseases.

10.4.5.3 Cerebrovascular Disease

It is one of the AIDS-related neurological diseases and can be combined with systemic vascular lesions. The imaging shows worm-eaten, multifocal patchy abnormalities in the brain parenchyma, and sometimes large infarcts in one side of the brain can be seen, which often distributed asymmetrically, with or without different degrees of enhancement, and MRA shows gross narrowing of the cerebral artery walls, interruption of the distal small vessels, and diminished or absent blood flow signals. In contrast, the pathology basis of PML is demyelinating change, which manifests as hypointense on T_1WI, and the lesions are disseminated, asymmetrical, and mostly without significant abnormal enhancement, and the disease is clinically progressive.

10.4.6 Status and Progress of Research

10.4.6.1 Hydrogen Proton Spectroscopy Imaging (^{1}H-MRS)

Typical ^{1}H-MRS of PML lesions shows a decrease in NAA, an increase in Cho levels, an increase in the Lac peak, an increase in mI in the early phase of PML and a decrease in the late phase, and eventually a decrease in all metabolites. The NAA/Cr ratio decreases and the Lac/Cr, Cho/Cr, and lipid /Cr ratios increase. One study found an increase in the NAA/Cr ratio and a decrease in the Cho/ creatine ratio after treatment. ^{1}H-MRS can be used to assess treatment efficiency [16].

10.4.6.2 Magnetic Resonance Diffusion-Weighted Imaging (DWI)

DWI shows poorly defined PML lesions with hyperintense and hypointense within the lesions, which are typical features of PML. The peripheral signal gradually decreases over time but remains hyperintense on conventional T_2WI. It has been shown that DWI presentation of PML patients may be related to the stage of the disease [17]. The edges of new lesions and large lesions show normal or low ADC values and hyperintense on DWI, while old lesions and large lesions have increased ADC values and low DWI signal in the center. These findings also help to differentiate PML from other similar diseases [18]. It has been suggested that $b = 3000$ improves the visualization of important imaging features in PML compared to $b = 1000$. When $b = 3000$, the contrast resolution between the lesion margins and interior and normal white matter increased, and the identification of marginal-core patterns improved and helps evaluate treatment response and assess prognosis in PML [19].

Both CT and MRI can be used to examine immunodeficiency-associated intracranial infections, with MRI being the mainstay. CT is the primary screening examination; however, MRI has a high resolution and can detect more lesions and their internal and peripheral structures without enhancement, which is of great clinical value to reflect the whole picture of immunodeficiency-associated intracranial infections and improve the detection rate of lesions. Therefore, MRI is clearly superior to CT.

10.5 Penicilliosis Marneffei Infection

Xiaodan Du, Yibanu, Jian Wang, and Min Luo

10.5.1 Overview

Penicilliosis marneffei (PSM) is a fungal disease caused by the conditional pathogen *Penicillium marneffei* (PM) infection, and PM is one of the most common opportunistic infection-causing pathogenic bacteria in patients with AIDS. It is mainly inhaled through the respiratory tract but can also be infected through the gastrointestinal tract, skin breaks, etc. It is phagocytosed and cleared by macrophages, and when the immune function of the infected person is reduced, PM proliferates in macrophages and causes disease. When HIV invades the human immune system, the number of $CD4^+$ T lymphocytes decreases, leading to a defect in the immune function of human cells, which makes them vulnerable to various opportunistic infections [20]. PSM can be clinically divided into progressive disseminated and limited forms, and PM can often lead to systemic disseminated lesions due to cellular immunodeficiency in AIDS patients. Localized penicilliosis is common in cutaneous and subcutaneous infections, while disseminated penicilliosis more often involves the lungs, liver, and lymph nodes. The respiratory system is the most commonly affected organ, while PM infections are very rare in the central nervous system [21].

AIDS-associated intracerebral PM infections are mainly delayed with $CD4^+$ T lymphocytes <50/μL, and their clinical symptoms often appear in the later stages of the disease [22]. The clinical manifestations are complex and varied due to multisystem involvement, with fever and weight loss being the most common clinical manifestations, sometimes with fever being the only symptom [23]. Acute onset often presents with fungemia and shock; papules on the face, upper trunk, and upper extremities; and infectious molluscum contagiosum-like necrotic papules which are the most characteristic manifestations of the disease. In the subacute stage, there may be systemic symptoms such as fever, headache, emaciation, malaise, and impaired mobility of one or both lower extremities. In immunologically active hosts, abscesses, osteolytic destruction, septic pneumonia, hepatomegaly, splenomegaly, and lymph node enlargement are more typical presentations and are rarely seen in patients with AIDS. A temperature of 37 °C for growth and vascular invasion are the main reasons for the spread of the disease and the high mortality rate. About 50% of patients have fungemia, especially HIV-positive patients, and PM often invades blood vessels and can produce fungal emboli [21]. For laboratory tests, PM can be cultured in blood, cerebrospinal fluid, or bone marrow.

10.5.2 Pathological Manifestations

PM is a temperature biphasic fungus, which exhibits mycelium phase at 25 °C and grows fast; the surface of colony is fluffy and can form folds, which is cerebral gyrus-like and its color can change from light green to gray during the differentiation process; and the production of soluble red pigment in 2–3 days is its characteristic performance. It grows slowly in the yeast phase at 37 °C. PM reproduces mainly by division, with blunt rounded ends, like "salami," forming a horizontal septum from the middle of the bacterium and dividing evenly. PM can cause granulomatous reaction, suppurative reaction, and nonreactive necrosis. PM spreads hematologically to the central nervous system, causing reactive proliferation of the mononuclear phagocyte system and purulent inflammation, mainly in the brain. When the immune system is relatively robust, liquefaction and necrosis of the tissue are the main features which lead to the formation of localized abscesses. PM infection in immunocompromised HIV-infected patients is often prone to disseminated lesions due to defective T-lymphocyte immunity [24].

10.5.3 Imaging

10.5.3.1 CT Findings

Multiple hypodense lesions can be seen in the brain parenchyma, mostly in the corticomedullary junction area, and single lesions are rare. In the early stage, lesions may not enhance on enhanced scan, and as the disease progresses, the typical lesions enhanced in a nodular or circular pattern (Fig. 10.8) [25].

10.5.3.2 MRI Findings

There are multiple lamellar lesions in the brain parenchyma with slightly hypointense on T_1WI, and slightly hyperintense on T_2WI, and the lesions are associated with obvious edema and occupying effects. The enhanced scan shows circular or target-like enhancement [25].

10.5.4 Diagnostic Key Points

1. Intracerebral infections are mostly secondary to systemic infections of PM, with $CD4^+$ T lymphocytes <50/μL.
2. It occurs mostly in the corticomedullary junction area, and papules on the face and trunk are the characteristic manifestations of the disease.
3. According to CT findings, multiple hypodense lesions are seen in the brain parenchyma, with significant edema and occupying effects and nodular or ring target sign enhancement on enhanced scan. On the other hand, on MRI findings, there are multiple lamellar abnormal signals in the brain parenchyma with slightly hypointense on T_1WI and slightly hyperintense on T_2WI, and the manifestation on enhanced scan is similar to that of CT, but the detection rate of the lesions is higher than CT.
4. Immunological examination and pathological histology can detect PM from cultured colonies and pathological sections.

10.5.5 Differential Diagnosis

10.5.5.1 Toxoplasma Encephalopathy

PSM and toxoplasmic encephalopathy are both common HIV-associated opportunistic infections, and enhanced scans demonstrate multiple ring-like or target enhancements. However, the foci of toxoplasmic encephalopathy are widely

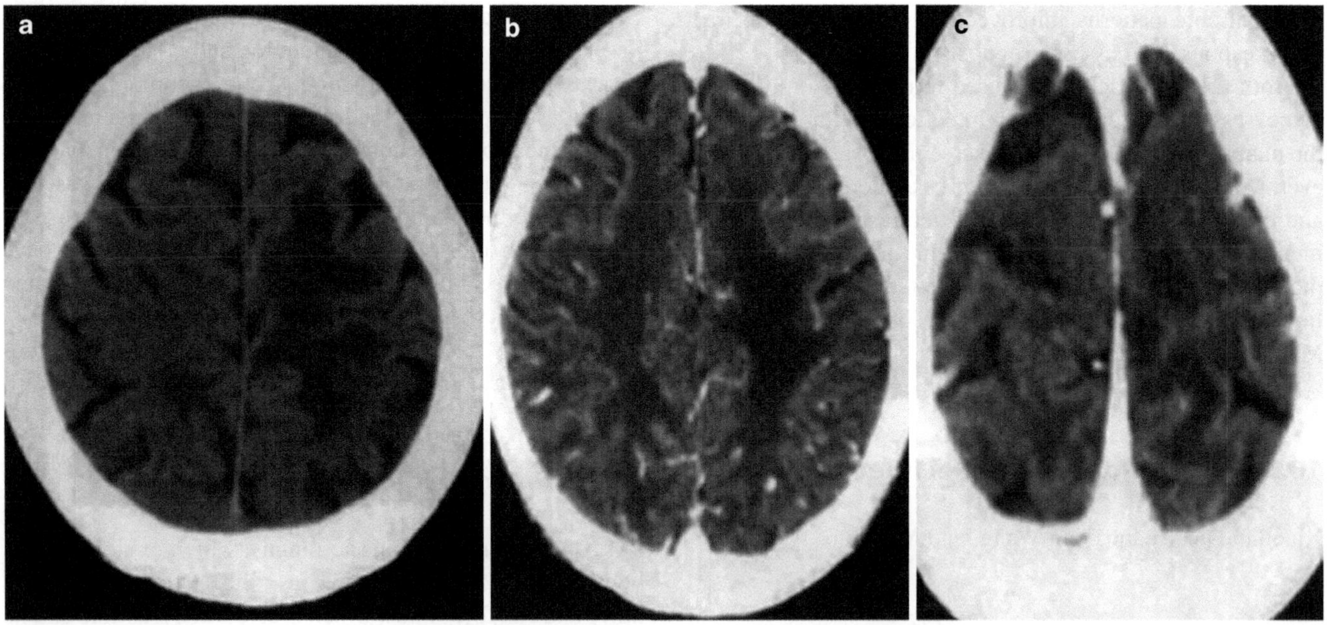

Fig. 10.8 AIDS-associated intracerebral penicillium marneffei disease. (**a**) CT plain scan shows irregular lamellar hypodense lesions in the frontal and parietal lobes bilaterally with obvious edema, mainly on the left side; (**b**, **c**) enhanced scan shows cerebral gyrus-like enhancement around the lesion and multiple small nodule-like abnormal enhancements. (Image courtesy of Professor Li Hongjun of Beijing Youan Hospital, Capital Medical University)

distributed and typically show a "concentric target sign" or "eccentric target sign," with a significant occupying effect and surrounding edema. PSM is found in the corticomedullary junction area and the imaging presentation lacks specificity. The diagnosis of PSM is confirmed by the bacterial culture of cerebrospinal fluid seen in PM.

10.5.5.2 Tuberculoma

Both PSM and tuberculoma show ring-like enhancement on enhanced scans, and both may show the circumferential target sign. Tuberculomas can be single or multiple, and the lesions tend to be calcified and caseous necrosis. Slightly hypointense on T_2WI is its characteristic feature, and tuberculomas tend to have a history of extracerebral tuberculosis. While the PSM is well located in the corticomedullary junction area, the lesions are mostly multiple and manifest as slightly hyperintense on T_2WI with obvious edema and occupying effects.

10.5.5.3 Cryptococcosis

Both PSM and cryptococcosis show ring-like enhancement on enhanced scans, but PSM has a target sign, whereas cryptococcosis does not. Cryptococcosis is found in the basal ganglia, around the cistern, and mostly in the perivascular space, while PSM is mostly located in the corticomedullary junction area. Cryptococcosis may form characteristic colloidal pseudocyst and cryptococcoma with hydrocephalus, meningeal thickening and enhancing in the mid to late stages, whereas PSM does not have this characteristic manifestation, and the two can be distinguished.

10.5.6 Status and Progress of Research

PM infections in the CNS are very rare and can be initially suggested by imaging manifestations. In some cases of advanced AIDS combined with CNS infection, the imaging manifestations are not typical and the cerebrospinal fluid changes may not be conventional. It is important to carefully analyze the medical history before the pathogenic and pathological findings are available, carefully identify the disease according to its spectrum, strictly follow the indications for diagnostic treatment, scientifically assess the effectiveness of diagnostic treatment, and actively search for other possible pathogenic evidence if the treatment is not effective. Brain tissue biopsy is an effective way to make a definitive diagnosis, and multidisciplinary cooperation can help improve diagnostic accuracy and patient prognosis. This disease needs to be further studied extensively.

10.6 *Rhodococcus equi* Infection

Xiaodan Du, Jinying Wang, Jian Wang, and Min Luo

10.6.1 Overview

Rhodococcus equi is a parthenogenic, anaerobic, intracellular, nonmotile, non-spore-forming parasite that is a zoonotic opportunistic pathogen, ingested by inhalation from infected soil, exposure to wounds or mucous membranes, ingestion through the gastrointestinal tract, and most commonly through the respiratory tract after contact. It is generally the causative agent of horses, pigs, and cattle, while human *Rhodococcus equi* infections are low; however, as HIV infections increase, human *Rhodococcus equi* infections appear to be on the rise. *Rhodococcus equi* can cause infections of the brain and respiratory tract in humans and can cause sepsis [26]. The lungs are the most common site of infection, and disease onset is usually insidious and slow, with transmission from the lungs to other sites through the bloodstream, leading to abscess formation. Brain abscesses caused by *Rhodococcus equi* often occur in the supratentorial area, mainly in the frontal, temporal, and occipital lobes. Cerebral symptoms can present in 63% of patients, including infiltrates, pustules, and cavitary lesions, suggesting a pulmonary-central nervous system syndrome [27].

The presentation varies by site of infection. The clinical manifestations may include symptoms of encephalitis such as prolonged illness, fever, and twitching of one limb; or symptoms of meningitis such as headache, vomiting, and fever; or no positive neurological symptoms. The laboratory investigation of the strain is positive for catalase test, and the cerebrospinal fluid culture of *Rhodococcus equi* is purple or pink.

10.6.2 Pathological Manifestations

Rhodococcus equi is an intracellular parthenogenic anaerobic pathogen that infects human macrophages and inhibits phagocytic lysosomal fusion, which is considered to be the basis of its pathogenicity and drug resistance mechanisms [28]. Pathological examination reveals basophilic inclusion bodies. It is difficult to diagnose in the laboratory due to its morphological similarity to diphtheroid bacilli, *Bacillus*, or *Micrococcus*. Depending on the growth conditions and the growth cycle, the microscopic morphology varies from spherical to rod-shaped, and the appropriate growth temperature for *Rhodococcus equi* is 10–40 °C, with an optimal temperature of 30 °C. It grows readily on nonselective media and forms smooth mucus colonies, and over time, the pigmented colonies increase, hence named *Rhodococcus rubrum* [29].

10.6.3 Imaging

CT and MRI demonstrate AIDS-associated intracerebral *Rhodococcus equi* infection as multiple round-like lesions in the brain parenchyma, with slightly hypointense on T_1WI and slightly hyperintense on T_2WI, with perifocal edema and significant occupying effects (Fig. 10.9). The focal area may show ring-like enhancement or ring target sign on enhanced scan. The extent of the lesion decreases after general treatment [29].

10.6.4 Diagnostic Key Points

1. The lesions are most often located deep in the brain and result from systemic dissemination, most often in combination with pulmonary *Rhodococcus equi* infection.
2. MRI shows multiple round-like abnormal signals in the brain, T_1WI shows slightly hypointense, T_2WI shows slightly hyperintense, there is a clear occupying effect, edema is seen around the lesion, and enhanced scan shows ring or ring target enhancement.
3. Reduction in the extent or disappearance of intracerebral lesions after anti-*Rhodococcus equi* infection treatment.
4. Laboratory tests with positive catalase test for the strain; the presence of *Rhodococcus equi* in cerebrospinal fluid culture confirms the diagnosis.

10.6.5 Differential Diagnosis

The disease needs to be differentiated from other infectious lesions, such as tuberculous encephalitis, cerebral toxoplasma encephalitis, gummatous neurosyphilis, staphylococcal encephalitis, cryptococcal encephalitis, etc. The imaging manifestations are similar [30], which are not easily distinguishable and mainly rely on laboratory tests for differentiation.

10.6.6 Status and Progress of Research

AIDS-associated intracerebral *Rhodococcus equi* infection is often secondary to pulmonary *Rhodococcus equi* infection, and the diagnosis relies primarily on laboratory tests. The diagnosis is confirmed by the presence of *Rhodococcus equi* in cerebrospinal fluid culture. There are few imaging studies, but there are case reports of AIDS-associated intracerebral *Rhodococcus equi* infection that have been treated with anti-inflammatory therapy to reduce the extent of the lesion and eliminate the surrounding edema.

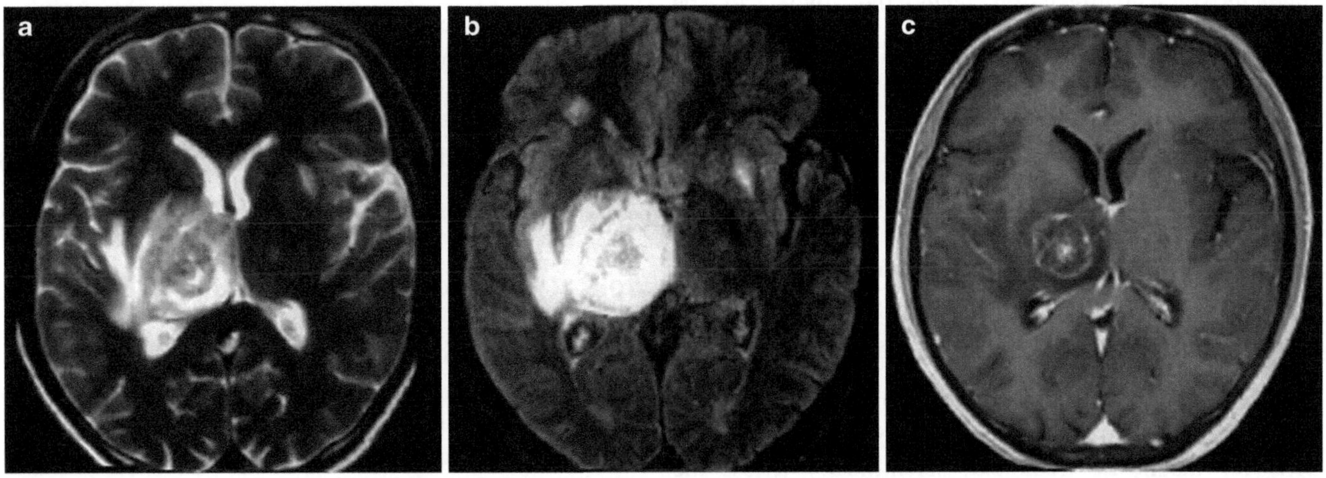

Fig. 10.9 AIDS-associated intracerebral *Rhodococcus equi* infection. (**a**) A round-like lesion in the right dorsal thalamus with slightly hyperintense on T_2WI, surrounded by edema; (**b**) the extent of edema is clearer on the FLAIR sequence; (**c**) enhanced scan shows a ring target-like enhancement of the lesion (Image courtesy of Prof. Li Hongjun of Beijing Youan Hospital, Capital Medical University)

10.7 Immune Reconstitution Inflammatory Syndrome

Yuxin Yang, Aniwar Ulam, and Xin Gao

10.7.1 Overview

Immune reconstitution inflammatory syndrome (IRIS) is a group of clinical syndromes in which clinical symptoms worsened despite improved immune function, increased $CD4^+$ T-lymphocyte counts, and decreased HIV viral load after treatment with highly active retroviral therapy (HAART) in an immunocompromised state following HIV infection. In view of the important role of the host inflammatory response in the pathogenesis, De Simone and others [31] first proposed the name "immune reconstitution inflammatory syndrome" for the disease. IRIS occurs in the early stage after antiviral therapy (commonly within 3 months) with a high incidence; 10–50% of patients can develop IRIS after receiving HAART. The pathogenesis of IRIS is not well understood, and the reestablishment of pathogen-specific immunity and inflammatory response induced by the remission of the immunosuppressed state is currently considered the most likely basis for the pathogenesis of IRIS. Antigenic stimuli in the organism (including clinically occult structurally intact pathogens, dead or dying pathogens and their residual antigens) are necessary for the occurrence of IRIS. The incidence of pathogen-associated IRIS is related to its ability to be cleared in vivo, e.g., *Streptococcus pneumoniae* can be cleared rapidly and the incidence of IRIS is low; in contrast, *Mycobacterium tuberculosis* and *Cryptococcus* are not easily cleared and the incidence of IRIS is high. It is now generally accepted that IRIS is due to the recovery of immune function after receiving HAART and that the body produces an excessive immune inflammatory response against the antigenic components of latent pathogens or treated pathogens in the body, resulting in worsening clinical symptoms. IRIS is divided into two types [32]: (1) the exposed type, i.e., no manifestation of the associated infection before the administration of HAART, which appears only after treatment, mainly in response to the active pathogen, and (2) the paradoxical type, i.e., the infection was present or treated before the administration of HAART, which instead worsens after treatment, mainly in response to the persistent antigenic component of the inactive pathogen [33].

IRIS of the CNS is relatively rare and most often occurs after treatment of a conditional pathogenic infection. The following pathogens are common causes of CNS IRIS: (1) *Mycobacterium tuberculosis*, which is the most common form of IRIS in a high HIV/TB mixed infection setting. CNS *Mycobacterium tuberculosis* (TB)-associated IRIS appears relatively late, usually 5–10 months after HAART treatment, and once it appears, symptoms are severe, so clinical vigilance is desirable. There is a lack of diagnostic criteria for the disease, and patients with $CD4^+$ T cells/$CD8^+$ T cells >0.33 have a relatively high probability of immune reconstitution [32]. (2) Cryptococcal IRIS has been found to be present in 9.4% of patients with cryptococcal infection. Risk factors include women; initial visits with brain manifestations or involvement of the brain, meninges, and lungs; and a high median $CD4^+$ T lymphocyte count. The onset of IRIS is 1–12 months after initiation of antifungal therapy. (3) Toxoplasmosis, a rare form of IRIS caused by *Toxoplasma gondii*, has a subacute onset and lacks specificity in clinical and imaging presentation. $CD8^+$ and $CD68^+$ T lymphocyte infiltration are often seen in the vascular periphery, leading to symptoms of diffuse brain damage. (4) Cytomegalovirus, the most common cause of IRIS due to cytomegalovirus infection, is a $CD8^+$ T lymphocyte infiltration, with the eye being the most vulnerable organ and the brain being another organ that can be attacked by an overreactive immune system. Cytomegalovirus encephalitis typically presents with ventriculitis and isolated focal lesions. (5) In PML, IRIS occurs in 10–20% of PML-HIV patients, usually 3–6 weeks after initiation of HAART [34].

There is no accepted gold standard for the diagnosis of IRIS, but at least these three following conditions must be met: (1) improvement in plasma HIV viral load and $CD4^+$ T lymphocyte count in HIV infection/AIDS patients treated with HAART; (2) presence of inflammatory process consistent with clinical signs and symptoms; and (3) exclusion of natural course of previous infection or adverse effects of drugs. The main risk factors for the occurrence of IRIS include the following: (1) the organism is in a dominant/subclinical opportunistic infection, or there is a residual inactive pathogen or its antigenic component in the body; (2) the organism has a low baseline $CD4^+$ T lymphocyte count, e.g., $CD4^+$ T lymphocyte count $<50 \times 10^6$/L, CD4/CD8 <0.15; (3) rapid decrease in viral load in patients treated with HAART; and (4) the starting time of HARRT is too short from the diagnosis or treatment of opportunistic infection. Therefore, patients with diffuse infections, low $CD4^+$ T-lymphocyte counts, and premature initiation of HAART are at higher risk of developing IRIS.

10.7.2 Pathological Manifestations

The main pathological manifestation of IRIS is the inflammatory infiltration of CD4+ and CD8+ T lymphocytes in the perivascular and parenchymal areas of the brain [34]. In addition, IRIS is often associated with the same pathology as HIV infection combined with opportunistic infections caused by different pathogens because the infection was present or treated prior to HAART treatment but worsened after treatment (see Sects. 10.2–10.4, Chap. 6, Sect. 6.2, and Chap. 12, Sect. 12.2 for details on the pathology of associated infections).

10.7.3 Imaging

The IRIS imaging presentation is not specific and is the same as that of HIV infection in combination with opportunistic infection (see Sect. 10.1 for details). However, imaging methods are an important tool for dynamic observation of disease changes. Therefore, the diagnosis of IRIS currently relies on the clinical history combined with the continuous dynamic changes in the imaging presentation. The typical imaging presentation of IRIS needs to be viewed dynamically in the context of clinical symptoms. In the early post-HAART period of HIV infection, new onset of infection, or recurrence or exacerbation of existing symptoms, the imaging presents a new onset of opportunistic infection or progression of an already improved opportunistic infection.

HIV infection combined with *Toxoplasma gondii* infection, for example, may present as focal or diffuse meningitis, with nonspecific speckle-like enhancement and markedly abnormal meningeal enhancement on enhanced scans. In early stage of infection, CT and MRI scans show single or multiple nodular lesions in the brain parenchyma, and CT scans show hypodense or isodense lesions, and multiple lesions may fuse to form sheets; MRI T_1WI shows isointense or slightly hypointense and T_2WI shows slightly hyperintense. DWI shows hyperintense and enhanced scan shows homogenous moderate enhancement with no or mild edema; in late stage of infection, edema around the lesions expands, and the lesion appears nodular, ring-shaped, ring target-shaped obvious abnormal enhancement on enhanced scan, with ring-shaped enhancement as more common. IRIS can be considered if the following conditions occur: compared with pre-HARRT treatment (Fig. 10.10), appearance of new lesions in the brain parenchyma (Fig. 10.11) or increases of lesions in the brain or increases of lesions in the brain parenchyma, or expansion and aggravation of meningeal enhancement after anti-HIV treatment, and the neurological changes of the patient gradually returned to normal after anti-Toxoplasma and antiviral treatment (Fig. 10.12).

10.7.4 Diagnostic Key Points

1. HIV-positive patients presenting with symptoms such as fever, exacerbation, or worsening of latent infection/pre-existing infection after HAART treatment.
2. Decrease in HIV viral load and/or increase in $CD4^+$ T lymphocyte count after HAART.
3. Imaging manifestations: patients with HIV who have no relevant infection before HAART and whose infection is detected on imaging after HAART; or HIV-infected patients who have an existing or improved pathogenic infection before HAART and who show signs of progression or exacerbation on imaging after HAART (within 3 months).
4. A definitive diagnosis requires the exclusion of opportunistic infections with adverse drug reactions.

10.7.5 Differential Diagnosis

Because the current understanding of IRIS is not sufficiently advanced, it needs to be analyzed in an integrated and dynamic way in the context of specific situations. The dif-

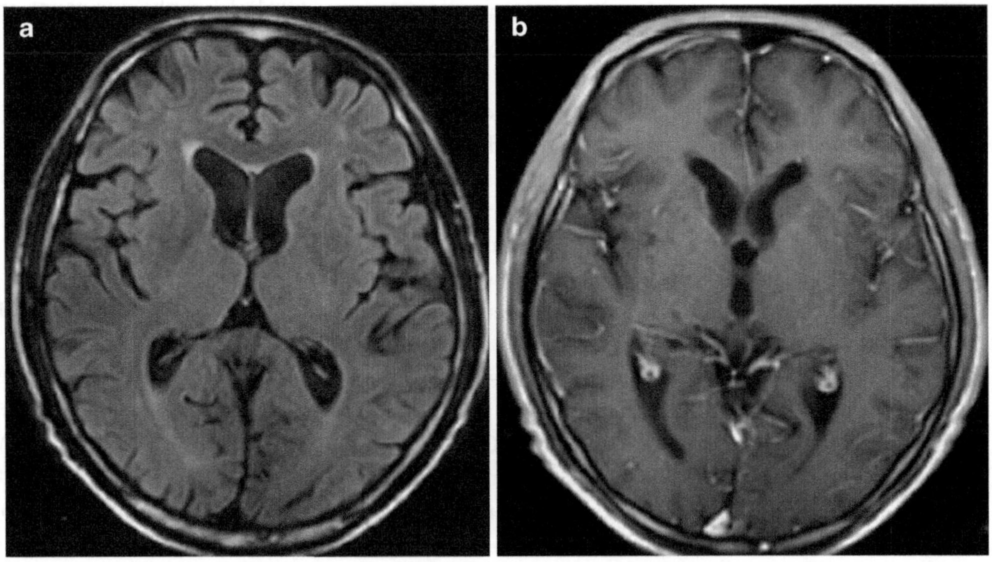

Fig. 10.10 HIV-positive male before HARRT treatment, 61 years old, HIV positive, cranial MRI before HAART treatment, with no intracranial lesion found. (**a**) T_2 FLAIR sequence; (**b**) T_1WI enhanced scan

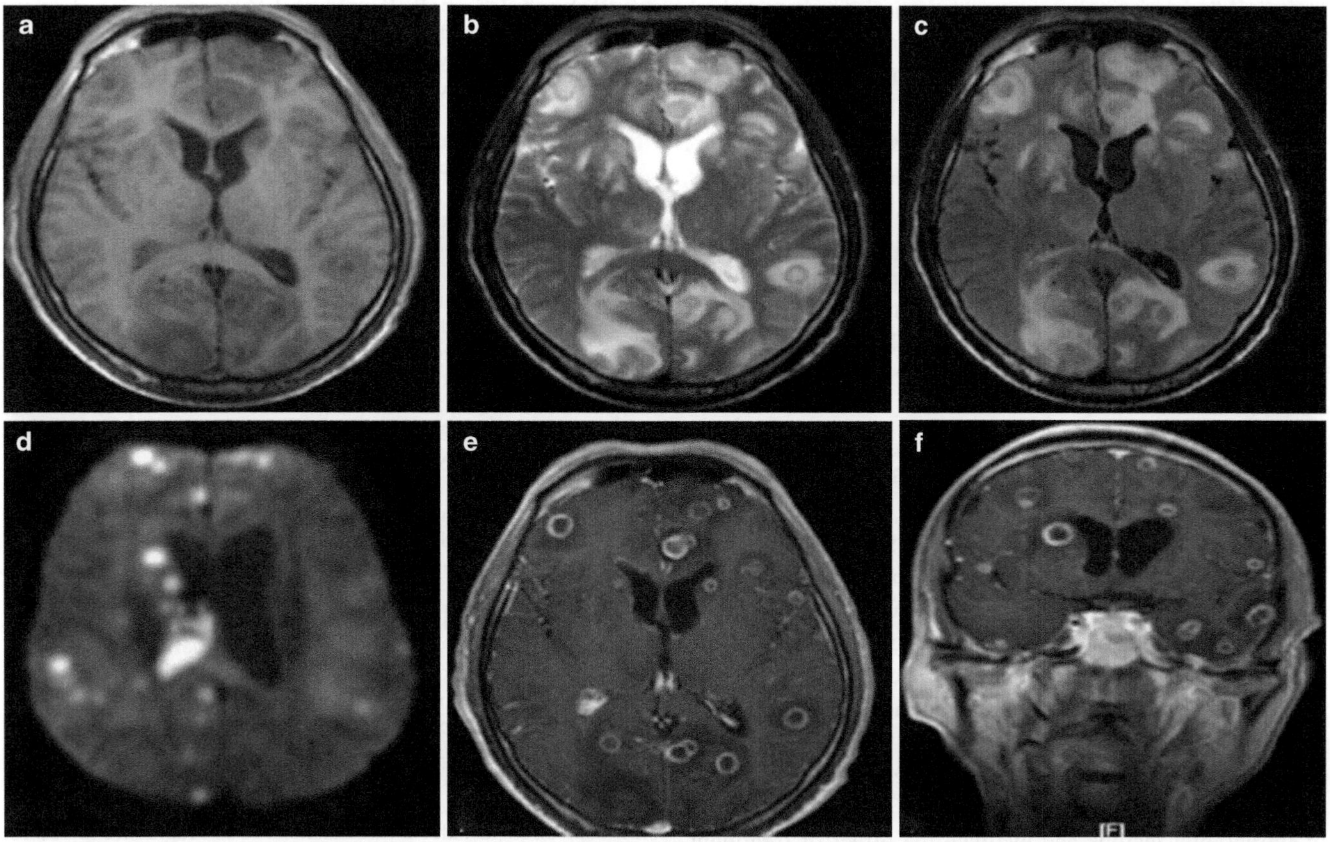

Fig. 10.11 Secondary toxoplasmic encephalopathy after 1 month of HARRT treatment. The same patient as in Fig. 10.10 was re-admitted 1 month after HARRT treatment for neurological symptoms such as headache and confusion. There are diffusely distributed round-like and ring-shaped lesions in the brain parenchyma. (**a**) T_1WI shows slightly hypointense inside the lesion and isointense in the wall; (**b**) T_2WI shows hyperintense inside the lesion and slightly hypointense in the wall, with a large patchy slightly hyperintense edema around the lesion; (**c**) FLAIR shows round-like slightly hypointense in the lesion; (**d**) DWI shows multiple round-like and ring-shaped hyperintense in the cerebral; (**e, f**) T_1WI enhanced scan showed the lesion with ring like enhancement (axial, coronal)

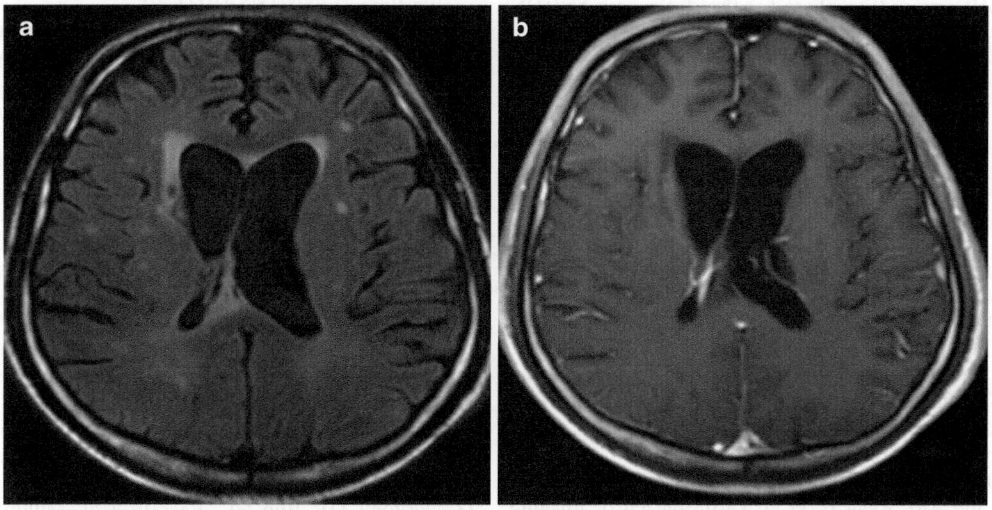

Fig. 10.12 After anti-Toxoplasma treatment and continuation of HAART therapy for 2 months. In the same patient as in Fig. 10.10, anti-Toxoplasma (compound sulfamethoxazole) and symptomatic support therapy were started and HAART was continued, and the patient's mind gradually cleared. (**a**) FLAIR shows scattered speckled hyperintense in the brain, compared with the previous one (Fig. 10.11), the number of lesions is significantly reduced, and the range of lesions is significantly reduced. (**b**) There is no abnormal enhancement in the brain

ferential diagnosis includes opportunistic infections (which can be secondary to HAART treatment failure), adverse reactions to antiviral drugs, etc. Patients who develop a pathogenic and immunologic response to HAART therapy with fever, tissue, and organ inflammatory responses are often misdiagnosed as secondary opportunistic infections, and the correct diagnosis is often not easily made. The period of high incidence of opportunistic infection is 0–3 months or more than 5 years after antiviral treatment for HIV-infected patients, which is different from the time of occurrence of IRIS. Bacterial pneumonia and tuberculosis are their main opportunistic infections.

10.7.6 Status and Progress of Research

Due to the critical condition of patients with neurological IRIS and the difficulty in obtaining pathological results, neuroimaging changes caused by immune reconstruction of the nervous system by some common pathogens are very important for clinical diagnosis. MRI and CT can be used to assist in the detection of IRIS to understand the size, morphology, location, number, and density of lesions, with MRI being the mainstay. MRI has a significant advantage over CT in detecting early lesions and can detect the size, shape, and location of intracranial lesions and evaluate the effect of treatment. MRI has good spatial resolution for HIV-associated inflammation and is sensitive for early detection of lesions and is suggestive of excessive neurological inflammation, with enhanced meningeal enhancement, hyperintense on DWI and FLAIR sequences, and clear occupying effects (especially for determining whether immune reconstitution is occurring in PML) providing clues for the diagnosis of IRIS [35]. The significance of imaging is that it allows dynamic observation of the disease process and provides a basis for clinical detection of intracranial infections.

References

1. Zhang Y, Song F, Wu H, et al. Pathological changes and imaging diagnosis of AIDS-associated dementia. Chin J Clin Infect Dis. 2012;5(5):318–20.
2. Li H. Practical AIDS imaging. Beijing: People's Health Publishing House; 2012.
3. Nakamoto BK, Jahanshad N, McMurtray A, et al. Cerebrovascular risk factors and brain microstructural abnormalities on diffusion tensor images in HIV-infected individuals. J Neurovirol. 2012;18(4):303–12.
4. Filippi CG, Ulug AM, Ryan E, et al. Diffusion tensor imaging of patients with HIV and normal-appearing white matter on MR images of the brain. Am J Neuroradiol. 2010;22(3):277–83.
5. Pomara N, Crandall DT, Choi SJ, et al. White matter abnormalities in HIV-1 infection: a diffusion tensor imaging study. Psychiatry Res. 2008;10(5):15–24.
6. Bladowska J, Knysz B, Zimny A, et al. Value of perfusion- weighted MR imaging in the assessment of early cerebral alterations in neurologically asymptomatic HIV-1-positive and HCV-positive patients. PLoS One. 2014;9(7):1–7.
7. Robert Y, Kelly K. Bacterial, fungal and parasitic infections of the central nervous system: radiologic-pathologic correlation and historical perspectives. Radiographics. 2015;35(2): 1141–69.
8. Masamed R, Meleis A, Lee EW, et al. Cerebral toxoplasmosis: case review and description of a new imaging sign. Clin Radiol. 2009;64(5):560–3.
9. Schroeder PC, Post MJD, Oschatz E, et al. Analysis of the utility of diffusion-weighted MRI and apparent diffusion coefficient values in distinguishing central nervous system toxoplasmosis from lymphoma. Neuroradiology. 2006;48(10):715–20.
10. Ernst TM, Chang L, Witt MD, et al. Cerebral toxoplasmosis and lymphoma in AIDS: perfusion MR imaging experience in 13 patients. Radiology. 1998;208(3):663–9.
11. Seok JH, Park HJ, Ahn K. Diffusion MRI findings of cytomegalovirus—associated ventriculitis: a case report. Br J Radiol. 2011;84(2):179–81.
12. Renard T, Daumas-Duport B, Auffray-Calvier E, et al. Cytomegalovirus encephalitis: undescribed diffusion-weighted imaging characteristics. Original aspects of cases extracted from a retrospective study. J Neuroradiol. 2016;43(6):371–7.
13. Midya V, Chakraborty U. A study of N-acetyl aspartic acid/creatine ratio in the white matter of HIV positive patients and its application. Amsterdam: European Meeting Statisticians; 2015.
14. Shah R, Bag AK, Chapman PR, et al. Imaging manifestations of progressive multifocal leukoencephalopathy. Clin Radiol. 2010;65(6):431–9.
15. Sahraian MA, Radue EW, Eshaghi A, et al. Progressive multifocal leukoencephalopathy: a review of the neuroimaging features and differential diagnosis. Eur J Neurol. 2012;19(8):1060–9.
16. Kasane N, Hiroki U, Mayu S, et al. Akinetic mutism caused by HIV- associated progressive multifocal leukoencephalopathy was successfully treated with mefloquine: a serial multimodal MRI study. Intern Med. 2012;51(2):205–9.
17. Cosottini M, Tavarelli C, Bono L, et al. Diffusion-weighted imaging in patients with progressive multifocal leukoencephalopathy. Eur Radiol. 2008;18(5):1024–30.
18. Yoon JH, Bang OY, Kim HS. Progressive multifocal leukoencephalopathy in AIDS: proton MR spectroscopy patterns of asynchronous lesions confirmed by serial diffusion-weighted imaging and apparent diffusion using coefficient mapping. J Clin Neurol. 2007;3(4):200–3.
19. Godi C, de Vita E, Tombetti E, et al. High b-value diffusion-weighted imaging in progressive multifocal leukoencephalopathy in HIV patients. Eur Radiol. 2017;27(9):3593–9.
20. Chastain DB, Henao-Martínez AF, Franco-Paredes C. Opportunistic invasive mycoses in AIDS: cryptococcosis, histoplasmosis, coccidiodomycosis, and talaromycosis. Curr Infect Dis Rep. 2017;19(10):36.
21. Ye F, Luo Q, Zhou Y, et al. Disseminated penicilliosis marneffei in immunocompetent patients: a report of two cases. Indian J Med Microbiol. 2015;33(1):161–5.
22. Thuy L, Nguyen HC, Ngo T, et al. AIDS-associated Penicillium marneffei infection of the central nervous system. Clin Infect Dis. 2010;51(12):1458–62.
23. Noritomi DT, Bub GL, Beer I, et al. Multiple brain abscesses due to Penicillium spp infection. Rev Inst Med Trop Sao Paulo. 2005;47(3):167–70.
24. Miao Z, Jue H. Clinicopathological analysis of nine cases of Penicillium marneffei misdiagnosed as histoplasmosis. J Gannan Med Coll. 2002;5(22):499–501.

25. Li H. Practical infectious disease imaging. Beijing: People's Medical Publishing House; 2014.
26. Velázquez BA, Tejero JC, Pérez LC, et al. Cerebral abscess due to Rhodococcus equi with pseudotumour presentation in an immunocompetent patient. Neurologia. 2013;28(8):522–5.
27. Roda RH, Young M, Timpone J, et al. Rhodococcus equi pulmonary-central nervous system syndrome: brain abscess in a patient on high-dose steroids—a case report and review of the literature. Diagn Microbiol Infect Dis. 2009;63(1):96–9.
28. Rallis G, Dais P, Gkinis G, et al. Acute osteomyelitis of the mandible caused by Rhodococcus equi in an immunocompromised patient: a case report and literature review. Oral Surg Oral Med Oral Pathol Oral Radiol. 2012;114(4):e1–5.
29. Li H. Practical infectious disease imaging. Beijing: People's Medical Publishing House; 2017.
30. Rahamat-Langendoen JC, van Meurs M, Zijlstra JG, et al. Disseminated Rhodococcus equi infection in a kidney transplant patient without initial pulmonary involvement. Diagn Microbiol Infect Dis. 2009;65(4):427–30.
31. DeSimone JA, Pomerantz RJ, Babinchak TJ. Inflammatory reactions in HIV-1-infected persons after initiation of highly active antiretroviral therapy. Ann Intern Med. 2000;133(6):447–54.
32. Bahr N, Boulware DR, Marais S, et al. Central nervous system immune reconstitution inflammatory syndrome. Curr Infect Dis Rep. 2013;15(6):583–93.
33. Shelburne SA, Hamill RJ, Rodriguez-Barradas MC, et al. Immune reconstitution inflammatory syndrome: emergence of a unique syndrome during highly active antiretroviral therapy. Medicine (Baltimore). 2002;81(3):213–27.
34. Post MJ, Thurnher MM, Clifford DB, et al. CNS-immune reconstitution inflammatory syndrome in the setting of HIV infection, part 2: discussion of neuro-immune reconstitution inflammatory syndrome with and without other pathogens. Am J Neuroradiol. 2013;34(7):1308–18.
35. Kozić D, Bjelan M, Boban J, et al. A prominent lactate peak as a potential key magnetic resonance spectroscopy (MRS)feature of progressive multifocal leukoencephalopathy (PML): spectrum pattern observed in three patients. Bosn J Basic Med Sci. 2017;17(4):349–54.

Part III

Special Infectious and Inflammatory Diseases of the Central Nervous System

11 Intracranial Purulent/Bacterial Infection

Hanqiu Liu, Weiwei Wang, Jianhua Ma, Chunhui Jiang, Shifeng Wang, Hongyan Chen, Yunling Wang, and Shuang Ding

11.1 Purulent Meningitis

Hanqiu Liu, Weiwei Wang, and Jianhua Ma

11.1.1 Overview

Purulent meningitis (PM) is a diffuse acute purulent bacterial infectious disease of the pia mater and arachnoid and subarachnoid spaces [1, 2]. PM is one of the serious intracranial infections that often coexist with purulent encephalitis or brain abscess. Pathogenic bacteria can be found in the cerebrospinal fluid, the most common pathogenic organisms being *S. meningitidis*, *S. pneumoniae*, and *H. influenzae*, followed by *S. aureus*, *Streptococcus*, *Escherichia coli*, *S. pyogenes*, and *P. aeruginosa*. *S. pneumoniae* meningitidis most commonly affects children, but adults can also be infected. *S. pneumoniae* meningitis occurs in the elderly and in infants and children. *B. influenzae* meningitis occurs in young children under the age of 6. Escherichia coli is the most common causative agent of neonatal meningitis. *Staphylococcus aureus* and *Pseudomonas aeruginosa* meningitis are often secondary to lumbar puncture and neurosurgery. Patients often present with acute infection, symptoms of intracranial hypertension, and focal brain symptoms. In the acute encephalitis stage, patients have fever, headache, vomiting, and elevated blood leukocyte counts. In the brain abscess formation stage, patients have increased intracranial pressure, headache, and optic disc edema. The detection of relevant pathogens in the cerebrospinal fluid is used as a basis for the diagnosis of this disease.

H. Liu (✉) · W. Wang
Huashan Hospital, Fudan University, Shanghai, China

J. Ma · C. Jiang · Y. Wang · S. Ding
The First Affiliated Hospital of Xinjiang Medical University, Urumqi, China

S. Wang
Tianjin Panorama Medical Imaging Diagnostic Center, Tianjin, China

H. Chen
Beijing Tiantan Hospital, Capital Medical University, Beijing, China

11.1.2 Pathological Manifestations

The pathological changes in acute septic meningitis caused by various pathogenic bacteria are essentially the same [3]. In the early stage, the pia mater and superficial blood vessels of the brain are congested and dilated, and the inflammation spreads along the subarachnoid space, with a large amount of purulent exudate covering the brain surface, often deposited in the cerebral sulcus and basal brain cistern, etc. It can also be seen in the ventricles of the brain. The color of the pus is related to the pathogenic organism species. As the inflammation spreads, both the superficial pia mater and the ventricular canal membranes become granular due to the fibrin exudate covering them. Late in the course of the disease, cerebrospinal fluid absorption and circulation are impaired due to meningeal adhesions, resulting in traffic or non-traffic hydrocephalus. Subdural fluid and pus accumulation are often seen in children and occasionally venous sinus thrombosis, brain abscesses, or cerebral softening and infarction due to endarteritis.

11.1.3 Imaging

11.1.3.1 CT

In early stages of septic meningitis, CT plain scan mostly shows no abnormal findings [4]. Further development of infection may show increased density or occlusion of the cerebral sulcus, cistern, cerebral fissure, and especially the basal pool of the brain due to meningeal congestion and arachnoid exudation. In complicated encephalitis, confined or diffuse hypodense areas appear in the brain parenchyma,

H. Li et al. (eds.), *Radiology of Infectious and Inflammatory Diseases - Volume 1*,
https://doi.org/10.1007/978-981-99-0039-8_11

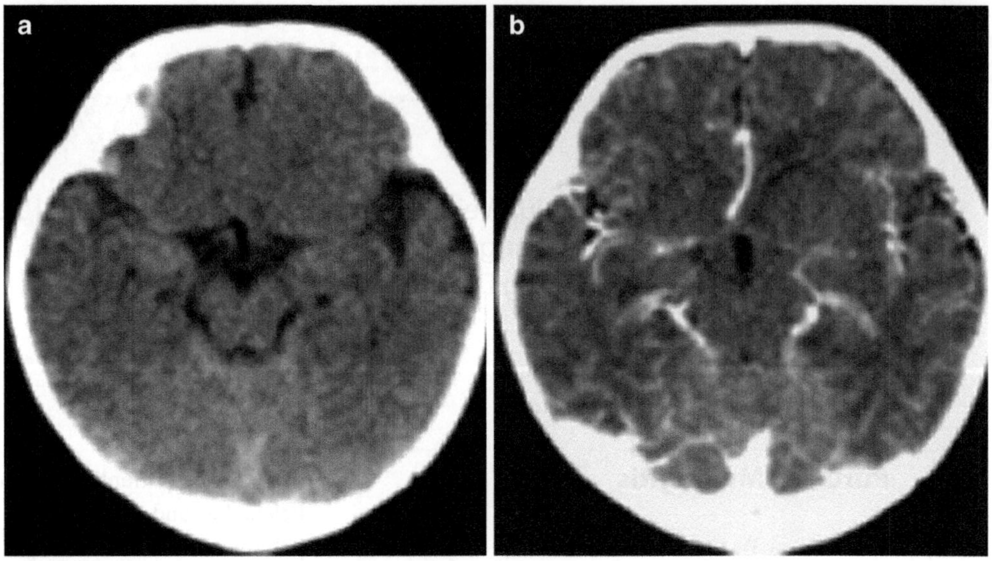

Fig. 11.1 Septic meningitis. (**a**) CT plain scan showing increased density in the cerebral sulci and brain cistern; (**b**) CT enhanced scan showing curve-like or gyral enhancement of the pia mater and brain surface

and diffuse cerebral edema may reduce the lateral and third ventricles on both sides symmetrically (Fig. 11.1a). Enhanced scans show curvilinear or gyral-like enhancement of the pia mater and brain surface, mostly in the frontal, parietal, longitudinal, and lateral fissures (Fig. 11.1b). In cases of ventriculitis caused by inflammation of the ventricular canal and choroidal plexus, extensive purulent fibrous exudate may occur, and patients may develop arachnoid space or aqueductal stenosis, resulting in a trafficked or obstructive hydrocephalus.

Meningitis may be associated with ventriculitis in 30% of cases and more than 90% of neonatal cases, and enhanced scans may show limited or diffuse thin linear enhancement of the ventricular wall, adhesions of the ventricular wall, and ventricular compartmentalized enhancement, often with concomitant choroid plexitis. In children under 1 year of age, 20–33% of intracranial infections can be combined with subdural and epidural pus, of which 10–15% are complications of meningitis, manifested as crescentic or pyknotic hypodense images beneath the cranial plate, also seen in the interhemispheric fissure, which can be strengthened if it forms an envelope. In adults with meningitis, 37% may be combined with cerebral ischemia and cerebral infarction due to cerebrovascular damage, which manifests as homogeneous hypodense foci, consistent with the distribution of blood vessels.

11.1.3.2 MRI

In the early stages of septic meningitis, most MRI plain scans are unremarkable. Positive findings may be a manifestation of the primary lesion or a manifestation of meningitis and its complications. However, MRI is more sensitive than CT, often showing earlier and more lesions than CT [4].

As the infection develops, a large amount of purulent exudate covers the brain surface and is often deposited in the cerebral sulcus and the basal brain pool. In T1WI, the signal of the subarachnoid space is slightly higher than that of the cerebrospinal fluid due to the accumulation of purulent exudate; in T2WI, a high signal is seen in the subarachnoid space; in the early stage, it may be accompanied by a widening of the subarachnoid space, and in the later stage, the subarachnoid space is often narrowed or occluded, and the basal pools are often occluded. On enhanced T1WI, pia mater enhancement is seen as a curvilinear intensification of the frontal, temporal, and parietal lobes extending into the sulcus (Fig. 11.2), and coronal or sagittal enhancement of the basal cisterns and lateral fissures is seen as thick lines. In contrast to enhanced CT, enhanced MR T1WI shows pia mater enhancement on the frontal, temporal, and parietal brain surfaces, as well as basal and lateral fissure cistern enhancement. In addition to enhancement of the frontal, temporal, and parietal brain surfaces and the basal and lateral fissure cistern, thicker lines of enhancement of the falx and tentorium of cerebellum can be seen on coronal or sagittal images. Enhanced T1WI shows pia mater enhancement. In late-onset bacterial meningitis occurring after 7 days of life, enhanced MR T1WI may show pia mater enhancement on the surface of the brain (including in the sulci), which may be accompanied by adjacent endocranium enhancement separated by subdural fluid; this endocranium enhancement may persist for months after full clinical recovery.

FLAIR imaging before and after enhancement shows the subarachnoid space, i.e., the cerebral sulcus, fissure, and/or brain cistern appearing as high signal (Fig. 11.2); enhanced T1WI shows pia mater enhancement, which is often not easily distinguished from the small cortical surface enhancement of veins. However, this is not a problem in those with enhanced T1 FLAIR imaging (as small cortical surface vein enhancement is rarely seen) [5, 6]. It has been found that a linear high signal in the cerebral sulcus is seen in DWI in

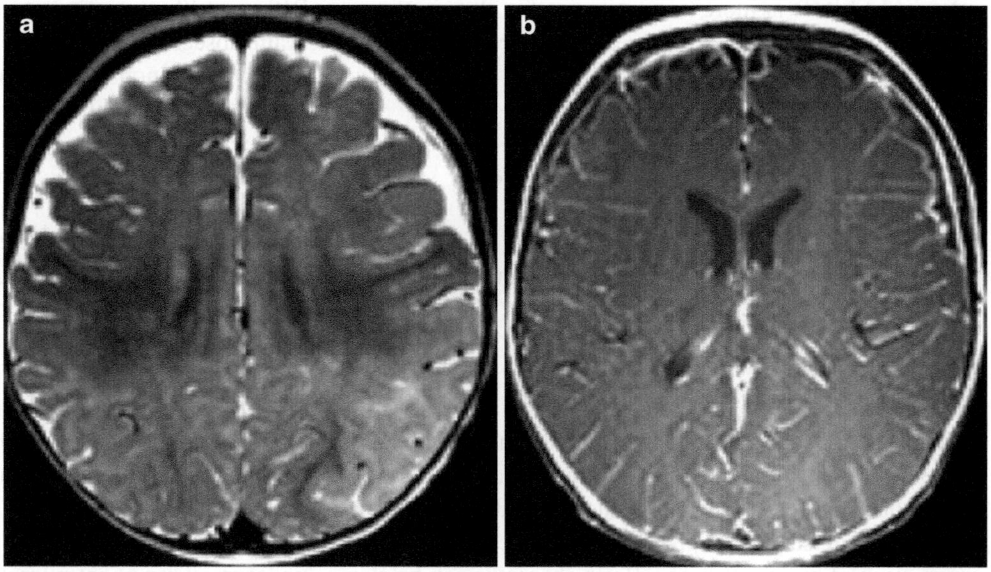

Fig. 11.2 Septic meningitis. (**a**) Enhanced FLAIR sequence shows extensive pia mater enhancement, and an extensive high signal band is seen under the dura on the surface of the other bilateral frontal lobes, suggesting possible subdural fluid and/or pus accumulation; (**b**) T_1WI enhanced scan shows extensive pia mater enhancement

patients with septic meningitis, and this sign helps in the diagnosis of septic meningitis [7].

Enhanced T1WI and MR FLAIR in bacterial (including septic), viral, tuberculous, and fungal meningitis show pia mater enhancement or subarachnoid enhancement, with enhanced FLAIR imaging being preferable compared to both. The presentation of bacterial (including septic), tuberculous, viral, and fungal meningitis was essentially similar, whether on enhanced MR T1WI, or enhanced MR FLAIR. However, the distribution of the meninges may vary in reinforcing them, with bacterial (including septic) meningitis mostly in the convex and lateral fissures of the brain, whereas tuberculous and fungal meningitis are mostly in the cistern, especially the basal cistern.

MRI and CT both reveal many complications of meningitis, such as ventriculitis, encephalitis, vasculogenic or cytotoxic cerebral edema, hydrocephalus, focal ischemic injury (e.g., cerebral infarction), infected venous sinus thrombosis, subdural effusion, subdural pus, epidural abscess, and brain abscess.

11.1.4 Diagnostic Key Points

1. Most often, there is a history of definite septic bacterial infection.
2. Imaging characteristics consist of meningeal enhancement. In CT scan, subarachnoid space is blurred and hypodense; in MR scan, T_1WI and T_2WI are normal, and FLAIR is isointense or slightly hyperintense; T_1 and FLAIR enhanced scans show linear enhancement of pia mater and meninges.
3. DWI sequences of the cerebral sulcus may show a significant hyperintense.
4. Cerebrospinal fluid examination: significantly higher white blood cell counts, increased protein, and decreased glucose. Associated pathogens can be detected in the cerebrospinal fluid.

11.1.5 Differential Diagnosis

1. Meningeal carcinomatosis. It is also known as carcinomatous meningitis, which can grow infiltratively along the meninges or form nodules or masses based on the meninges and can be combined with intracerebral metastases.
2. Tuberculous meningitis. In tuberculous meningitis, meningeal enhancement is linear, mainly in the brain cistern at the base of the brain, and sometimes nodular enhancement is seen in the brain as a result of tuberculoma lesions, but such tuberculomas are usually found only at the base of the skull and not on the convex surface of the brain or under the ventricles.
3. Viral meningitis. The clinical and imaging manifestations of bacterial meningitis and viral meningitis are often difficult to distinguish, relying mainly on laboratory tests and cultures of cerebrospinal fluid.

11.1.6 Status and Progress of Research

MRI and CT can be used for the examination of septic meningitis, with MRI being the recommended method of examination. MR sequence, FLAIR, and DWI are advantageous for detecting lesions. Enhanced CT and MRI scans are of great value for showing meningitis; especially MR enhanced FLAIR is more advantageous for showing meningeal changes and can be the recommended examination sequence.

11.2 Purulent Encephalitis and Brain Abscess

Hanqiu Liu, Chunhui Jiang, and Shifeng Wang

11.2.1 Overview

Invasion of the brain tissue by purulent pathogens causes limited purulent inflammation followed by abscess formation, called purulent encephalitis and brain abscess, respectively. Both are sequential processes in the development and progression of brain infections. Brain abscesses can be classified as four types according to the source of infection [8]: (1) Brain abscesses are caused by direct spread of adjacent foci of infection: the most common is otogenic brain abscess, accounting for 50% of all brain abscess cases, which is a complication of purulent otitis media [such as acute otitis media, acute mastoiditis of the auris media, chronic cholesteatoma otitis media (the most common), and chronic purulent otitis media]. Otogenic brain abscesses are mostly solitary, with 2/3 occurring in the temporal lobe and 1/3 in the cerebellar hemisphere. With regard to route of infection, auris media tympanitis leads to destruction of the paries tympanicus, tegmen tympani, mastoid roof, and posterior part of the petrous bone, invading and disrupting the meninges and invading the brain parenchyma, forming temporal brain abscesses upward and cerebellar abscesses downward. Nasogenic brain abscess is rare and accounts for 10–20% of brain abscesses, secondary to frontal sinusitis, often located in the anterior and base of the frontal lobe. Brain abscesses due to scalp and skull infections are caused by uncontrolled local infections, and abscesses occur in close proximity to these foci of infection. (2) The incidence of hematogenous brain abscess is second only to otogenic brain abscess, accounting for 25% of all brain abscesses. Infections in distant sites outside the brain cause bacteremia and spread the infection to the brain via arteries, veins, or the vertebral venous plexus, causing brain abscesses, also known as migratory brain abscesses or metastatic brain abscesses, which occur mostly in the middle cerebral artery supply area and are most common in the frontal and parietal lobes. About 50% of abscesses are multiple. Foci of infection in any part of the body can cause a hematogenous brain abscess, most commonly purulent inflammation of the pleura, lungs, and bronchi, such as lung abscess, chronic empyema, chronic bronchitis with bronchiectasis, and secondary infection from lung cancer, etc. Some call this pulmonary brain abscess. Patients with congenital atrial septal defect are prone to have brain abscess, because when patients develop bacteremia, most of the venous blood cannot be filtered through the lungs and enters the circulation directly to the brain; patients with congenital atrial septal defect tend to have polycythemia and hemoconcentration, which makes it easy to form small blood clots in the brain, and this is also one of the reasons why they are prone to have brain abscess, and the lack of oxygen in the brain weakens its ability to defend against infection. (3) Traumatic brain abscess accounts for about 10% of the brain abscesses and is caused by foreign bodies (broken bone fragments, hair, metal foreign bodies, glass fragments, etc.) entering the brain after craniocerebral trauma, especially open traumatic brain injury, or by secondary infection due to incomplete debridement. In recent years, early and complete debridement after trauma has become possible due to the widespread availability of neurosurgery. In addition, the widespread use of antimicrobial drugs has led to a significant decrease in the incidence of traumatic brain abscesses. (4) Cryptogenic brain abscess: 10% or so of brain abscesses cannot find the primary foci of infection, probably because the primary foci of infection are mild and controlled by antibacterial medication, but bacteria have already entered the brain via the bloodstream, and when the patient's immune resistance decreases, the foci in the brain gradually form brain abscesses. The primary foci of infection are deep insidious and not easily noticed, such as chronic pharyngeal infections and decubitus ulcer infections. The complications of cryptogenic brain abscesses are chronic and are often misdiagnosed as tumors preoperatively. Regarding cerebrospinal fluid examination, significantly higher white blood cell counts can be detected from the cerebrospinal fluid as a confirmation of the diagnosis of the relevant pathogen.

11.2.2 Pathological Manifestations

The development and progression of septic encephalitis and brain abscess is a continuous process and cannot be staged in a definite manner, but according to the pathological manifestations, it can be divided into three stages [9]: (1) Acute encephalitis stage: Brain abscesses of any cause initially cause a limited purulent encephalitis lasting 7–14 days, with limited inflammation, congestion, edema, and necrosis of brain tissue with small venous inflammatory emboli and meningeal reactions. Perivascular polymorphonuclear cell infiltration is seen microscopically. (2) Purulent necrotic stage: After 7–14 days, the encephalitis continues to spread, the malacia necrotic area of the brain gradually expanded and fused, forming a large pus cavity, surrounded by new blood vessels and a large amount of connective tissue proliferation gradually formed inconspicuous and irregular granulation tissue. A large infiltration of neutrophils can be seen microscopically. (3) Envelope formation stage: It lasts 3–4 weeks but can be as short as 12–14 days or as long as half a year or more. The abscess cavity and the surrounding connective tissue increase significantly, and the neuroglia increases, gradually thickening the abscess wall. Microscopically, the abscess wall is divided into three layers: the inner layer which is composed of purulent exudate, granulation tissue, and glial cells, with numerous neovascularization and neutrophil infiltration; the middle layer which is composed of a large amount of fibrous connective tissue; and the outer layer which is composed of gliosis and brain tissue edema, and increased vascularization and leukocyte infiltration.

11.2.3 Imaging

11.2.3.1 CT Findings

Brain abscesses have different CT findings depending on the stage of the abscess. It is very important for treatment to determine whether it is in the stage of encephalitis or in the stage of envelope formation according to the CT manifestation [10].

1. Encephalitis stage. Early CT plain scan may show normal or focal irregularly bounded hypodense shadow in the subcortical or corticomedullary junction area, or a heterogeneous hypodense, isodense mixed density shadow with a more pronounced occupancy effect (Fig. 11.3). Post-enhanced scans show no enhancement in the hypodense areas, or irregular speckle or gyrus-like enhancement, and rarely enhanced comprehensively. In the late stage, encephalitis continues to spread, the necrotic malacia gradually fuses, the lesion tends to be confined, and the enhanced scan may show an irregular, incomplete ring-like enhancement around the central hypodense area, and the delayed scan may show contrast "filling" of the central hypodense area. Peripheral brain tissue edema and occupying effects are evident, with narrowing, displacement, or even loss of adjacent brain sulci, brain cistern, brain fissures, and/or ventricles by compression.
2. Abscess stage: Early CT scan shows central abscess consisting of necrotic tissue and pus and manifests as a slightly hypodense shadow, with planes of gas and fluid visible in some pus cavities, and in about 50% of cases a complete or incomplete, regular or irregular isodense or slightly hyperdense ring around the hypodense foci (Fig. 11.4), with the ring of CT values averaged 34 HU and a thickness of approximately 5 mm, which is fibrous envelope layer.

   Enhanced scans show that the abscess inside remains hypodense, and the abscess wall is mildly enhanced, showing intact but irregular pale ring-like enhancement, which can be thick or thin, homogenous or heteroge-

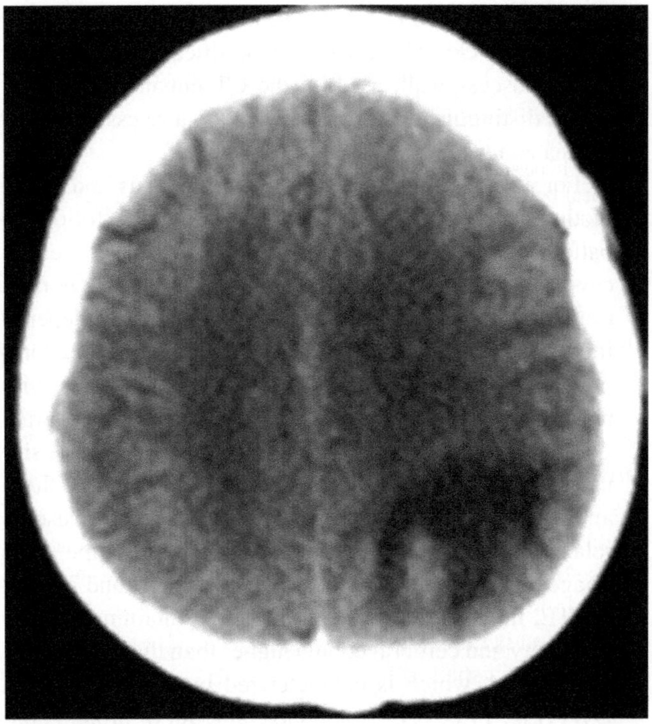

Fig. 11.3 Brain abscess encephalitis stage. CT scan shows a patchy iso-hypodense area under the left parietal cortex with marked surrounding edema and significant occupying effect

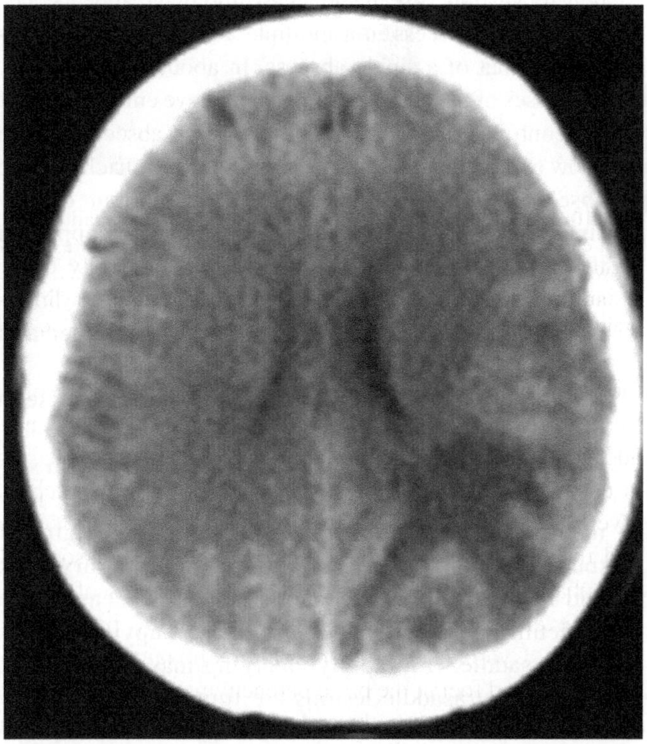

Fig. 11.4 Brain abscess (1). CT scan shows a nodular isodense foci with a central hypodense and a complete isodense ring around the left parietal cortex, with marked peripheral edema and mild occupying effect

neous, with blurred outer wall edges. As the abscess wall forms, enhanced scans reveal intact, thin-walled, uniform thickness and marked enhancement with wall CT values rising to 60 HU and thicknesses of 1–3 mm. In some cases, the enhanced ring is thicker on the gray matter side and thinner on the ependyma side, which is related with a lesser blood supply of the white matter and an abundant blood supply of the gray matter. At this stage, cerebral edema is relatively mild, and the peripheral hypodensity is less extensive than before. The abscess is gradually decreasing in extent, the fibrous envelope thickens, and the surrounding edema may decrease to disappear. CT plain scan shows central hypodensity, which is slightly higher than cerebrospinal fluid, of abscess, with intact envelope and slightly higher density. Enhanced scan shows ring-like enhancement with a more complete and smooth ring wall and increased wall thickness up to 3–6 mm with adjacent meningeal enhancement. The ring-like enhancement can persist for weeks to months, even up to 8 months after cessation of drug therapy.

The shape is usually round or oval, sometimes irregular. When abscesses are small, they may show nodular enhancement. In a few cases of open fractures or postoperative infection, the abscess wall may be thick and irregular. If there is gas formation in the abscess, a lower density shadow is seen and a gas-fluid plane appears. The CT of each abscess in a multiple abscess behaves similarly to that of a single abscess. In about 50% of cases, abscesses of the cerebral hemisphere have enlargement of the contralateral ventricle, and cerebellar abscesses often show enlargement of the lateral and third ventricles. If the abscess ruptures into the ventricle, abnormal density shadow and ventricular wall enhancement may appear in the ventricles. Brain abscesses treated medically or by surgical puncture can show reduced pus cavity, diminished ring enhancement, and reduced cerebral edema in follow-up CT.

Pituitary abscess is rare. Coronal CT scan of sella turcica shows enlarged or non-enlarged sella turcica, with hypodense shadow visible in the saddle, with significant enhancement on enhanced scan, which may manifest as substantial or ring-like. Limited bulging of the diaphragma sellae can be seen and pituitary stalk and adenohypophysis cannot be identified easily and difficult to differentiate from other occupying lesions in the saddle. If a rapidly enlarging mass and clinical signs of intrasaddle lesions are found, the possibility of an intrasaddle pituitary abscess should be considered in conjunction with a history of epidemic meningitis and cerebrospinal fluid nasal leakage. The diagnosis of pituitary tumors combined with abscesses remains difficult.

11.2.3.2 MRI Findings

MRI is superior to CT in showing brain abscesses and can help clinical treatment by providing early diagnosis of encephalitis [11–13].

1. Encephalitis stage: Early T_1WI shows isointense or slightly hypointense with irregular borders in the white matter. T_2WI shows hyperintense in both the central inflammation and the surrounding edema area, and sometimes the signal of encephalitis can be slightly lower than that of the surrounding edema with distinct occupying effect. After applying Gd-DTPA enhanced scan, there is no enhancement on T_1WI in most cases, and some may show patchy heterogenous enhancement. The earliest abscesses form a central area with hypointense on T_1WI and hyperintense on T_2WI after the necrotic areas of late stage have fused with each other; the periphery may show a thin irregular ring with isointense or moderately hyperintense on T_1WI and isointense or slightly hypointense on T_2WI. Enhanced scans show ring-shaped enhancement that lasts 30–60 min and often reveal more symptoms than plain scans. Peripheral cerebral edema may persist.
2. Abscess stage: The formation of a brain abscess is marked by the presence of an abscess wall, which manifest as a relatively iso- or slightly hyperintense on T_1WI and a relatively hypointense on T_2WI; the abscess cavity manifests as hypointense on T_1WI and hyperintense on T_2WI; and the surrounding brain edema manifests as hypointense on T_1WI and hyperintense on T_2WI. The scan after injection of Gd-DTPA shows a significant enhancement of the abscess wall, as does the CT enhancement ring, which distinguishes the abscess cavity, abscess wall, and edema zone (Fig. 11.5 and 11.6).

For a mature abscess with central necrosis and liquefaction, the signal intensity on T_1WI has the following pattern from low to high: cerebrospinal fluid $\leq$ central cavity < brain tissue of surrounding edema < normal brain tissue. The signal intensity on T_2WI varies depending on the echo time (TE) and the degree of protein composition and central liquefaction in the abscess, with normal brain tissue < cerebrospinal fluid < cavity $\leq$ brain tissue of surrounding edema. When TE <100 ms, the signal difference between cerebrospinal fluid, cavity fluid, and edema decreases when TE is prolonged because T_2 relaxation is maximized on long repetition time (TR) images and T_1 contrast is significant in short and moderate TE, making the signal of protein-containing fluid in the cavity and cerebral edema higher than that of cerebrospinal fluid, which is characterized by hyperintense on DWI (Fig. 11.6c) due to the large amount of protein content in the abscess resulting in local tissue viscosity and restricted diffusion of water molecules, which is characteristic and of some value in differential diagnosis.

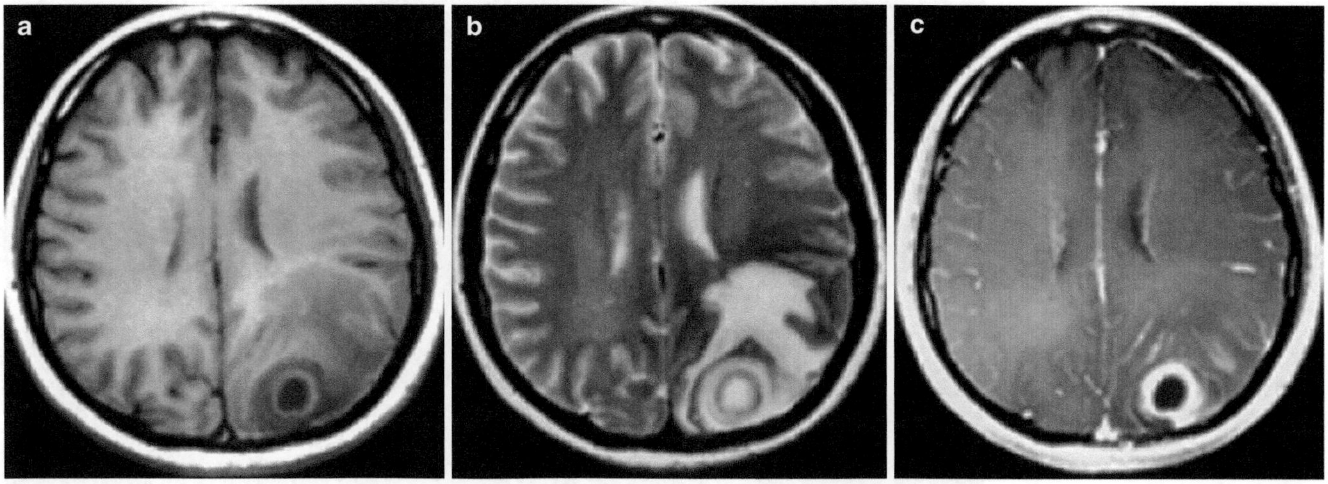

Fig. 11.5 Brain abscess (2). The left parietal subcortical round lesion clearly shows the abscess cavity, abscess wall, and edema zone of the brain abscess. (**a**) T1WI shows hyperintense in the abscess inner wall and hypointense in outer layer, hypointense in the abscess cavity and surrounding brain edema; (**b**) T_2WI shows relatively hypointense in the abscess wall, hyperintense in the abscess cavity and the surrounding brain edema; (**c**) T_1WI enhanced scan shows significant ring-like enhancement of the abscess wall

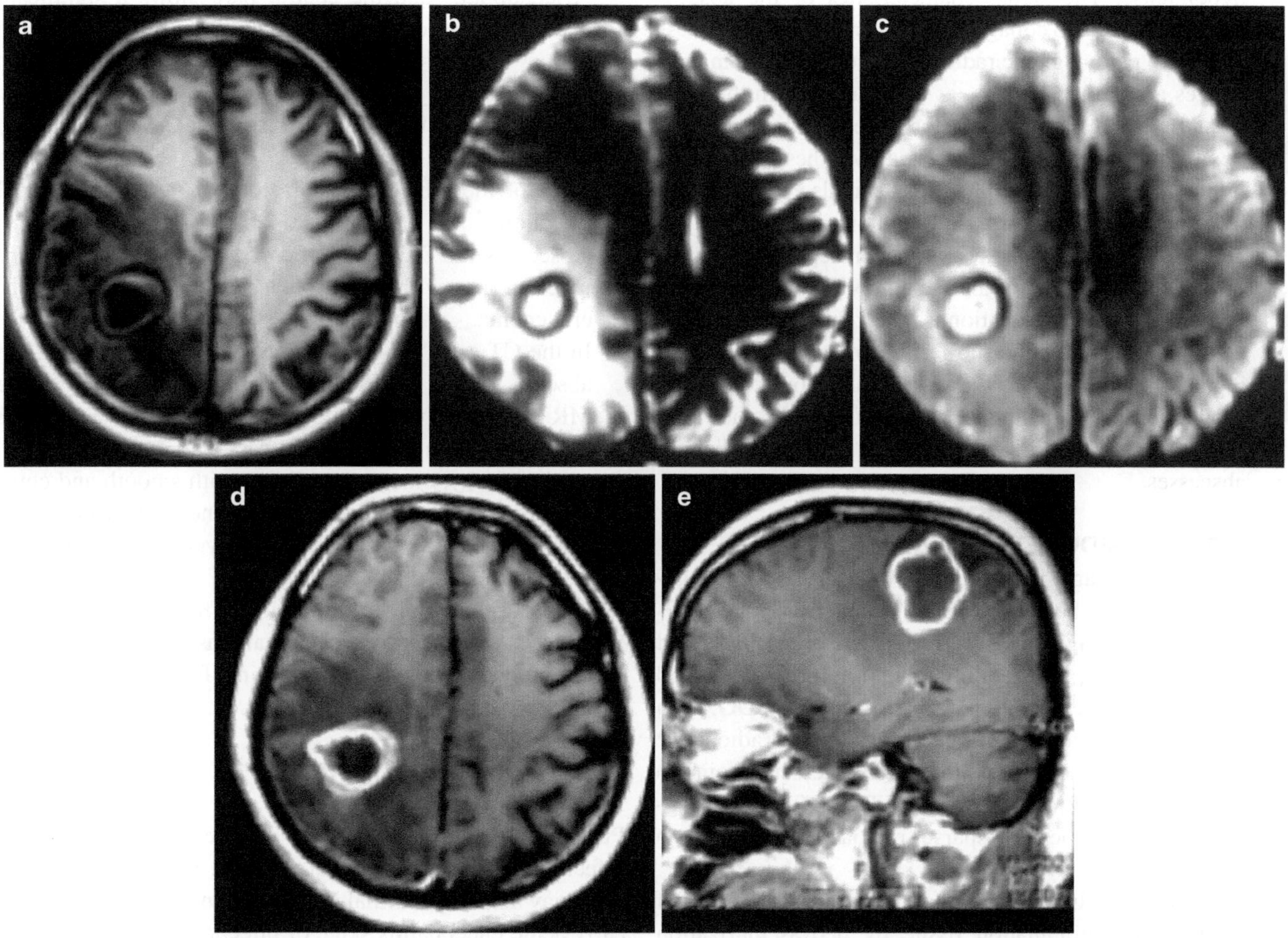

Fig. 11.6 Brain abscess (3). There is a circular lesion in the right frontal lobe. (**a**) T_1WI shows hyperintense in the inner layer of the abscess wall and hypointense in the outer layer, hypointense in the abscess cavity and surrounding cerebral edema; (**b**) T_2WI shows hypointense in the abscess wall, hyperintense in the abscess cavity and surrounding cerebral edema; (**c**) DWI shows relatively hypointense in the abscess wall and largely uniform hyperintense in the abscess cavity; (**d, e**) T_1WI enhanced scan shows a clear ring-like enhancement in the abscess wall

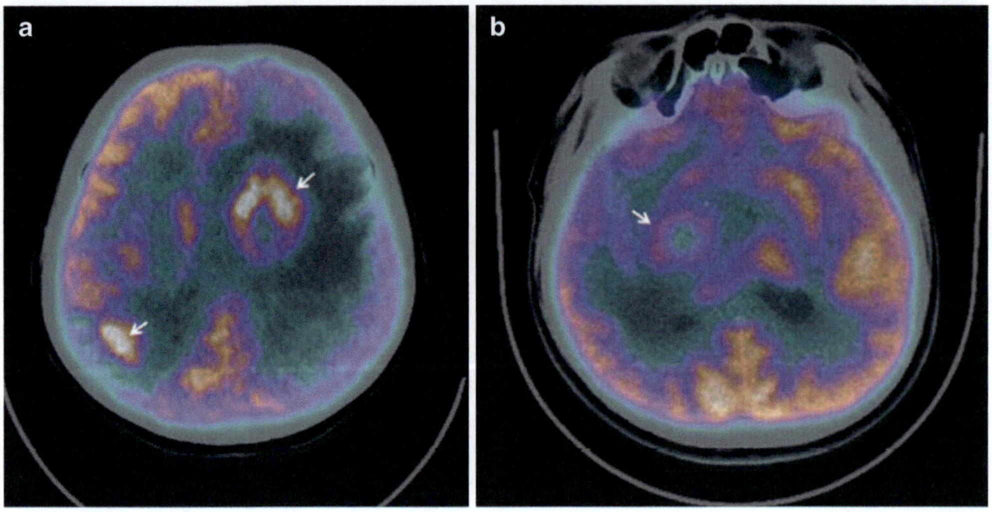

Fig. 11.7 Brain abscess in the right parietal, left frontal, and right basal ganglia regions. (**a**) Brain ^{18}F-FDG PET showing right parietal and left frontal masses or circular heterogenous foci of radioactive distribution; (**b**) brain ^{18}F-FDG PET showing circular foci of radioactive distribution in the right basal ganglia region

In the absence of proteins and other macromolecules, the signal of the cavity will be the same as that of the cerebrospinal fluid, with DWI as cerebrospinal fluid-like hypointense. The signal characteristics of the abscess wall may be due to collagen or hemorrhage in the abscess wall or to paramagnetic radicals phagocytized by macrophages around the abscess, as they can shorten the local T_1 and T_2 relaxation times to form the signal characteristics of the abscess wall which is a hypothesis supported by the following fact: granulomas can also show similar hypointensity rings on T_2WI without hemorrhage. In addition, some metastases have no iron deposits and hemorrhage but instead have a large number of macrophages. A more complex explanation is that free radicals contribute to the formation of ortho-ferric hemoglobin, so bleeding and free radicals may play a simultaneous role in the production of signaling characteristics. Air and fluid planes are seen in the abscess cavity which is typical in abscesses.

11.2.3.3 ^{18}F-FDG PET Findings

1. Encephalitis stage: Early ^{18}F-FDG PET may appear negative, or it may show an irregular, faintly marginated ^{18}F-FDG slightly high shadow of radioactive distribution at the lesion site, and as inflammation progresses and inflammatory cells continue to take up ^{18}F- FDG, then ^{18}F-FDG PET shows a further increase in the radioactive distribution at the lesion site, and as necrosis begins to appear in the central area, thus ^{18}F-FDG PET shows irregular small patches of sparse radioactive distribution reduced or defective.
2. Abscess stage: In the early stage, due to the formation of inflammatory granulation tissue by neovascularization and massive connective tissue proliferation, a large number of inflammatory cells continuously take up ^{18}F-FDG, thus PET manifesting as a confined mass-like radiolucent foci with clear boundaries (Fig. 11.7). With the formation of the abscess wall and cavity, the PET shows a ring-shaped foci of concentrated radioactivity in the form of "fried donut," and the central part shows a significant decrease in radioactivity distribution or even defect.

11.2.4 Diagnostic Key Points

1. Most of them had a clear history of purulent bacterial infection.
2. Abscesses are found in the cortical or corticomedullary junction area, with round-like lesions and marked peripheral edema.
3. In the CT scan, the abscess cavity is hypodense and the abscess wall is isodense or slightly hyperdense. In the MR scan, pus manifests as hypointense on T_1WI and hyperintense on T_2WI, and abscess wall manifests as iso- or slightly hypointense on T_2WI, with smooth and complete ring-like enhancement of the inner wall on enhanced scans; pus often has significant hyperintense on DWI sequences.
4. Cerebrospinal fluid examination: The white blood cell count is significantly elevated and associated pathogens can be detected in the cerebrospinal fluid.

11.2.5 Differential Diagnosis

Purulent infection is one of the more common intracranial infectious diseases in clinical practice. CT and MRI plain scan may not see abnormal manifestations in early stage. The early acute encephalitis stage of infection imaging manifestations lacks specificity; its qualitative diagnosis mainly relies on history, physical signs, and laboratory examination of cerebrospinal fluid; and imaging manifestations can assist in diagnosis and play a role in localization. Brain abscesses have a more typical imaging presentation and are not difficult to identify. Brain abscesses need to be differentiated from cerebral cysticercosis, high-grade astrocytomas, brain metastases, intracerebral hematomas, cerebral infarcts, and postsurgical residual cavities.

11.2.5.1 Cerebral Cysticercosis

They are often multiple cystic lesions with eccentrically growing cephalic segments within the cystic cavity, often with calcification, and relatively mild perilesion edema. In contrast, most of the brain abscesses are solitary, and the lesion is often surrounded by a more extensive acupressure edema, and the abscess wall shows a distinct and more regular ring-like enhancement in the enhanced scan.

11.2.5.2 High-Grade Astrocytomas

It shows ring-like enhancement because of the frequent combination of cystic changes and necrosis, similar to the enhancement pattern of brain abscesses, so the two need to be differentiated. The annular enhancement of high-grade astrocytoma is uneven in thickness and irregular in shape, and the central necrosis is often incomplete, with "luciferous" changes, while the annular enhancement in most brain abscesses is more complete and uniform, with a smooth inner wall. Central necrosis of high-grade astrocytomas generally manifests as hypointense on DWI, while the pus in the abscess cavity manifests as hyperintense.

11.2.5.3 Brain Metastases

It is susceptible to necrosis and cystic degeneration, mostly manifests as ring-like enhancement, similar to that of brain abscess. However, brain metastases are more common in middle-aged and elderly patients with a history of extracerebral malignancy, often with multiple foci, and some of the foci with ring-like enhancement have a poorly defined inner wall and can be seen as attached nodules. Brain abscesses, on the other hand, occur in adolescents and can also be seen in the elderly and are more often solitary, with smooth and intact inner walls of the lesions on enhanced scans with ring-like enhancement, mostly without attached nodules. On the DWI sequence, the central liquefied necrotic area of brain metastases mostly manifests as hypointense, while the central pus of brain abscesses mostly manifests as hyperintense.

11.2.5.4 Intracerebral Hematoma

During resorption, perihematoma envelope may appear as a ring-shaped enhancement, which needs to be differentiated from brain abscess. In addition to the typical history, the hematoma is often bean or kidney shaped on resorption, with a three-layer structure on CT, with a hyperdense in the center and a hypodense in the periphery, and a thin, uniformly enhancing envelope. In contrast, the three-layer structure of a brain abscess is hypodense centrally, slightly hyperdense peripherally in the fibrous envelope, and hypodense in the peripheral edema, which is very different from the intracerebral hematoma presentation.

11.2.5.5 Cerebral Infarction

A few cerebral infarctions may also show ring-like enhancement and occupying effect, but all cerebral infarcts have a clear history of sudden onset, mostly in hypertensive elderly patients. After follow-up review, the occupying effect will diminish and the enhanced effect will vary with the stage of the disease, making it easy to distinguish from brain abscess.

11.2.5.6 Postoperative Residual Cavity

It appears annular on enhancement and is generally thin walled. It is difficult to identify whether postoperative ring-like enhancement of the tumor is a normal surgical residual cavity or an infected residual cavity forming an abscess. If it is found that the residual cavity retains secretory function and worsens the clinical symptoms, it indicates abscess.

11.2.5.7 Radiation Encephalopathy

This is a history of radiotherapy with extremely irregular enhancement.

11.2.6 Status and Progress of Research

MRI and CT are available for purulent encephalitis and brain abscesses, wherein MRI is the predominant one.

MRI has high soft tissue resolution, and its multisequence, multimodal examination can provide a wealth of information for the localization, characterization, and even quantitative diagnosis of purulent meningitis, encephalitis, and brain abscess. In recent years, with the introduction of several MRI new techniques, their clinical applications have gradually become popular. MRI new techniques are widely used in the diagnosis, differential diagnosis, surgical plan development, and treatment follow-up of intracranial purulent infections [11–13].

11.2.6.1 MR Diffusion-Weighted Imaging (DWI)

It can provide important information for the diagnosis and differential diagnosis of brain abscess. DWI shows generally hyperintense in brain abscesses and ADC values are low. The conventional MRI varies between stages of brain abscess, with isointense on DWI during the encephalitis stage; when necrotic foci appear in the brain parenchyma, their spread within the brain abscess slows and ADC values decrease; as the abscess absorbs and shrinks, the DWI of central necrosis shows isointense and hypointense. In conclusion, the DWI of a brain abscess is not fixed but varies with the evolution of the abscess at each stage. Imaging plays an important role in the diagnosis of brain abscesses when the clinical presentation and laboratory tests are atypical. Some studies have reported that the ADC value of the abscess cavity increases after abscess treatment, and when the ADC value continues to decrease or decreases repeatedly, it can indicate recurrence of infection.

11.2.6.2 Magnetic Resonance Perfusion-Weighted Imaging (PWI) and Magnetic Resonance Susceptibility-Weighted Imaging (SWI)

PWI can also be used to differentiate between brain abscesses and necrotizing or cystic enhancing tumors. Recent studies have shown that the mean relative cerebral blood volume of cyst walls in brain tumor is significantly higher than that of brain abscesses.

SWI is not well reported in the literature for the diagnosis of brain abscess, but it has been shown that purulent brain abscess is characterized by the "ring sign" on SWI, i.e., an intact smooth hypointense ring is seen on the outer edge of the abscess lesion and a ring with higher signal than the abscess cavity is seen on the inner edge of the lesion, so SWI can be used to differentiate purulent brain abscess from necrotizing glioma.

11.2.6.3 Hydrogen Proton Spectrum Imaging (^{1}H-MRS)

It can be used as an important complementary imaging method to conventional MRI and DWI. Characteristic manifestations of the abscess cavity of an untreated purulent abscess are absence of the NAA peak, Cho peak, and Cr peak and elevation of the amino acids (AA, 0.9 ppm) and lactic acid (Lac, 1.3 ppm) level, with or without elevation of acetic acid (1.9 ppm) and succinic acid (2.4 ppm). ^{1}H-MRS can also be used to follow up the effects of intracranial abscess treatment by showing early abnormal changes. Some studies have shown that the amino acid peak disappears gradually during treatment and the acetate and succinate peaks may also disappear within 1 week, while the lactate peak may persist longer due to macrophage involvement. When doing a multi-voxel MRS examination, the same care should be taken to place the relative voxel in the center of the abscess cavity.

11.2.6.4 Diffusion Tensor Imaging (DTI)

It can be shown that the anisotropy fraction (FA) value of pus in the abscess cavity is positively correlated with the neuroinflammatory adhesion molecule of the pus. Nath et al. found increased FA values and decreased mean diffusivity (MD) values of pus in the abscess cavity, with sensitivity and specificity of 100% and 75%, respectively, for the diagnosis of brain abscess; after treatment the FA values of pus in the abscess cavity will decrease, while MD values will not, suggesting that FA values can be used to monitor the effectiveness of treatment of brain abscesses.

11.2.6.5 PWI Methods

There are two main types, dynamic susceptibility contrast-enhanced (DSC) method based on T_2WI technique and dynamic contrast-enhanced (DCE) method based on T_1WI technique. The majority of articles studying the differential diagnosis between the abscess wall of purulent brain abscess and the necrotic cavity wall of malignant brain tumor by MR PWI use DSC and a few use DCE. It was found that the enhanced T_1WI with ring-like enhancement of the wall of the necrotic cavity had a significantly higher rCBV value than the rCBV value of the enhanced abscess wall, thus facilitating the differentiation between the two.

In short, DWI and MRS can play a greater role in the diagnosis, differential diagnosis, and postoperative evaluation of purulent infection. Brain abscesses present as hyperintense on DWI, and MRS can detect specific metabolites, while DTI can show the relationship between fiber bundle and the lesion and can help to avoid surgical damage to important fiber tracts.

11.3 Epidural and Subdural Abscesses

Hanqiu Liu, Weiwei Wang, and Hongyan Chen

11.3.1 Overview

Intracranial pus accumulation is a purulent inflammatory condition that often results in intracranial epidural or subdural pus accumulation due to hematogenous spread or direct spread of adjacent purulent infected tissue [14–17]. According to the site of abscess, intracranial accumulation of pus can be classified as epidural and subdural abscesses. The most common cause is a chronic purulent infection of the otorhinolaryngology. It can also be caused by osteomyelitis occurring in the skull, septic meningitis, septicemia, and secondary infections after craniotomy. *Staphylococcus aureus* is the most common causative agent of epidural/subdural abscesses. Because of the small amount of connective tissue and venous plexus within the epidural space, pathogenic bacteria that enter that space spread within the epidural space and form cellulitis and then abscesses. Intracranial epidural abscess (IEDA), also known as epidural pus (intracranial epidural empyema, IEDE), is an epidural septic infectious disease of the interstitial space. The dura has a barrier effect on septic inflammation, which allows pus from cranial osteomyelitis, for example, to accumulate in the epidural space, causing limited stripping of cranial bone that is very tightly adherent to the dura and forming a single or multiple poke-shaped or spherical local accumulation of pus. Intracranial subdural empyema (intracranial subdural empyema, ISDE), also known as intracranial subdural abscess (ISDA), is a relatively rare, septic infection located between the intracranial dura mater and the arachnoid. The subdural space is not spaced, and septic material can easily spread when it accumulates in this space, often spreading to the entire convexity of the cerebral hemisphere, to the longitudinal fissure, or along the base of the skull; it is often accompanied by an intracerebral abscess. At the stage of acute encephalitis, patients have symptoms such as fever, headache, vomiting, and elevated blood leukocyte count. In the stage of brain abscess formation, patients have symptoms such as increased intracranial pressure, headache, and optic disc edema. According to laboratory test results, the peripheral blood picture is mostly normal or mildly increased after abscess formation, and the erythrocyte sedimentation rate is accelerated in some patients; pathogenic bacteria can be observed in pus or cerebrospinal fluid bacterial smear.

11.3.2 Pathological Manifestations

Pathologically intracranial pus accumulation can be divided into acute, subacute, and chronic phases. In epidural abscesses, the pathogenic organism forms cellulitis in the epidural space, followed by abscess formation, whereas in subdural abscesses, the septic material spreads more widely, often involving the entire convex surface of the cerebral hemisphere, the longitudinal fissure, or along the skull base; they may be accompanied by intracerebral abscesses.

11.3.3 Imaging

11.3.3.1 Epidural Abscess

1. CT. For CT plain scan, before the abscess envelope forms or reaches a certain thickness, the epidural abscess shows a pyknotic hypodense area with faint or clear borders under the intracranial plate, which may be aqueous or slightly above water density. In the case of gas-producing bacterial infections, fluid planes may be present. After the envelope has formed and reached a certain thickness, the borders of the pyknotic hypodense area under the inner plate of the skull are well defined, and its inner envelope is isodense or slightly hyperdense (Fig. 11.8a). In epidural abscesses complicated by hemorrhage, the density of fluid in the abscess cavity may be divided into two layers, with pus in the upper layer and blood in the lower. CT enhanced scan shows marked enhancement of the envelope of the epidural abscess as an arcuate band of high density, with a well-defined non-enhancing pyknotic hypodense area visible under the intracranial plate (Fig. 11.8b). Epidural abscesses can be complicated by subdural abscesses or subdural effusions, and CT enhanced scans can show them separately. Subdural effusion usually has no envelope formation or very thin envelope formation; very thin envelope may have mild enhancement on enhanced imaging [18, 19]. If the subdural abscess has an unformed or very thin envelope, it is difficult to distinguish it from a subdural effusion. Sometimes an epidural abscess and a subdural abscess are present at the same time.

   When epidural and subdural abscesses are present together, CT is more difficult to distinguish and MRI examination may be helpful. When an epidural abscess forms first, the wall of the abscess made of its envelope is often thicker, whereas the envelope of a later-forming

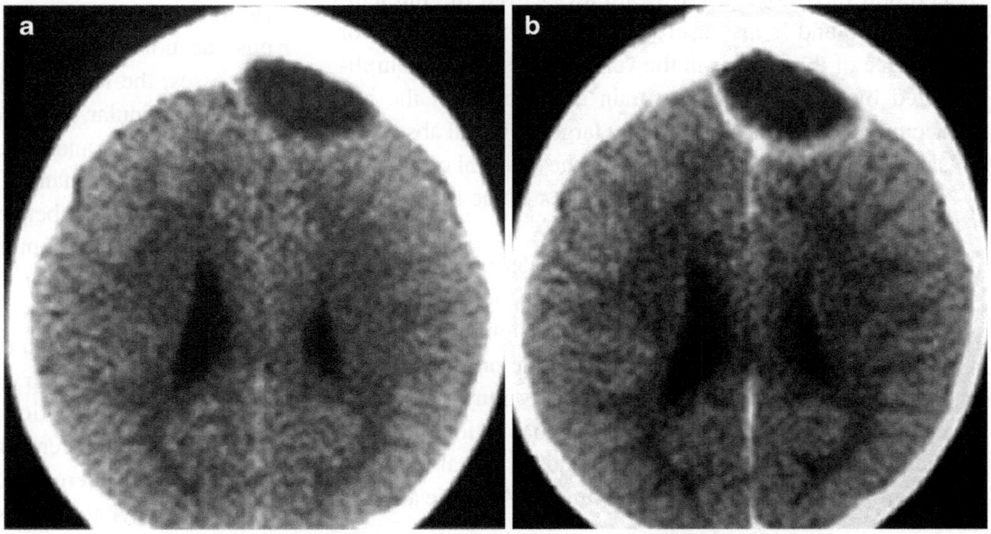

Fig. 11.8 Epidural abscess. (**a**) CT plain scan shows a spindle-shaped hypodense area between the left anterior frontal skull below and the surface of the brain, which is slightly hyperdense than the cerebrospinal fluid, and an arcuate slightly hyperdense band formed by an abscess envelope is seen at its inner edge; (**b**) the abscess envelope is significantly enhanced after enhancement

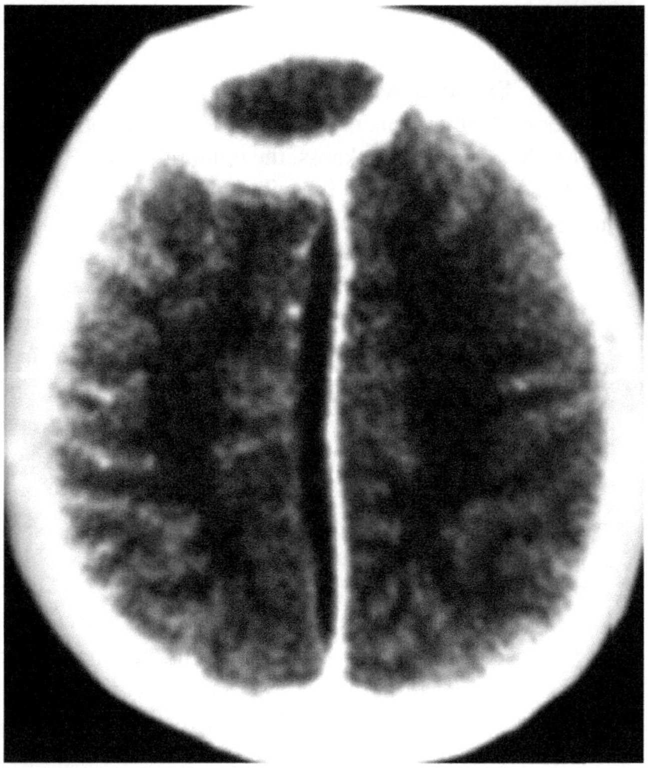

Fig. 11.9 Epidural abscess secondary to subdural abscess of the cerebral falx. CT enhanced scan shows a confined subcranial subplate pyknotic hypodense area in the forehead, with a thicker curved distinctly enhanced zone made up of an abscess envelope seen at its inner edge, suggesting an epidural abscess. A hypodense band is also seen within the longitudinal fissure, the left edge of which is an intensified cerebral falx, and the right edge of which is a mildly intensified fine linear shadow, the latter probably being the envelope of the subdural accumulation of pus in the cerebral falx

subdural abscess may not yet be formed or may be very thin, and the two may be distinguished (Fig. 11.9). When the abscess is located in the midline, a coronal scan can show the superior sagittal sinus at the attachment of the cerebral falx moving downward away from the intracranial plate and is also useful in showing the presence or absence of thrombosis in the venous sinus. If not complicated by encephalitis, the brain tissue beneath the pus accumulation behaves normally; larger epidural abscesses show compression and nudging of the cerebral cortex and displacement of the midline structures of the brain to the contralateral side.

2. MRI: On T_1WI scan, the pus cavity under the inner plate of the skull has a well-defined convex lens-shaped or shuttle-shaped low signal area, and its signal intensity is close to that of cerebrospinal fluid; if the protein content of pus is very high, its signal intensity may be significantly higher than that of cerebrospinal fluid. In T_2WI, the pus cavity shows high signal, and its signal intensity is similar to that of cerebrospinal fluid FLAIR; the abscess cavity shows high, equal, or low signal, or mixed-signal intensity, sometimes with signal intensity stratification, depending on the composition of the abscess, such as the presence of residue from incomplete necrosis, and the amount of protein content, etc. The abscess envelope appears as T_1WI and presents as a slightly low signal band on T_2WI and FLAIR, i.e., slightly below or equal to the signal intensity of the cerebral cortex. On T_2WI and FLAIR, it presents as a slightly high signal band, i.e., slightly above the signal intensity of the cerebral cortex, or as isointense. On enhanced T_1WI, abscess envelope is all significantly strengthened; envelope near the brain surface is generally strengthened, and envelope near the skull surface made of periosteum is generally not strengthened. If the periostitis is severe and the granulation tissue formation is high, it may also constitute an abscess and strengthen the envelope (Fig. 11.10). If the abscess contains gas, a fluid plane appears, and the gas above it is a black signal-free area on T_1WI. And on T_2WI and DWI, the abscess cavity appears as a high signal, indicating restricted diffusion [19]; the abscess envelope appears as a low signal or as an isointense.

Epidural abscesses can complicate meningitis, brain abscesses, and subdural abscesses, and MRI can show these intracranial conditions if they occur.

11.3.3.2 Subdural Abscess

1. CT: On CT plain scan, a typical subdural abscess shows a thin, widespread crescentic isodense or hypodense area spanning the cranial suture between the inner plate of the skull and the brain surface (Fig. 11.11a); its density correlates with the viscosity of the pus accumulation, with the thinner being less dense but often higher than that of the cerebrospinal fluid. On enhanced CT scan, the contrast injection is faster, and on parallel early scans, the inner surface of the pus accumulation area is seen to be composed of reinforced blood vessels and reinforced cerebral cortex, clearly showing the medial margin of the pus accumulation area. In chronic stage subdural abscesses, the lesion may appear as a single or multiple convex lenticular, round or round-like shape due to marginal adhesions and envelope formation around the pus cavity. On post-enhanced scans, the medial margin of the pus cavity located between the skull and brain surface reinforcement and sometimes a well-defined, uniformly thick, distinctly reinforced band on the lateral edge may be present, consisting of an enhanced abscess envelope. Subdural abscesses that occur in the subdural space of the falx and the cerebellar curtain differ in morphology, in addition to their location. Subdural abscesses in the subdural space of the cerebral falx, located between the two cerebral hemispheres, are striped in the acute phase and tend to be pyknotic or spherical in the chronic phase.

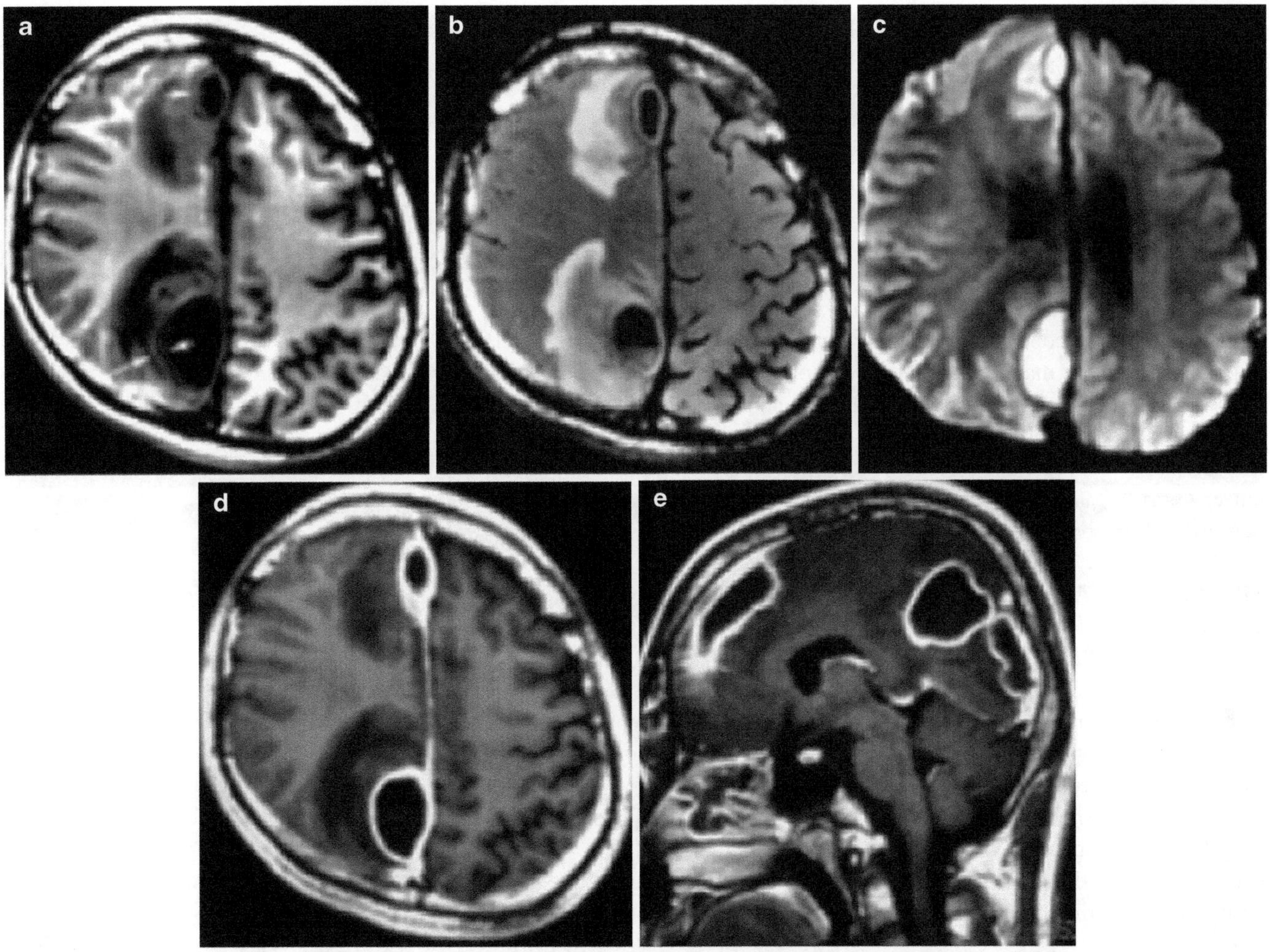

Fig. 11.10 Epidural abscess. A convex lens-shaped epidural abscess of variable size next to the right cerebral falx. (**a**) On T_1WI, the upper abscess envelope is slightly hypointense, and its signal intensity is lower than that of the compressed cerebral cortex; (**b**) FLAIR sequence shows more severe perifocal edema, more pronounced in those located in the white matter portion of the brain, and the pus in the abscess cavity is iso- or hypointense, and fluid planes are seen; (**c**) DWI on the pus cavity is hyperintense, and the envelope is hypointense; (**d**, **e**) with marked enhancement of the abscess envelope after enhancement

Subdural abscesses in the subdural space of the cerebellar curtain are best shown on coronal scans, which show a convex lenticular, round, or round-like shape; cross-sectional scans do not necessarily show a convex lenticular shape and may show an irregular round-like shape. Enhanced post-scan, too, shows envelope enhancement. Chronic subdural abscesses adjacent to the pia mater and cerebral cortex can become infected and inflammatory; on enhanced scan, cerebral gyrus-like enhancement is seen medial to the reinforcing envelope [18, 19]. As mentioned above, subdural abscesses can be complicated by cerebral thrombophlebitis and venous sinusitis, which can further lead to cerebral infarction; the corresponding CT manifestations are seen when these complications occur. Sometimes the subdural abscess is small in extent while the area of cerebral edema is large, with significant occupancy effects and significant displacement of midline structures.

2. MRI: MRI morphology of subdural abscesses in acute and chronic stages is the same as that seen on CT. The pus accumulation or pus cavity in the subdural space on the surface of the cerebral hemisphere appears as a low and high signal with signal intensity close to that of the cerebrospinal fluid covering the surface of the cerebral hemisphere on T_1WI and T_2WI images, respectively. On T_1WI, the signal intensity is often slightly higher than cerebrospinal fluid. The envelope made of connective tissue in the chronic phase appears as a low signal on T_1WI and T_2WI; on the enhanced T_1WI, the envelope is obviously strengthened.

The envelope near the surface of the brain is generally strengthened, and the envelope near the surface of the skull may or may not be strengthened. Subdural abscesses located in the subdural space of the falx and cerebellar curtain are best viewed in three dimensions to get a full picture because of their specific location. In addition, coronal and sagittal views are also useful to show subdu-

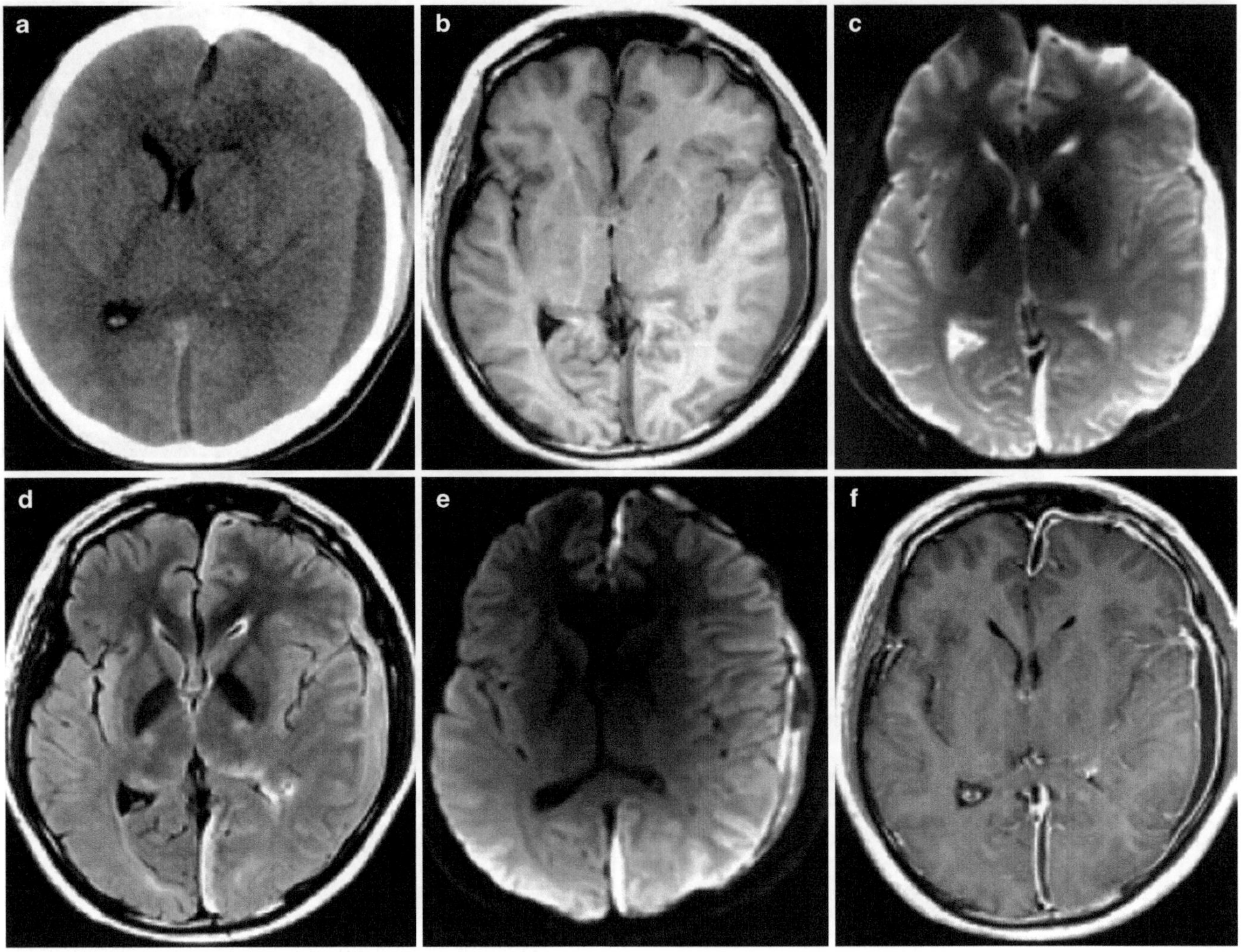

Fig. 11.11 Intracranial subdural abscess. (**a**) CT plain scan shows a thin, crescentic, hypodense area spanning the cranial suture visible between the left frontal and temporal skull and the brain surface and next to the midline falx cerebri with an inner surface morphology similar to that of the cerebral gyrus on the brain surface; (**b**) T_1WI is low signal; (**c**) T_2WI is more uniform high signal; (**d**) FLAIR sequence is high signal; (**e**) DWI is high signal (mostly T_1WI, signal intensity slightly higher than cerebrospinal fluid area); (**f**) enhancement shows marked enhancement of the envelope

ral abscesses in the cerebellar vermis and the base of the brain. Subdural abscesses in the subdural space of the cerebral fossa, located between the two cerebral hemispheres, are striped in the acute phase and are more often pyknotic or spherical in the chronic phase. Subdural abscesses in the subdural space of the cerebellar curtain are best shown on coronal scans, which show a convex lenticular, round, or round-like shape; cross-sectional scans do not necessarily show a convex lenticular shape and may show an irregular round-like shape. Subdural abscesses secondary to meningitis often show the MRI findings of meningitis, such as extensive dural and arachnoid enhancement and pia mater enhancement. If it shows limited dural or arachnoid enhancement or pia mater enhancement adjacent to the subdural abscess, it may be due to the spread of inflammation from the subdural abscess to the adjacent meninges. Similar to the brain abscess described above, the pus cavity of a subdural abscess shows high and low signal on DWI and ADC images, respectively, indicating restricted diffusion [20] (Fig. 11.11).

Subdural abscesses complicated by thrombophlebitis, venous sinusitis, and/or cerebral infarction corresponding MRI manifestations are seen.

11.3.4 Diagnostic Key Points

1. Most often there is a history of definite septic bacterial infection.
2. Abscesses are found in the intracranial epidural and subdural areas.
3. In the CT flat scan, the abscess cavity is hypodense and the abscess wall is isodense or slightly hyperdense. In the

MR plain scan, the pus shows hypointense and hyperintense in T_1WI and T_2WI, respectively. The abscess wall shows isointense or slightly hypointense in T_2WI, and enhanced scan shows smooth and complete circumferential enhancement of the inner wall; DWI sequence pus shows significantly hyperintense.
4. Cerebrospinal fluid examination: the white blood cell count is significantly elevated and associated pathogens can be detected in the cerebrospinal fluid.

11.3.5 Differential Diagnosis

11.3.5.1 Subdural Abscess

1. Intracranial subdural hematoma. Subdural hematoma has different signal performance at different times of MRI, which differs from the signal characteristics of abscess, and in the case of subdural abscess, the dura mater can be significantly enhanced, which can be distinguished by the typical feature of high signal in DWI.
2. Intracranial subdural effusion: both exhibit widening of the subdural space; subdural effusion approximates cerebrospinal fluid signal and differs from abscess signal characteristics, and in subdural abscess, the dura can be significantly enhanced and DWI shows significant high signal, which is not difficult to distinguish.

11.3.5.2 Epidural Abscess

1. Intracranial epidural hematoma. Most patients with epidural hematoma have a history of significant trauma and may present with a combination of cerebral contusion, intracranial hematoma, and skull or spine fracture, usually without a history of infection. The MRI signal of epidural hematoma differs in different periods, with hematoma wall enhancement seen in chronic phase, while epidural abscess always shows T_1WI with low signal and T_2WI with high signal, and DWI shows typical high signal and is not difficult to identify.
2. Intracranial epidural effusion. It is common to see chronic epidural hematoma liquefaction after craniocerebral trauma, with density or signal approximating cerebrospinal fluid, no localized cranial compression thinning, and no enhancement of adjacent meninges on enhanced scans; in addition, epidural effusion is rare.

11.3.6 Status and Progress of Research

MRI and CT can be used for epidural/subdural abscesses, with MRI being the preferred test.

MRI has high soft-tissue resolution with its multi-sequence, multi-modal state examination that can provide a wealth of information for the localization, characterization, and even quantitative diagnosis of septic meningitis, encephalitis, and brain abscess. DWI and MRS may play a greater role in the diagnosis and differential diagnosis of septic infection and postoperative evaluation, brain abscesses are hyperintense on DWI, and MRS may detect specific metabolites. CT can have a wide range of applications for screening intracranial lesions because of its fast and inexpensive scans, CT is superior to MRI in showing microcalcifications and bone cortical destruction. But CT has lower soft-tissue resolution and is less accurate in diagnosis than MRI.

11.4 Ventriculitis

Hanqiu Liu, Weiwei Wang, and Yunling Wang

11.4.1 Overview

Purulent ventriculitis is a type of ventriculitis characterized by the accumulation of purulent fluid in the ventricles of the brain as a result of septic bacterial infection [21–23]. Ventriculitis was once called ependymitis, intraventricular abscess, and ventricular empyema.

Infectious agents of septic ventriculitis can enter the ventricles through the following routes: (1) bloodstream infection, in which a distant septic bacterial infection spreads through the bloodstream to the subventricular canal or choroid and enters the ventricles; (2) direct implantation, secondary to septic bacterial infection from trauma or surgery, such as that brought on by intraventricular catheter implantation; (3) direct spread of infection adjacent to the ventricles, where an abscess adjacent to the ventricles breaks into the ventricles; and (4) cerebrospinal fluid from extraventricular infections that flows back into the ventricles, wherein septic ventriculitis secondary to septic meningitis is likely to come through this route.

The most common causative agent of septic ventriculitis is *Staphylococcus* [24], including *Staphylococcus aureus*, etc.; *Enterobacter*, including *Enterobacter aerogenes*, *Enterobacter cloacae*, etc.; and other bacteria such as *Escherichia coli*, *Streptococcus pneumoniae*, *Klebsiella pneumoniae*, *Pseudomonas aeruginosa*, and *Cryptococcus neoformans*. Because the pathogenic bacteria of most septic meningitis enter the brain through the choroid plexus, most septic meningitis has mild ventriculitis; 30% or more have ventricular-ventricular inflammation, most often in young patients, especially infants. In the last 30 years, there has been an increase in the occurrence of septic ventriculitis due to an increase in in-hospital infections of septic meningitis. The clinical signs and symptoms of septic ventriculitis are often fever, headache, nausea, vomiting, and impaired consciousness and signs of meningeal stimulation. Cerebrospinal fluid tests performed by lumbar puncture reveal increased neutrophil counts, increased protein levels, and decreased glucose levels in the cerebrospinal fluid; detection of relevant pathogens in the cerebrospinal fluid may confirm the diagnosis.

Septic ventriculitis often begins in the lateral ventricles and then gradually spreads to other ventricles, with an incidence of 0.2–4%; patients with septic ventriculitis are often in critical condition, with a mortality rate of 58%. Diabetes is one of the major risk factors for septic ventriculitis. Laboratory tests show elevated total peripheral blood leukocyte count, elevated reactive protein and calcitonin gene, decreased sugar levels, elevated protein levels, and increased nucleated cells in the cerebrospinal fluid, and cerebrospinal fluid cultures and smears can detect pathogenic bacteria.

11.4.2 Pathological Manifestations

Septic ventriculitis initially occurs mostly in the lateral ventricles. Due to the inflammatory reaction or the accumulation of septic material in this interstitial space that spreads easily, the inflammation involves the local ventricular canal, intraventricular adhesions, and septum formation, leading to abnormal cerebrospinal fluid absorption and secretion and impaired cerebrospinal fluid circulation, thus causing hydrocephalus and the formation of small infected compartmentalized cavities in the ventricles.

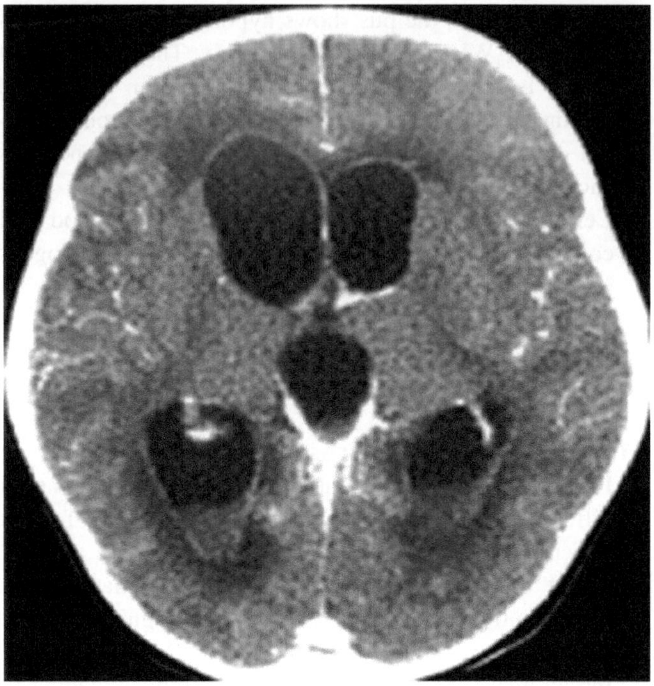

Fig. 11.12 Septic ventriculitis. Enhanced CT scan shows enlarged lateral ventricles and third ventricle, ventricular canal enhancement, and dense pus debris deposited in the occipital horn of both lateral ventricles. (Image courtesy of Professor Chen Xingrong, Huashan Hospital, Fudan University)

11.4.3 Imaging

11.4.3.1 CT Findings

Septic ventriculitis can often cause hydrocephalus and enlarged choroid plexus. The enlarged choroid plexus is shown on the pre-enhanced CT scan as ventricular enlargement and enlarged choroid plexus, respectively. If there is intraventricular pus debris deposition, it is shown in the lower part of the ventricle, such as in the lateral ventricular triangle or occipital horn, with higher density pus debris deposition; the post-enhanced CT scan, in addition to showing ventricular enlargement and higher density pus debris deposition, may also show ventricular canal enhancement and enlarged choroidal plexus enhancement [21, 23] (Fig. 11.12).

CT is less sensitive than MRI for demonstrating ventricular canal enhancement and pus debris deposition, etc. When CT is difficult to confirm the diagnosis, MRI should be performed immediately.

11.4.3.2 MRI Findings

MRI is valuable in the demonstration and diagnosis of septic ventriculitis [25–27]. MRI is sensitive to show ventricular enlargement and choroid plexus enlargement in septic ventriculitis and is also sensitive to show intraventricular signal abnormalities caused by ventriculitis. T_1WI can sometimes show low ventricular areas, such as the lateral ventricular triangle or within the occipital horn, with signal intensity higher than cerebrospinal fluid and pus debris deposits below the brain parenchyma; enhanced T_1WI may also show ventricular canal enhancement and enlarged choroidal plexus enhancement; T_2WI may show low ventricular sites with lower signal intensity than cerebrospinal fluid and higher than parenchymal pus deposits. On FLAIR, the pus debris in the low ventricular area appears to have a higher signal intensity than the signal intensity of the cerebrospinal fluid and white matter; the pus debris deposits appear as a high signal on DWI and a low signal on ADC (Fig. 11.13). Intracerebroventricular abscess is formed when there is an envelope formation around the pus accumulation in the ventricles, which shows abnormal signal intensity in the local ventricles. On T_1WI, the signal intensity is higher than the cerebrospinal fluid and lower than the brain parenchyma. On T_2WI, the abscess envelope appears as a low signal, and the pus in the abscess cavity appears as a high signal with similar signal intensity as the cerebrospinal fluid. Enhanced T_1WI showed enhancement of the abscess envelope.

MRI reveals many complications of ventriculitis, such as meningitis, encephalitis, vasogenic or cytotoxic brain edema, focal ischemic injury (e.g., cerebral infarction), infected venous sinus thrombosis, subdural effusion, subdural abscess, epidural abscess, and brain abscess. If these compli-

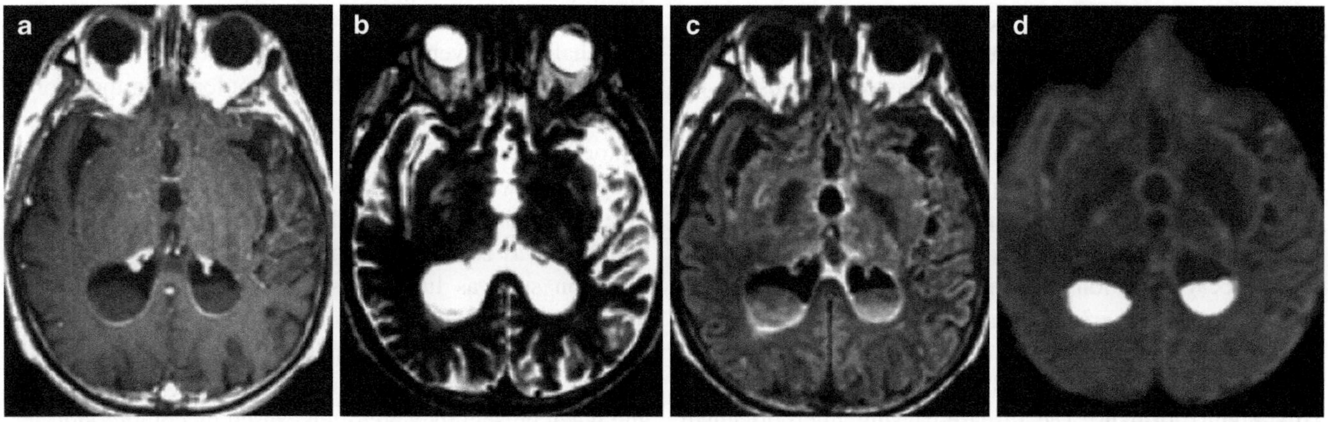

Fig. 11.13 Septic ventriculitis. The lateral ventricles and the third ventricle are enlarged. (**a**) T1WI enhancement shows ventricular canal enhancement in the lateral ventricular triangle; (**b**) T_2WI shows lower signal of pus debris deposition within the lateral ventricular triangle than cerebrospinal fluid; (**c**) FLAIR sequence shows that the signal intensity of pus debris deposition in the lateral ventricular triangle is higher than that of cerebrospinal fluid; (**d**) DWI shows that the pus debris deposition in the lateral ventricular triangle is high signal. (Image courtesy of Prof. Chen Xingrong of Huashan Hospital, Fudan University)

cations occur, MRI may show the appropriate presentation. In concurrent encephalitis, enhanced T1WI often shows focal enhancement, whereas in concurrent cerebral edema, enhanced T1WI fails to show focal enhancement.

11.4.4 Differential Diagnosis

1. **Hydrocephalus:** The ventricular system is enlarged, and in severe cases, interstitial hydrocephalus is seen. However, the ventricle is of density or signal of cerebrospinal fluid, and the ventricular wall is often has no abnormal enhancement on enhanced scan.
2. **Ventricular hemorrhage**: Patients often have a history and imaging of subarachnoid hemorrhage or intracerebral hemorrhage into the ventricles. The ventricles are often seen as fluid planes on MRI, and intraventricular deposits of iron-containing heme are seen on SWI. No significant enhancement of the ventricular wall can be seen after enhancement.

11.4.5 Diagnostic Key Points

1. Most often there is a history of definite septic bacterial infection.
2. The lesion occurs in the ventricles of the brain. Lesion occurs in the ventricles of the brain.
3. In the CT scan, enlarged ventricular system with increased cerebrospinal fluid density can be seen. In the MR flat scan, the pus shows hypointense on the T_1WI, hyperintense on the FLAIR, T_2WI shows a high signal and DWI shows high signal or mixed high and low signal in the superior ventricle, and linear enhancement is seen in the ventricular wall on enhanced scan.
4. Cerebrospinal fluid examination. The white blood cell count is significantly elevated and associated pathogens can be detected in the cerebrospinal fluid.

11.4.6 Status and Progress of Research

Imaging methods for septic ventriculitis include ultrasound, CT, and MRI, with MRI having the highest diagnostic value and being the first-line tool for the diagnosis of septic ventriculitis. Ultrasound is mainly used for infants with unclosed fontanelles. MR examination in DWI, FLAIR, and enhanced scans are important sequences for the diagnosis of septic ventriculitis. The study of Hong et al. [28] concluded that after a brain abscess breaks into the ventricle, both intraventricular abscess and brain abscess show a high signal on DWI, but on the corresponding ADC map, the signal intensity of intraventricular abscess is variable (medium to low signal), presumably attributed to the high concentration of macromolecules, the cells and cellular debris are diluted by cerebrospinal fluid, and the ADC plot (regional changes in ADC values) is more sensitive to showing subtle changes in the amount or concentration of pus compared to the DWI.

11.5 Choroid Plexitis

Hanqiu Liu and Weiwei Wang

11.5.1 Overview

The choroid plexus is an important portal of entry for many central nervous system infections [29, 30]. *Mycobacterium tuberculosis*, *Cryptococcus*, and *Nocardia* are the main infectious agents causing primary choroid plexitis. Among these, central nervous system infections caused by *Mycobacterium tuberculosis* and *Cryptococcus* mostly present as choroid plexus inflammation, while intracranial infections by *Nocardia* usually present as abscesses. Most infectious agents invade the central nervous system through bloodstream transmission. In contrast, the pathogenesis of cryptococcal infection has many similarities to that of *Mycobacterium tuberculosis* infection in that the infections are acquired by inhalation, and once the pathogen is inhaled, it is contained at the level of the lungs or lymph nodes and can remain dormant. The disease-causing microorganism proliferates only in the encapsulated strain, and when the dose of infection is so high as to overwhelm the host's defenses, or in the presence of an underlying disease that compromises the host's immunity, the lesion can rupture to drain the bacillus into the cerebrospinal fluid and cause meningitis. Similar to cryptococcosis, the fungus can reach the choroid plexus by hematogenous dissemination, colonize it, and then enter the cerebrospinal fluid, causing meningitis, encephalitis, or ventricular meningitis. *Cryptococcus* also enters the brain parenchyma through the perivascular spaces and expands within these cavities to form the pseudocystic lesions characteristic of this disease. Unlike tuberculous and cryptococcal intracranial infections (which usually present as meningitis), *Nocardia* infection most often presents as intracerebroventricular abscess formation. Therefore, *Nocardia* plexus chorioretinitis is more dangerous and requires more aggressive treatment. Primary choroid plexitis is a rare but serious condition, and early detection allows intervention before the infection extends further into the central nervous system. Neuroimaging may observe varying degrees of abnormality, but radiological findings alone are not specific to a particular pathogen; microbiologic diagnosis remains clinically dependent, including patient history, bacterial culture, or biopsy; detection of a relevant pathogen from cerebrospinal fluid may be the basis for a definitive diagnosis of this disease.

11.5.2 Pathological Manifestations

Nocardia is a partially acid-intolerant mycobacterium [20, 31]. It inhabits in the soil, and inhalation of airborne bacilli is the most common route of infection. The most common CNS infection with *Nocardia* presents as a brain abscess, mostly as an isolated lesion, while multiple lesions have been found in about 1/3 of cases, and meningitis, brain granulomas, diffuse parenchymal infiltrates, and spinal cord involvement may also be seen but are rare as isolated presentations.

Mycobacterium tuberculosis and fungi can reach the choroid plexus through hematogenous dissemination, colonize it, and then enter the cerebrospinal fluid, causing meningitis, encephalitis, or ventriculitis. Mycobacterium tuberculosis forms nodular tumors or nodular granulomas in the choroid plexus, which can develop into intraventricular nodular tumors by rupture into the ventricles. Polysaccharides of *Cryptococcus* are phagocytosis-blocking and impede leukocyte migration. Thus, the inflammatory response caused by *Cryptococcus* is minimal compared to other forms of nerve infection such as tuberculosis. In addition, *Cryptococcus* does not release any foreign toxins and therefore rarely causes tissue necrosis. Secondary changes such as fibrosis, calcification, infarction, or hemorrhage are also very rare, and when present they are often caused by compression.

11.5.3 Imaging

11.5.3.1 CT Findings

Plain scan may show choroid plexus unilaterally or bilaterally protrusion. Hydrocephalus is more common, and hypodense edema is seen around the lesion. After enhancement, the choroid plexus is significantly enhanced, bilateral ventricular canal may be enhanced, and the brain parenchyma adjacent to the lesion may be circumferentially enhanced [31].

11.5.3.2 MR Manifestation

In addition to displaying the above features, it is possible to find intraventricular cystic masses and perivascular gap enlargement. Bilateral lateral ventricular choroidal asymmetry or bilateral prominence and significant enhancement of the choroid plexus are the main characteristic imaging findings, but the degree of enlargement varies from subtle to severe abnormalities. Although the intensity of the signal on T_1WI and T_2WI is variable, enhanced images can indicate the severity of choroid plexus inflammation through enhancement. Due to adhesions between the inflammatory ventricular canal and choroid plexus, small cystic cavities form within the ventricles, and the inflammatory response also tends to extend into the ventricular wall, often with extensive edema in the adjacent brain parenchyma [32] (Fig. 11.14).

11.5.4 Differential Diagnosis

Choroid plexus tumors. In particular, choroid plexus papillomas and choroid plexus carcinomas have similar imaging presentations to choroid plexitis, showing an enlarged, enhancing mass with hydrocephalus centered on the choroid plexus. Choroid plexus carcinoma often presents with tumor extension into the parenchyma and surrounding edema. In identifying infection from tumor, DWI may be helpful, with high signal at the lesion suggesting an infection. Although parenchymal abscesses exhibit features of restricted spread,

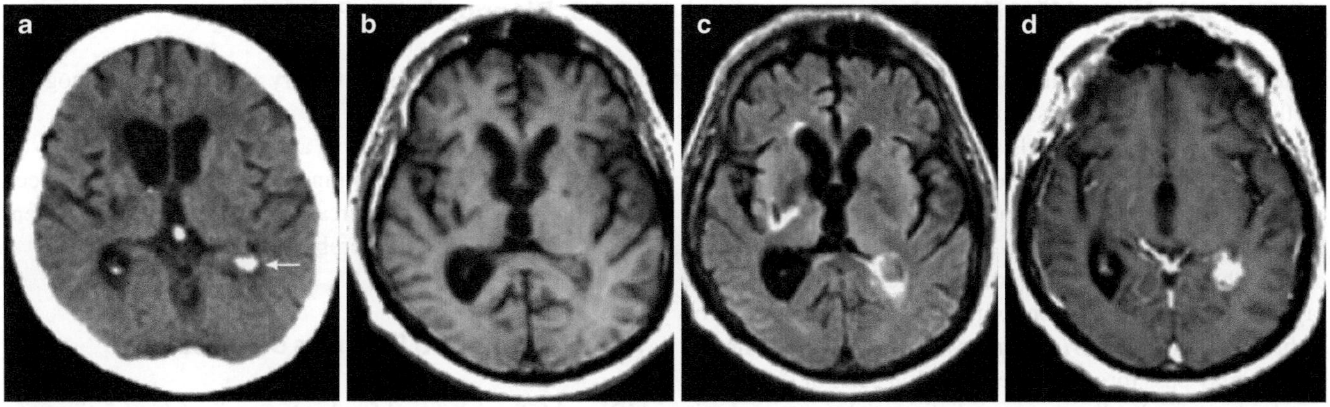

Fig. 11.14 Choroid plexitis. (**a**) CT plain scan showing calcification of the left choroid plexus; (**b**) T_1WI showing mild protrusion of the left choroid plexus with bilateral asymmetry of the choroid plexus within the posterior horn of the lateral ventricles; (**c**) FLAIR sequence showing significant periventricular edema; (**d**) T_1WI enhancement showing marked enhancement of the left choroid plexus. (Image courtesy of Prof. Li Hongjun, Beijing Youan Hospital, Capital Medical University)

the choroid plexus involved in many cases is not restricted in spread. Magnetic resonance spectroscopy is also of high value in the diagnosis of specific focal parenchymal lesions. In addition, the history is also discriminatory, with choroid plexitis progressing more rapidly.

11.5.5 Diagnostic Key Points

1. Most often there is a history of definite pathogenic infection.
2. CT and MR plain scan shows unilateral or bilateral ventricular choroid plexus prominence, hydrocephalus, and paraventricular edema in the posterior horn of the lateral ventricle, with localized abnormal choroid plexus enhancement and abnormal ventricular canal enhancement seen on enhancement; there may be a high signal at the lesion on the DWI.
3. Cerebrospinal fluid examination. The white blood cell count is significantly elevated and associated pathogens can be detected in the cerebrospinal fluid.

11.5.6 Status and Progress of Research

CT has a low detection rate for lesions that do not form abscesses. MR can detect the lesion early, and enhanced MR, DWI sequences, and MRS can play an important role in the diagnosis and differential diagnosis of the disease. MR shows certain specific signs that are suggestive for identifying different pathogens, but a definitive diagnosis still depends on clinical manifestations and laboratory tests.

11.6 Listeriosis

Hanqiu Liu, Weiwei Wang, and Shuang Ding

11.6.1 Overview

Cerebral listeriosis is a central nervous system lesion caused by infection with *Listeria monocytogenes* in brain tissue [33]. The route of infection is as follows: the pathogenic bacteria first enter the digestive tract and enter the central nervous system by hematogenous dissemination through the gastrointestinal tract. Patients affected are often immunocompromised elderly, patients undergoing oncological treatment, transplant patients, patients with chronic wasting diseases such as diabetes or cirrhosis, pregnant women, and newborns. However, some patients with brainstem encephalitis are often young people with no predisposing factors.

The most common clinical manifestations in patients with *Listeria monocytogenes* infection are gastroenteritis, bacteremia, and meningitis. Central nervous system involvement can cause meningitis, encephalitis, or brainstem encephalitis. Some patients present with ventricular dilatation, cerebral hemorrhage, or even cervical medullary involvement. Clinical manifestations include headache, fever, nausea, vomiting, and local neurological symptoms. Some patients may experience seizures, respiratory weakness, and disorientation. If it causes brainstem encephalitis, the patient may present with corresponding asymmetric involvement of the cerebellum, medulla oblongata, and superior pons. If the condition is severe, the patient may become unconscious or even comatose. Pathogens can be found in the cerebrospinal fluid.

11.6.2 Pathological Manifestations

Listeria can attack normally infection-resistant tissues such as the central nervous system, the pregnant uterus, or the fetus. The pathogen spreads hematologically through the gastrointestinal tract or reaches the central nervous system through the choroid plexus and causes meningitis [34, 35]. Listeria monocytogenes can also reach the brain parenchyma through brain capillary endothelial cells (a single layer of cerebrovascular endothelial cells characterized by tight junctions). *Listeria monocytogenes*-infected macrophages may pass through the endothelial cells of the middle cerebral artery, leading to encephalitis and, in turn, brain abscess formation. In addition, *Listeria monocytogenes* can invade the central nervous system via the peripheral dura mater route. And when bacteria enter the central nervous system through the peripheral nervous system, the infection also spreads along the axons. Because the disease spreads along the white fiber tracts of the brain, it creates unique anatomical features that provide important clues for early diagnosis on imaging.

11.6.3 Imaging

Cephalic CT abnormalities were present in only 1/4 of the patients. Cranial MR is more likely to detect intracranial lesions than cranial CT. The imaging presentation was noncharacteristic. CT may show diffuse hypodense foci around the lateral ventricles or in the white matter areas of the brain parenchyma. MRI shows hypointensity on T_1 and hyperintensity on T_2, and it is difficult to distinguish listeriosis from demyelinating, glioma or ischemic vascular disease. On enhanced CT scan, the lesion is mostly circumferentially enhanced. Enhanced MRI further reveals necrotic areas within the lesion with significant surrounding edema [35, 36].

11.6.4 Differential Diagnosis

1. High-grade astrocytoma. The central necrosis is often incomplete and has a "loofah" shape, and the ring-shaped strengthening area has a high signal on DWI sequence.
2. Brain metastases. Metastases are often multiple foci, mostly located cortical or subcortical, susceptible to necrosis and cystic degeneration, with some ring-enhanced lesions having a non-glossy interior and visible attached nodules with marked peripheral edema. Brain metastases tend to occur in middle-aged and elderly people and tend to have a history of primary malignancy.

11.6.5 Diagnostic Key Points

1. Most often there is a history of definite pathogenic infection.
2. Routine CT and MR exams are not characteristic.
3. Cerebrospinal fluid examination. The white blood cell count is significantly increased and associated pathogens can be detected in the cerebrospinal fluid.

11.6.6 Status and Progress of Research

MRI and CT can be used for the diagnosis of *Listeria* intracranial infection and MRI is the recommended test. CT may show intracranial abscesses due to *Listeria* infection but is of limited diagnostic value for specific lesions. MRI has high soft-tissue resolution and is particularly good at showing lesions that invade the nerve bundles and is also highly diagnostic of lesions involving the brainstem and spinal cord. MRI with conventional serial plain scan + enhancement and DWI provide important information for the differential diagnosis of intracranial *Listeria monocytogenes* and posttreatment follow-up. CT can be widely used in screening for the presence of intracranial lesions because of its fast and inexpensive scanning, but CT has a lower soft-tissue resolution and a lack of diagnostic accuracy.

References

1. Heckenberg SGB, Brouwer MC, van de Beek D. Bacterial meningitis. Handb Clin Neurol. 2014;121(3):1361–75.
2. Kim KS. Acute bacterial meningitis in infants and children. Lancet Infect Dis. 2010;10:32–42.
3. Barichello T, Generoso JS, Collodel A, et al. Pathophysiology of acute meningitis caused by Streptococcus pneumoniae and adjunctive therapy approaches. Arq Neuropsiquiatr. 2012;70(5):366–72.
4. Mohan S, Jain KK, Arabi M, et al. Imaging of meningitis and ventriculitis. Neuroimaging Clin N Am. 2012;22(4):557–83.
5. Kastrup O, Wanke I, Maschke M. Neuroimaging of infections of the central nervous system. Semin Neurol. 2008;28(4):511–22.
6. Kamran S, Bener AB, Alper D, et al. Role of fluid-attenuated inversion recovery in the diagnosis of meningitis: comparison with contrast-enhanced magnetic resonance imaging. J Comput Assist Tomogr. 2004;28:68–72.
7. Kawaguchi T, Sakurai K, Hara M, et al. Clinico-radiological features of subarachnoid hyperintensity on diffusion-weighted images in patients with meningitis. Clin Radiol. 2012;67(4):306–12.
8. Shen T, Chen X. Neuroimaging. Shanghai: Shanghai Science and Technology Press; 2004.
9. Woo Chung Pil. Pathology. Page 4 version. Beijing: People's Health Press; 1997.
10. Hughes DC, Raghavan A, Mordekar SR, et al. Role of imaging in the diagnosis of acute bacterial meningitis and its complications. Postgrad Med J. 2010;86(1018):478–85.
11. Teixeira J, Zimmerman RA, Haselgrove JC, et al. Diff Imag Neuroradiol. 2001;43(12):1031–9.

12. Ebisu T, Tanaka C, Umeda M, et al. Discrimination of brain abscess from necrotic or cystic tumors by diffusion weighted imaging. Magn Reson Imaging. 1996;14(6):1113–6.
13. Toh CH, Wei KC, Chang CN, et al. Differentiation of pyogenic brain abscesses from necrotic glioblastomas with use of susceptibility-weighted imaging. AJNR Am J Neuroradiol. 2012;33(8):1534–8.
14. Kanu OO, Ukponmwan E, Bankole O, et al. Intracranial epidural abscess of odontogenic origin. J Neurosurg Pediatr. 2011;7(3):311–5.
15. DeVries S. Metastatic epidural bacterial abscess in a 4-year-old boy. JAMA Neurol. 2013;70(5):648–9.
16. Seto T, Takesada H, Matsushita N, et al. Twelve-year-old girl with intracranial epidural abscess and sphenoiditis. Brain Dev. 2014;36(4):359–61.
17. Osborn MK, Steinberg JP. Subdural empyema and other suppurative complications of paranasal sinusitis. Lancet Infect Dis. 2007;7(1):62–7.
18. Salunke PS, Malik V, Kovai P, et al. Falcotentorial subdural empyema: analysis of 10 cases. Acta Neurochir. 2011;153(1):164–9.
19. Parmar H, Ibrahim M. Pediatric intracranial infections. Neuroimaging Clin N Am. 2012;22(4):707–25.
20. Wong AM, Zimmerman RA, Simon EM, et al. Diffusion-weighted MR imaging of subdural empyemas in children. AJNR Am J Neuroradiol. 2004;25:1016–21.
21. Fukui MB, Williams RL, Mudigonda S. CT and MR imaging features of pyogenic ventriculitis. AJNR Am J Neuroradiol. 2001;22(8):1510–6.
22. Kanamalla US, Ibarra RA, Jinkins JR. Imaging of cranial meningitis and ventriculitis. Neuroimaging Clin N Am. 2000;10(2):309–31.
23. Lambo A, Nchimi A, Khamis J, et al. Primary intraventricular brain abscess. Neuroradiology. 2003;45(12):908–10.
24. Fujikawa A, Tsuchiya K, Honya K, et al. Comparison of MRI sequences to detect ventriculitis. AJR Am J Roentgenol. 2006;187(4):1048–53.
25. Spanu T, Rigante D, Tamburrini G, et al. Ventriculitis due to staphylococcus lugdunensis: two case reports. J Med Case Reports. 2008;2:267.
26. Marinelli L, Trompetto C, Cocito L. Diffusion magnetic resonance imaging diagnostic relevance in pyogenic ventriculitis with an atypical presentation: a case report. BMC Res Notes. 2014;7:149.
27. Jorens PG, Voormolen MH, Robert D, et al. Imaging findings in pyogenic ventriculitis. Neurocrit Care. 2009;11(3):403–5.
28. Hong JT, Son BC, Sung JH, et al. Significance of diffusion-weighted imaging and apparent diffusion coefficient maps for the evaluation of pyogenic ventriculitis. Clin Neurol Neurosurg. 2008;110(2):137–44.
29. Hagiwara E, Nath J. Choroid plexitis in a case of systemic nocardiosis. Emerg Radiol. 2007;14(5):337–43.
30. Mogilner A, Jallo GI, Zagzag D, et al. Nocardia abscess of the choroid plexus: clinical and pathological case report. Neurosurgery. 1998;43(4):949–52.
31. Patronas NJ, Makariou EV. MRI of choroidal plexus involvement in intracranial cryptococcosis. J Comput Assist Tomogr. 1993;17(4):547–50.
32. Kovoor JME, Mahadevanb A, Narayana JP, et al. Cryptococcal choroid plexitis as a mass lesion: MR imaging and histopathologic correlation. Am J Neuroradiol. 2002;23:273–6.
33. Liu Y, Zhang W, Wang F. Severe listeria monocytogenes meningoencephalitis 1 example. Microorganisms Infect. 2011;6(3):153–7.
34. Xu D, Wu T, Zhou M. A case of severe meningoencephalitis-type listeriosis. Chin J Neuroimmunol Neurol. 2008;15(5):392–3.
35. Karlsson WK, Harboe ZB, Roed C, et al. Early trigeminal nerve involvement in listeria monocytogenes rhombencephalitis: case series and systematic review. Neurology. 2017;264(9):1875–84.
36. Kayaaslan BU, Akinci E, Bilen S, et al. Listeria rhombencephalitis in an immunocompetent young adult. Int J Infect Dis. 2009;13(2):e65–7.

Intracranial Viral Infection

12

Shuang Xia, Shaozhou Wang, Qiang Liu, Zi'ao Fu,
Yinhua Jin, and Qing Li

12.1 *Herpesvirus* spp. Infections

Shuang Xia, Shaozhou Wang, and Qiang Liu

12.1.1 Herpes Simplex Viral Infection

12.1.1.1 Overview

Herpes simplex virus (HSV) invades the central nervous system (CNS) and causes a series of inflammatory changes. When it mainly involves the brain parenchyma, it is called herpes simplex virus encephalitis (HSVE), which is the most common CNS viral infectious disease. The incidence of herpes simplex virus encephalitis abroad is 0.4–1/100000, accounting for 20–68% of all viral encephalitis. The virus most often attacks the temporal and frontal lobes and the limbic system and is also known as acute necrotizing encephalitis or hemorrhagic encephalitis because it often causes hemorrhagic necrosis and/or metabolic damage to the brain parenchyma.

Herpes simplex virus encephalitis is divided into neonatal and adult forms. In adults and older children, herpes simplex virus encephalitis usually involves the temporal and frontal lobes and is caused by the herpes simplex virus type 1. In neonates, herpes simplex virus encephalitis is usually caused by the herpes simplex virus type 2, acquired during delivery, and has diffuse brain involvement. The average incubation period for viral infection is 6 days, ranging from 2 to 21 days. Prodromal symptoms include headache, dizziness, nausea, vomiting, sore throat, myalgia, and general malaise. Herpes simplex virus encephalitis is most acute in onset, with an ultra-high fever of 40–41 °C for about 1 week, followed by a series of neurological symptoms, such as headache, nausea, and meningeal irritation; when it involves the nerve, it causes brain nerve dysfunction, such as ocular synergetic dysfunction, abducens nerve paralysis, etc. It can cause symptoms of focal nerve damage, such as hemiplegia, aphasia, hemiparesthesia, ataxia, etc. Patients may also experience partial or generalized epileptic seizures; psychiatric symptoms such as dullness, muteness, hallucinations, confusion of speech, paranoia, irritability, and abnormal behavior, etc., can be seen. Most patients may experience disorders such as confusion, drowsiness, delirium and confusion, or even coma. Severely ill patients can suffer from extensive brain tissue necrosis and edema leading to intracranial hypertension, brain herniation, and even death.

Serology showed increased neutrophilia in 35–50% of patients and hyponatremia in 40% [1]. Cerebrospinal fluid examination showed increased lymphocytosis in about 90% of patients, hypoglycemia in 25%, and elevated protein levels in 70% [1]. Cerebrospinal fluid herpes simplex virus DNA polymerase chain reaction (PCR) is the gold standard for the diagnosis of herpes simplex virus encephalitis; the presence of anti-herpes simplex virus IgG antibodies after 7–10 days of onset is of high diagnostic value.

12.1.1.2 Pathological Manifestations

The pathological changes of herpes simplex virus encephalitis include brain parenchymal edema, hemorrhage, necrosis, and encephalomalacia, with hemorrhagic necrosis being the most important pathological change, often asymmetrically distributed, with the temporal lobe, insula, frontal orbital gyrus, and limbic system being most frequently involved, as well as the occipital lobe, and also the bilateral cerebral hemispheres being diffusely involved. Microscopically, the

S. Xia (✉) · Q. Li
Tianjin First Central Hospital, Tianjin, China

S. Wang
Tianjin Third Central Hospital, Tianjin, China

Q. Liu
Shandong Provincial Hospital, Jinan, China

Z. Fu
Teda International Cardiovascular Hospital, Tianjin, China

Y. Jin
Xiamen Fifth Hospital (Xiang'an Hospital of the First Affiliated Hospital of Xiamen University), Xiamen, China

H. Li et al. (eds.), *Radiology of Infectious and Inflammatory Diseases - Volume 1*,
https://doi.org/10.1007/978-981-99-0039-8_12

nerve cells were diffusely degenerated and necrotic with hemorrhage, with massive lymphocytic and plasma cell infiltration around the focal necrotic vessels and glial cell proliferation. Eosinophilic stained inclusion bodies are seen in the nuclei of neurons and glial cells [2].

The pathological changes in herpes simplex virus encephalitis are broadly divided into two phases. The first stage is the initial onset, lasting about 1 week, mainly manifesting asymmetric temporal and frontal lobe inflammatory changes, edema, widening of the cerebral gyrus, narrowing of the cerebral sulcus, possible congested surface meninges, oozing, or even hemorrhagic necrosis and softening. The second stage is the necrohemorrhagic phase, which manifests as focal or patchy hemorrhage and necrosis in the frontal and temporal brain parenchyma. After the acute phase, gliosis or even atrophy of brain tissue occurs [3].

12.1.1.3 Imaging

The cranial CT is mostly normal within 1 week of onset, followed by asymmetric temporal, frontal, and insular hypointense shadows on one or both sides, which may have mild to moderate occupying effects and hyperdense shadows in the presence of hemorrhage; enhanced CT scans show linear enhancement of the temporal, frontal, and insular brain surfaces (Fig. 12.1).

MRI shows asymmetric lamellar hypointense on T_1WI and hyperintense on T_2WI and FLAIR sequence with blurred margins in unilateral or bilateral temporal, frontal, and insular, mostly involving cortical and subcortical white matter, mostly with hemorrhage. There may be mild to moderate occupancy effects. DWI sequence shows diffusion restriction, which manifest as hyperintense, with decreased ADC values (Figs. 12.2, 12.3 and 12.4). Enhanced scans may show linear or gyral-like enhancement of the brain surface in the lesion area and occasionally may show ring-like enhancement. Lesions show hyperperfusion on PWI [4, 5]. After antiviral therapy, patients may develop brain atrophy.

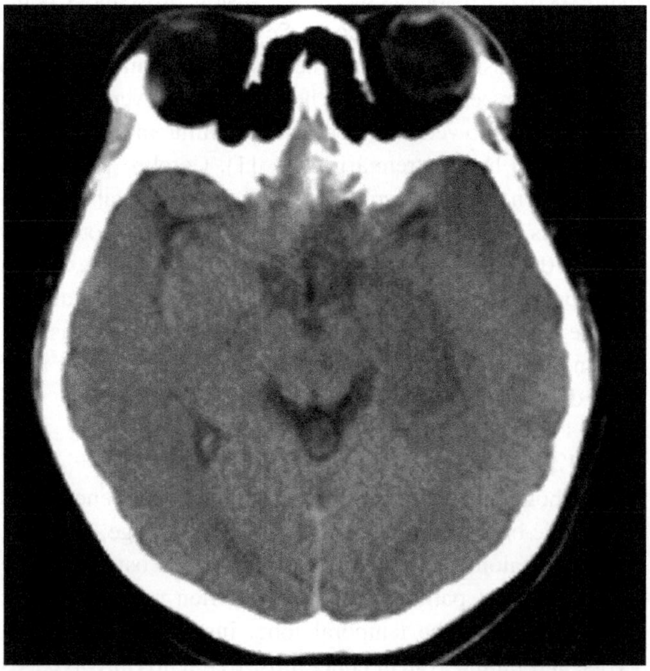

Fig. 12.1 Herpes simplex virus encephalitis (1). Head CT shows a lamellar hypodense shadow in the left medial temporal lobe and left parahippocampal gyrus

When the lesion invades the temporal lobe, frontal lobe, or insula cortical area, it may be manifested as a "knife-cutting sign," which is the most characteristic manifestation of the disease because the lesion does not involve the basal ganglia area, the nucleus pulposus is often not invaded, the lesion area is clearly demarcated from the nucleus pulposus, and the convexity is outward. When lesions invade the basal nucleus, thalamus, and brainstem, it can manifest as "basal nucleus protrusion sign" [6].

12.1.1.4 Diagnostic Key Points

1. The patient had symptoms of diffuse and focal brain damage such as hemianopia, hemiparesis, aphasia, oculomotor paralysis, ataxia, hyperactivity, meningeal irritation signs, and a clear history of herpes virus exposure and infection.
2. The lesions are asymmetrically distributed, mostly involving the medial aspect of the temporal lobe and the orbital surface of the frontal lobe, and may continue to involve the cingulate gyrus and the insula, but usually not the basal ganglia, and manifest as "knife-cutting sign."
3. T_2WI and FLAIR sequence show hyperintense in cortical and subcortical. Epithelial medullary demarcation is not clear on T_1WI and may have mild to moderate occupying effects.
4. Pathogenic examination of cerebrospinal fluid herpes simplex virus DNA polymerase chain reaction (PCR) is the gold standard for the diagnosis of herpes simplex virus encephalitis; the presence of anti-herpes simplex virus IgG antibodies after 7–10 days of onset is of high diagnostic value.

12.1.1.5 Differential Diagnosis

Enterovirus Encephalitis

It is common in autumn and summer, with gastrointestinal symptoms at the beginning of the disease, and imaging mainly shows lamellar hypodense shadowing in the cerebral cortex and paraventricular space, which is associated with inflammatory changes in the small cerebral arteries, meninges, and ventricular canal due to the invasion of the central nervous system by the enterovirus, especially the inflammatory response of the small paraventricular arteries; PCR detected the virus DNA in the cerebrospinal fluid.

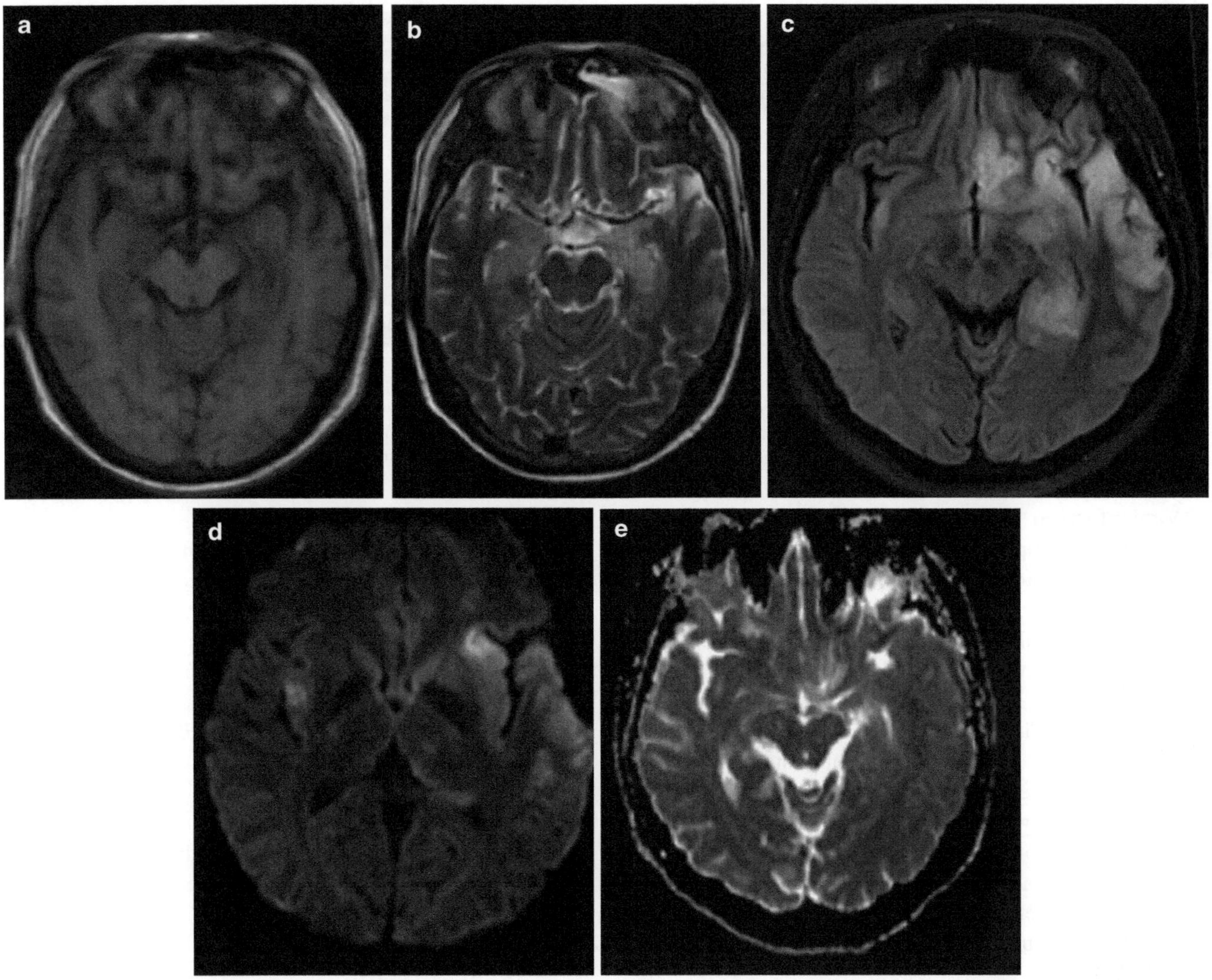

Fig. 12.2 Herpes simplex virus encephalitis (2). (**a**) T_1WI shows lamellar hypointense in the bilateral hippocampal region; (**b**) T_2WI shows lamellar hyperintense in the bilateral hippocampal region; (**c**) FLAIR sequence shows asymmetric distribution of the lesion, with large lamellar hyperintense seen in the left temporal lobe, left hippocampus, left insula, and left frontal orbital gyrus. On the right side, only small patches of hyperintense are seen in the hippocampus; (**d**) DWI shows asymmetric distribution of the lesion, with lamellar hyperintense seen in the left temporal lobe and left insula. On the right side, only small patches of hyperintense are seen in the hippocampus; (**e, a, c, d**) diagrams show varying degrees of signal reduction in the above lesions (hyperintense areas on the DWI sequence)

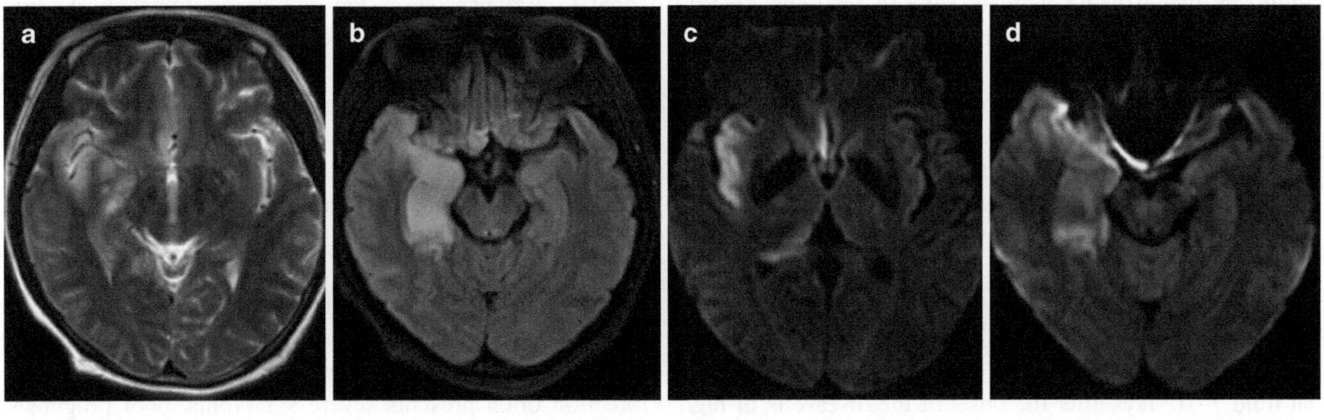

Fig. 12.3 Herpes simplex virus encephalitis (3). (**a**) T_2WI shows patchy hyperintense in the right temporal lobe, insula, and hippocampus with indistinct lesion borders; (**b**) FLAIR sequence shows hyperintense; (**c, d**) DWI shows patchy hyperintense in the right temporal lobe, right insula, right hippocampus, and right thalamus

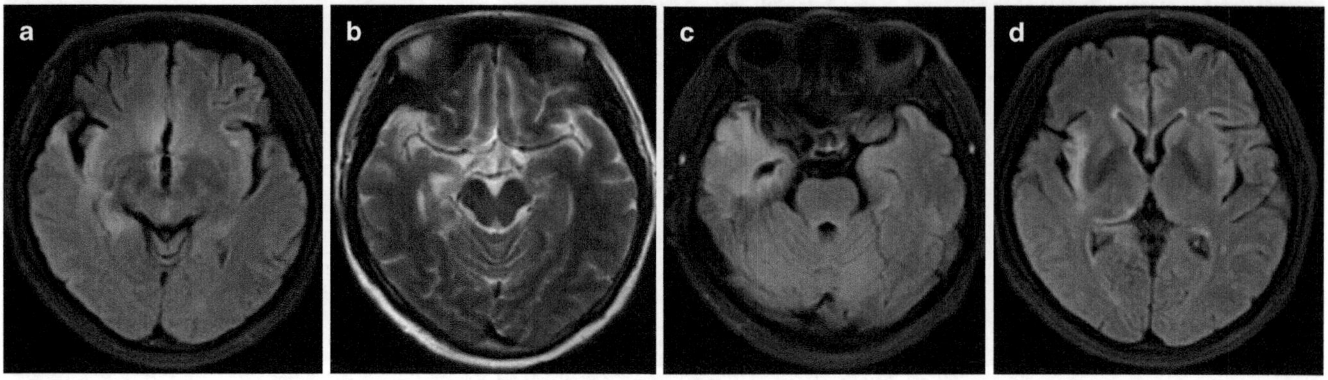

Fig. 12.4 Herpes simplex virus encephalitis after 1 month of treatment. The above patient, after 1 month of treatment for herpes simplex virus encephalitis. (**a**, **c**, **d**) FLAIR sequence: compared with before (Fig. 12.3), the extent of patchy hyperintense in the right temporal lobe, right insula, and right hippocampus is significantly reduced. (**b**) T_2WI: the extent of patchy hyperintense in the lesion area is significantly reduced, the adjacent temporal lobe brain sulcus is widened, and the temporal horn of the right lateral ventricle is dilated

EB Viral Infection

For single or multiple hypodense foci in the mass, calcification in the basal ganglia area, and traffic hydrocephalus with intracranial hemorrhage and demyelination-like changes, EEG showed mainly diffuse bilateral leads with continuous high-amplitude slow waves or delta waves.

Varicella: Zoster Viral Infection

Brain CT shows multifocal ischemic and hemorrhagic infarcts in the white matter of the lesion area, mostly concentrated in the gray-white matter junction area. DSA shows a beaded stenosis of the proximal middle cerebral artery, mostly due to intracranial arterial endarteritis due to herpes zoster causing cerebral infarction. Cerebrospinal fluid detection of antibodies to varicella-zoster virus is used to identify this infection.

Glioma

Malignant gliomas of the frontotemporal lobe should be differentiated from herpes simplex virus encephalitis when local necrosis and hemorrhagic changes are present. Malignant gliomas of the brain are often accompanied by significant hemorrhagic necrosis. CT and MRI show a heterogeneous lesion with significant occupancy effects [6].

12.1.1.6 Status and Progress of Research

The Diagnosis of Herpes Simplex Virus Encephalitis

It needs to be closely combined with the clinical situation. Fever and headache with psychiatric symptoms should be differentiated from this disease.

Laboratory Tests

The detection of anti-HSV IgG antibodies in the cerebrospinal fluid 7–10 days after the onset of the disease is of high diagnostic value for herpes simplex virus encephalitis [7].

Image

MRI is the most sensitive and specific imaging method for herpes simplex virus encephalitis, especially in the early stage of the disease, which typically shows T_2WI asymmetric hyperintense lesions in the mesial temporal lobe, orbitofrontal lobe, and insula. DWI demonstrated diagnostic advantages in detecting lesions in early stage, showing restricted diffusion, but was inferior to FLAIR in detecting involvement of thalamic lesions.

Neurophysiological Examination

It can detect diffuse discharge abnormalities, or frontotemporal lobe epileptiform discharges. The severity of the condition and prognosis can be assessed.

12.1.2 Varicella-Zoster Viral Infection

12.1.2.1 Overview

Varicella encephalitis occurs most often in children under 15 years of age, and herpes zoster encephalitis often occurs in middle-aged and older adults, and neither onset is seasonal. Central nervous system symptoms are not always synchronized with the onset of herpes, occurring days to weeks after herpes, but also before or during the onset of the rash, or in patients without varicella-herpes [8].

Central nervous system symptoms include headache, vomiting, seizures, altered consciousness, neurological abnormalities and focal neurological deficits, and, rarely, agitation, delirium, and even coma and death. Involvement of the brainstem may result in cerebral nerve palsy, often with fever. Infections in healthy children or adults tend to be mild and have a good prognosis. In the presence of immune deficiency, or the use of immunosuppressive therapy, the infection often presents severe symptoms, poor prognosis, and even death [9].

The cerebrospinal fluid examination may show mononucleosis; an increased cerebrospinal fluid/serum albumin ratio is often indicative of a disruption of the blood-brain barrier. The pathogenic examination can be performed in the acute phase of the lesion by cerebrospinal fluid varicella-zoster virus DNA PCR examination and/or intrathecal varicella-zoster virus DNA antibodies. With the appearance of central nervous symptoms for 1–3 weeks, the level of DNA in the cerebrospinal fluid decreases, and antibodies to viral DNA become the main indicator of diagnosis. Enzyme-linked immunosorbent assay (ELISA) for varicella-herpes zoster virus IgG serum/cerebrospinal fluid ratio may be helpful in diagnosis.

12.1.2.2 Pathological Manifestations

Pathology showed extensive necrosis of sensory ganglia and destruction of neuronal structures during herpes zoster, manifesting as multifocal necrotizing encephalomyelitis, brain parenchymal swelling, diffuse inflammatory reaction, phagocytic infiltration, and massive lymphocytic and plasma cell infiltration around the meningeal vessels, and neuronal degeneration, eosinophilic inclusion bodies in the nuclei of neuronal cells in the focal area, and glial cell hyperplasia with demyelination damage. Viral particles are visible in the envelope under electron microscopy [10].

Varicella-herpes zoster virus, in addition to direct intracranial invasion which causes brain tissue damage, can also cause inflammatory reactions in different intracranial vessels, resulting in hemorrhagic or ischemic changes in the corresponding brain parenchyma, mostly in the cortical and subcortical gray-white matter junction areas and deep gray matter nuclei in the white matter.

12.1.2.3 Imaging

Head CT shows multifocal ischemic and hemorrhagic infarction with hypodense shadow, mostly in cortical and subcortical white matter, deep nuclei, and brainstem, with gyral-like enhancement in enhanced scan [11].

MRI shows multifocal hypointense on T_1WI and hyperintense on T_2WI. In acute phase, lesion shows restricted diffusion on DWI with hyperintense signal and decreased ADC value. Enhancement characteristics are similar to CT enhancement which shows gyrus-like enhancement (Figs. 12.5, 12.6, 12.7 and 12.8).

DSA may show beaded stenosis of the proximal middle cerebral artery, most often caused by intracranial arterial endocarditis due to herpes zoster.

12.1.2.4 Diagnostic Key Points

1. The central nervous system symptoms are mainly headache, vomiting, seizures, neurological abnormalities, altered consciousness, and, in a few cases, irritability, delirium, and even coma and death, often with fever.
2. Multifocal ischemic and hemorrhagic infarct foci, mostly in the cortical and subcortical white matter, deep nuclei, and brainstem, were seen, and the lesions showed cerebral gyrus-like enhancement on enhanced scans.
3. DSA may show a beaded stenosis of the proximal middle cerebral artery [12].
4. Serology varicella-herpes zoster virus IgG serum. An elevated cerebrospinal fluid ratio is the more common test used to diagnose this disease.

12.1.2.5 Differential Diagnosis

EB Virus Infection

Single or multiple hypodense foci can be seen in the brain parenchyma, calcification of basal ganglia area, and traffic hydrocephalus with intracranial hemorrhage and demyelination-like changes; EEG showed mainly diffuse bilateral leads with continuous high-amplitude slow waves or delta waves.

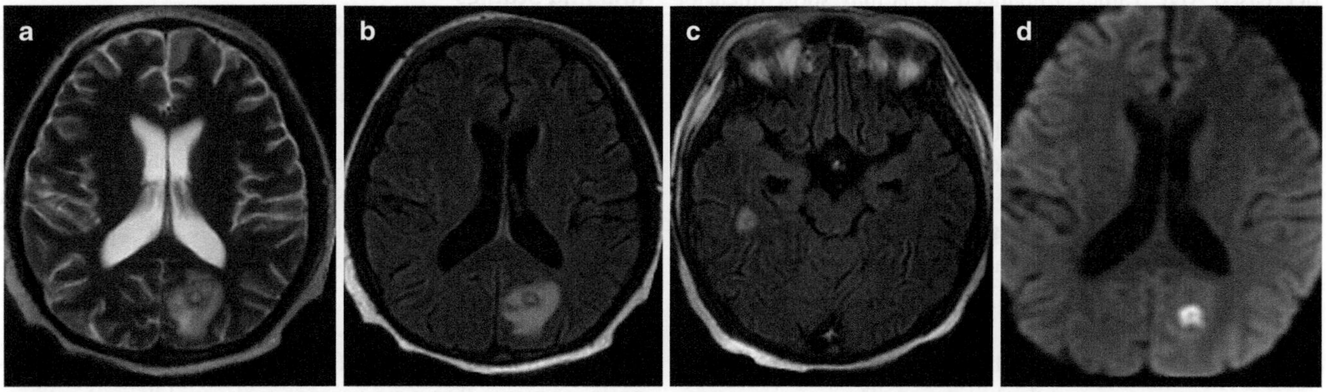

Fig. 12.5 Varicella-zoster encephalitis (1). (**a**) T_2WI shows speckled hyperintense visible in the left occipital lobe; (**b**, **c**) FLAIR sequence shows speckled hyperintense visible in the left occipital lobe with large surrounding edema and speckled hyperintense visible in the right medial temporal lobe. (**d**) DWI shows a hyperintense lesion in the left occipital lobe

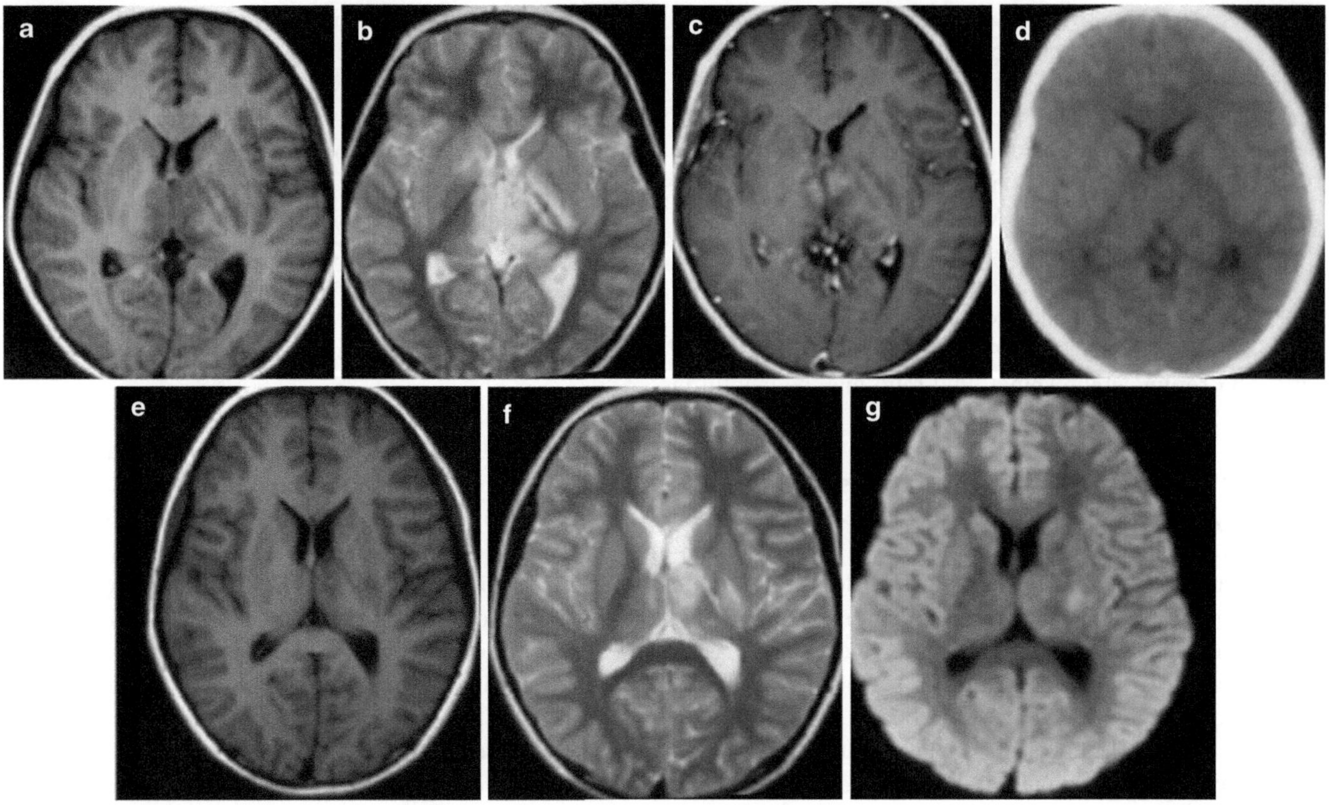

Fig. 12.6 Varicella-zoster encephalitis (2). Multiple patches and strips of abnormal signal are seen in the bilateral thalamus and basal ganglia areas. (**a**) T_1WI showing hypointense; (**b**) T_2WI showing hyperintense with compression of the anterior horn of the right lateral ventricle; (**c**) enhanced T_1WI shows that some of the lesions have mild patchy enhancement; (**d**) CT shows slightly hypo- to isodense in the above lesions with blurred edges and slightly shifted midline structures to the right; (**e**, **f**) reexamination after 3 weeks of treatments, T_1WI and T_2WI showed a significant reduction in the extent of the lesion compared to before (Fig. 12.6a, b); (**g**) DWI shows a hyperintense lesion in the left basal ganglia area

Herpes Simplex Virus Infection

Typical signs are asymmetric temporal, frontal, and insula-like abnormal density or signal on one or both sides, mostly involving the cortex and subcortical white matter, mostly with hemorrhage; may have mild to moderate occupancy effects; and show restricted diffusion on DWI sequence with decreased ADC values. Enhanced scans may show linear or gyral-like enhancement of the brain surface in the lesion area and occasionally may show ring-like enhancement. When the lesion invades the temporal lobe, frontal lobe, or insula cortical area, it may be manifested as the "knife-cut sign," which is because the lesion does not involve the basal ganglia area and the nucleus pulposus is often not invaded. When the lesion invades the basal ganglia, thalamus, and brainstem, it is characterized as "basal nucleus protrusion sign."

Enterovirus Encephalitis

It is common in summer and autumn, and gastrointestinal symptoms may appear at the beginning. The imaging manifestations are mainly lamellar hypodense in cerebral cortex and paraventricular area. This is associated with inflammatory changes in the small cerebral arteries, meninges, and ventricular canal due to enterovirus invasion of the central nervous system, especially the inflammatory response of the small paraventricular arteries.

12.1.2.6 Status and Progress of Research

Imaging Studies

CT and MRI can show abnormalities, and the latter is more sensitive. The lesions were cortical and deep, both occurring in the gray and white matter and gray-white matter junction areas. Most lesions are ischemic, but they may also be hemorrhagic. For ischemic lesions, the detection of the MRI DWI sequence is more sensitive, and when it occurs at the blood-brain barrier, the lesion area can be detected better by MRI.

Vascular Imaging Technique

DSA examination can detect involvement of the multiple stenotic segments that were present in the middle and anterior arteries of the brain. If vasculitis is suspected, CTA or MRA can be used, but they are less sensitive than conventional angiography, especially in distal vessels, and newer methods

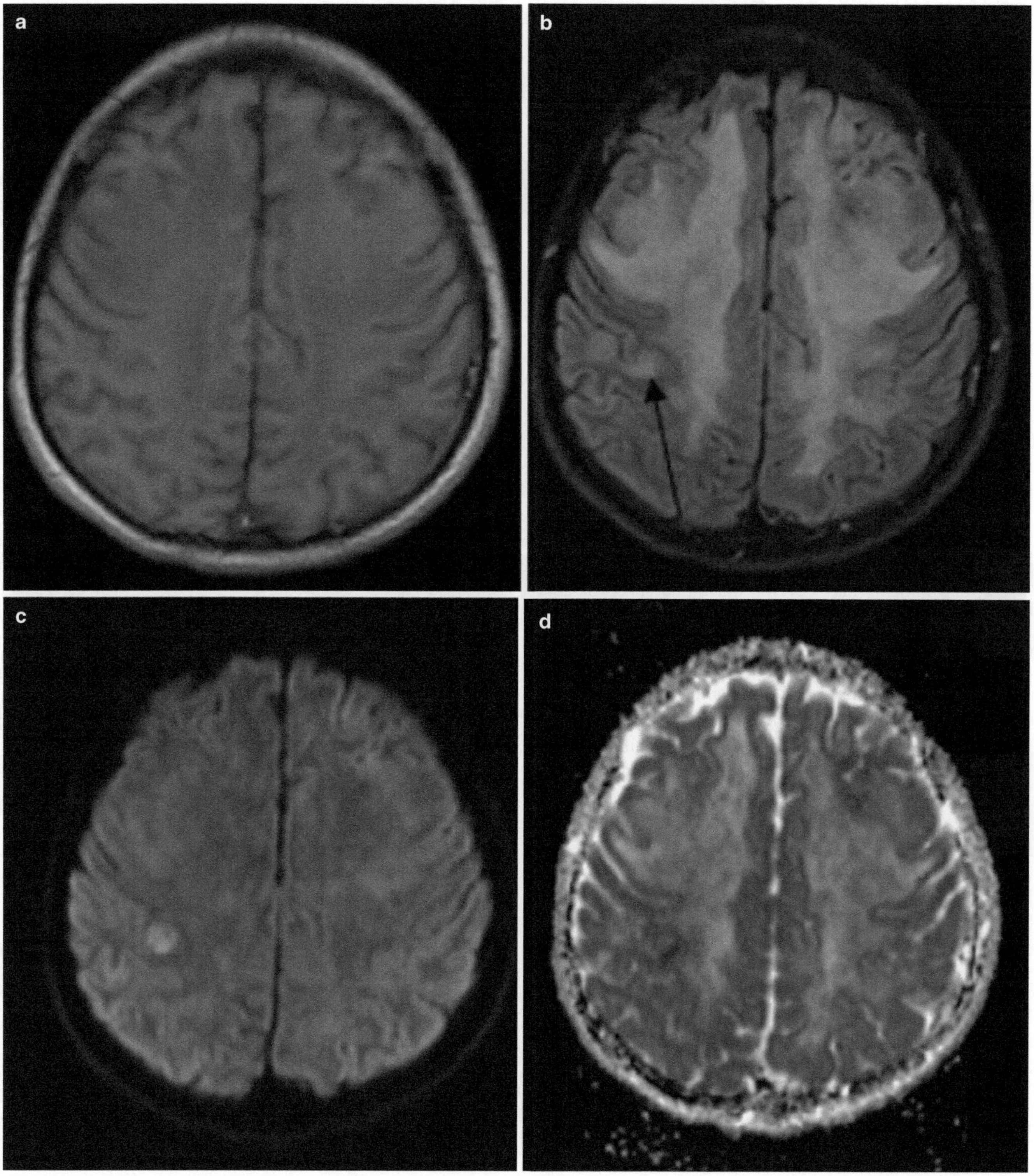

Fig. 12.7 Varicella-zoster encephalitis (3). (**a**) T_1WI shows a diffusely distributed lamellar slightly hypointense visible in the bilateral fronto-parietal white matter area; (**b**) FLAIR sequence shows a slightly hyper-intense lesion in the bilateral frontoparietal white matter area, and a nodular hyperintense (arrow) is visible in the right parietal lobe; (**c**) DWI shows a slightly hyperintense in the right parietal node; (**d**) ADC shows a right parietal nodule with mixed hypointense, and signal of bilateral frontoparietal white matter area lesion is increased

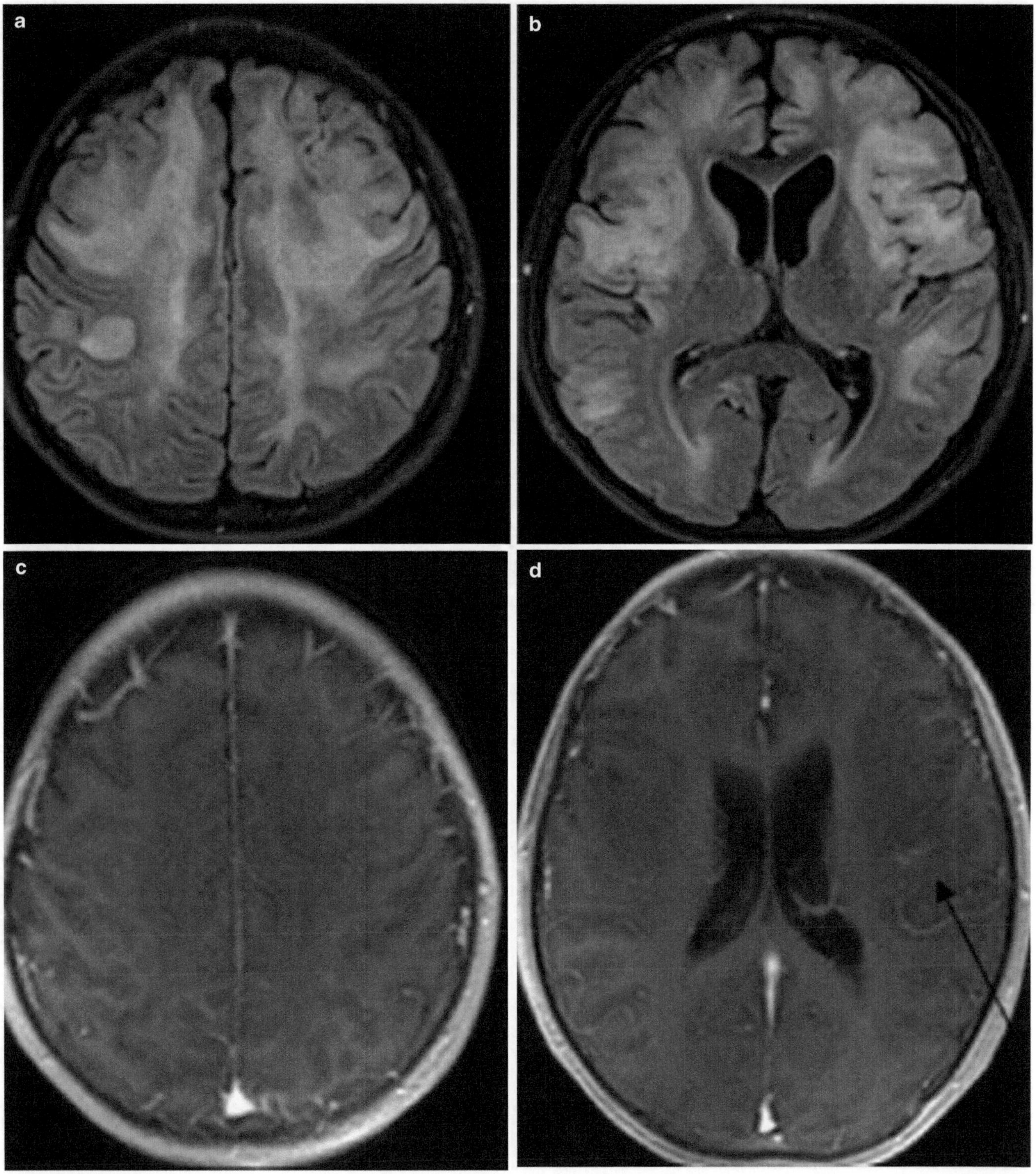

Fig. 12.8 Varicella-zoster encephalitis (4). (**a**, **b**) FLAIR sequence shows multiple lamellar hyperintense visible in the subcortical white matter area of the frontoparietal temporal insula bilaterally, suggesting diffuse swelling of the frontoparietal temporal insula gyrus bilaterally, and a round-like hyperintense visible in the right parietal lobe; (**c**, **d**) T_1WI enhancement shows hypointense lesions in the subcortical white matter area of the frontoparietal temporal insula bilaterally, with small patchy foci of enhancement (arrows) visible in the left frontal lobe

such as high-resolution MRI (HRMR) are increasingly being used [13].

Serology

Varicella-herpes zoster glycoprotein IgE may make the diagnosis of varicella-herpes zoster encephalitis.

12.1.3 EB Virus Infections

12.1.3.1 Overview

EB virus (Epstein-Barr virus, EBV) is one of the common pathogens that trigger viral infections of the central nervous system in children. EBV is widespread in nature and transmitted via saliva to the body and disrupts B lymphocyte surface-related receptors and stimulates corresponding metabolic reactions. It involves the brain parenchyma and/or meninges, resulting in Epstein-Barr virus encephalitis (EBE).

Most patients present with enlarged lymph nodes, pharyngitis, and splenomegaly, and about 10% of patients have hepatomegaly, jaundice, palatal mucosal rash, and skin rash. Any region of the brain parenchyma can be involved by EBE, with the cerebellum being the most susceptible, in which patients mostly start with gait abnormalities and can die in severe cases due to acute cerebellar swelling leading to cerebellar tonsillar herniation. EBE can cause acute hemiparesis in children and young adults. The EEG examination mainly showed diffuse bilateral leads with continuous high-amplitude slow waves or delta waves. EBV serology or cerebrospinal fluid PCR positive result is the gold standard for the diagnosis of the disease, and cerebrospinal fluid tests show increased cellularity and near-normal protein and glucose levels.

12.1.3.2 Pathological Manifestations

EBV multiplies in pharyngeal lymphoid tissue and is subsequently released into the bloodstream, where it enters the circulation and reaches brain tissue and meninges, causing inflammation.

Acute EBE is mostly a direct viral invasion of brain tissue and neural axons in the spinal cord, meninges, and multiple parts of the peripheral nerves, causing cerebral edema, hemorrhage, perivascular leukocyte infiltration, and glial cell hyperplasia, which can also manifest as diffuse foci of necrosis and perivascular hemorrhage, forming acute hemorrhagic leukoencephalitis, often involving the brainstem, mesencephalon, and cerebellum.

Chronic EBE is associated with a viral autoimmune response, with immune complex deposition, infection-induced inflammatory response resulting in demyelination of brain tissue, and perivascular lymphocytic infiltration with atypical lymphocytes.

12.1.3.3 Imaging

CT shows single or multiple hypodense foci in the brain parenchyma with hyperdense shadowing in the presence of intracranial hemorrhage. MRI often shows symmetrical hyperintense in the caudate and shell nuclei on T_2WI, which may involve the thalamus, dermatomedullary, brainstem, and corpus callosum pressure and increased or decreased signal on DWI and ADC [14, 15]. MRS imaging shows a decrease in NAA and an increase in amino acid and inositol levels (Figs. 12.9 and 12.10).

12.1.3.4 Diagnostic Key Points

1. Patients had a clear history of viral infection, mostly with pharyngitis, generalized lymph node enlargement, hepatosplenomegaly, and skin rash.

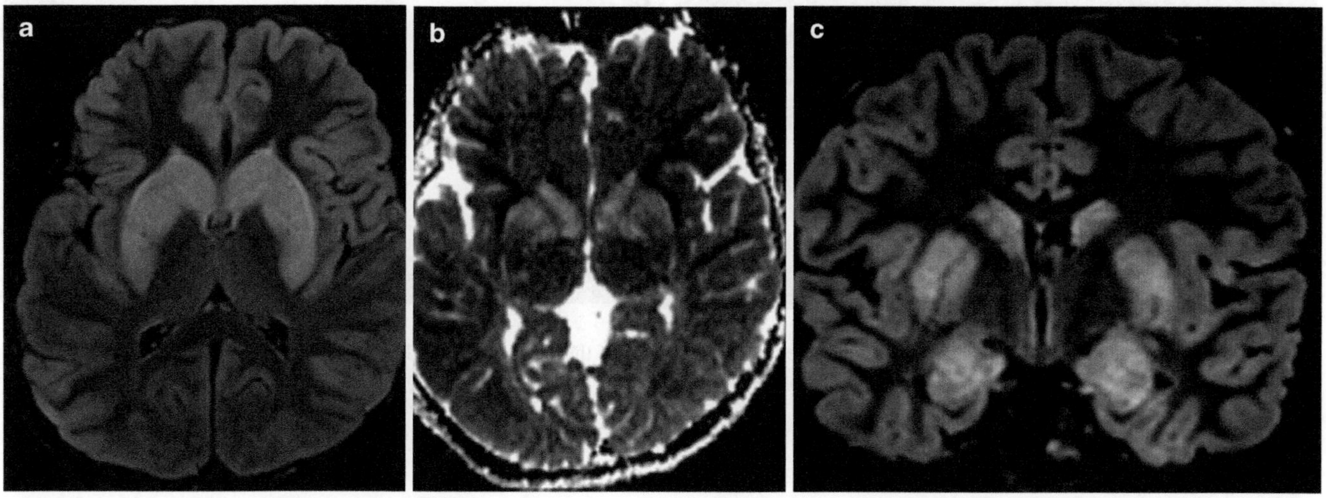

Fig. 12.9 EB viral encephalitis (1). (**a**, **c**) FLAIR sequence shows that symmetrical patchy hyperintense can be seen in the striatum (caudate and cisternal nuclei) and hippocampus bilaterally; (**b**) ADC image shows no decrease in signal in the above lesion

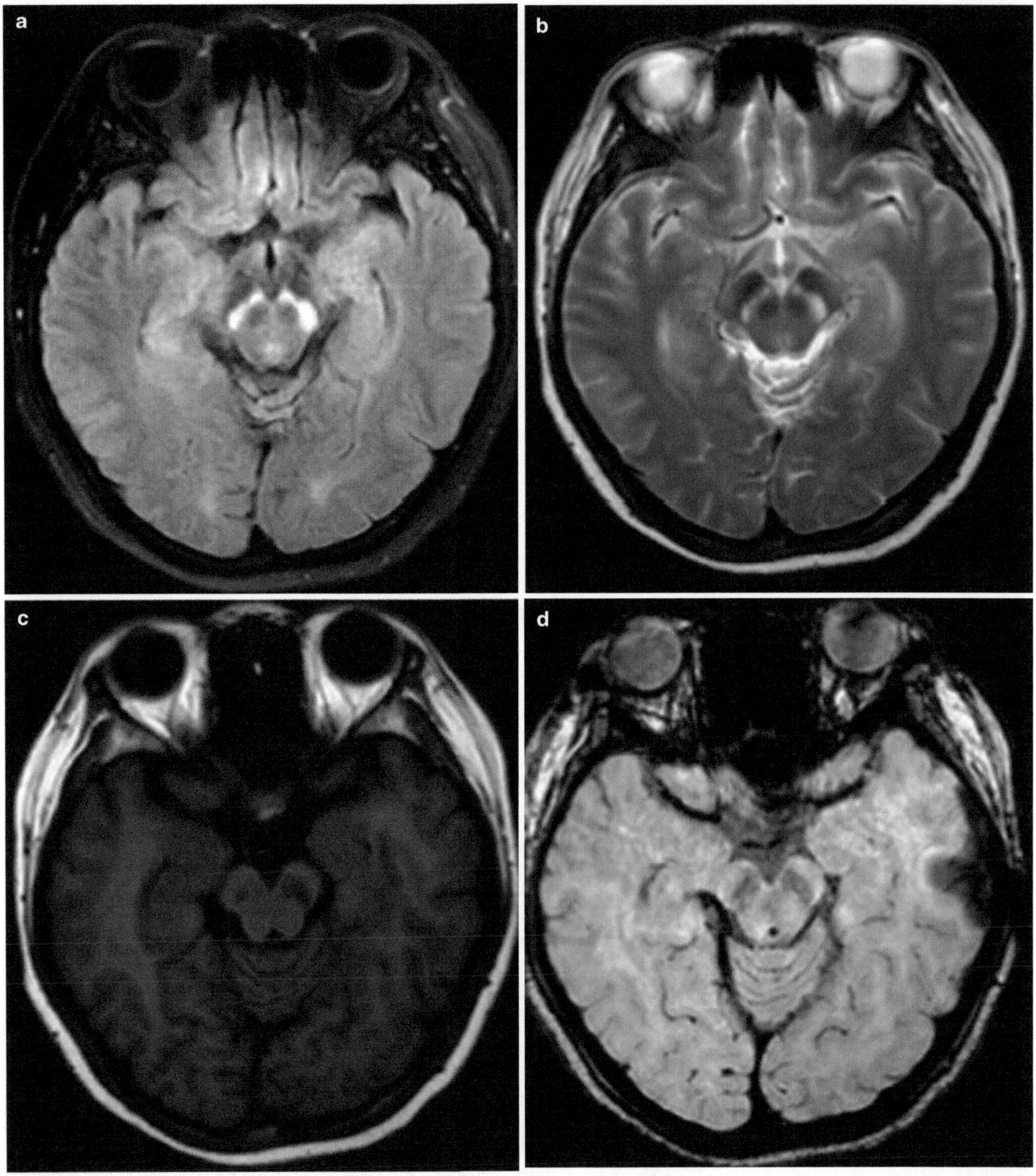

Fig. 12.10 EB viral encephalitis (2). (**a**) Bilateral symmetrical strip lesions of the cerebral peduncle with hyperintense on FLAIR sequence; (**b**) T_2WI shows slightly hyperintense; (**c**) T_1WI shows hypointense; (**d**) SWI with no signal abnormality

2. Imaging. CT shows a nonspecific hypodense lesion; MRI T_2WI often shows symmetric hyperintense on the caudate and shell nuclei, which may involve the thalamus, cortex and medulla, brainstem, and splenium of corpus callosum.
3. Laboratory tests. Positive in phagocytic agglutination antibody test, EBV viral load test, and EBV-specific antibody.

12.1.3.5 Differential Diagnosis

EBV often involves the basal ganglia region, so EBE needs to be differentiated from other diseases that can cause abnormalities in the basal ganglia region, and clinical history and first symptoms can be helpful in the differentiation.

Mitochondrial Encephalopathy

In granulomatous encephalopathy and other organic aciduria, imaging manifestations resembling EBE can be seen, but these disorders are often associated with symptoms of progressive psychomotor retardation and no other neurological deficits.

Ischemia and Hypoxia Damage

Ischemia and hypoxia damage, carbon monoxide poisoning, or hypoglycemia need to be differentiated from EBE, which is facilitated by medical history and usually accompanied by diffuse white matter involvement, exhibiting marked restricted diffusion.

Sinus Thrombosis

It also causes brain tissue swelling and signal changes on DWI and ADC. MRV helps to exclude the diagnosis [16, 17].

12.1.3.6 Status and Progress of Research

Imaging diagnosis of EBE is difficult. MRI often shows symmetrical hyperintense in the caudate and shell nuclei on T_2WI, but it is not specific. A positive phagocytic agglutination antibody test, a positive EBV viral load test, and a positive EBV-specific antibody were used to confirm the diagnosis. Therefore, a combination of molecular, serological, and imaging techniques should be used in the study of childhood encephalitis [18].

12.1.4 Human Herpes Virus 6 Infections

12.1.4.1 Overview

Human herpesvirus type 6 (HHV- 6) is a double-stranded DNA virus that is lymphophilic for human T lymphocytes and belongs to the beta subfamily of herpesviruses. HHV-6 has significant lymphophilic and neurophilic properties, and its infections have been associated with many pediatric diseases, such as posttransplant infections and early childhood acute rash. HHV-6 can invade the central nervous system and can cause potentially permanent damage or even life-threatening in severe cases [19].

Serum anti-HHV-6 IgG and/or IgM indirect immunofluorescence assays are widely used methods for the diagnosis of HHV-6 infections. Detection of viral nucleic acids via PCR and reverse transcription (RT)-PCR has become the method of choice for the identification of HHV-6 in plasma, serum, and cerebrospinal fluid specimens.

12.1.4.2 Pathological Manifestations

The virus reactivation occurs after acute infection, and HHV-6 is in long-term incubation in various parts of the host's salivary glands, liver, lymphatic system, central nervous system, etc. and causes disease when the body is immunocompromised or suppressed, especially when the host is immunodeficient; some studies have shown that HHV-6 has the potential to reactivate even when the host is immunocompetent. This is because HHV-6 infection itself selectively hinders the maturation of dendritic cells and affects the production of some cytokines, leading to immune suppression [20].

12.1.4.3 Imaging

The lesions are often located in the medial temporal lobe and the entorhinal cortex, with particular involvement of the hippocampus and thalamus; in contrast to herpes simplex virus encephalitis, the lesions are more limited and less likely to involve the insular cortex. Lesion showed clearly on FLAIR. The lesion may be mildly enhanced or not enhanced on enhancement scan.

12.1.4.4 Diagnostic Key Points

1. It is most often seen in infants and young children with a clear history of viral exposure and infection, as well as mononucleosis, and presents with fever and bilateral enlarged cervical lymph nodes without attachment tenderness.
2. Imaging. The lesions are often located in the medial temporal lobe and entorhinal cortex, particularly involving the hippocampus and thalamus, and less frequently in the insular cortex. Lesion showed clearly on FLAIR. Enhanced examination of the lesion may be mildly enhancing or non-enhancing.
3. Laboratory tests. Detection of anti-HHV-6 IgM in infants and children is a reliable indicator for the diagnosis of initial infection. Initially negative for antibodies in *E. coli*, antibody titers begin to rise after 7 days and are measurable after 2 weeks. Viral culture is the method for confirming active HHV-6 infection. HHV-6 DNA was detected in the blood specimen, supporting the active replication of HHV-6 [21, 22].

12.1.4.5 Differential Diagnosis

EB Viral Infection

Isolated or multiple hypodense foci can be seen in the brain parenchyma, calcification of basal ganglia area, and traffic hydrocephalus with intracranial hemorrhage and demyelination-like changes; EEG showed mainly diffuse bilateral leads with continuous high-amplitude slow waves or delta waves.

Herpes Simplex Virus Infection

Typical signs are asymmetric temporal, frontal, and insular lamellar abnormal density or signal on one or both sides, mostly involving cortical and subcortical white matter, mostly with hemorrhage, and may have mild to moderate occupying effects, showing restricted diffusion on DWI sequences with decreased ADC values. Enhanced scans may show linear or gyral-like enhancement of the brain surface in the lesion area and occasionally may show ring-like enhancement. When the lesion invades the temporal lobe, frontal lobe, or insular cortical area, it may be manifested as the "knife-cut sign," which is the most characteristic manifestation of the disease. Lesions invading the nucleus basalis, thalamus, and brainstem present as "basal nucleus protrusion sign."

Enterovirus Encephalitis

It is common in summer and autumn, and gastrointestinal symptoms may appear at the beginning. The imaging manifestations are mainly lamellar hypodense in cerebral cortex and paraventricular area. This is associated with inflammatory changes in the small cerebral arteries, meninges, and ventricular canal due to enterovirus invasion of the central nervous system, especially the inflammatory response of the small paraventricular arteries.

12.1.4.6 Status and Progress of Research

HHV-6 infection occurs most often in immunocompromised patients but can also occur in immunocompetent patients and is associated with central nervous system diseases (e.g., meningitis, multiple sclerosis, medial temporal lobe sclerosis, posttransplant limbic encephalitis).

HHV-6 central neurological infection imaging is characterized by a specific distribution, with lesions often located in the medial temporal lobe and entorhinal cortex with a particular tendency to involve the hippocampus and thalamus and, less frequently, the insular cortex. Lesion showed clearly on FLAIR. The lesion may be mildly enhanced or not enhanced on enhancement scan. However, a combination of clinical signs, serum and cerebrospinal fluid of anti-HHV-6 IgG and/or IgM antibodies, and viral DNA PCR tests is required for diagnosis [23].

12.1.5 Monkey B Virus Infection

12.1.5.1 Overview

Monkey B virus, also known as monkey herpesvirus type 1, belongs to the family *Herpesviridae*, subfamily alpha herpesvirus. It is the member of herpes simplex virus along with human herpes simplex virus type 1 (HSV-1) and human herpes simplex virus type 2 (HSV-2). Macaques are the natural host of Monkey B virus, which is naturally infectious among apes and monkeys, in Asia. It is the most potentially dangerous zoonotic virus carried by non-human primates and can cause virulent infections in both humans and monkeys. Monkey B virus is transmitted to humans mainly through bites and scratches of infected macaques, and airborne droplet transmission is not an important route of transmission.

Infected apes and monkeys only have oral herpes simplex; however, when humans were bitten or scratched by infected monkeys, it causes monkey b virus disease. The incubation period is 2–30 days, with pain, redness, swelling, herpes, and exudate in the local area of the injury site, often complicated by lymphangitis and lymphadenitis, followed by episodic myelitis or encephalomyelitis. The vast majority die within 3 weeks after the onset of the disease, with a small percentage of patients who were cured in acute stage need to take effective antiviral drugs for a long time [24, 25].

The monkey B virus is far more pathogenic to humans than to monkeys. The incubation period of the virus is 2–10 years after infection, and the disease is severe once it attacks. Human infection with monkey B virus is mainly due to direct contact with infectious saliva or tissue cultures of monkeys, such as bites or scratches by infected monkeys, or contamination from laboratory operations.

Diagnostic methods include enzyme-linked immunoassay, polymerase chain reaction (PCR), protein blotting, etc. The specificity and sensitivity of the PCR for serological samples is now close to 100%. For symptomatic patients, the skin wounds should be cultured for the virus. In laboratory tests, B virus can be isolated from cerebrospinal fluid, B virus-specific antibodies and antigens can be detected in cerebrospinal fluid, and B virus nucleic acid tests are positive.

12.1.5.2 Pathological Manifestations

The mechanism of monkey B virus is similar to that of HSV, in that initial viral replication occurs at the site of mucosal infection, transported via nerve axons to sensory neurons, and latent in sensory ganglia, where the virus no longer replicates during the latency period. The B virus can be activated from a latent state and re-replicate by passing through neuronal axons to mucosal epithelial cells. The B virus can cause swelling of the brain parenchyma, lymphocytic meningitis, and the accumulation of lymphocytes around the blood vessels, forming vascular sleeves, often with extensive hemorrhage. Inflammation is more extensive and can involve the cerebral hemispheres, cerebellum, brainstem, and spinal cord.

12.1.5.3 Imaging

CT has a low detection rate for early B viral encephalitis. The lesion on MRI manifested as hypointense on T_1WI and hyperintense on T_2WI. The lesions are wide ranging, often involving the cerebral hemispheres, cerebellum, brainstem, and spinal cord.

12.1.5.4 Diagnostic Key Points

1. History of exposure and infection with monkey B virus.
2. Imaging. The lesion manifested as hypointense on T_1WI and hyperintense on T_2WI. The lesion is widespread, often involving the cerebral hemispheres, cerebellum, brainstem, and spinal cord.
3. Laboratory tests. The B virus can be isolated from the cerebrospinal fluid, and B virus-specific antibodies and antigens can be detected in the cerebrospinal fluid.

12.1.5.5 Differential Diagnosis

Acute Disseminated Encephalomyelitis

The time of onset is days or weeks after viral infection or vaccination. The pathologic basis is demyelinating changes involving the white matter of the brain and manifests as asymmetrical multiple punctate lesions in the white matter of the brain, with foci of necrosis and occasionally small hemorrhagic foci in the center of the lesions. Simultaneous involvement of the cortex, brainstem, or basal ganglia can be seen. During acute phase there may be perifocal edema and marked enhancement of the lesion.

Herpes Simplex Virus Encephalitis

Typical sign is asymmetric temporal, frontal, and insular lamellar abnormal density or signal on one or both sides, mostly involving cortical and subcortical white matter, mostly with hemorrhage, may have mild to moderate occupying effects, and shows restricted diffusion on DWI sequences with decreased ADC values. Enhanced scans may show linear or gyral-like enhancement of the brain surface in the lesion area, and occasionally may show ring-like enhancement. When the lesion invades the temporal lobe, frontal lobe, or insular cortical area, it may be manifested as the "knife-cut sign," which is the most characteristic manifestation of the disease. Lesions invading the nucleus basalis, thalamus, and brainstem present as "basal nucleus protrusion sign" [26, 27].

12.1.5.6 Status and Progress of Research

Current national and international reports indicate a low incidence of the disease, which is mostly seen in case reports. The existing imaging methods are still in the preliminary stage of research for the diagnosis of this disease, and the diagnosis needs to be integrated with clinical history, symptoms, and laboratory tests.

12.2 Papova Virus Infections

Shuang Xia, Shaozhou Wang, and Zi'ao Fu

12.2.1 Overview

The family *Papillomaviridae* consists of the first letters of the virus names of the papillomavirus, polyoma virus, and vacuolavirus, that is, "papova" consists of the first two letters of "papillom," "polyoma," and vacuolating agent.

Human papilloma virus (HPV) is an epitheliophilic virus that is widely distributed in humans and animals and often induces benign tumors and warts in humans, such as human common warts, condyloma acuminatum, and papillomas. Polyoma virus is also known as murine subauricular tumor virus. Ape vacuolating agent is an oncogenic virus found in both humans and monkeys.

HPV often has cutaneous symptoms, such as rashes and warts, before causing central nervous system symptoms, which are often mild at onset, with headache and fever predominating, and some patients may have other symptoms of nerve damage. Confirmation of diagnosis requires cerebrospinal fluid detection of HPV [28, 29].

12.2.2 Pathological Manifestations

Papillomavirus transforms cells of the squamous epithelium or basal lamina of the mucosa, causing tumors in the host, hyperkeratosis with incomplete keratinization, hypertrophy of the spinous layer, and ectoplasmic papillomatous hyperplasia. Focal vacuolated cells are seen in the upper part of the sphenoid layer and in the granular layer, with the basement membrane intact. Fibropapilloma viruses transform both skin keratinocytes and dermal fibroblasts, whereas other papilloma viruses do not transform into fibroblasts [30].

12.2.3 Imaging

Cranial CT and MRI (including enhanced MRI) have a low detection rate for lesions and often have no positive findings. When the cerebrospinal fluid viral load is high, the blood-brain barrier can be disrupted and focal enhancement can occur. The lesion is patchy-like, often involving the frontal-

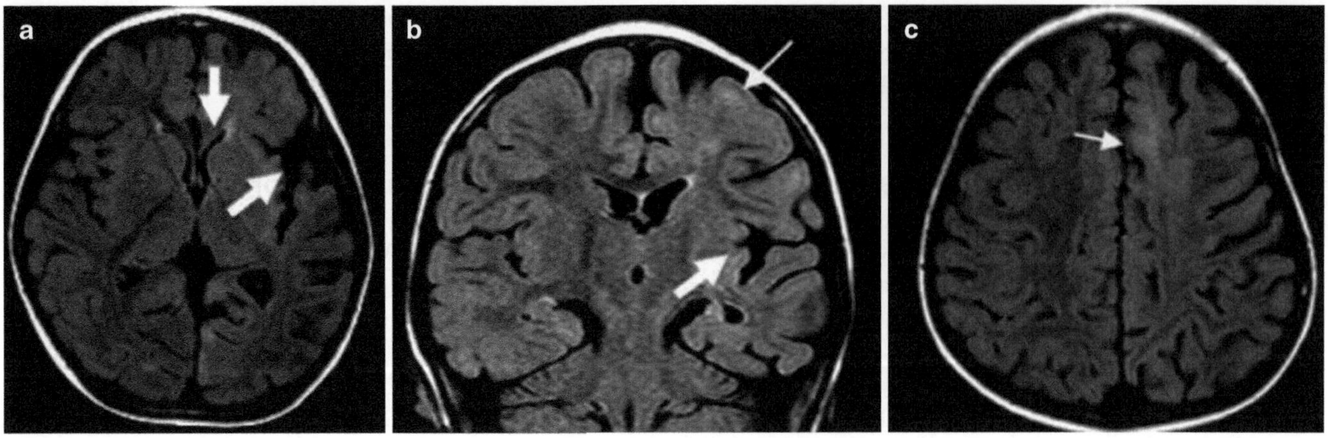

Fig. 12.11 Human papilloma virus encephalitis (1). (**a**) FLAIR sequence showing atrophy around the genu of corpus callosum, left lateral fissure, and widening of the adjacent cerebral sulcus; (**b**) FLAIR sequence showing increased signal in the left frontal lobe (thin arrow), left insula (thick arrow). (**c**) FLAIR sequence showing multiple patchy-like mild hyperintense in the left frontal lobe (thin arrow)

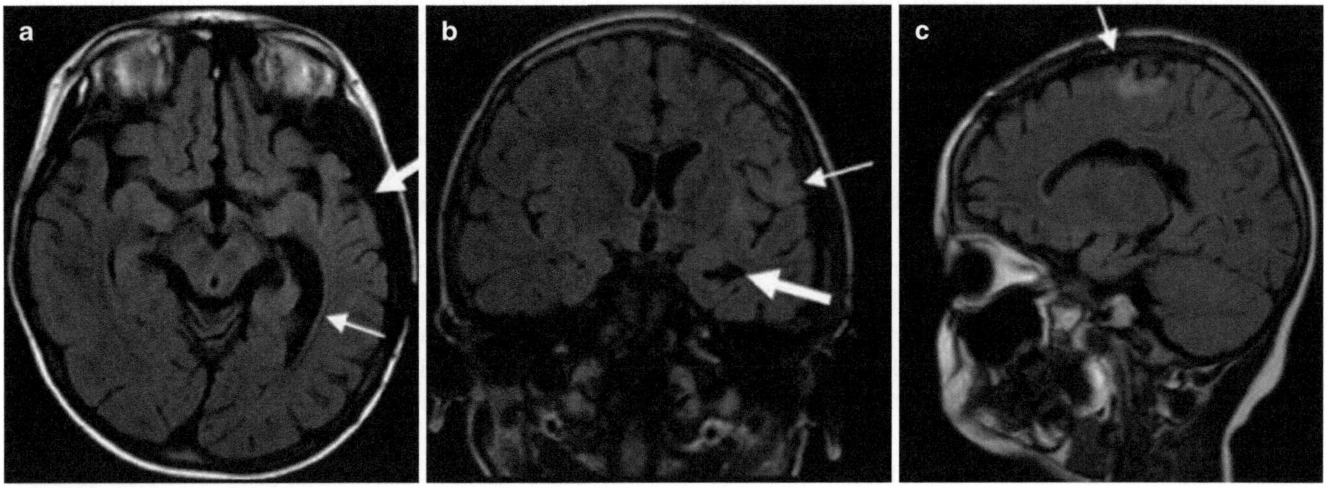

Fig. 12.12 Human papilloma virus encephalitis (2). (**a**) FLAIR sequence shows cortical atrophy of the left cerebral hemisphere (thick arrow) and enlargement of the temporal horn of the left lateral ventricle (thin arrow); (**b**) FLAIR sequence shows enlargement of the temporal horn of the left lateral ventricle (thick arrow) and patchy-like mild hyperintense under the frontal cortex around the left lateral fissure (thin arrow); (**c**) FLAIR sequence shows patchy like mild hyperintense under the left frontal cortex (thin arrow)

parietal cortex. FLAIR shows the lesion sensitively with hyperintense, and no or mild enhancement can be seen (Figs. 12.11 and 12.12).

12.2.4 Diagnostic Key Points

1. History of virus-related exposures and infections, mucosal surface infections, and skin infections.
2. Imaging is often unremarkable but can also appear as patchy-like, often involving the frontal-parietal cortex. FLAIR shows the lesion sensitively with hyperintense, and lesions are non- or mildly enhanced.
3. Pathogenic examination. Depending on the specimen, HPV DNA is detected by spot hybridization or in situ hybridization; IgG antibodies in the patient's serum are detected by applying recombinant techniques to express antigens, or immune sera or monoclonal antibodies are prepared from antigen-immunized animals to detect HPV antigens in tissues or local mucus [31].
4. Pathological microscopy. The initial determination of HPV infection can be made by taking tissue sections of warts or collecting local mucus smears from the genital tract and observing characteristic vacuolated cells or dyskeratotic and hyperkeratotic cells under light microscopy.

12.2.5 Differential Diagnosis

Herpes simplex virus encephalitis. The typical sign is asymmetric temporal, frontal, and insular lamellar abnormal density or signal on one or both sides. The lesion mostly involves cortical and subcortical white matter, mostly with hemorrhage, and may have mild to moderate occupying effects, showing restricted diffusion on DWI sequences with decreased ADC values. Enhanced scans may show linear or gyral-like enhancement of the brain surface in the lesioned area and occasionally may show ring-like enhancement. When the lesion invades the temporal lobe, frontal lobe, and insular cortical area, it may be manifested as "knife-cut sign," which is the most characteristic manifestation of the disease. When the lesion invades the basal nucleus, thalamus, or brainstem, it shows a "basal nucleus protrusion sign."

12.2.6 Status and Progress of Research

Currently available imaging examinations have no specific diagnostic value for this disease and need to be combined with medical history, clinical symptoms, and laboratory tests for a comprehensive analysis.

12.3 Flavivirus Infection

Shuang Xia, Zi'ao Fu, and Yinhua Jin

12.3.1 Overview

Flaviviruses are viruses that transmit diseases through hematophagous arthropods (mosquitoes, ticks, white flies, etc.) and include mainly encephalitis B virus, dengue virus, yellow fever virus, forest encephalitis virus, West Nile virus, and Murray Valley encephalitis virus. The inflammatory disease caused by a flavivirus entering the brain is known as flavivirus encephalitis. The main flaviviruses in our country are epidemic B encephalitis virus, dengue virus, and forest encephalitis virus. Encephalitis B caused by epidemic B encephalitis virus is described in Chap. 8, Sect. 8.1, and is therefore not described here. West Nile virus, which is most commonly found in Africa, Europe, North America, and Central Asia, is described in Part II of this section. Murray Valley encephalitis virus, which is mostly found in Australia, is described in the third part of this section.

12.3.1.1 Common Flavivirus Infections

Dengue virus (DENV), which has *Aedes aegypti* mosquitoes as the main vector, is mostly found in southern regions of China and can cause dengue fever, dengue hemorrhagic fever, and dengue shock syndrome. Central nervous system involvement is relatively rare in dengue virus-infected patients, and central nervous system lesions can be encephalopathy secondary to hepatic and renal insufficiency, hypotension, or encephalitis due to direct viral invasion, as well as immune complex-mediated vasculitis and demyelinating lesions. Diagnosis was confirmed by detection of anti-DENV IgM antibodies, viral RNA, or nonstructural protein 1 (NS1) in the cerebrospinal fluid.

Forest encephalitis virus uses ticks as a vector, so it is also called tick-borne forest encephalitis virus (TBFEV), which can cause forest encephalitis. The onset is predominant in spring and summer, mostly in Russia and in the northeastern and northwestern forest areas of China. Most patients show occult infection, and a few patients suddenly develop high fever, headache, nausea, neck tonicity, impaired consciousness, limb paralysis, and other symptoms after an incubation period of 1–2 weeks, and severe cases may develop respiratory and circulatory failure or even death due to medulla oblongata paralysis. Durable immunity is acquired after infection. Confirmation of the diagnosis was made by serological or cerebrospinal fluid isolation of TBFEV or detection of specific IgM or IgG antibodies [32].

Yellow fever virus uses *Aedes aegypti* as the main vector and can cause yellow fever, mostly in Africa and South America. Patients may present with high fever, headache, jaundice, proteinuria, relatively slow pulse, and hemorrhage. CNS symptoms tend to be epilepsy or hepatic encephalopathy due to the severity of the disease, with no significant abnormalities on imaging.

12.3.2 Pathological Manifestations

Dengue virus infections tend to have systemic involvement, with degenerative changes in the liver, kidneys, heart, and brain. Subarachnoid hemorrhage and focal brain parenchymal hemorrhage, cerebral edema, and cerebral tenderness are seen in those with central nervous system involvement.

Forest encephalitis has a wide range of pathological changes, with gray matter, white matter, and meninges involved, mostly inflammatory exudative changes, manifested as hemorrhage, congestion, perivascular lymphocytic set infiltration, neuronal cell degeneration and necrosis, glial cell proliferation, and also degenerative lesions.

12.3.3 Imaging

Dengue encephalitis usually presents as isolated or multiple patchy shadows in the brain parenchyma. On CT images it is mostly hypodense. MRI T_1WI shows hypointense or isointense and T_2WI shows hyperintense. FLAIR sequences show hyperintense. DWI and ADC have diffusion-limited changes and mild enhancement can be seen. Sometimes intra-focal hemorrhage is seen in SWI. Lesions mostly involve the cerebellum, basal ganglia area, internal capsule, and brainstem [33].

Forest encephalitis. CT mostly shows patchy-like hypodense lesions, usually without enhancement or mildly enhanced. MRI T_1WI shows hypointense or isointense and T_2WI shows hyperintense. FLAIR shows hyperintense. DWI and ADC show diffusion-limited changes with no or mild enhancement. The lesions are mostly found in the basal ganglia area and thalamus [34, 35].

12.3.4 Diagnostic Key Points

1. Patients have a corresponding history of mosquito bites and may present with flu-like symptoms during the incubation period, followed by high fever, impaired consciousness, convulsions, and even limb paralysis.
2. Imaging. MRI plain scan shows single or multiple patchy hypointense on T_1WI and hyperintense on T_2WI in the brain parenchyma which shows hyperintense on FLAIR sequence. The lesion manifests hyperintense in DWI and ADC, mostly in the basal ganglia, thalamus, and cerebellum.
3. Laboratory tests. Virus-specific IgM and IgG antibodies were detected, and RT-PCR amplification found viral nucleic acid sequences, confirming the diagnosis.

12.3.5 Differential Diagnosis

MRI differential diagnosis includes thalamic infarction, tumor, Wilson disease, and Wernicke encephalopathy. Although MRI examinations can also reveal abnormal signal changes in the bilateral pedunculopontine, thalamic, and basal ganglia regions, they all have their own imaging features, such as tumors that generally include primary tumors and metastases, most of which present with peripheral brain tissue edema and significant occupancy effects, and metastases that generally have a primary focus. Enhanced scans often reveal signs of abnormal enhancement. Symmetrical bilateral thalamic and brainstem lesions in patients with Wernicke encephalopathy are characterized by symmetrical T_2WI high signal around the third ventricle and midbrain aqueduct, and papillary atrophy is typical of the acute phase of Wernicke encephalopathy. Wilson disease is characterized by bilateral symmetrical basal ganglia area, cerebellar dentate nucleus, internal capsule and thalamus involvement, with characteristic hypointense in the pallidum on T_2WI as a characteristic feature, along with corneal K-F rings. Combined with clinical presentation and laboratory tests, Wilson disease can be differentiated from flavivirus encephalitis. However, the imaging manifestations of several flavivirus encephalitis lack specificity, and differentiation requires a combination of clinical manifestations and laboratory tests.

12.3.6 Status and Progress of Research

MRI DWI may show characteristic changes in the thalamus from punctate to homogeneous, from left to right with a low apparent diffusion coefficient, suggesting that flavivirus may first affect one side of the thalamus and then spread to the other side. The characteristic pattern from punctiform to homogeneous is consistent with the manifestation of cytotoxic edema [36].

Flavivirus infection of the central nervous system can result in neuronal dysfunction and decreased metabolism, as seen on ^{18}F-FDG PET/CT examination with decreased ^{18}F-FDG uptake. PWI may show a local decrease in cerebral blood flow in the area of the lesion.

12.3.7 West Nile Virus Infection

12.3.7.1 Overview

West Nile virus enters the brain and causes an inflammatory disease which transmitted by mosquitoes and called West Nile virus encephalitis. West Nile virus was first discovered in the West Nile region of Uganda, Africa, in 1937 and hence the name [37–40]. So far, no West Nile virus has been found in animals in China, and there have been no cases of West Nile virus infection.

West Nile virus is a RNA virus, with a virus size of approximately 40 nm. Birds are the primary hosts, and the virus maintains and expands transmission in the bird-mosquito-bird cycle. Humans and other vertebrates, such as horses, are incidental hosts and are thought to play a secondary role in the transmission cycle. In addition, the virus can be transmitted from person to person through blood transfusions or organ transplants, but person-to-person contact does not result in the spread of the disease. It belongs to the *Flaviviridae* family. The diagnosis is primarily confirmed by positive serology and cerebrospinal fluid IgM antibodies or cerebrospinal fluid nucleic acid amplification tests [37–40].

12.3.7.2 Pathological Manifestations

Patients with West Nile virus meningitis may have focal cerebral nerve or medulla oblongata injury, and some patients have acute limb paralysis (flaccid paralysis) with loss or weakening of tendon reflexes and bladder dysfunction due to damage to the anterior horn cells of the spinal cord. Some patients may have specific clinical symptoms, such as Parkinson's syndrome, symptomatic myospasm, flaccid paralysis, etc., suggesting an association with viral invasion and damage to its basal ganglia, thalamus, pons, and anterior horn cells [41].

12.3.7.3 Imaging

1. **CT findings**: Usually no significant abnormalities can be found.
2. **MR findings:** MR FLAIR and T_2WI usually manifest patchy hyperintense shadow with irregular borders in gray matter, white matter, cerebellum, basal ganglia region, thalamus and internal capsule, pons, midbrain region, or restricted DWI diffusion in white matter, corona radiata, and internal capsule only. The lesions may also involve the meninges, spinal cord, cauda equina, and nerve roots. In some cases, there may also be no abnormal manifestations [41].

12.3.7.4 Diagnostic Key Points

1. Patients present with severe clinical symptoms such as high fever, severe headache (severe in the frontal and retro-orbital areas), cervical tonicity, myoclonus, convulsions, balance disturbances and gait disorders, resting and motor tremors or convulsions, personality or behavioral changes, and coma.
2. The lesion appears as a patchy hyperintense shadow with irregular borders on T2WI/FLAIR imaging, with no enhancement of the lesion on enhanced scan and limited diffusion on DWI. The lesions can also involve the midbrain, corpus callosum, temporal lobe, cerebellum, and spinal cord.
3. Laboratory tests can detect virus-specific IgM and IgG antibody or RT-PCR amplification to discover viral RNA.

12.3.7.5 Differential Diagnosis

Typical signs of herpes simplex virus encephalitis are unilateral or bilateral asymmetric temporal, frontal, and insular lamellar abnormal density or signal, mostly involving cortical and subcortical white matter, mostly with hemorrhage, and may have mild to moderate occupying effects, showing restricted diffusion on DWI sequences with decreased ADC values. Enhanced scans may show linear or gyral-like enhancement of the brain surface in the lesion area and occasionally may show ring-like enhancement. When the lesion invades the temporal lobe, frontal lobe, or insular cortical area, it may be manifested as the "knife-cut sign," which is the most characteristic manifestation of the disease. When the lesion invades the basal nucleus, thalamus, or brainstem, it shows a "basal nucleus protrusion sign."

12.3.7.6 Status and Progress of Research

Imaging of West Nile virus encephalitis is nonspecific and may appear normal or appear abnormal on DWI only or may show hyperintense in the involved portion on T_2WI and FLAIR. There was no tendency for the distribution of lesions. Therefore, the diagnosis needs to be considered in conjunction with the history, clinical symptoms, and laboratory tests.

12.3.8 Murray Valley Encephalitis Virus Infection

12.3.8.1 Overview

The inflammatory disease caused by the Murray Valley encephalitis virus entering the brain is known as Murray Valley encephalitis virus infection of the brain. Murray Valley encephalitis occurs mainly in the Murray Valley region of New South Wales and Victoria, Australia, and the main vector of the disease is the *Culex* mosquito. In addition, viruses were isolated from *Aedes aegypti*, *Culex tritaeniorhynchus*, and *Culex aculeatus*. Large water birds (e.g., herons and egrets) are the main hosts for the spread of the virus, and mammals (e.g., rabbits and wallabies) also play an important role in maintaining the circulation of the virus. The mechanism of virus overwintering and the origin of the continuing epidemic are not known. Year-round epidemics of the disease are uncommon even in tropical Australia, and experimental studies have shown that the virus can be transmitted via eggs in *Aedes aegypti* [42].

Murray Valley encephalitis can be detected by detecting serum-specific IgM and IgG antibodies or confirming the diagnosis by PCR test for Murray Valley encephalitis virus.

12.3.8.2 Pathological Manifestations

Murray Valley encephalitis virus multiplies in many vertebrate and mosquito cells, forms empty spots in primary chicken embryo cells, and passaged porcine kidney cells, monkey kidney cells, and vole kidney cells, and the addition of macrophages containing the Fc receptor to primary chicken embryo fibroblasts promotes virus growth. All routes of inoculation of newborn mice can cause disease. The pathogenesis of the disease is similar to that of epidemic B encephalitis [43].

12.3.8.3 Imaging

MRI T_2WI shows hyperintense on thalamus, which may involve the red nucleus, substantia nigra, and cervical medulla. These findings precede the serological diagnosis, which is similar to that of epidemic B encephalitis. In the right context, thalamic T_2WI hyperintense suggests flavivirus infection [44].

12.3.8.4 Diagnostic Key Points

1. The patient was from an infected area and had been in close contact with a person infected with the Murray Valley encephalitis virus for 2 weeks before the onset of the disease.

2. MRI T2WI hyperintense on thalamus, which may involve the red nucleus, substantia nigra, and cervical medulla.
3. Laboratory tests. Diagnosis can be confirmed by detection of virus-specific IgM and IgG antibodies or viral RNA by RT-PCR amplification.

12.3.8.5 Differential Diagnosis

Epidemic B encephalitis. Also known as Japanese encephalitis, it is an acute infectious disease of the central nervous system caused by the encephalitis B virus. The disease is predominant in children and is endemic and seasonal. MRI T_1WI showed hypointense or mixed signal lesions, which manifest as hyperintense on T_2WI and FLAIR, in the midbrain, thalamus, and basal ganglia regions.

12.3.8.6 Status and Progress of Research

The imaging of Murray Valley encephalitis is poorly reported, and studies have shown that MRI can be used to observe the extent and severity of lesions, but the diagnosis still needs to be confirmed with a history of life in the affected area, clinical symptoms, and relevant laboratory tests.

12.4 Nipah Virus Infection

Shuang Xia, Shaozhou Wang, and Zi'ao Fu

12.4.1 Overview

Nipah virus encephalitis is a zoonotic infection caused by the Nipah virus (NiV) of the genus *Henipavirus* of the family *Paramyxoviridae*. Nipah virus is a new human-animal virus isolated in the late twentieth century from a fatal case in the village of Nipah, Perak, Malaysia. The virus is found mainly in and around Malaysia and Bangladesh in South Asia and is not pathogenic to bats, is somewhat pathogenic to pigs, and is highly pathogenic to humans. Nipah virus can cause severe encephalitis and respiratory disease in animals and humans, with high morbidity and mortality rates. The mortality rate is 40–70% in humans after infection with Nipah virus. Nipah virus is classified as the most dangerous biosafety 4 (P4) level pathogen. The incubation period for humans is 4 days to 2 months. Patients present with fever, headache, dizziness, and vomiting and even develop severe encephalitis. Neurological involvement is diverse and multi-focal, including aseptic meningitis, diffuse encephalitis, and focal brainstem involvement. Cerebellar symptoms are relatively common. Patients may also experience psychiatric symptoms, including depression and personality changes, as well as persistent cognitive impairment, etc. [45, 46].

Nipah virus infection can be detected via virus-specific IgM antibody or RT-PCR amplification revealed viral nucleic acid sequences to confirm the diagnosis.

12.4.2 Pathological Manifestations

Nipah virus infection can involve all systems of the body. The basic pathological changes of Nipah virus infection are multi-organ vasculitis and endothelial cell inflammation. CNS infections exhibit extensive and spreading small necrotic lesions. Postoperative examination shows that the brain is the most severely infected organ and that the gray matter, white matter, basal ganglia, cerebellum, brainstem, and spinal cord may be invaded, as well as other organs such as the lungs, heart, and kidneys. Nipah virus antigen can be detected in central nervous system tissues, especially in vascular endothelial cells and parenchymal cells. Small amounts of viral antigens can also be detected in other tissues. Vasculitis occurs mainly in small arteries, capillaries, and small veins and manifests as necrosis of the vessel wall and thrombosis and infiltration of inflammatory cells such as leukocytes and monocytes. The main cause of death in patients with Nipah virus infection is the massive death of virus-infected nerve cells and extensive focal infarction of brain tissue.

12.4.3 Imaging

In the acute and late stages of the lesion, MRI shows lesions mostly located in the peripheral areas of the brain parenchyma (subcortical), around the basal pool, brainstem, gray-white matter junction area, and periventricular areas, with multiple small focal lesions of 2–7 mm in diameter, round or strip-like, with hyperintense T_2WI and FLAIR and no edema around the lesion. Even when extensive disseminated lesions throughout the brain parenchyma are present, larger masses rarely appear, and cortical damage is present in nearly half of patients. In advanced stages of the lesion, some patients may see signs of old hemorrhage. No hyperintense changes in the subarachnoid space can be found on the FLAIR sequence. Enhanced scans in the acute phase show no enhancement of the lesion and no significant meningeal enhancement. The main pathological manifestation is thrombosis due to vasculitis, which in turn causes extensive microinfarct formation throughout the brain. In some patients, there is no significant difference in the performance of MRI in the acute and late stages of the lesion, while recurrent and delayed encephalitis may show significant fusion lesions in the cortex on MRI, indicating that the performance of MRI in recurrent and delayed Nipah virus encephalitis is significantly different from that of early Nipah virus encephalitis (Fig. 12.13) [46].

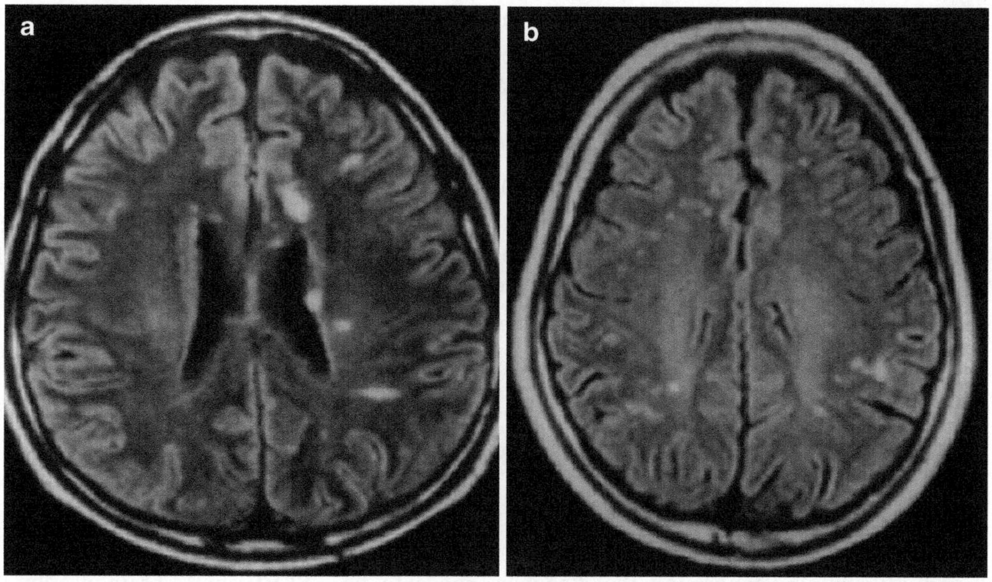

Fig. 12.13 Nipah virus infection. (**a**, **b**) FALIR sequence showing multiple irregular hyperintense lesions in the deep white matter of the bilateral frontal and parietal subcortical and lateral periventricular lobes

12.4.4 Diagnostic Key Points

1. The patient was from an infected area and had been in close contact with a Nipah virus-infected person or pig for 2 weeks before the onset of the disease or had consumed food that might have been contaminated with fruit bats, etc.
2. Patients have fever, vertigo, headache, vomiting, varying degrees of confusion, and significant brainstem dysfunction.
3. Imaging. In acute and late stage, MRI shows multiple small focal lesions in the subcortex and deep white matter, etc., T2WI and FLAIR show hyperintense, and recurrent and delayed viral encephalitis shows continuous cortical damage.
4. Laboratory tests. The diagnosis can be confirmed by detection of Nipah virus-specific IgM, IgG antibodies, or RT-PCR amplification to discover the viral nucleic acid sequence.

12.4.5 Differential Diagnosis

Nipah virus encephalitis has a variety of imaging presentations and should be differentiated from other viral encephalitis, cerebral infarction, and multiple sclerosis.

1. Herpes simplex virus encephalitis. The typical sign is one side or bilateral asymmetric temporal, frontal, and insular lamellar abnormal densities or signals, mostly involving cortical and subcortical white matter, mostly with hemorrhage, may have mild to moderate occupancy effects, showing diffusion restriction on DWI sequences with decreased ADC values. Enhanced scans may show linear or gyral-like enhancement of the brain surface in the lesioned area and occasionally may show ring-like enhancement. When the lesion invades the temporal lobe, frontal lobe, or insular cortical area, it may be manifested as the "knife-cut sign," which is the most characteristic manifestation of the disease. When the lesion invades the basal nucleus, thalamus, or brainstem, it shows a "basal nucleus protrusion sign."
2. Epidemic B encephalitis. It also known as Japanese encephalitis and is a type B acute infectious disease of the central nervous system caused by encephalitis virus. The disease is predominant in children and is endemic and seasonal. MRI T1WI shows hypointense or mixed signal lesions, which manifest as hyperintense on T2WI and FLAIR, in the midbrain, thalamus, and basal ganglia regions.
3. Multiple sclerosis. It is the most common demyelinating disease, characterized by multiple focal spreads and a disease course that often alternates between remission and relapse. It occurs in young and middle-aged women. Intracerebral lesions are predominantly located in the ventricles and deep white matter surrounding the cerebral hemispheres and, to a lesser extent, the brainstem and cerebellum. The lesions are predominantly round, with plaques prevalent and some lesions fused. CT plain scan shows homogeneous or hypodense lesions with blurred borders, most of which have no obvious occupying effect and most of which are multiple and vary in size. In the acute or active phase, the lesions show ring-like or nodular enhancement, while in the chronic phase and after hormone therapy, there is no enhancement. The MRI presentation of multiple sclerosis lesions varies depending on the stage, with hypointense on T1WI, hyperintense on T2WI in active lesions, and hyperintense on DWI. In

silent period, changes on T1WI are inapparent and T2WI shows hyperintense with iso- or hypointense on DWI. Most lesions enhanced during the active phase in the enhanced scan, but no enhancement or mild enhancement was seen during the silent phase or after hormone therapy. Enhanced lesions may be lamellar, nodular, annular, semicircular, and arcuate in shape. The degree of enhancement is related to the disruption of the blood-brain barrier and the repair response. Nodular enhancement is a new lesion, while ring-like enhancement often indicates reactive of an old lesion [47].

12.4.6 Status and Progress of Research

Nipah virus encephalitis imaging manifestations are diverse; MRI is more conducive to observe the extent and severity of lesion distribution, confirming the diagnosis needs to be combined with the history of life in the infected area, clinical symptoms, and laboratory related tests.

12.5 St. Louis Virus Encephalitis

Shuang Xia and Zi'ao Fu

12.5.1 Overview

Zoonotic central nervous system infections caused by St. Louis encephalitis virus (SLEV) and transmitted by mosquito vectors are called St. Louis viral encephalitis (SLVE). The basic transmission of the virus is the bird-mosquito-bird cycle; in nature, humans are only occasional hosts. According to the study, the only animal that became ill after a natural infection was a human. SLEV is transmitted by many mosquitoes in the genus *Culex* and amplified by passerine birds. Phylogenetic analysis based on the full-length E gene sequence divided the SLEV strain into eight genotypes. Genotypes I and II are common in the United States, while genotype V is widely distributed in South America. Other genotypes have a limited distribution. Genotype III is located in southern South America, IV is restricted to Colombia and Panama, VI is located in Panama, VII is located in Argentina, and VIII has been detected only in the Brazilian Amazon. The disease is diagnosed by molecular detection of SLEV RNA in serum or cerebrospinal fluid [48].

12.5.2 Pathological Manifestations

After a patient is bitten by an infected arthropod, the virus replicates in local lymph nodes and local tissues and reaches the central nervous system through the bloodstream. The onset and persistence of viremia depends on the stage of virus replication in local tissues outside the nervous system, the emergence of specific antibodies, and the rate of virus clearance by the monocyte macrophage system, so the clinical presentation varies considerably. Signs of cerebral congestion and edema are visible to the naked eye. Microscopically, neuronal cells, monocytes, lymphocytes, and polymorphonuclear leukocytes infiltrate the perivascular area, forming a "perivascular" structure, with some glial cells proliferating and polymorphonuclear leukocytes aggregating to form nodules. The lesions mainly located in gray matter and white matter of brainstem and basal ganglia and could invade cerebellum and spinal cord.

12.5.3 Imaging

SLVE shows brain atrophy or chronic ischemic changes on CT with or without abnormalities, T_2WI usually shows hyperintense in the substantia nigra, and T_1WI plain or enhanced scan shows no abnormal signal [49].

12.5.4 Diagnostic Key Points

1. The patient was from an infected area and had been in close contact with a SLEV-infected person for 2 weeks before the onset of the disease.
2. CT shows brain atrophy or chronic ischemic changes; MRI T_2WI shows hyperintense in nigrostriatal.
3. Laboratory tests. Detectable SLEV-specific IgM and IgG antibodies or RT-PCR amplification to discover viral RNA.

12.5.5 Differential Diagnosis

Murray Valley encephalitis. MRI T_2WI shows hyperintense on thalamus, which may involve the red nucleus, substantia nigra, and cervical medulla. These findings preceded the serologic diagnosis and were similar to those of epidemic B encephalitis.

12.5.6 Status and Progress of Research

The MRI presentation of SLVE has some features, such as hyperintense in the substantia nigra usually seen on T_2WI, but for diagnosis, it still needs to be combined with a history of life in the infected area and relevant laboratory tests.

12.6 Enteroviral Encephalitis

Shuang Xia, Qing Li, Zi'ao Fu, and Yinhua Jin

12.6.1 Overview

Enteroviral encephalitis is caused by enterovirus infection. Human enteroviral encephalitis accounts for 10–20% of viral encephalitis. Enteroviruses include polioviruses, coxsackieviruses, echoviruses, and neo-intestinal viruses. Different types of viruses can cause different types of disease. The same type of virus can cause different clinical symptoms, and the same clinical symptoms may be caused by different types of viruses.

Infectious diseases caused by enteroviruses are distributed worldwide and are seen year-round in tropical and subtropical regions. In temperate regions, they are more common in the summer. The incidence of infectious diseases is higher in warm, unhygienic, humid, and crowded areas. Children are susceptible to enterovirus infection due to immature immune system development. Patients usually have acute or subacute symptoms such as fever, impaired consciousness, headache, vomiting, apathy, and drowsiness and are more likely to develop cervical spondylosis and typical meningeal irritation. In severe cases, neuropsychiatric symptoms, such as confusion, coma, and sometimes focal or generalized convulsions, may occur [50].

Enteroviral encephalitis can be diagnosed by real-time fluorescent polymerase chain reaction (RT-PCR) for detection of viral nucleic acids and enzyme-linked immunosorbent assay (ELISA) for detection of cerebrospinal fluid-specific IgM antibodies.

12.6.2 Pathological Manifestations

Enterovirus particles are small, shaped like icosahedrons, with a diameter of 24–30 nm, do not contain lipid-like bodies, have a single-stranded ribonucleic acid in their core, are resistant to fat-soluble solvents such as ether, are acid-resistant, and are resistant to various antibiotics, antivirals, and decontaminants. Most viruses produce cytopathic effects in cell culture. Enteroviruses are usually parasitic in the intestinal tract and, in only a few cases, enter the blood circulation or nerve tissue. Normal carriers of the virus are rare, and occult infection is more common, with a few people showing clinical signs immediately after infection. The enterovirus enters the central nervous system through the bloodstream causing an inflammatory response in the meninges, ventricular canal, and small cerebral arteries [51].

12.6.3 Imaging

Cranial CT mainly shows lamellar hypodense shadow in cerebral cortex and paraventricular area, which is associated with inflammatory reaction of meninges, ventricular canal, and small cerebral arteries caused by enterovirus entering central nervous system through blood circulation, especially small vascular inflammatory lesions in paraventricular area.

MRI of the spinal cord showed hypointense on T_1WI and hyperintense on T_2WI from the neck to the spinal cord cone, with the lesion concentrated at the level of the cervical, lower thoracic, and lumbosacral segments of the spinal cord. Axial scan shows bilaterally or unilaterally anterior horn of the spinal cord as hypointense on T_1WI and hyperintense on T_2WI. MRI of the brain shows dotted or fuzzy laminar hypointense on T_1WI and hyperintense on T_2WI in the midfoot of the cerebellum bilaterally, and MRI of the spinal cord shows mild enhancement in the anterior horn of the spinal cord and significant enhancement in the ipsilateral anterior roots [52]. MRI shows that the lesion is mainly located in the middle peduncle of the cerebellum, and the boundary of the lesion is indistinct and often occurs symmetrically bilateral (Figs. 12.14 and 12.15).

12.6.4 Diagnostic Key Points

1. In the early stage, there is fever and gastrointestinal and respiratory herald symptoms, and headache, photophobia, signs of meningeal irritation such as neck stiffness, nausea, vomiting, and rash may occur.
2. CT shows a lamellar hypodense shadow in the cerebral cortex and paraventricular space.
3. MRI may show symmetrical hyperintense shadow in the midfoot of the cerebellum and anterior horn of the spinal cord bilaterally, FLAIR shows lesion sensitivity. Mild enhancement is seen on enhancement scan.
4. Cerebrospinal fluid pathogenesis. Disease-causing enterovirus-specific antibodies and antigens can be detected.

12.6.5 Differential Diagnosis

1. EB viral infection. Single or multiple hypodense foci in the brain parenchyma, calcifications of the basal ganglia, traffic hydrocephalus with intracranial hemorrhage, and demyelination-like changes; EEG mainly shows diffuse continuous high-amplitude slow waves or δ-waves in bilateral leads.
2. Herpes simplex virus. The CT is normal for 1 week, followed by hypodense shadowing from the temporal lobe to the insula on one or both sides, occupancy effect, hyperintensity with hemorrhage, and linear enhancement of the temporal and insular lobes. MRI of the brain shows mild hypo- and hyperintense in the temporal lobe, orbitofrontal surface, insula, and angular gyrus. T_1WI and T_2WI show mixed hyper- and hypointense when hemorrhage occurs, with cerebral edema and occupational effects. Enhanced scans may reveal meningeal or gyral enhance-

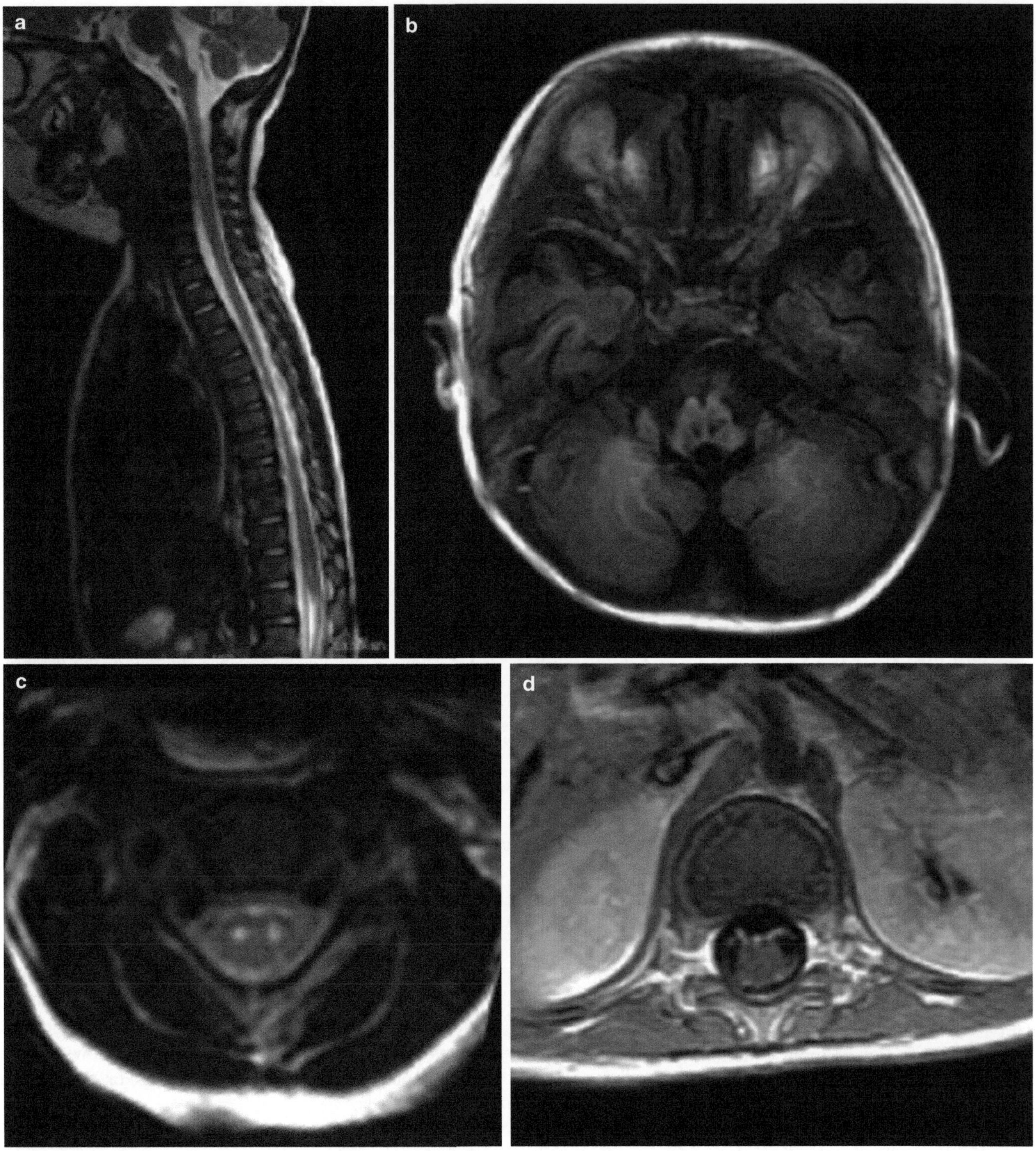

Fig. 12.14 Enteroviral encephalitis, myelitis. (**a**) T_2WI shows long strip-like hyperintense (sagittal) visible in the cerebral bridge, medulla oblongata, and cervical segment to conus spinalis; (**b**, **c**) symmetrical punctate abnormal signal visible in the anterior horn of the cervical segment spinalis, and T_1WI shows hypointense and T_2WI shows hyperintense (axial); (**d**) enhanced T_1WI shows marked enhancement of the bilateral anterior roots of the spinal nerve (image courtesy of Prof. Chen Feng, Hainan Provincial People's Hospital)

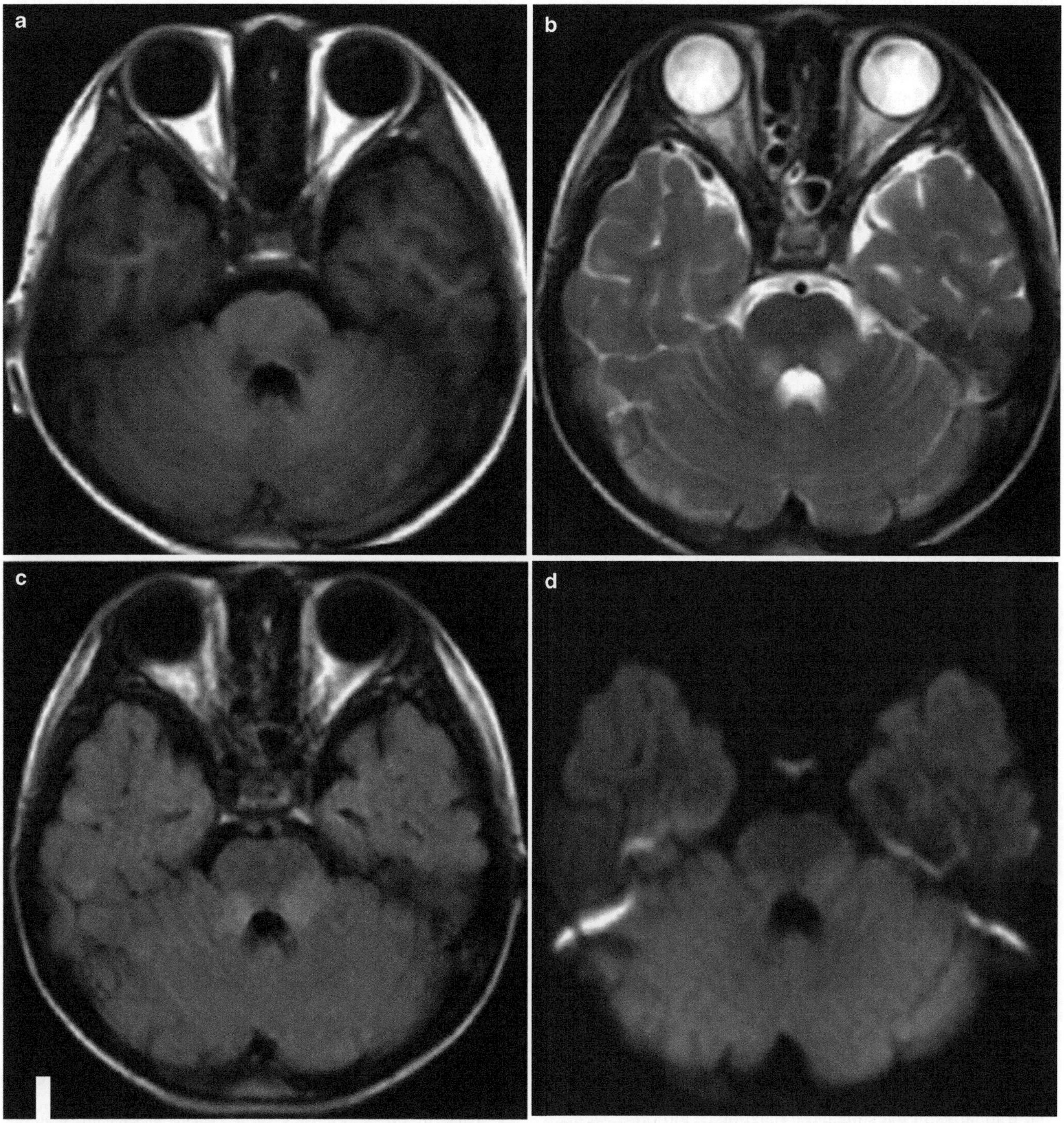

Fig. 12.15 Enteroviral encephalitis. Child, male, 6 years old, intermittent fever for 7 days, weakness in both lower extremities; physical examination, decreased muscle tone in all four extremities; MRI plain scan, patchy lesions visible in the midfoot of the cerebellum bilaterally. (**a**) T_1WI shows hypointense; (**b, c**) T_2WI and FLAIR sequences show slightly hyperintense; (**d**) DWI shows slightly hyperintense with indistinct lesion borders

ment. However, some patients do not show any abnormalities on cranial MRI.

3. Varicella-herpes zoster virus encephalitis. Head CT shows multifocal ischemic and hemorrhagic infarcts in the white matter of the focal area, mostly concentrated in the gray-white matter junction, and DSA shows bead-like stenosis of the proximal middle cerebral artery, most likely caused by herpes zoster-induced intracranial artery endarteritis.

12.6.6 Status and Progress of Research

1. It occurs in children and often presents with vomiting, headache, fever, and central nervous system damage, increasing the risk of HFMD in children.
2. Imaging. MRI allows more sensitive observation of the extent and severity of lesions in the brain parenchyma and spinal cord, providing a basis for clinical assessment of the condition.
3. Pathogenic examination. RT-PCR is an important tool for the detection of viral nucleic acids, allowing rapid detection of trace-specific nucleic acid sequences with high accuracy.

References

1. Sili U, Kaya A, Mert A, et al. Herpes simplex virus encephalitis: clinical manifestations, diagnosis and outcome in 106 adult patients. J Clin Virol. 2014;60(2):112–8.
2. Wu H. Early diagnostic and prognostic value of electroencephalography in herpes simplex virus encephalitis. Chin J Pract Neurol Disord. 2015;18(2):141–2.
3. Wang X, Zou Q, Pu T. Herpes simplex virus encephalitis 60 clinical analysis of cases. Sichuan Med. 2012;33(8):1433–5.
4. Zhang Y, Li Y, Wang X, et al. Herpes simplex virus encephalitis CT and MRI manifestations. Radiol Pract. 2014;29(3):276–8.
5. Kataoka H, Ueno S. Herpes simplex virus and acute fulminant disseminated encephalitis with extensive white matter lesions. J Infect. 2009;59(1):70–2.
6. Leib DA. Herpes simplex virus encephalitis: toll-free access to the brain. Cell Host Microbe. 2012;12(6):731–2.
7. Linde A, Klapper PE, Monteyne P, et al. Specific diagnostic methods for herpesvirus infections of the central nervous system: a consensus review by the European Union concerted action on virus meningitis and encephalitis. Clin Diagn Virol. 1997;8(2):83–104.
8. Ge M, Jin Z. Anti-varicella—advances in research on herpes zoster virus drugs. Foreign Med Dermatol Venereol Div. 1996;06:344–8.
9. Shen Y, Chen J. Anti-varicella- advances in research on herpes zoster virus drugs. Anhui Med. 2012;16(1):4–6.
10. Kennedy PG, Barrass JD, Graham DI, et al. Studies on the pathogenesis of neurological diseases associated with varicella-zoster virus. Neuropathol Appl Neurobiol. 1990;16(4):305–16.
11. Yu H, Zhu Q. Varicella—current status of research on herpes zoster virus infection. China's Plan Immun. 2001;7(2):59–62.
12. Qi J, Li Y. Varicella—recent research in the treatment of herpes zoster virus infection. Int J Dermatol Venereol. 1996;22(2):83–6.
13. Grahn A, Studahl M. Varicella-zoster virus infections of the central nervous system. Prognosis, diagnostics and treatment. J Infect. 2015;71(3):281–93.
14. Hu DJ, Yan JC, Zhang WD. Viral encephalitis CT diagnosis. Radiol Pract. 2001;16(6):405–7.
15. Li S. Children EB viral encephalitis 24 clinical analysis of cases. Chin J Pract Pediat. 2004;19(3):172–3.
16. Zhang M, Yang M. Children EB advances in viral encephalitis research. Med Rev. 2010;16(16):2444–6.
17. Spagnolo F, Ceppi D, Cardamone R, et al. Frontotemporal dementia with parkinsonism presenting as posterior cortical atrophy. Mov Disord. 2011;26(11):2131–2.
18. Hagemann G, Mentzel HJ, Weisser H, et al. Multiple reversible MR signal changes caused by Epstein-Barr virus encephalitis. Am J Neuroradiol. 2006;27(7):1447–9.
19. Wang C, Zhan X. Progress in the study of human herpesvirus 6 infection. J Pediatr Pharm. 2014;20(8):62–5.
20. Zhao M, Jiang SC. Status of research on human herpes virus 6 type. Infect Dis Info. 1999;12(4):165–6.
21. Hill JA, Venna N. Human herpesvirus 6 and the nervous system. Handb Clin Neurol. 2014;123:327–535.
22. Harberts E, Yao K, Wohler JE, et al. Human herpesvirus-6 entry into the central nervous system through the olfactory pathway. Proc Natl Acad Sci U S A. 2011;108(33):13734–9.
23. Caserta MT, Hall CB, Schnabel K, et al. Diagnostic assays for active infection with human herpesvirus 6(HHV-6). J Clin Virol. 2010;48(1):55–7.
24. Ryo B, In Yeol T. Ape herpes B viral infection. Jpn Med Present. 2006;27(9):398.
25. Li J, Xiang Z. Brief analysis of the lethality of monkey B virus in humans. Chin J Comp Med. 2017;27(9):98–103.
26. Li X, He J. Monkey B advances in virus detection technology research and application. Lab Anim Sci. 2007;24(4):59–62.
27. Davenport DS, Johnson DR, Holmes GP, et al. Diagnosis and management of human B virus (herpesvirus simiae) infections in Michigan. Clin Infect Dis. 1994;19(1):33–41.
28. Amalfitano A, Martin LG, Fluck MM. Different roles for two enhancer domains in the organ and age specific pattern of polyomavirus replication in the mouse. Mol Cell Biol. 1992;12(8):3628–35.
29. de La Roche Saint André C, Mazur S, Feunteun J. Viral genomes maintained extrachromosomally in hamster polyoma virus induced lymphomas display a cell specific replication in vitro. J Virol. 1993;67(12):7172–80.
30. Andrews DW, Gupta J, Abisdris G. Evidence that the middle T antigen of polyomavirus interacts with the membrane skeleton. Mol Cell Biol. 1993;13(8):4703–13.
31. Baker TS, Newcomb WW, Olson NH, et al. Structures of bovine and human papillomaviruses. Analysis by cryoelectron microscopy and three-dimensional image reconstruction. Biophys J. 1991;60(6):1445–56.
32. Yang Y, Du Y. Advances in tick-borne encephalitis research. Chin J Epidemiol. 2016;37(10):1435–8.
33. Hegde V, Aziz Z, Kumar S, et al. Dengue encephalitis with predominant cerebellar involvement: report of eight cases with MR and CT imaging features. Eur Radiol. 2015;25(3):719–25.
34. Zawadzki R, Garkowski A, Kubas B, et al. Evaluation of imaging methods in tick-borne encephalitis. Pol J Radiol. 2017;82:742–7.
35. Pichler A, Sellner J, Harutyunyan G, et al. Magnetic resonance imaging and clinical findings in adults with tick- borne encephalitis. J Neurol Sci. 2017;375:266–9.
36. Arahata Y, Fujii K, Nishimura T, et al. Longitudinal magnetic resonance imaging changes in Japanese encephalitis. Brain Dev. 2019;41(8):731–4.
37. Chu SX. West Nile virus encephalitis. World core medical journal abstracts. Neurol Fascicle. 2006;2(6):1–2.

38. Jin S, Zhang H. Advances in the study of West Nile virus. Chin J Pathog Biol. 2009;4(8):623–5.
39. Turell MJ, Dohm DJ, Sardelis MR, et al. An update on the potential of north American mosquitoes (diptera: culicidae) to transmit West Nile virus. J Med Entomol. 2005;42(1):57–62.
40. Hayes EB, Sejvar JJ, Zaki SR, et al. Virology, pathology, and clinical manifestations of west nile virus disease. Emerg Infect Dis. 2005;11(8):1174–9.
41. Ali M, Safriel Y, Sohi J, et al. West nile virus infection: MR imaging findings in the nervous system. Am J Neuroradiol. 2005;26(2):289.
42. Evans IA, Hueston L, Doggett SL. Murray Valley encephalitis virus. N S W Public Health Bull. 2009;20(11/12):195.
43. Lee E, Lobigs M. Mechanism of virulence attenuation of glycosaminoglycan-binding variants of Japanese encephalitis virus and Murray Valley encephalitis virus. J Virol. 2002;76(10): 4901–11.
44. Einsiedel L, Kat E, Ravindran J, et al. MR findings in Murray Valley encephalitis. Am J Neuroradiol. 2003;24(7):1379–82.
45. Lamp B, Dietzel E, Kolesnikova L, et al. Nipah virus entry and egress from polarized epithelial cells. J Virol. 2013;87(6):3143–54.
46. Ang BSP, Lim TCC, Wang L. Nipah virus infection. J Clin Microbiol. 2018;56(6):e01875–17.
47. Li H. Practical infectious disease imaging. Beijing: People's Health Press; 2014.
48. Diaz LA, Coffey LL, Burkett-Cadena ND, et al. Reemergence of St. Louis encephalitis virus in the Americas. Emerg Infect Dis. 2018;24(12):2150–7.
49. Wasay M, Diazarrastia R, Suss RA, et al. St Louis encephalitis: a review of 11 cases in a 1995 Dallas, Tex, epidemic. Arch Neurol. 2000;57(1):114.
50. Dourmashkin RR, Dunn G, Castano V, et al. Evidence for an enterovirus as the cause of encephalitis lethargica. BMC Infect Dis. 2012;12(1):136.
51. Wang SM, Lei HY, Huang KJ, et al. Pathogenesis of enterovirus 71 brainstem encephalitis in pediatric patients: roles of cytokines and cellular immune activation in patients with pulmonary edema. J Infect Dis. 2003;188(4):564–70.
52. Lei Z, Jie Y, Ojcius DM, et al. Novel and predominant pathogen responsible for the enterovirus-associated encephalitis in eastern China. PLoS One. 2013;8(12):e85023.

Intracranial Fungal Infections

13

Bailu Liu, Zhehao Lv, Yulin He, Huimin Li, Lili Liu,
Tingting Chen, and Liwei Fu

13.1 Cryptococcosis

Bailu Liu, Zhehao Lv, and Yulin He

13.1.1 Overview

Cryptococcal infection of the central nervous system is caused by intracranial invasion of *Cryptococcus novelis* from the respiratory tract, which can present with an acute, subacute, or chronic fungal infection. It tends to occur in young people and predominant in males. New *Cryptococcus* species has a worldwide distribution and is commonly found in the feces of birds such as pigeons and soil and humic matter. Inhalation of aerosols containing cryptococci is the most common route of infection in humans. *Cryptococcus neoformans* and *Cryptococcus guttatus* are the main pathogens of human cryptococcosis. *Cryptococcus neoformans* can be classified serologically into A, B, C, D, and A/D 5, of which serotypes B and C are *Cryptococcus neoformans* var gattii, A is the Cryptococcus neoformans var grubbi, and D is the var neoformans.

There are one million new cases of cryptococcal infection in the world. In immunosuppressed patients, incidence of cryptococcosis is 5–10%. In AIDS patients, the incidence of cryptococcal infection can be as high as 30%, while in immunocompetent people, the rate of cryptococcal infection, although only about 1/10 million, is now also on the rise year by year. Cryptococcal infections is most common in patients with impaired immune function, including patients with HIV infection, organ transplants, malignancies, diabetes mellitus, and some chronic respiratory diseases. The greatest risk factors for the development of cryptococcosis in patients who weren't HIV infected include malignancy, diabetes, steroid therapy, parenchymal organ transplantation, and chronic diseases such as liver and renal failure.

Clinical symptoms of cryptococcosis vary including fever, progressive headache, and psychiatric and neurological symptoms (confusion, agitation, disorientation, behavioral changes, drowsiness, etc.). As the disease progresses, patients can develop cerebral nerve palsy, motor and sensory impairment, cerebellar dysfunction, seizures, and dementia. The disease tends to attack the central nervous system causing meningitis and occasionally focal intracranial granuloma, known as cryptococcomas. The clinical symptoms of meningitis include headaches that can last for weeks to months, accompanied by changes in mental status and personality.

It can also manifest as fever, drowsiness, and coma. Other symptoms include hydrocephalus, sudden sensorineural deafness, cerebral nerve palsy, motor and sensory deficits, cerebellar dysfunction, and epilepsy. In addition, due to increased intracranial pressure, patients may develop ocular symptoms, which manifest as oculomotor palsy, optic disc edema, and complete loss of vision.

13.1.2 Pathological Manifestations

1. Gross pathology: congestion of meningeal vessels, cerebral edema, gelatinous exudate in the subarachnoid space, opacity, diffuse or focal thickening of the soft meninges,

B. Liu (✉) · L. Liu · T. Chen
The Second Hospital of Harbin Medical University, Harbin, China

Z. Lv
The First Hospital of Harbin Medical University, Harbin, China

Y. He
The First Affiliated Hospital of Nanchang University, Nanchang, China

H. Li
People's Hospital of Inner Mongolia Autonomous Region, Huhhot, China

L. Fu
The Second Affiliated Hospital of School of Medicine, Zhejiang University, Harbin, China

H. Li et al. (eds.), *Radiology of Infectious and Inflammatory Diseases - Volume 1*,
https://doi.org/10.1007/978-981-99-0039-8_13

especially near the base of the brain and the lateral fissure, and small nodules in the interpeduncular fossa and sulcus. In the brain slice, there are numerous cystic gaps scattered around the lateral fissure and striatum, lined with gelatinous material, and similar lesions are seen in the cerebellum and spinal cord. There was moderate enlargement of the ventricles. Approximately 50% of cases show multiple intracerebral parenchymal cysts, similar to soap bubble-like changes, formed by the fusion of enlarged perivascular spaces, diameter > 5 mm, single or multiple, may be aggregated into clusters of cysts, dilated by filling with mucus and gelatinous material produced by cryptococcal pods, forming small cystic cavities containing large numbers of cryptococci, usually soap bubble-shaped, characteristic, cryptococcal cysts most pronounced in the basal ganglia.

2. Microscopically cryptococcus showed a single yeast form with a round body, 4–7μm in diameter, surrounded by 3–5-μm-thick vesicular sheaths. The cystic sheath is strongly positive on PAS stain or mucous carmine stain. Sometimes the staining of cryptococci is similar to amyloid vesicles in the brain parenchyma and can be easily confused. Early lesions were seen in the lumen of the subarachnoid space or cyst with large numbers of cryptococcal organisms suspended in a gelatinous mass, some in phagocytes and foreign body giant cells. PAS stain and ink stain reveal *Cryptococcus*. *Cryptococcus* in HE stain is pale purplish-red or uncolored (same color as background), similar to erythrocytes, round or ovoid, solid body without nuclear structure, smaller or slightly larger than lymphocytes, partially similar in size to crinkled erythrocytes, bodies of various sizes, arranged singly or in clusters, circular translucent areas visible around the body, some bodies with outgrowth, and gourd-shaped or dumbbell-shaped (Fig. 13.1).

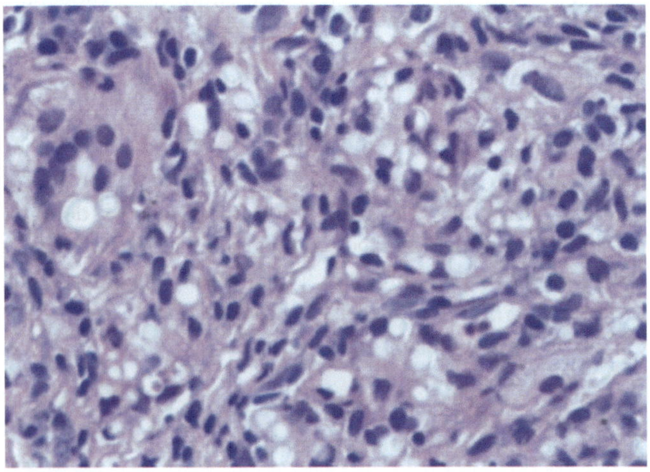

Fig. 13.1 Pathological manifestations of cryptococcosis. HE staining shows a large number of histiocytes, multinucleated giant cells, and epithelioid histiocytes aggregated with slow granuloma; the organism is within the multinucleated giant cells, and the organism is light blue in color and surrounded by transparent areas

Diagnosis of cryptococcal infection can be conducted through examination of ink stain of cerebrospinal fluid, but with low sensitivity. Blood and/or cerebrospinal fluid latex agglutination tests for detecting cryptococcal polysaccharide antigens are more sensitive but having false positive in immune disorders.

13.1.3 Imaging

1. **Enlarged perivascular gaps.** The perivascular spaces (VR spaces) are fluid-filled spaces that surround small arterioles, capillaries, and venules in the brain. The enlarged VR spaces were mainly distributed in the anterior commissure and subcortical centrum semiovale of the brain but appear less at the polar external capsule, cerebellum, and thalamus and generally do not appear in the cortex. T_1WI shows iso- or hypo-intensity, T_2WI shows hyperintensity, no significant enhancing after enhancement scan, generally ≤3 mm in diameter, similar to lacunar cerebral infarction.
2. **Colloid pseudocyst.** The lesion shows hypointensity on T_1WI and peripheral hypointense rim (the hypointense ring on T_2WI, which may be the result of the cyst wall with high iron hemoglobin or activated free radicals and paramagnetic artifacts produced by macrophages; diffusion restriction may be related to acidic mucopolysaccharide production by cryptococci and high protein content and viscosity); pseudocysts are devoid of vascular structures and have well-defined borders with partial diffusion restriction; enhanced scans show mostly unreinforced or lamellar; large pseudocysts may evolve into abscesses with enhancement and diffusion restriction. The main reason for non-enhancement is that colloid pseudocysts, unlike other inflammatory or malignant tumors, do not disrupt the blood-brain barrier.
3. **Meningeal enhancement.** The involved meninges show hyperintensity on T_2WI and more commonly located at the brain ganglial, cerebellar vermis, and the other surfaces of the brain, often involving the arachnoid and soft meninges. In severe cases, even the whole meninges are involved, and the meninges are linearly thickened and strengthened, which may be accompanied by edema of the adjacent brain tissue (Fig. 13.2).
4. **Hydrocephalus.** The main manifestation is enlargements of bilateral ventricular and cistern.
5. **Cryptococcal granuloma**
   (a) MRI findings. The lesion is mainly located in the bilateral basal ganglia and paraventricular area, T_1WI shows isointensity and slight hypointensity, T_2WI shows hyperintensity, and the lesion is surrounded by visible edema. Enhanced nodular and beaded uniform enhancement is evident, which may

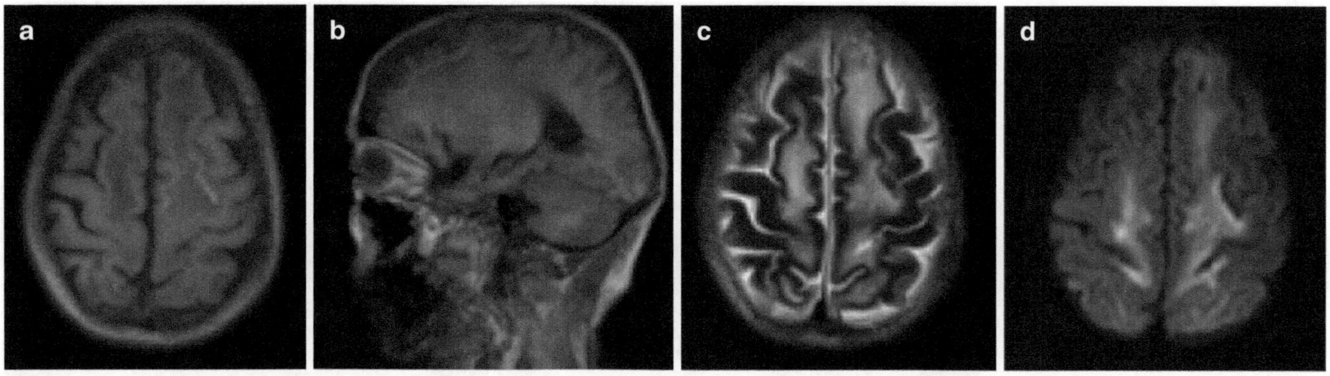

Fig. 13.2 Cryptococcus cerebri infection (1). Male, 54 years old, with a history of hepatitis B for more than 30 years. (**a**) T_1WI enhancement shows linear thickening and intensification of the meninges and patchy slightly hypointensity (axial) of the adjacent brain tissue edema; (**b**) sagittal enhanced T_1WI image; (**c**) T_2WI shows large patchy hyperintensity (axial) in bilateral frontal brain parenchyma; (**d**) DWI shows patchy hyperintensity, which shows restricted diffusion of water molecules in cerebral edema. (Image courtesy of Yulin He, The First Affiliated Hospital of Nanchang University)

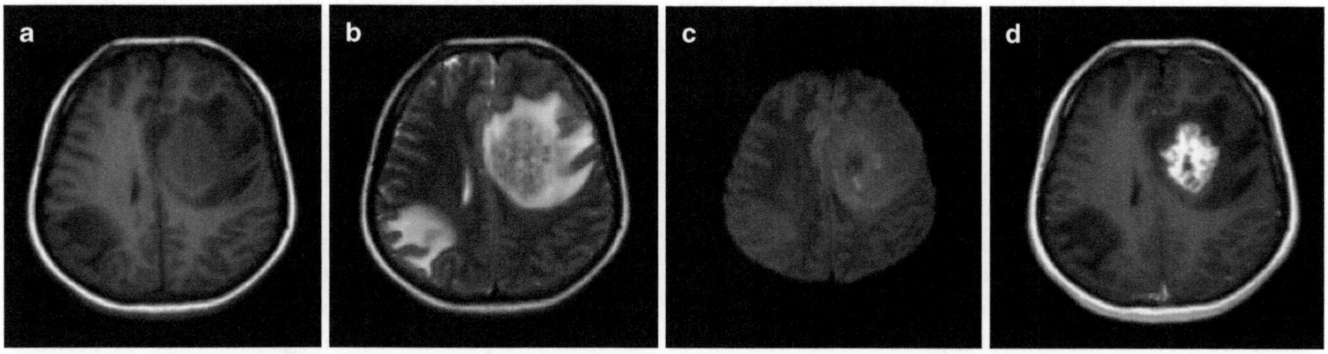

Fig. 13.3 Cryptococcal granuloma of the brain. Multiple lesions with round, nodular shape and varying sizes, located in the left corona radiata area and right parietal lobe. (**a**) MRI scan shows isointensity on T_1WI; (**b**) T_2WI shows slightly hypointensity, surrounded by patchy high-signal edema; (**c**) DWI sequence shows slightly hyperintensity; (**d**) enhanced scan shows obvious nodular enhancement of the lesion

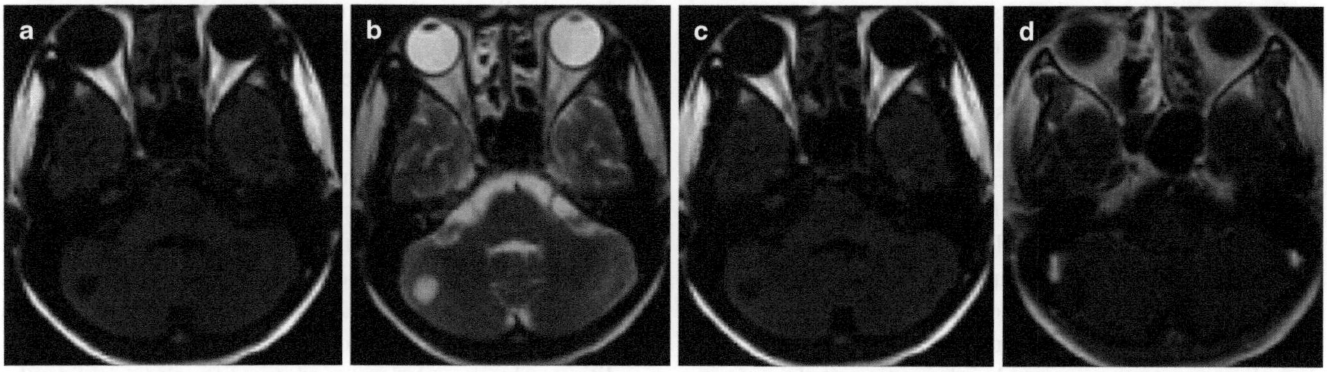

Fig. 13.4 Cryptococcus cerebri infection (2). (**a**) A 31-year-old female patient who is HIV negative. (**a**) T_1WI shows a rounded hypointensity shadow with well-defined borders and homogeneous intensity in the right cerebellar hemisphere (axial); (**b**) T_2WI shows a hyperintensity lesion (axial); (**c**) FLAIR sequence shows a hypointensity lesion (axial); (**d**) T_1WI enhanced scan shows no significant enhancement (axial)

also be circumferential or no significant enhancement (Figs. 13.3 and 13.4).

(b) ^{18}F-FDG PET. Cryptococcal infections of the CNS often present as gelatinous pseudocysts and granulomatous lesions. Because granulomatous lesions are pathologically characterized by a chronic granulomatous response, including infiltration of macrophages, lymphocytes, and foreign body giant cells, these inflammatory cells can continuously uptake ^{18}F-FDG, manifesting as well-defined mass-like foci

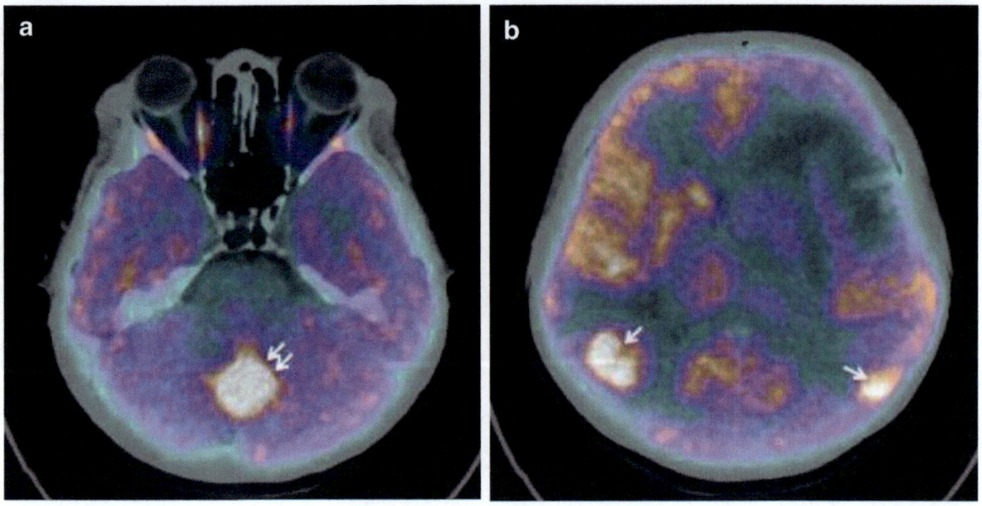

Fig. 13.5 Cryptococcal granuloma of the brain. (**a**) ^{18}F-FDG PET shows a well-defined mass of radiolucent foci of distribution in the cerebellar vermis; (**b**) ^{18}F-FDG PET shows a well-defined mass of radiolucent foci of distribution in the bilateral occipital lobes

of radiolucent distribution. Some patients also show a "fried doughnut"-like ring-shaped radiolucent foci, with a markedly reduced or even absent radiolucent distribution in the center (Fig. 13.5). In contrast, PET with gelatinous pseudocysts shows significantly reduced or absent radioactive distribution

6. **Other inspections.** Some patients may present with cerebral atrophy, mostly mild; intracranial calcification is rare; cryptococcal infection of the CNS may also present with cerebral infarction secondary to vasculitis, thrombosis, and vascular occlusion [1–3].

13.1.4 Diagnostic Key Points

1. Patients with early clinical signs of intracranial hypertension, accompanied by progressive exacerbation. The systemic inflammatory response is not severe, usually without fever or other signs of infection.
2. Imaging diagnosis should be closely integrated with clinical data and laboratory tests. In the imaging examination, the detection rate of MRI was significantly higher than that of CT and provides more information, such as enlarged perivascular gaps, gelatinous pseudocysts, hydrocephalus, cerebral atrophy, and meningeal enhancement in the brain parenchyma.
3. Laboratory tests can provide information on the presence or absence of *Cryptococcus neoformans* in cerebrospinal fluid in patients with confirmed treatment.

13.1.5 Differential Diagnosis

1. **Tuberculous meningitis.** Mycobacterium tuberculosis invades the skull via the blood and first deposited in the soft meninges and ventricular canal at the base of the skull. It is more common in the skull base, usually in the early stage. MRI shows blurred brain pools at the base of the brain and long T_1 or mixed T_2 signals in the subarachnoid space of the medulla oblongata, optic cross, cerebral bridge, interpeduncular pool, and anterior pontine pool. Some patients show meningeal enhancement, which is more significant than cryptococcal infection. The incidence of hydrocephalus in patients with tuberculous meningitis is significantly higher than that of novel cryptococcal meningitis, and the severity is moderate to severe, with [4] appearing early in the course of the disease.
2. **Viral encephalitis.** The imaging findings are predominantly brain parenchymal lesions. MRI shows abnormal signal areas with poorly defined borders, which may be accompanied by hemorrhage in the acute phase and mainly involve bilateral or unilateral temporal lobes, and irregular linear enhancement of the meninges is seen on enhanced scans when combined with meningitis.
3. **Brain abscesses due to other pathogens.** After enhancement, the abscess shows typical circumferential enhancement with complete, smooth, and uniform wall. It can be seen on DWI with obvious diffusion restriction.
4. **Tumor lesions.** Metastases show small subcortical lesions and large edema; gliomas show enhancement with uneven wall thickness and may be associated with cystic changes, hemorrhage, and necrosis. If vasculitis is secondary, other causes of cerebral infarction and vasculitis need to be ruled out, and it is difficult to confirm the diagnosis by a single imaging examination alone; radiologists need to conduct comprehensive analysis in combination with clinical and laboratory examination.

13.1.6 Status and Progress of Research

1. Real-time fluorescent quantitative PCR (FQ-PCR). It is a new technique that combines PCR technology, DNA probe hybridization technology (labeled with fluorescent reporter

groups and fluorescent quenching groups), and advanced spectroscopic detection technology. The FQ-PCR assay technique has the advantage of higher sensitivity and specificity and prevents the strong carcinogenic properties of the dye ethidium bromide used in the assay from leading to a greater safety risk problem for the assayer [5].

2. MRI has better diagnostic information than CT, which is significantly more sensitive than CT and other imaging methods for the demonstration of white matter lesions. On diffusion-weighted images, pseudocysts exhibit diffusion restriction, hyperintensity on DWI and hypointensity on ADC sequences due to the viscosity of their contents; there is no enhancement on enhanced scans. And these cysts could explain the DWI features of the central cavity of cryptococcal infections as opposed to those of pyogenic abscesses. It is inferred that the contents of the central cavity of a cryptococcal infection are much less viscous than pus and exhibit unrestricted diffusion, more like free water molecules [6].
3. Magnetic resonance spectroscopy (MRS)-observed amino acids can be used as a diagnostic basis for intracranial infectious lesions; MRS images of intracranial cryptococcal infections show elevated lipid peaks; pseudocystic lesions show peaks in acetate, alanine, and lipid; and lesions with intact capsule show succinate, alanine, lactate, and lipid peaks. The morphology of *Cryptococcus* is complex and the application of MRS is very promising [6, 7].
4. Blood colloidal gold immunochromatography: The sensitivity and specificity of cryptococcal polysaccharide antigen test for the diagnosis of pulmonary cryptococcal infection in immunodeficient patients can reach 98–100% [8, 9], which is a simple, rapid, and effective method for early diagnosis.
5. Latex agglutination test (LAT). Comparative analysis with ink-stained smears and fungal cultures revealed that the latex agglutination test had a high detection rate for cryptococcal meningitis, indicating the advantage of the latex agglutination test for early diagnosis of cryptococcal meningitis. And latex agglutination test is a test for detecting cryptococcal capsular polysaccharide antigen in the cerebrospinal fluid of patients with high sensitivity and specificity [10] by using high-potency anti-cryptococcal antibodies adsorbed on standard-size latex as antibodies.

13.2 Aspergillosis

Bailu Liu, Zhehao Lv, and Huimin Li

13.2.1 Overview

Aspergillus is ubiquitous in the natural environment, accounting for about 12% of airborne fungi and feeding on mainly dead plants, animal excrement, and animal carcasses as a nutrient source and as a parasitic saprophytic fungus in the soil. It is often inhaled by humans and is morphologically characterized by an acrosome at the head of the conidium, and there are at least 170 or more known species of *Aspergillus*, only a few of which can cause human disease. The most important factor in *Aspergillus* infection is the host's ability to resist tissue invasion by the pathogen, but inhalation of pathogen load is also associated with the development of infection. *Aspergillus* is an opportunistic pathogen and occurs in patients with severe immunosuppression, including HIV infection, organ transplantation, alcoholism, and hematologic malignancies; it can also occur in patients who are not immunosuppressed but have chronic underlying disease (e.g., diabetes). It can even occur in immunocompetent individuals. *Aspergillus* infections of the central nervous system are relatively rare, and the route of infection is mostly from the primary foci of the lung to the brain and meninges via the blood circulation; in a few patients, it can also be caused by direct invasion and spread of infection from adjacent tissues (eyes, ears, nose, etc.).

The clinical symptoms of CNS *Aspergillus* infection are less specific. Headache is often the first symptom, which can be gradually aggravated, but also mental abnormalities, agitation, and other symptoms. In severe cases, there can be varying degrees of consciousness disorders and intracranial hypertension symptoms. Headache in the corresponding location can occur when localized meningitis is formed. *Aspergillus* is prone to invade blood vessels causing hemorrhage or obstruction. The clinical symptoms of focal neurological deficits are related to the occupying effect of the lesion, the location of the hematoma after rupture and bleeding of the lesioned vessel, and cerebral infarction.

The positive culture result of blood and cerebrospinal fluid examination is very low, so it is difficult to only examine the infection of *Aspergillus* in the central nervous system. In addition, *Aspergillus* can be isolated from human skin, eyes, ears, and gastrointestinal tract. The positive result of the culture of specimens from these parts should be considered carefully, and the pathological examination is still diagnostic with the specimen tissue taken from sterile parts. There is no *Aspergillus* in human blood, cerebrospinal fluid, or brain tissue; therefore, the positive result can confirm the diagnosis of *Aspergillus* infection. Laboratory tests for *Aspergillus* infection in the central nervous system are as follows.

1. Routine blood tests. Elevated total peripheral blood leukocyte count, predominantly neutrophils.
2. Cerebrospinal fluid routine and biochemical tests. Lymphocytes were significantly increased, protein levels were mildly elevated, and sugar levels were normal or decreased.
3. Cerebrospinal fluid and diseased tissue were taken for direct microscopic examination or inoculated on the medium. Most cerebrospinal fluid cultures were negative

and only a few were positive. The positive rate may increase when the disease invades the ventricles of the brain or causes meningitis.
4. Serological tests, including detection of *Aspergillus* antigens and antibodies. This method is simple and effective but can only be used in non-immunosuppressed patients. Immunosuppressed patients often have undetectable relevant antibodies due to poor immune response, for which detection of circulating antigens of *Aspergillus* is more reliable.
5. Pathological examination. Pathological sections of coughing up material and pathological tissues in the lungs are feasible, and the diagnosis is confirmed by HE staining for mycelium, spores, and conidia. PAS staining or silver staining if necessary.
6. Techniques such as molecular biology. The application of nucleic acid probes, for example, is still on the exploratory stage.

13.2.2 Pathological Manifestations

There are many pathological types of *Aspergillus* infection in the central nervous system, including hemorrhagic or ischemic brain injury, brain abscess, intracranial granuloma, meningitis, and encephalitis. *Aspergillus* selectively infiltrates and destroys the elastic tissue of the main intracranial vessels, sometimes causing inflammation, leading to tissue necrosis and disintegration, dilatation of large blood vessels with hemorrhage, infarction, and even the formation of *Aspergillus* aneurysms. *Aspergillus* cerebral abscesses are often multiple lesions and mostly involve the gray-white matter junction of the brain and accompanied by cerebral edema. *Aspergillus* can invade the skull through nasal sinus and tympanic chamber, which can lead to skull base bone destruction, localized epidural abscesses, dural meningitis, granuloma formation, and localized skull base nerve involvement.

13.2.3 Imaging

Because *Aspergillus* can invade and destroy the perforating arteries, the early findings of *Aspergillus* infection in central nervous system is cerebral infarction or cerebral hemorrhage; the predilection sites are the basal ganglia area, thalamus, and corpus callosum. As the lesion progresses, intracranial abscess can be formed. In addition to the common imaging findings of brain parenchymal abscess, there are two specific morphological features in CT and MRI of CNS *Aspergillus* infection:

1. Imaging shows multifocal and polymorphic damage in the brain parenchyma, including cerebral infarction, cerebral hemorrhage, cerebral abscess, intracranial granuloma, meningitis, and encephalitis, which can occur simultaneously.
2. Localized epidural abscess and dural enhancement can be seen. Besides, soft tissue of the surrounding paranasal sinus and orbit is also visible. The lesions invading the optic nerve, the optic nerve sheath, and optic nerve enhancement can be seen.

13.2.3.1 CT Findings

1. Cerebral infarction. In most cases, they present as poorly defined hypodense lesions that may have mild or no occupying effects.
2. Cerebral hemorrhage. It mostly presents as an irregular, dense foci with clear intracranial borders, and subarachnoid hemorrhage can occur when rupture of a mycotic aneurysm is caused by *Aspergillus* invasion and destruction of arteries.
3. Meningitis. The cerebral sulcus and gyrus become shallow, the brain pool is isointense or slightly dense, and limited meningeal thickening may be present. Contrast enhanced CT scan shows heterogenous and diffuse thickening of the meninges.
4. Brain abscess. On non-contrast CT scan images, abscesses are mostly characterized by single or multiple hypodense foci with well-defined borders and certain occupancy effect. Enhanced scans of the lesions tend to show circumferential enhancement. Some patients may be complicated with intracerebral hemorrhage. Further mechanization and fibrosis of the abscess may form a granuloma. Non-contrast CT shows a nodular isodense or slightly hypodense lesion. The central part of the lesion appears to be necrotic and shows heterogeneous enhancement on enhanced scan.

13.2.3.2 MRI Findings

1. Infarctive changes. T_1WI shows heterogeneous hypointensity and T_2WI shows inhomogeneous hyperintensity, which may be accompanied by hypointensity in case of combined bleeding.
2. Meningitis. It shows hypointensity in T_1WI, and iso- to hyperintensity in T_2WI, and the FLAIR sequence is more sensitive to show the lesion. The meninges are seen to be unevenly thickened and abnormally enhanced after intensity scanning.
3. Brain abscess changes. MRI shows foveal mixed abnormal signals, mostly hypointense on T_1WI and hyperintense on T_2WI, with an unsmooth abscess wall and a ring-shaped edema zone at the edge. The lesions show circumferential enhancement or grape bunch enhancement after an enhanced scan. The irregular hypointensity shadow between the abscess wall and the central necrotic foci on T_2WI indicates that *Aspergillus* multiplication is in active stage. This hypointensity feature has a certain

value in the diagnosis of *Aspergillus* infection in the central nervous system. In addition, MRI enhanced scans of patients with normal immune function show clear and distinct foci of enhancement, while patients with poor immune function show foci of faint enhancement. Therefore, the different enhancement of the lesion may also reflect the immune status of the patients [11–13].

13.2.4 Diagnostic Key Points

1. *Aspergillus* encephalopathy is easily induced by a variety of susceptibility factors, and the clinical symptoms are mainly fever, headache, hemiparesis, and impaired consciousness.
2. The early imaging features are cerebral infarction or cerebral hemorrhage, with the prevalent sites in the basal ganglia, thalamus, and corpus callosum. MRI mostly shows foveal mixed signal shadow, and most of the lesions are predominantly hypointense in T_1WI and hyperintense in T_2WI, and the lesions show circular or grape bunch enhancement on enhanced scans. When the meninges are invaded, the meninges show heterogeneous diffuse thickening and abnormal enhancement.
3. The diagnosis of this disease mainly relies on biopsy or cerebrospinal fluid culture to detect *Aspergillus* mycelium, spores, or conidia.

13.2.5 Differential Diagnosis

Cerebral aspergillosis is rare in clinic and lacks of specific imaging features. Qualitative diagnosis mainly relies on the history of *Aspergillus* infection, physical signs and laboratory examination of cerebrospinal fluid, etc. Imaging findings can be used as one of the auxiliary diagnostic tools. This disease needs to be differentiated from cryptococcal brain infection and mucormycosis.

1. **Cryptococcal brain infection.** The CT and MRI findings of novel cryptococcal meningoencephalitis are mainly gelatinous pseudocysts formed by enlarged perivascular spaces in the brain parenchyma, hydrocephalus, cerebral atrophy, and meningeal enhancement. The detection rate of MRI is significantly higher than that of CT, which can provide more information.
2. **Mucormycosis.** Once trichinella invaded the brain, it can quickly cause encephalitis and meningitis. Most of them are acute onset, and a few are subacute or chronic. Cranial CT or MRI shows brain abscess, cerebral infarction, sinus clouding, bone destruction, and cerebral hemorrhage, and other changes occurred in a few cases, and histopathology was the best to determine the pathogen.

13.2.6 Status and Progress of Research

1. Susceptibility-weighted imaging (SWI): Phase and amplitude data are used to enhance sensitivity differences between adjacent tissues and produce enhanced contrast. There is no double-ring sign in SWI of intracranial fungal infection, but a ring-shaped hyposignal shadow combined with a central hyposignal is often seen, which can be distinguished from typical bacterial brain abscess. It may be due to the presence of paramagnetic substances such as iron and magnesium in the ring. The hypointensity on T_2 and T_2^* gradient echo sequences may be associated with pathological hemorrhagic necrosis [14, 15].
2. The foci of intracranial *Aspergillus* infection show hyperintensity on DWI, reflecting diffusion restriction in the central part of the lesion, which is consistent with abscess formation. MRS of the abscess cavity shows elevated acetate (1.92 ppm), succinate (2.4 ppm), amino acids (0.9 ppm), and lactate, which is significantly different from the cystic or necrotic spectrum of brain tumors [14]. The importance of using MRS clinically to evaluate intracranial *Aspergillus* infections also lies in the monitoring of treatment outcome through the metabolic status of the infection lesion. With appropriate treatment, acetate, amino acids, and succinate are usually catabolized within 1 week, whereas lactate may remain elevated due to the involvement of macrophages [14, 15].
3. PCR: The specific amplification method can rapidly and accurately detect the DNA component of *Aspergillus*. The systematic evaluation has shown that PCR has good diagnostic value for invasive *Aspergillosis* in blood and bronchoalveolar lavage fluid [16]. For the diagnosis of *Aspergillus* infection in central nervous system, PCR of cerebrospinal fluid is superior to blood PCR and cerebrospinal fluid GM assays [17].

13.3 Mucormycosis

Bailu Liu, Zhehao Lv, and Lili Liu

13.3.1 Overview

Mucor is a conditionally pathogen, existing in the air, soil, and rotten food. Mucor can enter the human body through spores in the air, ingestion, or direct skin contact. Mucor can rapidly invade the mucosa, blood vessels, and bone and further lead to tissue necrosis when the human immune system is weakened. It can spread to neighboring tissues and result in serious consequences in a short time, if lacking of effective and timely treatment. It is a relatively rare but extremely serious fatal fungal infection caused by a fungus of the phycomycetes, which can be classified as nasal-cerebral, pulmonary, gastrointestinal, or cerebral depending on the site of infection. The nasal-brain-type cases predominate in clinical work and the simple brain type is rare. The pathogenic bacteria are *Rhizopus* and *Mucor* in the order Mucorales, wherein the former invades the nose, sinuses, brain, and digestive tract, and the latter invades the lungs. Mycelium of this class of fungi is 10–20μm thick, not separated, and branches out at right angle with fungal cell wall unevenly thick and thin, and cross-section resembling a spore.

Cerebral mucormycosis (CM) is mostly hematogenous infections, in which the pathogenic bacteria enters the bloodstream and then seeds directly into the brain tissue. The disease is characterized by invasion of the cerebral arteries with arterial wall invasion that produces septic arteritis, which then leads to cerebral embolism, resulting in tissue infarction and the formation of deep brain confined encephalitis and/or abscesses. In the case of infections in organs that do not have direct contact with the outside world, such as the cranium and heart, blood-borne transmission should be considered. Patients with transvenous infections present with cranial lesions only, usually mostly basal ganglia lesions.

Rhinocerebral mucormycosis is the most common type; patients with diabetic ketoacidosis are most susceptible, often spreading through the blood vessels to the sinuses, eyes, or brain; infection is usually fulminant and has a high mortality rate; necrotic tissue lesions often occur in the nasal mucosa, sometimes seen in the palate; and invasion of blood vessels by mycelium can cause progressive tissue necrosis of the nasal septum, palate, and bones around the orbit or sinuses. Clinical manifestations are fever, headache, lethargy, facial or orbital pain, nerve palsy, cranio-orbital edema, cellular tissue necrosis, etc. Nasal symptoms are purulent nasal discharge and recurrent rhinorrhea, easily misdiagnosed as sinusitis and missed, and the infection can spread intracranially within days leading to nasopalatine crusting, retinal artery, internal carotid artery, cavernous sinus vascular embolism, ischemic necrosis of brain tissue, etc. Clinical manifestations are persistent headache, impaired consciousness, signs of meningitis, blindness, hemiparesis, and epilepsy. Sinusitis combined with painless black crust formation on the face, nasal cavity, or palate is a characteristic manifestation of nasal cerebral trichomycosis but is seen only in 20–40% of patients, suggesting a poor prognosis.

Because of the lack of specificity of early symptoms of trichomycosis, diagnosis is difficult, and most patients are often first seen in ophthalmology or otorhinolaryngology for ocular or nasal symptoms, or in internal medicine for fever. Fungal culture is mostly negative, not suitable for the rapid diagnosis of mucormycosis; direct microscopic examination is more meaningful than culture, can be examined with tissue with 10% potassium hydroxide solution soaked and dissolved or treated with fluorescent binding antibody. In addition, direct microscopic examination to find the morphological characteristics of the fungus consistent with the characteristics of *Trichinella* mycelium is the gold standard for the diagnosis of mucormycosis.

13.3.2 Pathological Features

Mucor has a very strong affinity for blood vessels. Once the organism grows and multiplies at the site of infection, it can produce elastase and rapidly invade the peripheral blood vessels (especially arteries), the hyphae invade the endothelium and produce septic arteritis, and the spores can proliferate in the elastic layer of the artery, causing it to detach from the intima, leading to vasculitis, thrombosis, vascular obstruction, and tissue infarction. The most prominent histopathological changes in cerebral trichomycosis are thrombosis and adjacent tissue ischemia, infarction, and necrosis due to fungal invasion of blood vessels, especially large and small arteries, where hyphae are visible within the vessel walls and lesions can become septic and even form granulomas. Gross pathology shows large sheets of coagulative necrosis of tissue, fungal granulomas, fungal vasculitis, thrombosis, and bone destruction. The typical granuloma pattern is centered on mycelium and neutrophils, surrounded by epithelioid cells and multinucleated giant cells and then peripherally by a variable number of plasma cells, lymphocytes, and eosinophils, with mycelium visible in the cytoplasm of the multinucleated giant cells. These pathological manifestations further reveal the local response mechanism of the organism against *Mucor* invasion, i.e., neutrophils as the first-line force, multinucleated giant cells and epithelioid cells as the second-line force, and lymphocytes and plasma cells as the third-line force. The overall morphology of the mycelium could not be observed under transmission electron microscopy, coupled with the small size of the specimens taken, which was not as good as light microscopic observation.

13.3.3 Imaging Features

13.3.3.1 CT Findings

1. Acute cerebral infarction. The blood vessel affinity nature of *Mucor* causes infectious thrombosis or infectious arteritis causing vascular occlusion, which manifests as poorly defined hypodense lesions in the brain parenchyma and may have a predominant effect when the infarct size is large. CTA shows a spiral, serpentine filling defect or occlusion of the internal carotid and intracranial arteries.
2. Brain abscess. Further necrosis in the infarcted area may form a limited septic focus; CT plain scan shows multiple hypodense intracranial shadows with a dominant effect

and edematous bands visible at the edge of the lesion. Most patients may have nodular-like thickening of the turbinate mucosa and punctate destruction of the sinus bone wall.

3. Granuloma. CT mostly shows hypointense with poorly defined borders or mixed-density mass shadow with heterogeneous enhancement of the lesion on enhanced scan, with non-enhancing cavities within the area of enhancement in some lesions.

13.3.3.2 MRI Findings

In acute cerebral infarction, the infarct area shows T_1WI inhomogeneous low signal and T_2WI inhomogeneous high signal, and the site of involvement is mostly in the lobes, followed by the meninges and the basal ganglia. The lesion is mostly T_1WI low signal and T_2WI high signal at the time of abscess formation, with an unsmooth abscess wall and edges with edematous bands, and nodule-like enhancement at the edge of the lesion on enhanced scan.

The MRI scan of granuloma formation shows nodular foci of irregular size in deep white matter, T_1WI with equal and low mixed signal, T_2WI with inhomogeneous high signal, after enhancement. The nodal foci are significantly heterogeneously enhanced, with significant cut marks on the lateral edges. It is surrounded by multiple foci of scattered poorly defined punctate and lamellar enhancement (Fig. 13.6). This sign may be due to the formation of necrotic, predominantly inflammatory granulomatous tissue in the brain and the direct spread of necrotic and granulomatous foci and pathogenic pathogens to the periphery, resulting in the appearance of multiple subfoci around the main foci; the main foci are connected to the subfoci by striations of enhancement, which also reflect the spread of pathogens from the main foci to the periphery. The margins of the lesion are invaginated and may show a sharp angle sign, which is not tense, unlike intracranial tumors that show swelling or infiltrative growth [18–20].

13.3.4 Diagnostic Key Points

1. The high affinity for invading blood vessels predisposes to infectious thrombosis or infectious arteritis causing vascular occlusion, which manifests as irregular foci of infarction in the brain parenchyma.
2. Intracranial lesions are predominantly involved in the lobes of the brain, followed by the meninges and the basal ganglia region.
3. Identifying the fungus with the morphological characteristics consistent with the mycelial characteristics of *Mucor* via direct microscopic examination is the golden standard for the diagnosis of mucormycosis.

13.3.5 Differential Diagnosis

1. **Cerebral aspergillosis.** Most often secondary to pulmonary aspergillosis, with symptoms of pulmonary infection and hematogenous dissemination to the brain, usually presenting with headache, nausea, and vomiting, but fever is mostly unremarkable. *Aspergillus* invades the skull and forms inflammatory granulomas or purulent changes in the anterior and middle cranial fossa meninges and brain parenchyma. And cerebral mucormycosis first appears as sponge symptoms of internal carotid artery lesions in the sinus and sinus, followed by manifestations of meningeal and parenchymal brain damage.
2. **Gliomas.** It can be found anywhere in the brain, preferably in the deep white matter, with a distribution unrelated to the arterial supply area, rarely with scattered enhance-

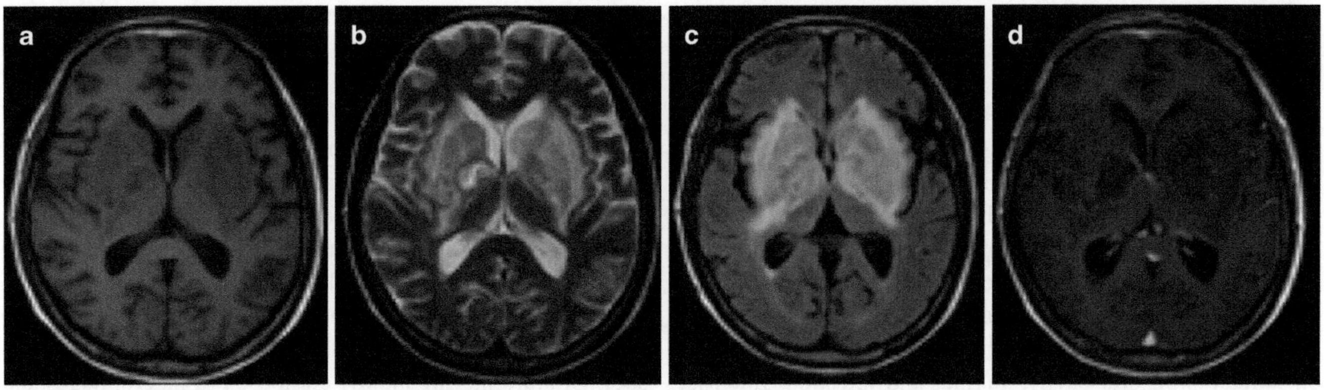

Fig. 13.6 Trichophyton cerebral infection. A 60-year-old male was hospitalized with "sudden onset of left-sided limb weakness for 9 days, aggravated with impaired consciousness for 5 days." (**a**) T_1WI shows multiple nodular-like low signals in the bilateral basal ganglia area with slightly low signal in the surrounding edema zone; (**b**) T_2WI shows multiple nodular-like mixed high signal in the bilateral basal ganglia area with slightly high signals in the surrounding edema zone; (**c**) FLAIR sequence shows heterogeneous high signals in the bilateral basal ganglia area with obvious occupying effects; (**d**) T_1WI enhanced scan shows circular enhancement of the lesion, which represents the enhancement of the abscess wall. (Image courtesy of Wensheng Wang, Guangdong Sanjiu Brain Hospital)

ment, and without sharp angles and incisive signs of inward depression of the lesion margins.
3. **Metastases.** History of malignant tumor with lesions in the corticomedullary junction area, intracranially multiple, small tumors, and may be surrounded by large edema.
4. **Bacterial abscesses.** Smooth, tense interior walls.
5. **Chronic inflammatory granulomatous lesions.** The differential diagnosis of chronic inflammatory granulomatous lesions is difficult, and the morphology of *Mucor* infection of the central nervous system is not significantly specific. In MRS, the lack of leucine, isoleucine, and valine resonance spectra can be distinguished from general intracranial bacterial infections.

13.3.6 Status and Progress of Research

1. ^{1}H-MRS is useful in the diagnosis of central nervous system *Mucor* infection, with significantly elevated peak of succinate (2.4 ppm), acetate (1.9 ppm), and alanine (1.5 ppm) in necrotic/ hemorrhagic lesions of the basal ganglia within the brain mucor, accompanied by depletion of NAA and decreased creatine and inositol levels. Cho significantly elevated, consistent with histologically apparent acute granulomatous inflammatory changes [21].
2. ^{18}F-FDG PET/CT scan is a tool that can monitor intracranial *Mucor* infection, overcoming the limitations of CT and MRI. It is possible to detect active functional/metabolic changes in the lesion before morphological changes are detected by conventional imaging methods, as evidenced by increased ^{18}F-FDG uptake in the lesion [22].

13.4 Candidiasis

Bailu LiuZhehao Lv, and Tingting Chen

13.4.1 Overview

Candida is the most common conditional pathogenic fungus, which is ovoid shaped, with budding spores and pseudomycorrhizae formed by cell germination and elongation. *Candida* is heat-sensitive and dies after 1 h of exposure to heat although it is resistant to dryness, sunshine, ultraviolet radiation, and chemical agents. *Candida* is mostly parasitic on human skin, oral cavity, vagina, and intestinal mucosa. Candidiasis is easily triggered when the body's immune system is impaired or the micro-ecological milieu of the typical host site is disrupted. The susceptible population for candidiasis includes premature infants, low birthweight infants, newborns with various underlying diseases that result in immune deficiency, neutropenia, after long-term intravenous infusion or peripheral central venous placement, and patients on long-term cytotoxic drugs and corticosteroids.

Candida meningitis is rare and is mainly caused by hematogenous dissemination or ventricular drainage. The onset of the disease is insidious and the clinical manifestations are mostly chronic or subacute processes. Candidiasis of the central nervous system is similar to septic meningitis in age, both in infants and young children, presenting with fever, convulsions, irritability, vomiting, cough, diarrhea, and lack of appetite. However, central nervous system candidiasis also has its own characteristics. (1) The disease's course is mostly prolonged, the psychiatric response is relatively good, and the symptoms of infection and toxicity are mild. (2) The symptoms of increased intracranial pressure are not obvious. (3) The cerebrospinal fluid changes are similar to those of septic meningitis, but they are easily recurrent, showing a mild to moderate elevation of leukocytes, mostly multinucleated, a considerable decrease in sugar content, and a significant increase in protein content. (4) Inflammatory markers have not increased significantly. Leukocytes in the peripheral blood are normal or slightly increased. The levels of C-reactive protein and erythrocyte sedimentation rate were not abnormally high. (5) Antibiotics don't work. These features may be related to the low virulence of *Candida albicans* and the tendency to form restricted foci of suppuration or granulomas. Since *Candida* is one of the normal flora in the human body, a positive sputum, stool, and vaginal secretion can only indicate the presence of *Candida* but cannot confirm the diagnosis of candidiasis. Therefore, to confirm the diagnosis, several cultures of the same species are necessary in addition to the clinical signs of cerebral candidiasis.

13.4.2 Pathological Manifestations

Candida infection can spread to the cerebral cortex, cerebellum, and spinal cord. *Candida* infection of the brain and meninges often manifests as purulent inflammation or granuloma formation, while small abscesses of *Candida* infection of the central nervous system contain hyphae and necrotic inflammatory cells in the center, surrounded by proliferating endothelial cells, reactive glial cells, and astrocytes with edema-like changes. Capillary hyperplasia and leukocyte infiltration are seen around larger abscesses (granulation tissue). Granulomas are mainly composed of macrophages and foreign body giant cells, and sometimes tuberculous nodules or caseous necrosis are seen, and they can also be complicated by brain abscesses, cerebral thrombosis, and parenchymal softening and necrosis.

13.4.3 Imaging

Candida infections of the central nervous system are widely invasive. The subcortical white matter, deep periventricular, and semi-oval central white matter, as well as the cerebellum and brainstem, are the most common sites of onset. The most common imaging presentations are multiple cerebral parenchymal ring lesions and periventricular white matter fusion lesions, which are multiple microabscesses and larger abscesses formed by fusion. CT shows multiple punctate, round-like hypointense shadows, while MRI may shows diffuse corn-like nodular shadows widely distributed in the subcortex, periventricular white matter, basal ganglia, and cerebellum. The intensity on T1WI or T_2WI is associated with early cell destruction, increased protein and lipid level within the abscess, etc. MRI enhanced scans show significant circumferential enhancement. Soft meninges are also seen to be enhanced, and the dura mater and falx surface are now clearly striped and reinforced (Fig. 13.7). Early abscesses or small abscesses show hyperintense on T_1WI. Recovering lesions are smaller in size and still hyperintense on T_1WI, hypointense on T2WI, and hyperintense on FLAIR, which may be associated with glial cell hyperplasia. T1C+ scans usually show lesions with ring enhancement. About 2 weeks later, lesions show iso-/hyperintense on T_1WI, hypo-/isointense on T_2WI with peripheral hypointense signal, iso-/hyperintense on FLAIR, and "starry" enhancement on T1C+ (Fig. 13.8), which corresponds to different imaging features at different pathological stages.

As per DWI of brain abscesses in central nervous system, *Candida* infections are mostly hyperintense and show different intensities at different stages with different ADC values. The hyperintense signal on DWI indicates restricted movement of water molecules in the lesion resulting from the

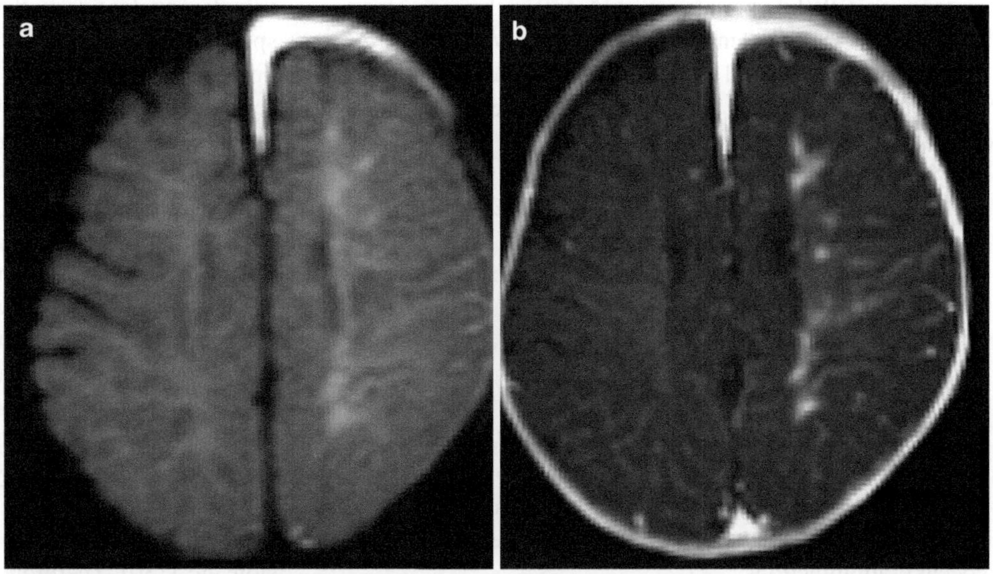

Fig. 13.7 Cerebral *Candida* infection (1). A Female patient, 3 months old, with recurrent abdominal distension for 3 months. (**a**) FLAIR shows lamellar slightly hyperintense lesions with blurred margins in the left lateral ventricular parietal white matter and semi-oval center; (**b**) T_1WI enhancement shows obvious enhancement in the left lateral ventricular parietal white matter and semi-oval center, linear enhancement in the left frontal soft meninges, as well as strip enhancement in the left frontal dura and falx cerebri. (Image courtesy of Li Hehong of Guangzhou Women and Children's Medical Center)

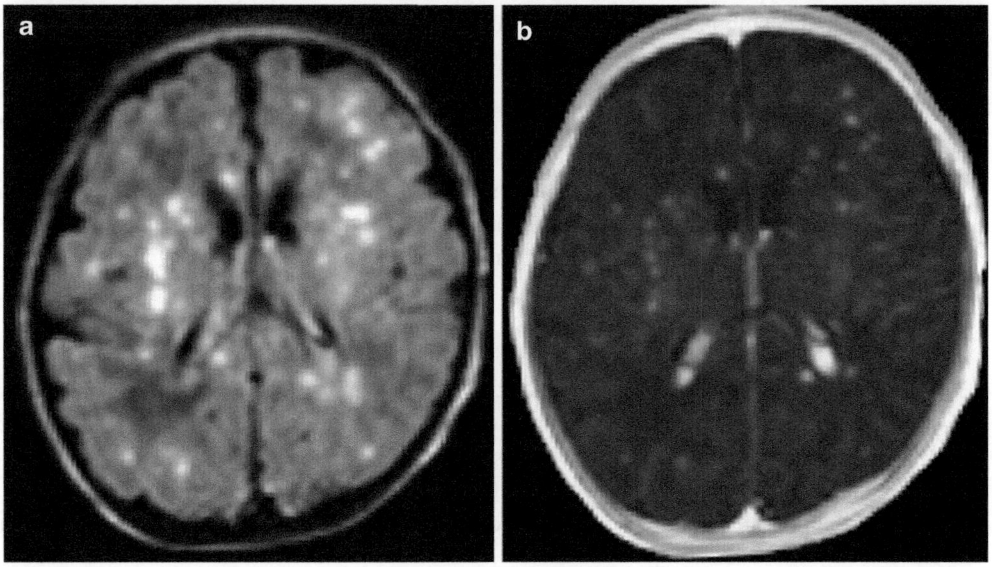

Fig. 13.8 *Candida* cerebralis infection (2). The patient, a newborn male. Abdominal bulge was found at birth for 1 h. (**a**) FLAIR shows diffuse small foci in both cerebral hemispheres, most of which are hyperintense and some are slightly hypointense; (**b**) T_1WI enhancement shows "starry sky"-like enhancement in bilateral cerebral hemispheres. (Image courtesy of Li Hehong, Guangzhou Women and Children's Medical Center)

swelling endothelial cell, increased proteins and lipids, and abscess wall formation. The dynamic changes on MRI are closely related to clinical treatment regression, and extensive white matter involvement may be a major cause of neurodevelopmental delay. MRI dynamic examination can provide a direct and objective basis for prognostic determination and post-injury brain development. Multifocal hyperintense signals on DWI combined with the manifestation of systemic fungal infection contributes to the early diagnosis of *Candida* infection in the CNS [23–26].

13.4.4 Diagnostic Key Points

1. *Candida albicans* infections of the central nervous system lack specific clinical manifestations, especially in infants and children.
2. The lesions mostly show hyperintense on T_1WI, hypointense on T2WI, hyperintense on FLAIR in the early stage, while iso-/hyperintense on T_1WI, hypo-/isointense on T_2WI with peripheral hypointense signal, and iso-/hyperintense on FLAIR 2 weeks later. Enhanced scans show "starburst"-like enhancement.
3. Multiple microabscesses may be a characteristic pathological change in neonatal CNS *Candida albicans* infections.
4. Direct microscopic examination reveals pseudomycelia and budding spores, and the presence of mycelia indicates a pathogenic state.

13.4.5 Differential Diagnosis

Candida albicans infections of the central nervous system need to be differentiated from brain abscesses and cryptococcal brain infections.

1. Brain abscess. Typical abscesses tend to be ring enhancement with intact, smooth, homogeneous walls and marked diffusion restriction on DWI.
2. Cryptococcal brain infection. The CT and MRI manifestations of novel cryptococcal meningoencephalitis are mainly gelatinous pseudocysts formed by enlarged perivascular spaces in the brain parenchyma, hydrocephalus, cerebral atrophy, and meningeal enhancement. MRI remains more sensitive imaging tool than CT and can provide more information.

13.4.6 Status and Progress of Research

1. Microscopic brain abscesses, meningitis, giant brain abscesses, and vascular complications are the main pathological changes in cranial *Candida* infections and are closely associated with poor patient prognosis. Imaging features can provide important information for diagnosis and prognosis. MRI shows fine intracranial lesions with more details better than CT. DWI shows multifocal hyperintense signals in the early stage, and DWI combined with the manifestation of systemic fungal infection helps the clinical diagnosis of this disease. The dynamic MRI changes are closely related to the clinical treatment regression, providing a direct and objective basis for the evolution of the disease process. Therefore, MRI-DWI and MRI dynamic examinations are of clinical importance for the diagnosis and prognosis of *Candida* infections in the central nervous system [27, 28].
2. Gene chip technology. All sequences suitable as probes were identified in the internal-transcribed spacer-2 (ITS-2) universal primer and ERG11 gene-specific primer amplification region. Then the candidate sequences were submitted to the gene database for blast comparison, and the oligonucleotide with the closest T*m* value and best specificity was selected for probe synthesis. The oligonucleotide microarrays were prepared by dotting sequence-specific oligonucleotides (amination probes) on aldehyde glass microarrays and hybridized with single-stranded DNA of 205 clinical isolates of ITS-2 gene amplified by asymmetric fluorescence PCR, and five common clinical pathogenic *Candida* and novel *Cryptococcus* species were accurately identified indicating that the test method has high specificity [29].
3. Plasma 1,3-beta-D glucan assay. Glucose is widely present in the fungal cell wall. After the fungus enters the deep tissues or blood of human body, the 1,3-beta-D glucose can be released from the fungal cell wall after phagocytosis and digestion by macrophages, elevating the 1,3-beta-D glucose level in blood or other body fluids (such as urine, cerebrospinal fluid, ascites, pleural effusion, etc.) [30]. Therefore, the early diagnosis of invasive fungal infections can be aided by the quantitative detection of plasma 1,3-beta-D glucose.

13.5 Paracoccidioidomycosis

Bailu Liu, Zhehao Lv, and Liwei Fu

13.5.1 Overview

Paracoccidioidomycosis is a chronic purulent granulomatous disease caused by *Paracoccidioides*, mostly affecting the mucous membranes, skin, lungs, and lymphatic system. *Paracoccidioides* infections of the central nervous system are characterized by the presence of granulomas with

Brucella brasiliensis, with a predilection for immunosuppressed individuals and a pathogen that can infect the lungs through the blood or lymphatic tract with subsequent involvement of the central nervous system called central nervous system paracoccidioidomycosis. *Coccidioides* is a dimorphic fungus that grows in a mycelial state in a saprophytic environment, manifesting as infectious arthrospores separated into segments, also known as arthrospores, and in human and animal tissues as spherical thick-walled sporangia containing many endospores, also known as sporangia or microspheres. The genus *Coccidioides* includes *C. immitis* and *C. posadasii*, all of which can cause disease. *C. immitis* and *C. posadasii* differ at the genomic and transcriptomic levels, but the morphology, phenotypic characteristics, and pathogenicity of the species are so similar that they are generally not subdivided clinically and are collectively referred to as *Coccidioides*.

Coccidioides are mainly found in soil, air, water, and animal fur and feces and are ingested by inhalation through the respiratory tract and also through the skin after trauma. After infection, 50–60% of patients have asymptomatic occult infection, 40% have self-limiting cold or flu-like symptoms, 10% develop pneumonia, and < 1% develop disseminated infection. In the early stages of infection, patients also often present with reactive symptoms such as erythema nodosum, erythema multiforme, and symmetrical polyarthralgia. The most frequent sites of disseminated infection are the skin, bones, and central nervous system, but practically any organ can be involved. Clinical manifestations vary depending on the organ involved and may be accompanied by systemic symptoms such as fever, chills, night sweats, weight loss, muscle pain, and fatigue. Severe cases can lead to infectious shock. Signs and symptoms of *Coccidioides* meningitis are nonspecific due to the complex and variable clinical presentation of disseminated infections, which can be easily misdiagnosed. In addition, the onset of symptoms is usually subacute, or even chronic, and it is not uncommon for the diagnosis to be established weeks or months after the onset of meningitis symptoms [31]. Direct microscopic examination of sputum, secretions or mucosal scrapings, microscopic visualization of budding thick-walled spores, positive fungal cultures, and serological tests are used to detect antibodies and antigens.

13.5.2 Pathological Manifestations

Special stains commonly used for pathological examination include Gomori's hexamine silver (GMS), calcofluor white (CFW), and PAS staining. However, the positive rate of culture and pathology is low, and serology is still needed to aid in the diagnosis as it is invasive and not widely available.

Paracoccidioides are dimorphic, rounded within the tissue, thick-walled, 20–80μm in diameter, containing several to hundreds of rounded or irregularly shaped endospores at maturity, arranged peripherally inward, and releasing endospores to form new spheres as the spheres mature. Direct microscopy reveals sporangia with spores inside, and fungal culture reveals mycelium and arthrospore balls. Primary cutaneous coccidioidomycosis is a chronic granuloma with neutrophil, eosinophil, lymphocyte, and plasma cell infiltration, and sometimes small abscesses containing endospores are seen. In progressive disseminated sporotrichosis, abscess formation is seen, caseous necrosis is visible, and endospore capsules are seen within the heterogeneous giant cells.

13.5.3 Imaging

Paracoccidioides infections of the central nervous system occur mostly in episodes. Neuroimaging may reveal hydrocephalus, basal meningitis, cerebral infarction, and granulomatous lesions. Hydrocephalus is the most common complication of coccidioidomycosis meningitis and is seen in 30–50% of patients. Vascular inflammatory infarcts are usually caused by inflammation of small- and medium-sized vessels. Aneurysm of the vertebral artery is an uncommon but serious complication, and suspected patients need to be excluded with MRA.

13.5.3.1 CT Findings

1. Meningitis. The cerebral sulcus gyrus became shallow and the brain pool manifests isodense or slightly hyperdense, and the leptomeninges and dura mater were significantly enhanced in most patients on enhanced scans.
2. Infarctive changes. Mostly, they present as poorly defined hypodense lesions with morphology related to cerebrovascular distribution and may have mild or no occupying effect.
3. Abscesses and granulomatous lesions. On the CT scan image, the lesion is hypodense with relatively clear borders, and the lesion generally has some occupying effect. Enhanced scans of the lesion tend to show circumferential enhancement with hypointense central portions of the lesion.

13.5.3.2 MRI Findings

1. Meningitis. T_1WI and T_2WI show abnormal signal; T_1WI shows isointense and hypointense; and T_2WI shows isointense, hypointense, hyperintense, and often hypointense; and FLAIR shows the lesion is more obvious. Leptomeninges and dura mater were significantly enhanced on enhanced scan.
2. Infarctive changes. T_1WI shows heterogenous hypointense and T_2WI shows heterogenous hyperintense, and in the case of combined bleeding, hypointense is seen at the edge of the lesion. Lesions are generally not enhanced on enhanced scans.

3. Abscesses and granulomatous lesions. A typical coccidioidomycosis brain abscess lesion mostly shows a central hyperintense and peripheral hypointense ring on T_2WI and just the opposite on T_1WI, with ring enhancement of the lesion seen on enhanced scans. *Coccidioides* brain abscess cavity may show restricted diffusion and DWI shows hyperintense. Further mechanization and fibrosis of chronic abscesses can form granulomas, most often in those with normal immune function or mild to moderate immune deficiency. The MRS of coccidioidomycosis granulomatous disease is characterized by the presence of high lipids and on the MRS 0.9 ppm, 1.3 ppm, 2.0 ppm, and 2.8 ppm can show lipid peaks, probably due to the methyl component within the fatty acids in the center of the granuloma.

   Magnetic resonance multi-sequence methods have considerable definite advantages in identifying granulomas and inflammatory lesions, such as enhanced scanning, expanded scatter-weighted imaging, and magnetic resonance spectroscopy. A typical coccidioidomycosis brain abscess lesion mostly shows a central hyperintense and peripheral hypointense ring on T_2WI and just the opposite on T_1WI, with ring enhancement of the lesion seen on enhanced scans. The same can be observed for the altered white matter signal in the brain surrounding the lesion. MRS can be used to distinguish septic abscesses from fungal granulomas, and DWI is more valuable in identifying necrotic components originating from tumors or abscesses than in determining the etiology of abscesses [32–35].

13.5.4 Diagnostic Key Points

1. Paracoccidioidomycosis is an endemic fungal disease, and patients often have a history of residence in endemic areas.
2. Signs and symptoms of *Coccidioides* meningitis are nonspecific and may be accompanied by systemic symptoms such as fever, chills, night sweats, weight loss, muscle pain, and fatigue.
3. The imaging shows a central hyperintense and peripheral hypointense ring on T_2WI, which is just the opposite on T_1WI, enhanced scan shows ring-like enhancement of the lesion; MRS may show lipid peak; DWI shows restricted diffusion.
4. Direct microscopic examination of sputum, secretions, or mucosal scrapings with microscopic visualization of budding thick-walled spores confirm the diagnosis.

13.5.5 Differential Diagnosis

1. **Cysticercosis** appears as a single or multiple cystic lesions, typically with punctate or nodular enhancement of the appendages (cephalic nodes) on enhanced scans, but no significant wall enhancement.
2. **Cystic metastases** mostly have a history of the primary tumor and the lesions are mostly located in the corticomedullary junction area, often multiple, with thick walls and irregular interiors, and small lesions that may be surrounded by large edema. In diffusion-weighted images, the central area of liquefied necrosis is not diffusion-limited (low signal), and the peripheral capsule wall is diffusion-limited.
3. **Miliary cerebral tuberculosis.** The majority of the lesions are located in the gray-white matter junction area, and the early stage is dominated by inflammatory exudate. MRI scan mainly shows a wide distribution of long T_1 and long T_2 signal edema areas in the brain of varying sizes, and the enhanced scan shows small nodules of close size, uniform distribution, and obvious enhancement. The MRI shows T_2WI "target sign" nodules with circumferential enhancement on enhanced scans.

13.5.6 Status and Progress of Research

1. Magnetic resonance multisequence methods offer considerable definitive advantages in identifying granulomas and inflammatory lesions, such as enhanced scans, diffusion-weighted imaging, and magnetic resonance spectroscopy. MRS can be used to distinguish septic abscesses from fungal granulomas; granulomatous disease characterized by the presence of high lipids, on MRS 0.9 ppm, 1.3 ppm, 2.0 ppm, and 2.8 ppm, can show lipid peaks, probably due to the methyl component within the fatty acids in the center of the granuloma. In addition, succinate (2.4 ppm), acetoacetate (1.9 ppm), and alanine (1.4 ppm) are seen in pyogenic abscesses rather than in *Paracoccidioides* granulomas.
2. DWI has more application in identifying the necrotic component as originating from a tumor or abscess than in determining the etiology of the abscess. Tumor necrosis usually spreads unrestrictedly. Although septic abscesses exhibit restricted spread, they are also seen in fungal abscesses [32].
3. Tests for the detection and diagnosis of *Coccidioides* antigen (CAg): The current kit for detecting CAg uses an enzyme-linked immunosorbent assay with a high positivity rate (70.8%) and its antigen titer correlates well with the disease, but this method has a high cross-reactivity rate with other diagnostic methods for fungal diseases (10.7%). The correctness of diagnosis may be improved if antigens and antibodies are tested in combination [36].

13.6 Actinomycosis

Bailu Liu and Zhehao Lv

13.6.1 Cerebral Actinomycosis

13.6.1.1 Overview

Actinomycosis is a progressive, septic, granulomatous, chronic infectious disease caused by actinomycetes. *Actinobacteria* are prokaryotes, the vast majority of which are anaerobic or partly anaerobic. Actinomycosis is an endogenous disease that is not contagious from person to person or person to animal, and it mostly affects men, with a male to female ratio of 3:1, and is more frequent in rural areas (incidence 5/10,000) than in urban areas (1/10000). The incidence in developed countries is 1–6/1 million people. In recent years, there has been a declining trend in actinomycosis in developed countries, probably related to improved sanitation and the application of broader-spectrum antibiotics.

Actinomyces belongs to the normal flora and may be present in the oral cavity, tonsillar crypt, upper respiratory tract, gastrointestinal tract, and genitourinary tract (female external genitalia) in normal individuals and is not normally pathogenic; in cases of weakened immunity and poor oral hygiene, it can cause endogenous infection, leading to suppurative inflammation of soft tissues and, in the absence of secondary infection, to chronic granulomas with multiple fistulae formation, and sulfur-like particles can be detected in the pus. *Actinomyces* invades the head and neck (55%), abdomen (20%), lungs (15%), and other parts (10%). Clinical features are multiple nodules, abscesses, and extensive fibrosis. *Actinomyces* facial and cervical infections account for the majority of cases, mostly with recent stomatitis, swelling of the neck behind extractions, ongoing production of new nodules, multiple abscesses, and fistula formation. Pathogenic bacteria can involve the chest or cause inhalation lung infections that form foci in the lungs. Actinomycotic infections of the central nervous system are very rare, accounting for 2–3% of all actinomycoses, and are highly misdiagnosed and missed.

The signs and symptoms of cerebral actinomycosis resemble those of a septic infection, but the symptoms are usually mild and slow, so the duration of symptoms before presentation is usually longer than that of a typical septic brain abscess. Brain actinomycosis presents as fever in no more than 50% of cases, and in addition there is very little evidence to suggest that it is an infectious lesion, so that brain actinomycosis is often initially misdiagnosed as a tumor. Both the Gram-positive filamentous microorganisms and the histological findings of sulfur granules strongly support the diagnosis of actinomycosis. Confirmation of the diagnosis of actinomycosis requires direct isolation of actinomycetes from clinical specimens or from sulfur pellets.

13.6.1.2 Pathological Manifestations

Classification of brain actinomycosis by pathological process: (1) the limited type, which may present as an abscess (67%), and generally characterized by a single abscess in the cerebral hemisphere, which may have varying degrees of envelope formation or fibrous lesions, or a very thick fibrous abscess wall and a small amount of granulation tissue, plasma cells, epithelioid cells, and giant cells are rare. The abscess wall is mainly infiltrated by mononuclear cells and a large number of polymorphonuclear leukocytes, with congestion, edema and astrocytosis of surrounding brain tissue and present with the usual features of a chronic brain abscess. It is of diagnostic value to see gram-positive mycelium or actinomycete particles in the abscess in which Gram-staining positive mycelium or actinomycete granules are seen with diagnostic value. Sometimes the actinomycetes invade the ventricular wall and the lesion resembles a tumor with an envelope and a central gelatinous substance, in which typical sulfur granules can be seen, and the diagnosis of such tumor-like cases depends mainly on histological findings. (2) the diffuse type mainly manifests as meningitis or meningoencephalitis (13%); others may have granulomas (7%), subdural abscess (6%), and epidural abscess (6%). Actinomycotic meningitis is easily confused with tuberculous meningitis, and both have similar cerebrospinal fluid findings (normal or decreased glucose levels, increased protein levels, and increased monocytes). Actinomycotic granulomas can form harder nodular or granulomatous lesions in various parts of the central nervous system due to the high fibrous component, making it difficult to diagnose actinomycosis until a pathologic biopsy is performed on the surgical specimen. Sometimes meningitis and brain abscesses occur in combination, and meningitis at the base of the brain can spread to the pituitary region, leading to serious consequences.

13.6.1.3 Imaging

1. **Angiographic manifestations.** *Actinomyces* cerebri abscesses may show occupying changes of vascular compression displacement or irregular stenotic changes in the superior siphon of the internal carotid artery, middle cerebral artery, and proximal anterior artery due to meningitis and cerebral arteritis, and cerebral ischemia, and hypoxia leading to anaerobic bacterial brain abscess formation in brain tissue.
2. **CT Findings**
   (a) Actinomycotic meningitis. The cerebral sulcus gyrus becomes shallow, the brain pool is isodense or slightly dense, and some show limited meningeal

thickening or soft meningeal nodule formation. Enhanced scans of the soft meninges and dura mater were significantly enhanced.

(b) Actinomycotic brain abscess. It is usually solitary and often involves the temporal or frontal lobes. CT plain scan shows a slightly hypodense central abscess with an intact or incomplete, regular or irregular ring of equal or slightly dense density around the hypodense foci visible as a fibrous envelope layer. The abscess remained hypodense on enhanced scans, with thick-walled, irregular, nodular, distinct enhancement of the abscess wall and linear enhancement of the adjacent meninges visible, with a hypointense edematous zone around the lesion. These manifestations can also be seen in brain abscesses and malignancies caused by other causes.

(c) Subdural abscesses and epidural abscesses. A subdural abscess presents as a crescentic hypodense shadow under the dura mater, with compression of adjacent brain tissue and displacement of midline structures, sometimes with adjacent brain tissue edema and brain abscess. Enhanced scans reveal envelope enhancement, especially in the lateral envelope of brain tissue. Epidural abscesses present as poorly defined biconvex lesions that are hypodense or isodense. The medial convexity of the lesion is enhanced on enhanced scan. Usually, the lesion does not significantly compress the brain parenchyma unless it is very large.

3. MRI Findings

(a) Actinomycotic meningitis. Abnormal signals can be seen on both T_1WI and T_2WI and manifest as hypointense on T_1WI and iso- or hyperintense on T_2WI, and FLAIR sequence shows the lesion more distinctly. The soft meninges and dura mater were significantly enhanced on the enhanced scan.

(b) Actinomycotic brain abscess. The abscess wall is isointense or slightly hyperintense on T_1WI, and "grape cluster" hypointense on T_2WI; the pus in the abscess cavity manifests as hypointense on T_1WI and hyperintense on T_2WI; perifocal edema manifests slightly hypointense on T_1WI and slightly hyperintense on T_2WI. The abscess wall was significantly enhanced on the enhanced scan. The DWI sequence shows significant hyperintensity due to the high protein content within the pus of the abscess, which can lead to local tissue viscosity and restricted diffusion of water molecules. The higher value of ADC in the abscess wall may be due to increased extracellular fluid in the abscess wall as a result of inflammation.

(c) Subdural abscesses and epidural abscesses. The pus of a subdural abscess manifests hypointense on T_1WI and hyperintense on T_2WI, and the wall of the abscess is seen to be significantly enhanced on enhanced scans. MRI can clearly show adjacent brain tissue edema and can effectively differentiate between epidural and subdural abscesses. The epidural abscess is similar to the subdural abscess on MRI, and the enhanced scan shows that the abscess is located in the epidural [37–39].

13.6.1.4 Diagnostic Key Points

1. Brain actinomycosis is often associated with mucosal barrier disruption or co-infection with other bacteria.
2. Actinomycete meningitis shows hypointense on T_1WI and isointense on T_2WI, and FLAIR sequence shows a more pronounced lesion. The leptomeninges and dura mater are significantly enhanced on the enhanced scan; the wall of the actinomycotic brain abscess displays isointense or slightly hyperintense on T_1WI, and "grape cluster"-like hypointense on T_2WI with obvious enhancement on the enhanced scan. The pus cavity manifests as significant hyperintense on DWI, which can be used as a characteristic imaging sign.
3. Both the Gram-positive filamentous microorganisms and the histological findings of sulfur granules strongly support the diagnosis of cerebral actinomycosis.
4. Confirmation of brain actinomycosis requires direct isolation of actinomycetes from clinical specimens or sulfur pellets.

13.6.1.5 Differential Diagnosis

The diagnosis of cerebral actinomycosis has been a challenge, with the qualitative diagnosis relying on history, signs, and histological examination. Although cerebral actinomycosis often lacks specific clinical and imaging manifestations, signs of low T_2 signal in the abscess wall may be helpful in the diagnosis of cerebral actinomycosis. This particular infection should be associated with a cystic brain tumor (e.g., high-grade astrocytomas, cystic metastases, etc.), or chronic granulomatous diseases (e.g., tuberculosis) are distinguished.

1. **Astrocytomas** can occur anywhere in the brain but often occur in the deep white matter and tend to have mixed signal on MRI plain scan and high signal on T_2WI. High-grade astrocytomas have significant occupying effects and marked edema. Enhanced scans of the lesion show wreath-like intensification or circumferential intensification with an irregular capsule wall, and significantly reinforced wall nodules can be observed. In the diffusion-weighted image, the central liquefied necrotic area is not diffusion-limited (low signal), the peripheral capsule wall is diffusion-limited (high signal) (low signal), and the peripheral cyst wall is diffusion-limited (high signal).

2. **Cystic metastases** mostly have a history of the primary tumor and the lesions are mostly located in the corticomedullary junction area, often multiple, with thick walls and irregular interiors, and small lesions that may be surrounded by large edema. In diffusion-weighted images, the central area of liquefied necrosis is not diffusion-limited (low signal), and the peripheral capsule wall is diffusion-limited.
3. **Tuberculoma** mainly shows thin-walled annular enhancement, with the typical "target sign" within the ring and a large target center.

13.6.1.6 Status and Progress of Research

1. **Magnetic resonance diffusion tensor imaging (DTI)** can be used as an aid in the diagnosis of brain actinomycosis. The high FA values for cerebral actinomycosis may be due to the fact that cerebral actinomycosis presents as granulomas and abscesses, histologically containing inflammatory cells, capillaries, necrotic debris, proteins, and amino acids. Cytoarchitecture and vascular components have a strong influence on the FA values, and brain actinomycosis containing a high cellular and vascular component and a high fibrous component of the abscess wall results in high FA values in brain actinomycosis.
2. **Magnetic resonance brain perfusion weighted imaging (PWI) and hydrogen proton spectroscopy imaging (^{1}H-MRS)** has been used in the preoperative evaluation of actinomycotic brain abscesses. Local blood volume is reduced in actinomycotic brain abscesses, suggesting a reduced blood supply. The local CBF was reduced, suggesting a lesser blood supply in actinomycotic brain abscesses compared to normal brain tissue. The MRS features of actinomycotic brain abscesses include elevated amino acids due to increased protein hydrolase activity resulting in protein breakdown. The presence of acetate and succinate in the spectrum may indicate enhanced glycolytic and fermentation processes in the pathogenic bacteria, and the presence of acetate and succinate helps to identify anaerobic and aerobic abscesses, and the presence of succinate and acetate in MRS suggests an anaerobic infection. The non-enhanced portion of the lesion showed elevated FA values, decreased ADC, decreased CBF values, and elevated amino acids, with elevated acetate and succinate peaks, suggesting a hypoperfused abscess cavity. In contrast, the ring-enhanced portion exhibits elevated FA, ADC, and CBF values, suggesting an abscess wall [40].

13.6.2 Nocardiosis

13.6.2.1 Overview

Nocardia actinomycetes belong taxonomically to a group of morphologically similar microorganisms in the domain Bacteria, phylum thick-walled Bacteria, class Actinomycetes, and order Actinomycetes. Its distribution in nature is widespread, but the vast majority (85% or more) are not yet known due to the limitations of the isolation and classification methods. Nocardia actinomycetes are an important class of natural resources, and some species can produce antibiotics, such as rifamycin, some species produce important metabolites that can be used, such as 2,3-dihydroxybenzoic acid, cyclohexylacetic acid, hydroxyphenylketone butyric acid, L-histidine, 16α- hydroxysteroids, etc. In addition, some species produce important enzymes, such as cholesterol oxidase, glucose isomerase, lysozyme, etc. Moreover, some species are used in the biological treatment of wastewater (substances). There are also some species that cause nocardia and podoconiosis in humans and animals.

In 1967, Prauser first introduced the concept of "Nocardia-type actinomycetes" to generalize a group of Gram-positive actinomycetes with morphological primordial prefilaments that break regularly into spherical- or rod-shaped vesicles.

About 1/3 of patients are asymptomatic at the beginning of the infection; as the disease progresses, patients may also have symptoms such as diffuse headache, vomiting, blurred vision, or drowsiness, which can last for several weeks, and symptoms such as sensory ataxia and unsteady gait may occur if the spinal cord is involved. If the patient is in poor health, *Nocardia* infection of the central nervous system may progress or recur, with a cure rate of 50% and a mortality rate of 55% for brain abscess. Sputum, pus, cerebrospinal fluid, tissue blocks, etc. for pathogenic examination were first digested and then centrifuged to collect bacteria which can be filmed for direct microscopic examination. Gram staining can be seen in the thin, curved, and branched mycelium, inoculated in antibiotic-free medium, under aerobic conditions, and then, according to the characteristics of the colony, combined with biochemical characteristics to identify.

13.6.2.2 Pathology Diagnosis

Nocardia brain abscesses may be ovoid and contain abundant green, dull, light brown purulent material. Microscopy showed multiple necrosis, consisting mainly of lymphocytes and neutrophils, with gliosis visible in the surrounding brain parenchyma. Silver staining reveals abundant right-angled branching bacteria and Gram staining shows bead-like features.

13.6.2.3 Imaging

Imaging is nonspecific, and MRI shows diffuse thickening of the dura mater, falx and cerebellar curtain, with significant nodule-like low signal seen in T_1WI, and T_2WI image shadow and marked edema. DWI may not reveal significant diffusion restriction. Enhanced scan shows heterogeneous mild enhancement with marginal enhancement of the lesion.

13.6.2.4 Diagnostic Key Points

1. Most often migrates from pulmonary lesions and rarely can be primary; patients present with symptoms of meningeal irritation such as headache, dizziness, nausea, vomiting, and irregular fever.
2. Invasion of the meninges causes meningitis, invasion of the brain parenchyma forms multiple abscesses, or they can fuse with each other to form large abscesses.
3. MRI shows diffuse thickening of the dura mater, falx, and cerebellar curtain.
4. Sputum, pus, cerebrospinal fluid, and tissue masses are taken for pathogenic examination to confirm the diagnosis.

13.6.2.5 Differential Diagnosis

Nocardia brain abscesses are similar to cerebral actinomycosis and should be differentiated from cystic brain tumors (e.g., high-grade astrocytomas, cystic metastases, etc.) or chronic granulomatous disease (e.g., tuberculosis).

1. **Astrocytomas** can occur anywhere in the brain but often occur in the deep white matter and tend to have mixed signal on MRI plain scan and high signal on T_2WI. High-grade astrocytomas have significant occupying effects and marked edema. Enhanced scans of the lesion show wreath-like enhancement or circumferential enhancement with irregularity in its capsule wall, and significantly enhanced wall nodules are seen. In diffusion-weighted images, there is no diffusion limitation in the central liquefied necrotic area (low signal), and the peripheral capsule wall shows diffusion restriction (high signal).
2. **Cystic metastases** mostly have a history of the primary tumor and the lesions are mostly located in the corticomedullary junction area, often multiple, with thick walls and irregular interiors, and small lesions that may be surrounded by large edema. In diffusion-weighted images, the central area of liquefied necrosis is not diffusion-limited (low signal), and the peripheral capsule wall is diffusion-limited.
3. **Tuberculoma** mainly shows thin-walled annular enhancement, with the typical "target sign" within the ring and a large bull's eye.

13.6.2.6 Status and Progress of Research

1. There are few studies related to *Nocardia*-type brain abscess, which is similar to brain actinomycosis, and magnetic resonance diffusion tensor imaging can assist in the diagnosis. FA values are also high in *Nocardia* type, probably due to its histological presence of inflammatory cells, capillaries, necrotic debris, proteins, and amino acids, resulting in elevated FA values in brain actinomycosis, and imaging diagnosis remains a significant challenge [40].
2. Polymerase chain reaction (PCR). The rpoB, secA1, and 16S rRNA genes are the more conserved gene sequences of *Nocardia* with little variability. However, a comparison of the sequences of *Mycobacterium*, *Actinomyces*, and *Nocardia* 16S rRNA genes showed that they have some homology, and it is difficult to distinguish them using 16S rRNA. The simultaneous detection of the rpoB, secA1, and 16S rRNA genes of *Nocardia* by multiplex PCR is of good diagnostic value, and no non-*Nocardia* strains have been found to contain these three genes at the same time, so multiplex PCR with these three bands at the same time can be determined as *Nocardia* [41].

13.7 Histoplasmosis

Bailu Liu and Zhehao Lv

13.7.1 Overview

Histoplasmosis is a primary fungal disease caused by the *Histoplasma capsulatum*, with an incubation period of generally 3–21 days after exposure. Histoplasmosis is highly contagious, with the source of infection being naturally bearing avian species such as chickens, bats, and pigeons or their feces-contaminated soil and dust, and infected animals such as horses, dogs, cats, and rats. Histoplasma can be introduced from the respiratory tract, skin mucosa, and gastrointestinal tract, invading first the lungs and then other mononuclear macrophage systems such as the liver and spleen, but also the kidneys, central nervous system, and other organs. Excreta such as feces from patients and infected animals in endemic areas can carry the bacteria, but no direct transmission between animals or between humans has been reported. Activities such as going to caves with bats and passing through large bat-strewn mountain tunnels and operations and tourists in mines are susceptible to infection and cause outbreaks. Disseminated infections are most often seen in infants and young children, patients with Hodgkin's disease, patients with lymphocytic leukemia, and patients treated with immunosuppressive drugs and patients with AIDS.

About 95% of patients with primary histoplasmosis may be asymptomatic. Initially, the symptoms may be upper respiratory tract infection or flu-like symptoms, with dry cough, weakness, emaciation, night sweats, hemoptysis and other symptoms similar to tuberculosis, or high fever, shortness of breath, and other symptoms similar to acute pneumonia, often with hepatosplenomegaly and lymph node enlargement, anemia, leukopenia, and thrombocytopenia. In the endemic population, many foci of calcification are seen in the lungs, but the history of the disease is unremarkable.

Clinically, 5–10% disseminated histoplasmosis may reveal central nervous system invasion, histoplasmosis of the brain is usually a manifestation of disseminated histoplasmosis, and isolated histoplasmosis of the brain is rare, especially in immunodeficient patients. Clinical signs of histoplasmosis of the brain include subacute or chronic meningitis, focal brain symptoms, stroke syndrome, and encephalitis, with the most common manifestation being subacute or chronic meningitis and other manifestations including granulomatous lesions and ischemic cerebral vasculitis. Patients with chronic encephalitis or meningitis lesions for which no etiology has been found should be suspected of histoplasmosis infection, especially if the patient has traveled to an area where histoplasmosis is endemic. Serologic testing and antigen testing can help diagnose histoplasmosis, and the detection of Histoplasma capsulatum in patients is the gold standard for the diagnosis of histoplasmosis capsulatum.

13.7.2 Pathological Manifestations

The pathological changes in the invasion of different organs by *Histoplasma capsulatum* were essentially the same. The early stage is a central partial hyperplasia with more or less fungus in the phagocytes. Subsequently, tissue necrosis occurs with granuloma-like changes around it, and finally it heals or fibrosis. Primary contact histoplasmosis presents as a nonspecific inflammatory infiltrate with intermittent areas of giant cells and necrosis.

13.7.3 Imaging

13.7.3.1 CT Findings

1. Meningitis. The cerebral sulcus gyrus becomes shallow, the brain pool is isodense or slightly dense, and some show limited meningeal thickening or soft meningeal nodule formation. Enhanced scans show marked enhancement of the soft and hard meninges, with only mild enhancement of the meninges seen in some immunocompromised patients.
2. Infarctive changes. Mostly, they present as poorly defined hypodense lesions with morphology related to cerebrovascular distribution and may have mild or no occupying effect.
3. Abscesses and granulomatous lesions. In immunocompetent or mildly to moderately immunocompromised individuals, intracranial infections often form fungal abscesses, indicating that the body's normally functioning immune system is sufficient to confine the lesion to a certain area. On the CT scan image, the lesion is hypodense with relatively clear borders, and the lesion generally has some occupancy effect. On enhanced scans, the lesion is mostly circumferentially enhanced, while the abscess is not significantly enhanced by the protrusion or nodule. Further mechanization and fibrosis of chronic abscesses can form granulomas, most often in those with normal immune function or mild to moderate immune deficiency. CT The lesion may be nodularly isointense or slightly hypointense and may be single or multiple in plain scan. The lesion may appear significantly uniformly enhanced on enhanced scans, and some lesions appear to be heterogeneously enhanced by necrosis in the central portion of the lesion.

13.7.3.2 MRI Findings

1. Meningitis. T_1WI and T_2WI are abnormal signals of which T_1WI is low signal and T_2WI shows isosignal or high signal; FLAIR sequence shows more pronounced lesions. The soft meninges and dura mater were significantly enhanced on enhanced scan.
2. Infarctive changes. T_1WI shows inhomogeneous low signal and T_2WI shows inhomogeneous high signal. In the case of combined bleeding, low signal is seen at the edge of the lesion. Enhanced scan lesions are generally not strengthened.
3. Abscesses and granulomatous lesions. T_1WI lesion is low signal, T_2WI lesion is mostly isosignal or slightly high signal, the inner wall of abscess is not smooth and may be accompanied by irregular wall protrusion or wall nodular shadow, and the edge of abscess can be seen ring-shaped low signal. Some lesions within T_2WI low signal foci may appear in some lesions, which are related to the paramagnetic material contained in the fungal hyphae and may also be caused by hemorrhage and hemoglobin rupture products due to vascular involvement. On enhanced scan, the lesion is mostly seen to be circumferentially enhanced, whereas the abscess inner wall protrusions or wall nodules are mostly not significantly enhanced. This sign occurs because the fungal abscess cavity contents are mostly liquefied and necrotic components, and the inner wall structures are mainly infarcted brain tissue and fungal mycotic and mycelial components. The fungal abscess on DWI shows low signal in the lumen and high signal in the protrusion of the inner wall, while the lesion on ADC shows high signal in the lumen and low signal in the protrusion of the inner wall, suggesting unrestricted diffusion in the lumen and restricted diffusion in the wall of the abscess. This sign can be differentiated from bacterial and tuberculous brain abscesses. Granuloma lesion T_1WI is mostly isosignal or slightly low signal, T_2WI is mostly isosignal or slightly high signal, and the lesion may be surrounded by T_2WI high-signal edema band. On

enhanced scan, the lesion may show significant uniform enhancement or may show inhomogeneous enhancement due to the presence of necrosis in the central portion. MR spectral imaging shows elevated lipid and lactate peaks and elevated choline (Cho), indicating that it contains purulent contents, while the ventricles may be dilated with fluid [42–44].

13.7.4 Diagnostic Key Points

1. *Histoplasma* infection should be suspected when there are chronic encephalitis or meningitis lesions and no other etiology is found, especially if the patient has traveled to an area where *Histoplasma* is endemic; it is often combined with multisystem invasion, such as the lung, liver and spleen, and lymph nodes.
2. The imaging presentation is mostly meningitis and granulomatous lesions. Abscess DWI shows low signal in the abscess cavity and high signal in the inner wall protrusion, while ADC shows high signal in the lesion cavity and low signal in the inner wall protrusion, a relatively specific presentation.
3. Serologic tests and antigen testing help diagnose histoplasmosis, and the detection of *Histoplasma capsulatum* in patients is the gold standard for the diagnosis of *Histoplasma capsulatum*.

13.7.5 Differential Diagnosis

Histoplasmosis of the brain is clinically rare and lacks specific imaging. The qualitative diagnosis of *Histoplasma capsulatum* in the brain relies on history, signs, and laboratory tests of cerebrospinal fluid, and imaging manifestations can aid in the diagnosis and serve as localization. This disease needs to be differentiated from astrocytomas, metastases, and bacterial brain abscesses.

1. **Astrocytomas** can occur anywhere in the brain but often occur in the deep white matter and tend to have mixed signal on MRI plain scan and high signal on T_2WI. The occupying effect and edema of high-grade astrocytoma are obvious. Enhanced scan lesion shows wreath-like or ring-like intensification with irregular capsule wall and marked wall nodules.
2. **Typical bacterial brain abscess.** Enhanced scans of typical bacterial brain abscess lesions show circumferential enhancement and smooth abscess walls both inside and outside. Bacterial brain abscesses have high signal in the pus cavity on DWI and low signal on ADC due to the rich inflammatory cells and large amount of proteins in the pus, resulting in restricted diffusion of water molecules.
3. **Metastases.** Most often have a history of a primary tumor, and the lesions are located in the corticomedullary junction area, often multiple and small, and may be surrounded by large edema. Enhanced scans present enhancement in a variety of ways, often in a circular fashion.

13.7.6 Status and Progress of Research

1. MRI has a high resolution of soft tissues and has the advantage of clearly showing intracranial lesions and detailed signs, even reflecting to some extent the pathological features and the evolution of the disease, providing important information for the diagnosis, differential diagnosis, and posttreatment follow-up of this disease. In recent years, with the introduction of several MRI new techniques, their clinical application has gradually become popular. DWI and MRS can play a greater role in the diagnosis and differential diagnosis of septic infection, DWI shows low signal in the lumen and high signal in the inner wall protrusion on MRS which can detect specific metabolites [42, 44].
2. Polymerase chain reaction (PCR). It can be used to diagnose histoplasmosis, but the effectiveness still needs to be verified. Mayo Medical Center [45] detected two positive results in six culture-positive bronchoalveolar lavage (BAL) specimens. In another study, less than 10% of antigen-positive urine specimens were PCR positive [46].

References

1. Wang YB, Shi YS, Zhang CY. A controlled clinical and imaging study of AIDS and non-AIDS associated novel cryptococcal meningoencephalitis. Radiol Pract. 2012;27(9):932–6.
2. Qiu T, Zhu H, Wen H. Advances in the study of mechanisms associated with Cryptococcus invasion of the blood-brain barrier. Chin J Mycol. 2016;11(3):190–2.
3. Shih RY, Koeller KK. Bacterial, fungal, and parasitic infections of the central nervous system: radiologic-pathologic correlation and his- torical perspectives. Radiographics. 2015;35(4):1141–69.
4. Xiao H, Wang X, Xie F, et al. Differentiation of MRI signs of tuberculous meningitis from novel cryptococcal meningitis. J Tradit Chin Med. 2015;35(5):53–5.
5. You X. Application of a novel cryptococcus FQ-PCR detection system in an animal model of bloodstream infection (Master's thesis). Shijiazhuang: Hebei Medical University; 2016.
6. Orlowski HLP, McWilliams S, Mellnick VM, et al. Imaging spectrum of invasive fungal and fungal-like infections. Radiographics. 2017;37(4):1119–34.
7. Kawaguchi T, Sakurai K, Hara M, et al. Clinico-radiological features of subarachnoid hyperintensity on diffusion-weighted images in patients with meningitis. Clin Radiol. 2012;67(4):306–12.
8. Vidal JE, Boulware DR. Lateral flow assay for cryptococcal antigen: an important advance to improve the continuum of HIV care and reduce cryptococcal meningitis-related mortality. Rev Inst Med Trop Sao Paulo. 2015;57(Suppl 19):38–45.

9. Huang HR, Fan LC, Rajbanshi B, et al. Evaluation of a new cryptococcal antigen lateral flow immunoassay in serum cerebrospinal fluid and urine for the diagnosis of cryptococcosis: a meta-analysis and systematic review. PLoS One. 2015;10(5):e0127117.
10. Tang X, Wang Y. Latex agglutination test in the early diagnosis of cryptococcal infections. Chin J Hosp Infect. 2018;28(17):2561–3.
11. Li Y, Li H. A case of AIDS-associated intracerebral aspergillus infection. Radiol Pract. 2012;27(9):1038–9.
12. Liu X, Lu S. Changing strategies for the diagnosis and management of aspergillosis from an evidence-based medical perspective—2016 interpretation of the new edition of the American College of Infectious Diseases guidelines for the diagnosis and management of aspergillosis. Chin J Antituberculosis. 2017;39(1):16–21.
13. Liu Q, Yin S, Yi L, et al. Clinical and imaging features of Aspergillus encephalopathy. J Clin Neurol. 2014;27(2):130–2.
14. Oner AY, Celik H, Akpek S, et al. Central nervous system aspergillosis: magnetic resonance imaging, diffusion-weighted imaging, and magnetic resonance spectroscopy features. Acta Radiol. 2006;47(4):408–12.
15. Antulov R, Dolic K, Fruehwald-Pallamar J, et al. Differentiation of pyogenic and fungal brain abscesses with susceptibility-weighted MR sequences. Neuroradiology. 2014;56(11):937–45.
16. Sun W, Wang K, Gao W, et al. Evaluation of PCR on bronchoalveolar lavage fluid for diagnosis of invasive aspergillosis: a bivariate metaanalysis systematic review. PLoS One. 2011;6(12):e28467.
17. Liu Z, He G, Dong W, et al. Diagnostic value of cerebrospinal fluid PCR assay for invasive Aspergillus infection of the central nervous system—a systematic evaluation and bivariate meta analysis. Int J Cardiovasc. 2017;15(9):1041–5.
18. Yu H, Dong M, Cao S. Acute cerebral infarction due to nasal orbital cerebral trichomycosis 1 case. Chin J Stroke. 2013;8(4):281–4.
19. Wang Y, Wang Y, Chen J, et al. A typical case of mucor nasalis oculo-cerebralis and review of the literature. Chin J Pract Neurol Disord. 2014;17(18):141–2.
20. Li WD, Li YJ, Wang AP, et al. Isolated cerebral mucormycosis 1 case report and review of the literature. J Clin Neurosurg. 2013;10(6):371–2.
21. Ghuman MS, Kaur S, Bhandal SK, et al. Bilateral optic nerve infarction in rhino-cerebral mucormycosis: a rare magnetic resonance imaging finding. Neurosci Rural Pract. 2015;6(3):403–4.
22. Altini C, Niccoli-Asabella A, Ferrari C, et al. ^{18}F-FDG PET/CT contribution to diagnosis and treatment response of rhino-orbital-cerebral mucormycosis. Hell J Nucl Med. 2015;18:68–70.
23. Mao J, Li J, Chen D, et al. Significance of magnetic resonance imaging in the diagnosis of brain abscesses in premature infants with Candida albicans infection. Chin J Contemp Pediatr. 2011;13(8):621–6.
24. Zhu S, Han X, Qu Z, et al. Report of a case of intracranial Candida albicans infection and review of the literature. Chin Foreign Med. 2012;31(14):8–9.
25. Hu B, Chen H, Li S, et al. Candida albicans of the central nervous system in infants 5 examples and review of the literature. Chin J Pediatr. 2011;6(5):386–90.
26. Gao Y-Y, Yang S, Zhong W, et al. Candida albicans infections of the central nervous system 3 clinical features, imaging analysis and literature review of cases. Chin Clin Neurosci. 2016;24(3):311–7.
27. Zhang SC. Cerebral candidiasis in a 4-year-old boy after intestinal Surgery. J Child Neurol. 2015;30(3):391–3.
28. Lin DJ, Sacks A, Shen J, et al. Neurocandidiasis: a case report and consideration of the causes of restricted diffusion. J Radiol Case Rep. 2013;7(5):1–5.
29. Wang J, Yu P, Ge P, et al. Experimental analysis of gene microarray technology for the detection of clinically common pathogenic Candida and novel cryptococcus and ERG11 gene point mutations. Lab Med. 2018;8(33):742–8.
30. Su KC, Chou KT, Hsiao YH, et al. Measuring (1, 3)-beta-D-glucan in tracheal aspirate, bronchoalveolar lavage fluid, and serum for detection of suspected Candida pneumonia in immunocompromised and critically ill patients, a prospective observational study. BMC Infect Dis. 2017;17(1):252.
31. Wu J, Zhu L. Advances in the epidemiology, clinical presentation and diagnosis and management of coccidioidomycosis. Microbes Infect. 2017;12(1):44–9.
32. Reis F, Collier PP, Souza TF, et al. Neuroparacoccidioidomycosis (NPCM). Magnetic resonance imaging (MRI) findings. Mycopathologia. 2013;175(1/2):181–6.
33. Souza PV, Pinto WB, Matas SL. Paracoccidioidomycosis: a rare cause of infectious encephalomyelopathy. Arq Neuropsiquiatr. 2014;72(11):904–5.
34. Silva-Vergara ML, Rocha IH, Vasconcelos RR. Central nervous system paracoccidioidomycosis in an AIDS patient: case report. Mycopathologia. 2014;177(1/2):137–41.
35. Shih RY, Koeller KK. Bacterial, fungal, and parasitic infections of the central nervous system: radiologic-pathologic correlation and historical perspectives. Radiographics. 2015;35:1141–69.
36. Kassis C, Zaidi S, Kuberski T, et al. Role of coccidioides antigen testing in the cerebrospinal fluid for the diagnosis of coccidioidal meningitis. Clin Infect Dis. 2015;61(10):1521–6.
37. Wang S, Wolf RL, Woo JH, et al. Actinomycotic brain infection: registered diffusion, perfusion MR imaging and MR spectroscopy. Neuroradiology. 2006;48(5):346–50.
38. Xiong Y, Liu D, Wu X, et al. A case of intracranial infection after traumatic brain injury caused by actinomyces septicum. J Clin Radiol. 2012;31(9):83.
39. Zheng Y, Chu R, Tan S. Actinomycosis of the cerebral type. Chin J Dermatol Venereol. 2002;16(6):59–60.
40. Heo SH, Shin SS, Kim JW, et al. Imaging of actinomycosis in various organs: a comprehensive review. Radiographics. 2014;34(1):19–33.
41. Sun W, Hou X, Xu S, et al. Establishment of a multiplex polymerase chain reaction for the rapid identification of Nocardia spp. Microbes Infect. 2014;9(2):107–11.
42. Eid AJ, Leever JD, Husmann K, et al. Compartmentalized Histoplasma capsulatum infection of the central nervous system. Case Rep Infect Dis. 2015;2015:581415.
43. Trelkeld ZD, Broughton R, Khan GQ, et al. Isolated Histoplasma capsulatum meningoencephalitis in an immunocompetent child. J Child Neurol. 2012;27(4):532–5.
44. Ramireddy S, Wanger A, Ostrosky L. An instructive case of CNS histoplasmosis in an immunocompetent host. Med Mycol Case Rep. 2012;1(1):69–71.
45. Babady NE, Buckwalter SP, Hall L, et al. Detection of Blastomyces dermatitidis and Histoplasma capsulatum from culture isolates and clinical specimens by use of real-time PCR. J Clin Microbiol. 2011;49(9):3204–8.
46. Tang YW, Li H, Durkin MM, et al. Urine polymerase chain reaction is not as sensitive as urine antigen for the diagnosis of disseminated histoplasmosis. Diagn Microbiol Infect Dis. 2006;54(4):283–7.

Intracranial Parasitic Infections

14

Hanqiu Liu, Weiwei Wang, Mi Chen, Xuening Zhang, and Longlin Yin

14.1 Cerebral Cysticercosis

Hanqiu Liu, Weiwei Wang, and Mi Chen

14.1.1 Overview

Cerebral cysticercosis is the most common cerebral parasitic disease, caused by larvae of the pig tapeworm parasitizing the brain, and is also known as cysticercosis. The tapeworm larvae enter the bloodstream through the duodenal intestinal wall and evolve into cysticercus larvae in the skull. The disease is endemic in many countries and regions of the world and is a global health problem. It is endemic in north, northeast, northwest, and northeast China, and diseases are caused by intracranial parasitosis of cysticercus larvae.

Cerebral cysticercosis varies from months to 30 years from infection to the appearance of clinical symptoms. (1) Cerebrospinal fluid examination. Increased pressure; leukocytosis with eosinophilia; increased protein; sugar and chloride mostly in the normal range. (2) Immunological examination of cysts. Positive results of indirect hemagglutination test, enzyme-linked immunosorbent assay, and cysticercus complement binding test with high sensitivity and specificity. (3) Positive serum and cerebrospinal fluid cysticercus antibodies. (4) Fecal examination reveals tapeworm eggs or nodules.

14.1.2 Pathological Manifestations

The characteristic pathological manifestation of cerebral cysticerci is the identification of cysticercosis nodules. Live cysticerci often do not cause obvious organismal reactions, being round cysts of 4–20 mm diameter, containing live cecal larvae, and their head segments appear as small nodules with clear cystic fluid. When cysticerci degenerate and die, the death of cecal larvae causes the cystic fluid to become turbid, the cystic wall to thicken, and the cystic lumen to shrink. Due to the strong immune response of the host to the parasite's allogeneic protein, it causes local brain tissue inflammation, edema, and necrosis, often accompanied by thickened meningeal and ventricular canal adhesions and impaired cerebrospinal fluid circulation, resulting in hydrocephalus. Eventually, the dead cysticercus may undergo calcification with gliosis of the surrounding brain tissue.

Depending on where the cysticercosis lesions occur, they can be classified as parenchymal, ventricular, meningeal, and mixed [1]. Some scholars have divided the brain cysts into four stages [2] according to their different stages of pathological changes: (1) the live cyst stage, referred to as the cyst stage, the cyst fluid is clear and mostly does not cause the body to react; (2) the degenerative death stage, or the gelatinous cyst stage, the metabolites of cysticercus metabolites cause inflammatory reactions in humans; (3) the granulomatous phase, also known as the granulomatous nodular phase, in which the cyst wall thickens, the cystic lumen shrinks further, and the cephalic nodes calcify due to massive inflammatory cell infiltration; and (4) the complete calcification phase, in which the cystic foci shrink and calcify completely.

H. Liu (✉) · W. Wang
Huashan Hospital, Fudan University, Shanghai, China

M. Chen
The First Affiliated Hospital of Xinjiang Medical University, Urumqi, China
e-mail: lixin@cspm.com.cn

X. Zhang
Department of Radiology, The Second Hospital of Tianjin Medical University, Tianjin, China

L. Yin
Sichuan Provincial People's Hospital, Chengdu, China

H. Li et al. (eds.), *Radiology of Infectious and Inflammatory Diseases - Volume 1*,
https://doi.org/10.1007/978-981-99-0039-8_14

14.1.3 Imaging

14.1.3.1 CT Findings

1. Brain parenchymal type. The CT presentation of parenchymal cysticercosis varies according to the stage of the pathology. The lesions are often located in the corticomedullary junction area of the cerebral hemispheres and are often multiple.
   (a) Acute phase.
   - Encephalitis type. CT plain scan resembles other encephalitides, showing diffuse bilateral cerebral white matter edema, sometimes interspersed with scattered small cystic hypodense foci, and in severe cases, marked occupying effects with narrowing or occlusion of the ventricles, sulci, brain pools, and fissures. The hypodense foci do not enhance on enhanced scans.
   - Vesicular type. The CT scan of multiple vesicles shows multiple scattered round or ovoid hypodense shadows in the brain parenchyma, 3–10 mm in diameter, unevenly distributed, mostly located in the corticomedullary junction area; typical hypodense vesicles can be seen within the eccentric isodense dot-like nodular shadow, that is, the cephalic shadow of the cysticercus, forming typical "target sign" or "bull's-eye sign" (Fig. 14.1).

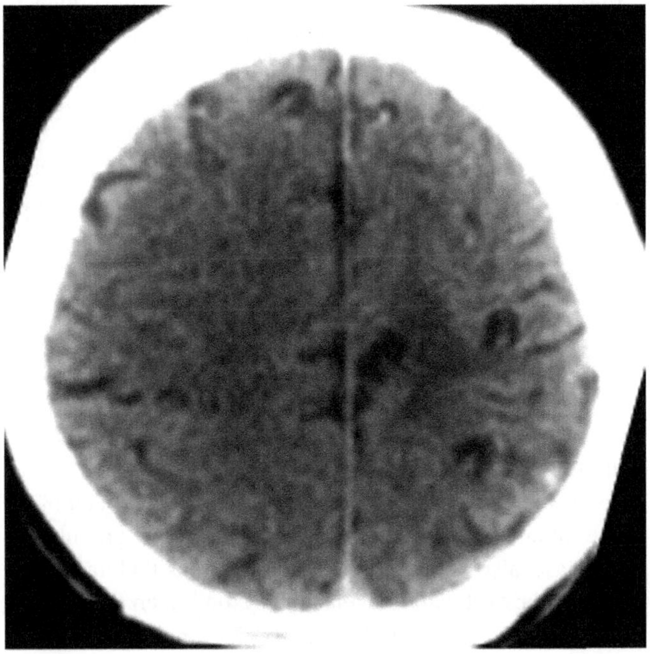

Fig. 14.1 Multiple cerebral cysticercosis in the brain (1). CT plain scan shows multiple scattered round or ovoid hypodense shadows in the brain parenchyma, mostly located in the corticomedullary junction area, with eccentric isodense cysticercal head nodules visible within typical hypodense vesicles

   - Most hypodense foci are non-enhancing on enhanced scans, while a few show nodular or small ring-like enhancement. Sometimes there is peripheral edema, and the ventricles are compressed to a smaller size. Single vesicular type, CT plain scan shows a single round-like or slightly lobulated large hypodense nodule in the brain parenchyma, CT value approximates cerebrospinal fluid, usually 4–10HU with clear borders. Enhanced scans of the lesion are mostly unreinforced, and some may show mild circumferential enhancement of the cyst wall.
   - Multiple nodular type CT scan shows multiple hypodense foci with occasional isodense or slightly dense foci with irregular morphology and significant peri-focal edema. Enhanced scans reveal multiple nodular or ring-like strong intensification, also seen as ring-like intensification around the periphery and dot-like intensification in the center, diameter 2–5 mm.

   (b) Chronic phase (calcified type). The cysts die, the cyst fluid is absorbed, and the cysts are ossified to form fibrous tissue and calcify. CT plain scan shows a single or multiple, 1–2 mm diameter, dot-like, dense calcified shadow. When the wall and part of the contents of the cysticercus are calcified, the lesion is circular or oval with a circular calcification of 3–10 mm in diameter, with a central calcification of the cysticercal head segment of 1–2 mm visible (Fig. 14.2), with no edema in the surrounding brain tissue. There was no enhancement of the lesion on the enhanced scan.
2. Ventricular type. Cysticerci are parasitic within the ventricular system, with the fourth ventricle being the most common, followed by the lateral and third ventricles. Typically the size is 1–2 cm, and the lesions are often larger than those in the brain parenchyma. Because of the thin wall of cysticercosis, the density of intracapsular fluid approximates that of cerebrospinal fluid, and there is no enhancement; CT examination is often not easily revealed, and the diagnosis is easily missed. Therefore, when intracerebroventricular cysticercosis is suspected, attention should be paid by adjusting the appropriate CT window width and window position for observation, as well as with the help of indirect signs, such as local asymmetric enlargement of the ventricles or nudged choroid plexus, and cerebrospinal fluid due to hydrocephalus due to impaired circulation. Very few cysticercosis deaths may show homogeneous isodense foci, ring enhancement, or calcification within the ventricles.
3. Meningeal type. In the meningeal type of cysticercosis infection CT plain scan, the lesions are mainly in the subarachnoid space, single or multiple, occasionally grape bunch-like, up to several centimeters, often lacking wall

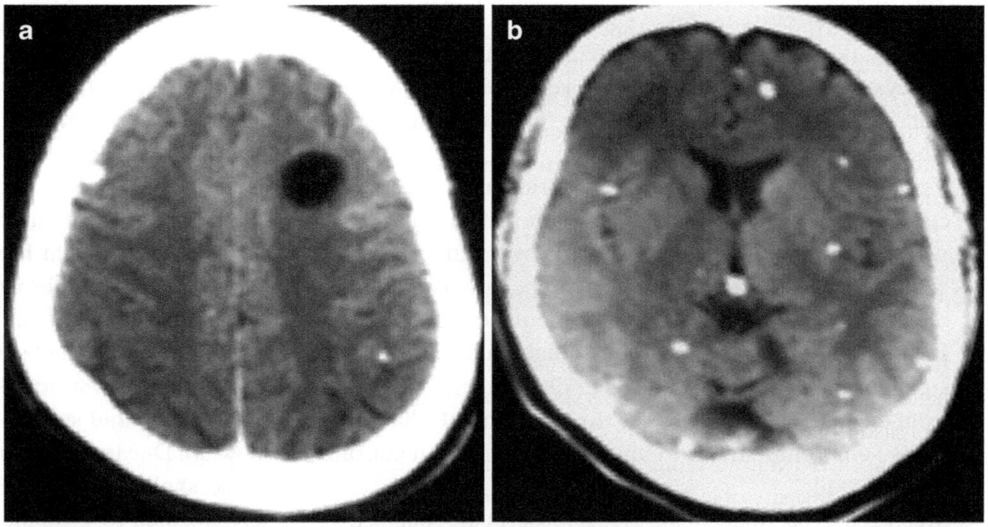

Fig. 14.2 Multiple cerebral cysticercosis in the brain (2). (**a**) CT scan shows scattered calcified nodules in the gray–white matter junction area of the brain parenchyma, and one cystic hypodense nodule in the left frontal corticomedullary junction area; (**b**) CT scan at different levels shows multiple calcified nodules in the gray–white matter junction area of the brain parenchyma, a calcified cephalic shadow of a cysticercus

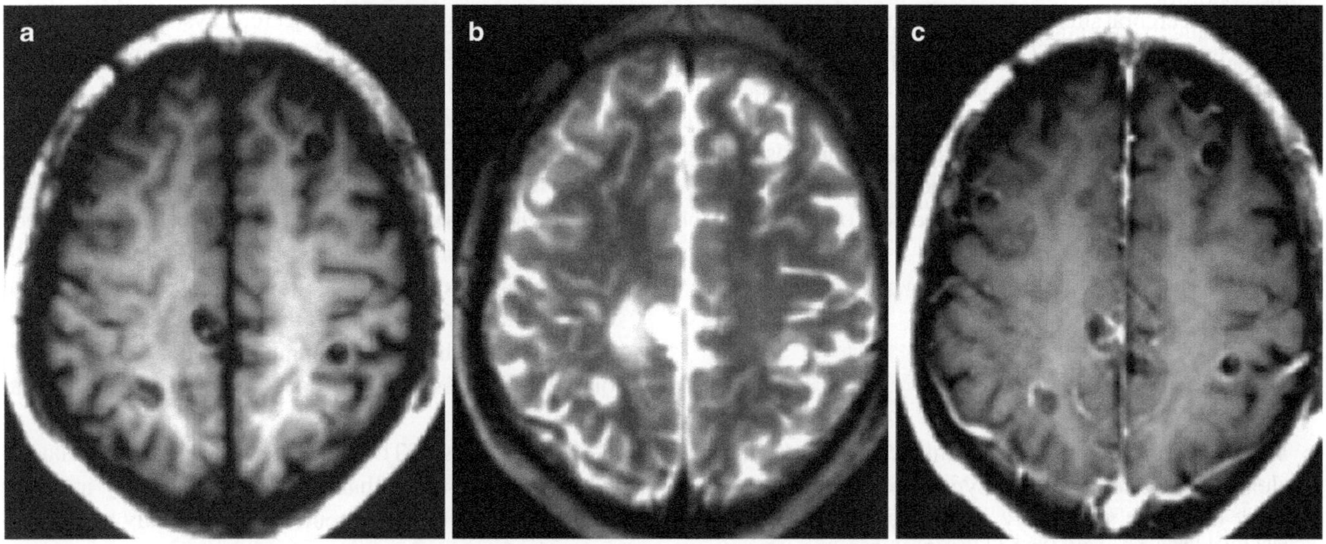

Fig. 14.3 Multiple encephalocysticercosis. Multiple round-like cystic lesions in the gray–white matter junction area of the brain parenchyma. (**a**) T_1WI shows a round-like cystic lesion with a low signal; (**b**) T_2WI cystic lesion with a high signal, no edema around most lesions, cysticercus head nodes in T_1WI, and T_2WI shows isointense; (**c**) T_1WI enhancement shows circumferential enhancement of the cyst wall

nodules or cephalic nodes, and often fail to show cysticercosis due to differences with cerebrospinal fluid, showing only asymmetric or restricted enlargement of the subarachnoid space, or inflammatory reaction of adjacent brain tissue. It is often associated with traffic hydrocephalus. Occasional meningeal enhancement is seen on enhanced scans.

4. Mixed type. A lesion with a mixture of two or more of these types, or a mixture of acute and chronic phases, with simultaneous imaging of different periods, is characteristic [3].

14.1.3.2 MRI Findings

MRI diagnosis of active stage brain cysts is significantly better in CT [4–6].

1. Brain parenchymal type. In the capsule stage, the T_1 and T_2 signals of the capsule contents are similar to those of the cerebrospinal fluid, T_1WI is a low signal, T_2WI is a high signal, FLAIR is a low signal, and most lesions are not surrounded by edema. Cysticercus cephalicus is isointense on T_1WI, and T_2WI is often not shown (Fig. 14.3). In the collagenous capsule stage, edema may be present around the cyst, forming a high signal area on the T_2WI, and the fluid within the capsule becomes cloudy and thick, FLAIR showing a high signal. In some cases, the cyst may become isointense and similar to the surrounding brain tissue MRI signal. Granulomatous stage cysts show punctate calcification, which MRI often fails to reveal. Enhanced scans of the acute phase of inflammatory brain lesions and edematous areas do not

enhance, and cysts in the cystic phase do not enhance; after the death of the cysticercus, circular enhancement of the cyst wall is seen, and the thickness of the intensified wall increases. It ceases to enhance until the late stage when the cyst calcifies.
2. Ventricular type. Intracerebroventricular cysts are clearly visualized on MRI, slightly hypointense on T_1WI with a thin ring of high signal in the cyst wall, and the cephalic nodes of the cyst caudate appear as isointense or slightly hyperintense punctate nodules against the surrounding low signal cerebrospinal fluid. The high signal of the cyst on T_2WI is generally indistinguishable from the high signal of the cerebrospinal fluid. Enhanced scans sometimes show circumferential enhancement of the cyst wall.
3. Meningeal type. Many of the cysticercosis in the subarachnoid space are formed by adhesions of cysts to the meninges in the cerebral sulcus. Similar to intracerebroventricular cysts, they show on the T_1WI, but mostly without cephalic segments, and because cysts in the subarachnoid space are mostly located at the cranial bony prominence, they are more sensitive on MRI than on CT. MRI may also reveal signs of infection, such as concomitant arachnoiditis. Enhanced scans often show enhancement of the basal pool due to granulomatous meningitis.
4. Hybrid. Two or more of the above types can co-exist.

14.1.4 Diagnostic Key Points

1. Young and middle-aged farmers in areas with a high prevalence of cysticercosis with symptoms of epilepsy, headache, dizziness (especially seizures), mild sensorimotor disorders, and intracranial hypertension, especially those with these symptoms.
2. Brain CT or MRI. There are some characteristic manifestations of cerebral cysticercosis on CT and MRI. The cephalic stage is seen as a cephalic node on one side of the cystic foci. The degenerative stage will show the disappearance of the cephalic nodes, thickening of the cystic wall, marked edema, and circular enhancement after enhancement; The granulomatous stage or complete calcification stage of cysticercosis may form calcifications; it is more valuable if the cysticercotic foci of different stages can be seen during the simultaneous examination. The diagnosis is more valuable if the cysticercosis foci of different periods can be seen during the same examination.
3. CT and MRI can show more clearly for ventricular or meningeal type and enables staging and accurate localization of the lesion.
4. Diagnosis is confirmed by palpation of subcutaneous cyst nodules, positive immunological examination for cysts, or a history of tapeworm expulsion.

14.1.5 Differential Diagnosis

1. **Brain abscess.** Enhanced scans mostly show single or multiple thin- or thick-walled distinctly reinforced annular lesions in the brain, with DWI-restricted diffusion within the abscess cavity and significant peripheral edema. It is not difficult to differentiate them by combining the acute clinical history and biochemical examination of blood or cerebrospinal fluid.
2. **Arachnoid cysts** are often located in the lateral fissure, parasagittal sinus, and subarachnoid space on the convex side of the brain, which shows a localized enlargement of the subarachnoid space, and the cyst wall often does not show up. Due to the prolonged growth, localized thinning of the skull bone by pressure is often seen, sometimes accompanied by atrophic changes in the brain tissue surrounding the cyst. No enhancement on the enhanced scan. Solitary meningeal-type cysticercus cysts are difficult to distinguish from arachnoid cysts on imaging. Cephalic nodes, although rare, are highly suggestive of cerebral cysticercosis when found. Multiple meningocele cysts can be found distributed in adjacent clusters of multiple cysts, which helps in the diagnosis.
3. **Epidermoid cysts.** It occurs in the subarachnoid space such as the fourth ventricle, cerebellopontine cistern, or suprasellar cistern, and has the biological characteristic of penetrating when it meets the crevices. CT scan shows lower density than cerebrospinal fluid density, and DWI on MRI with restricted diffusion of cystic fluid helps to differentiate.
4. **Brain metastases.** The occupancy effects and edema are often obvious, and enhanced scans are mostly irregular ring or nodular enhancement. Patients usually have a history of primary tumors.

14.1.6 Status and Progress of Research

MRI, CT, and X-ray can be used to examine for cerebral cysticercosis, with CT and MRI predominating.

X-ray may show indirect signs such as calcification of cerebral cysticercosis, but is of limited value in the diagnosis of specific intracranial lesions. MRI has high soft tissue resolution, and the multi-sequence and multimodal examination can provide informations about the localization, characterization and even quantitative diagnosis of cerebral cysticercosis. Among them, the lesion's T_2 values can reflect the lesion center and peripheral gliosis [7, 8] and continuous follow-up T values change, which can be used for follow-up and assessment of treatment effect and prognosis.

In recent years, with the widespread use of various new techniques of MRI, such as SWI, DWI, MRS, and PWI, MRI has provided important information for the diagnosis, differential diagnosis, and post-treatment follow-up of the disease.

14.2 Cerebral Paragonimias

Hanqiu Liu and Weiwei Wang

14.2.1 Overview

Cerebral paragonimiasis is also known as cerebral pulmonary schistosomiasis. Schistosomiasis is a zoonotic parasitic infection. The life history of the lung fluke is as follows: The eggs discharged by human or animal hosts hatch into trichariae in water, then the trichariae develop into cecal larvae in the Kawarau snail, and the cecal larvae develop into cysts in intermediate hosts such as freshwater stone crabs or clarkfish. Humans become infected by accidental ingestion of these stone crabs or clarkfish. The cysts decapsulate into child worms in the human duodenum and migrate to invade the abdominal cavity, penetrate the diaphragm, and reside in the lungs to develop into adults. There are many variants and subspecies of pulmonary schistosomes, and in China they are mainly caused by *Schistosoma weissei* and *Schistosoma* sp. The Kawasaki snail and stone crabs or clark mayflies mostly inhabit mountain streams and rivers, so they are common in mountainous areas and are mostly infected with *Schistosoma weissei* [9].

Cerebral pulmonary schistosomiasis is caused by the upward migration of lung flukes from the mediastinum in the abdominal or thoracic cavity through the loose surrounding soft tissue of the carotid artery and into the middle fossa of the skull via the carotid canal or the superior orifice of the rupture port [10]. The brain is damaged by the mechanical or immunopathological reaction of the brain tissue as a result of migration, oviposition, and breakdown of metabolites in the brain.

Clinically, most of them are accompanied by lesions in the lungs and other sites. Patients have a history of chronic cough or pulmonary schistosomiasis, and pulmonary schistosome eggs can be found in sputum or cerebrospinal fluid. Peripheral blood eosinophil sorting and absolute counts and cerebrospinal fluid sorting counts were significantly elevated, and the skin test for lung schistosome antigen was positive.

14.2.2 Pathological Manifestations

Child and adult worms of cerebral lung flukes penetrate and reside in the brain, causing mechanical damage to the tissue, damaging the blood vessels, and leading to brain tissue oozing and infarction [11] and fibrinous inflammation. The lesions first invade the temporal lobe and migrate to the parietal and occipital lobes and are mostly located deep in the white matter of the brain in these areas. There are three stages according to the course of the lesion.

1. Tissue destruction period. The worm migrates through the brain tissue and causes tunnel damage or linear hemorrhage, and the worm stays in the brain and destroys tissue, forming cave-like lesions and causing surrounding inflammatory reactions.
2. Granuloma or cystic stage. Higher egg deposition causes granuloma and foreign body giant cellularity reaction with surrounding connective tissue hyperplasia and inflammatory cell infiltration. The central tissue of the lesion is necrotic and liquefied. This cyst-like lesion is often multiply connected and interconnected by irregular tunnels.
3. Fibrous scar phase. When the worm dies or wanders away, the material in the cystic cavity is gradually absorbed, the eggs die and are calcified, and the cystic wall is gradually thickened and fibrotic and has calcium deposits. All of these stages can occur simultaneously, and eventually the lesions mechanize to form a scar and the brain parenchyma atrophies.

14.2.3 Imaging

1. CT findings: the plain scan shows large patches of hypodense areas, often accompanied by varying degrees of multiple irregular hemorrhagic changes; the enhanced scan shows aggregated multiple ring-enhancing lesions with peripheral edema [12, 13].
2. MRI findings: (1) irregular edematous areas in the white matter of the brain, such as the temporal lobe or occipito-parietal lobe, with varying degrees of central hemorrhagic changes; (2) after the hemorrhage is absorbed, the central part of the abnormal edematous area may show "tunnel"-like changes of long T_1 and long T_2 signals; (3) enhanced scans may show "tunnel signs" of variable length in different directions, with enhancement on both sides but no central enhancement. The "tunneling sign," with enhancement on both sides and no central enhancement, is often seen on perpendicular scans with multiple clustered ring-shaped foci of enhancement (Fig. 14.4) [13].

14.2.4 Diagnostic Key Points

1. History of living in infected areas, eating raw crabs and drinking raw water from infected waters.
2. Patients have a history of chronic cough or pulmonary schistosomiasis, and pulmonary schistosome eggs can be found in sputum or cerebrospinal fluid.

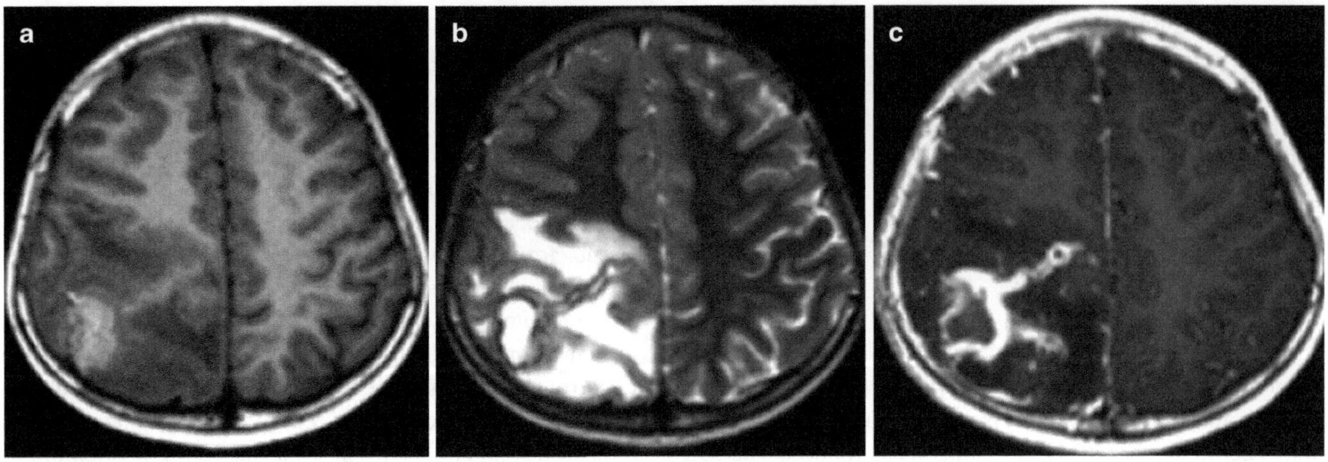

Fig. 14.4 Right frontoparietal cerebral pulmonary schistosomiasis. (**a**) T_1WI shows a low signal "tunnel"; (**b**) T_2WI shows a high signal "tunnel" with irregular surrounding edema; (**c**) T_1WI enhancement shows no central enhancement of the tunnel and the lesion is aggregated with multiple rings of unequal size

3. Cranial CT or MRI shows multiple, irregular intracerebral lesions and hemorrhage, which, if accompanied by the "tunnel sign," appears on enhancement as a cluster of multiple ring-enhancing lesions with peripheral edema.
4. Peripheral blood eosinophil sorting and absolute counts and cerebrospinal fluid sorting counts were significantly elevated, and the skin test for lung schistosome antigen was positive.

14.2.5 Differential Diagnosis

1. Cerebral cysticercosis. It appears to be a multifocal cystic lesion. Eccentric growths of cephalic nodes are seen in the cystic cavity, and the cephalic nodes are often calcified. The edema around the lesion is relatively mild and may not be enhanced or mildly circumferentially enhanced on enhanced scans.
2. High-grade astrocytoma. It usually combines with cystic degeneration and necrosis to cause wreath-shaped enhancement, the central necrosis is often incomplete, with loofah-like changes and high signal in the circular enhancement area DWI, and hemorrhage is rare.
3. Brain metastases. It is prone to necrosis and cystic degeneration, and the enhancement pattern is mostly circumferential enhancement. However, brain metastases tend to occur in middle-aged and elderly patients. Most of the patients have a history of primary malignant tumor, and they are often multiple foci. Some of the lesions with circumferential enhancement are not smooth, and nodules can be seen in the attached wall.
4. Tuberculous granuloma. Single or multiple caseous necrotizing granulomas are seen in the brain, with small circular enhancement or compartmentalized signs after enhancement. In the case of combined meningeal granuloma, cast or multiple nodular cluster-like enhancement along the subarachnoid space and hydrocephalus are characteristic signs after enhancement.
5. Lesions with hemorrhage need to be differentiated from cerebrovascular malformation brain. The characteristic manifestation of vascular malformation on MRI is a mass-like or foveal vascular flow-void shadow, CTA and MRA can directly show the blood supplying arteries and draining veins of cerebral vascular malformation, and DSA is the gold standard test for the diagnosis of cerebral vascular malformation.

14.2.6 Status and Progress of Research

MRI, CT, and X-ray can be used to examine for cerebral pulmonary schistosomiasis, with CT and MRI predominating.

CT and X-ray may show indirect signs such as calcification of brain-type pulmonary schistosomiasis but is of limited diagnostic value for specific intracranial lesions. MRI has high soft tissue resolution, and its multi-sequence and multimodal examination can provide a lot of information for localization and qualitative and even quantitative diagnosis of cerebral pulmonary schistosomiasis; in particular, SWI is valuable for the demonstration of mechanical injury, hemorrhage, and sinus tracts caused by pulmonary schistosomiasis. There are case reports of brain-type pulmonary schistosome abscess cavities showing significant low signal on DWI and high signal on ADC indicating unrestricted spread, suggesting that DWI is useful in identifying brain abscesses caused by pulmonary schistosomiasis abscesses with those caused by septic brain abscesses or necrotizing brain tumors, providing some confidence [14].

14.3 Cerebral Sparganosis

Hanqiu Liu, Weiwei Wang, Xuening Zhang, and Longlin Yin

14.3.1 Overview

Cerebral sparganosis (cerebral sparganosis mansoni) is a disease caused by infection with the second-stage larvae of the cestode *Mannheimia mansoni* [15]. The life history of *Cestoda mansoni* is as follows: adult worms are parasitic in the intestinal tract of cats and dogs, and their eggs are excreted in the feces. They hatch into larvae in contaminated water; then the larvae are ingested by cyclops and continue to develop into protozoa. The protozoa are parasitized through the food chain in frogs, snakes, and other wildlife. The majority of patients with lymphatic larvae are young adults, and the routes of infection are broadly three species [16]. (1) Apply raw frog meat or snakeskin directly to the wound. (2) Swallow raw or undercooked frog meat. (3) Drink raw water contaminated with this procercoid. Through these three pathways, larvae can infect humans through the skin of wounds, mucous membranes, or the digestive tract. The risk of human parasitism is much greater than that of adult larvae, which can invade any part of the body because of the tissue damage they cause as they migrate. Serological parasite antibody test: positive IgG antibody to cerebral schistosoma confirms the diagnosis.

14.3.2 Pathological Manifestations

The larval state and migration of the larvae in the human body cause mechanical damage to the body tissues and induce an immune response in the local organism, resulting in the formation of eosinophilic granulomas. The larvae were scattered with concentric round or oval limelets and single muscle fibers; the tunnel or cyst wall consisted of granulation tissue, with the outermost layer being fibrous tissue. There are multiple small abscesses of varying ages in the brain [17].

14.3.3 Imaging

The lesions are mainly distributed in the cerebral hemispheres, especially in the frontal and parietal lobes. It occasionally involves the capsula externa, capsula interna, and basal ganglia, and the cerebellum is rarely involved. The cerebellum is rarely involved, and about 1/4 of the lesions occur bilaterally. "Tunnel sign," "knot sign," and "wandering" are the three main imaging features of cerebral schistosomiasis.

1. CT findings: patches of old and new hypodense foci are seen in the white matter of the brain, and areas of old lesions are accompanied by enlargement of the adjacent ventricles and sulci. New lesions with marked edema and irregular or nodular enhancement on enhanced scans; sometimes, small pinpoint calcifications are present.
2. MRI findings: (1) mixed-signal in the focal area, visible around irregular areas of white matter edema of varying severity can be seen; FLAIR may show old and new lesions; the abnormal signal in the shape of bars or tubes, track-like changes, and enhancement of the edge of the tube wall reinforcement, shaped like a tunnel, cross-sectional small ring reinforcement, called "tunnel sign." (2) Enhanced scans show multiple rings, loops, and irregular twisted foci of enhancement, similar to "knot-like" enhancement (Fig. 14.5) [18] in areas with significant edema. (3) Dynamic observation of imaging data at different stages, the location and morphology of lesion enhancement can change, suggesting a migratory charac-

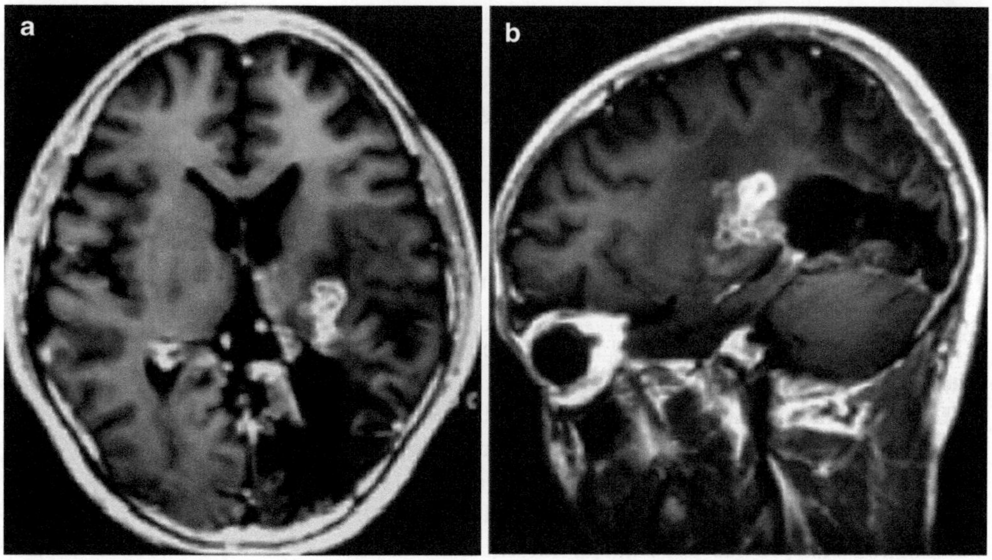

Fig. 14.5 Single schizothorax in the left ventricular triangle. (**a**, **b**) T_1WI enhancement of the left posterior horn of the lateral ventricle shows multiple rings, loops, and irregularly twisted foci of enhancement, similar to "knot-like" enhancement, surrounded by edema with low signal and soft foci of non-enhancement, suggesting that the lesion is displaced forward from the left occipital lobe (axial, sagittal)

ter, also called "wandering," suggesting that the larvae are still alive [19, 20]. (4) Negative occupancy effects. The focal occupancy effect is generally milder than that of the tumor, with a negative occupancy effect in later stages, partial tissue fibrosis, dilatation of the adjacent ventricles, and limited brain atrophy; this sign can be an important basis for differentiation from other brain tumors [21].

14.3.4 Diagnostic Key Points

1. It is common in young adults, living in areas with a dense water network, with a history of raw river and pond water, aquatic products, or frog or snake meat; the disease is prolonged, sometimes mild and sometimes severe, with variable symptoms; the foci are characterized by migration or multiple occurrences; history of parasitism in other parts of the body, such as the eye or subcutaneous schistosomes.
2. The "tunnel sign," "knot sign," and "wandering" are the three main imaging features of cerebral lissencephaly.
3. With a serological parasite antibody test, positive IgG antibodies can confirm the disease.

14.3.5 Differential Diagnosis

1. Bacterial brain abscess. Brain abscess in the cellulitis stage, showing multiple rings or compartments are separated and altered, and the enhancing polycyclic foci are mostly rings against rings and rarely form rings over rings, i.e., knotted. In contrast, the enhanced rings of the schizothoracic larvae are smaller and are multiple small rings set together.
2. Cerebral cysticercosis is often a multiple cystic lesion, with degenerating cerebral sacs caused by worm lesions that show ring enhancement, but not the ring-over-ring sign.
3. Tuberculous granuloma. Single or multiple with caseous necrotizing granulomas are seen in the brain, which tend to show small circular enhancement after enhancement or signs of compartmentalization.
4. High-grade astrocytomas show wreath-like enhancement because of frequent combined cystic changes and necrosis, and central necrosis is often incomplete, with filumi-noid changes rather than ring-over-ring changes.

14.3.6 Status and Progress of Research

MRI, CT, and X-rays can be used to examine for cerebral Mann's lytic disease, with CT and MRI predominating.

The X-ray may show indirect signs such as calcification of cerebral Mannich's disease but is of limited diagnostic value for specific intracranial lesions. MRI has high soft-tissue resolution, and its multisequence and multimodal examination can provide a wealth of information for the localization, characterization, and even quantitative diagnosis of cerebral Mann's lymphadenopathy. Although it is difficult for MRS to distinguish malignant tumors from granulomatous lesions, neurocysticercosis shows alanine peaks at 1.4 ppm and 1.8 ppm, with some degree of differential diagnosis [22].

References

1. do Amaral LL, Ferreira RM, da Rocha AJ, et al. Neurocysticercosis: evaluation with advanced magnetic resonance techniques and atypical forms. Top Magn Reson Imaging. 2005;16(2):127–44.
2. Guo Z, Yue Q, Guo Z, et al. A study of the relationship between epilepsy due to brain cysticerci and imaging and survival status of cysticercus. J Brain Neurol Disord. 2000;8(2):101–3.
3. Zhang C, Yang Q, Ouyang T, et al. Brain parenchymal cysts CT manifestations in relation to epilepsy. Chin J Clin Med Imaging. 2005;16(4):181.
4. Chang KH, Lee JH, Han MC. The role of contrast-enhanced MR imaging in the diagnosis of neurocysticercosis. Am J Neuroradiol. 1991;12:509–12.
5. Zhang Y, Cheng JL, Yang YJ, et al. Magnetic resonance imaging diagnosis of ventricular-type cysticercosis. J Clin Radiol. 2005;24(6):484–7.
6. Silbert PL, Gubbay SS, Khangure M. Distinctive MRI findings in a case of neurocysticercosis. Med J Aust. 1993;3:185–6.
7. Nalini A, de Souza A, Saini J, et al. Quantitative serial T_2 relaxometry: a prospective evaluation in solitary cerebral cysticercosis. Neuroradiol J. 2014;27(3):339–49.
8. de Souza A, Nalini A, Saini J, et al. T_2 relaxometry helps prognosticate seizure outcome in patients with solitary cerebral cysticercosis. J Neurol Sci. 2017;376:1–6.
9. Zhang QS, Hu JZ, Li LL, et al. A survey and analysis of pulmonary schistosomiasis infection in rural populations in mountainous areas. Pract Prev Med. 2007;14(6):1795–6.
10. Shen TC, Chen SR, Wu EH, et al. Neuroimaging. Shanghai: Shanghai Science and Technology Press; 2004.
11. Yang G. Pathology. Beijing: People's Health Press; 2002.
12. Zhang GY, Ren XF, Yang RH, et al. 5 Head of a case of cerebral-type schistosomiasis CT dynamic observation. Chin J Parasitol Parasit Dis. 1999;17(6):398.
13. Cha SH, Chang KH, Cho SY, et al. Cerebral paragonimiasis in early active stage: CT and MR features. Am J Roentgenol. 1994;162(1):141–5.
14. Xia Y, Chen J, Ju Y, et al. Characteristic CT and MR imaging findings of cerebral paragonimiasis. J Neuroradiol. 2016;43(3):200–6.
15. Fan KJ, Pezeshkpour GH. Cerebral sparganosis. Neurology. 1986;36(9):1249–51.
16. Wu Z, Yan C, Qiu X, et al. Investigation of frog lymphatic larvae infection in farmers' markets in Guiyang city and 104 clinical case analysis of. J Guiyang Med Coll. 2007;32(2):140–1.
17. Tsai MD, Chang CN, Ho YS, et al. Cerebral sparganosis diognosed and treated with stereotactic technique. J Neurosurg. 1993;78(1):129–32.
18. Lv T, Li K, Chen H. Characteristic MRI manifestations of cerebral Mannichia. Chin J Med Comput Imaging. 2007;13(2):78–80.
19. Chang KH, Chi JG, Cho SY, et al. Cerebral sparganosis: analysis of 34 cases with emphasis on CT features. Neuroradiology. 1992;34(1):1–8.
20. Gong C, Wang X, Liu H, et al. MRI of cerebral schistosomiasis diagnosis. Chin J Radiol. 2006;40(9):913–7.
21. Ding Y, Jian L. CT, MRI diagnosis of cerebral schistosomiasis. Jiangxi Sci. 2017;35(5):698–701.
22. Pandit S, Lin A, Gahbauer H, et al. MR spectroscopy in neurocysticercosis. J Comput Assist Tomogr. 2001;25(6):950–2.

Intracranial Spirochete Infection (Lyme Disease)

15

Yongxiao You, Yan Wang, and Wenxiao Jia

15.1 Overview

Lyme disease is a tick-borne natural focus disease caused by infection of *Borrelia burgdorferi*, also known as Lyme borreliosis [1], named for the widespread occurrence of juvenile idiopathic arthritis in 1975 in Lyme, Connecticut, USA. The disease can involve multiple organs and systems, with the skin, joints throughout the body, the heart and the central nervous system being the most prominent [2]. The disease usually develops in summer and early autumn, and the population is generally susceptible, with slightly more males than females, mostly young adults, and a higher rate of infection among field workers and forestry workers. The disease was first discovered in 1985 in the forest area of Heilongjiang Province, China.

The incubation period for Lyme disease is 3–32 days, with an average of 7 days. When a tick bites a person, the spirochete enters the microvasculature of the human skin by refluxing into the sucking cavity, where it enters the bloodstream and travels to various organs and tissues throughout the body.

Lyme disease is clinically divided into three phases, which may occur sequentially or overlap. Stage I is the skin damage phase, characterized by wandering erythema, usually in the axillae, thighs, groin, and other areas, lasting about 7 days, and may fade on its own without treatment. The most typical neurological symptoms are meningitis, cerebral neuritis, and radiculitis after the erythema has subsided, and atrioventricular block is the most common cardiac symptom. The bladder biopsy may show spirochetes. Stage III is a period of persistent infection, dominated by arthritis, chronic atrophic limb dermatitis, and advanced neurological manifestations.

Laboratory tests. Specimens of the patient's synovial membrane, skin, lymph nodes, and other tissues and cerebrospinal fluid are taken and examined with silver stain or dark field, allowing for a rapid pathogenic diagnosis, but the detection rate is low. The application of specific direct fluorescent antibody staining provides lesion detection rates. Detection of specific antibodies or *Borrelia* spirochetes from infected tissue or body fluids can confirm the diagnosis.

15.2 Pathological Manifestations

The main pathological changes of *Borrelia* spirochetes brain infection are demyelination of the white matter of the brain, meningitis, and in late stages, brain atrophy with cerebral nerve invasion as the characteristic manifestation.

Lyme disease is divided into three phases. Stage I is dominated by localized primary skin damage with plasma cell and lymphocyte infiltration around the superficial and deep vessels of the damaged skin, the presence of wandering erythema, microscopic thickening of the skin, mild keratinization with mononuclear cell infiltration, and edema of the epidermis without septic or granulomatous reaction. After the spirochete enters the blood circulation and travels to the tissues and organs and causes infection, it enters stage II, where the central nervous system is predominant and nerve damage may be caused by retrograde invasion of nerve roots along the peripheral nerves from the site of infection. Infection plays an important role in stage I and II neuro-Lyme disease, where patients have serum cultures of *Borrelia* spirochetes, which stimulate macrophage production of various cytokines

Y. You
Beijing Shunyi Maternal and Child Health Hospital, Beijing, China

Y. Wang
People's Hospital of Xinjiang Uygur Autonomous Region, Urumqi, China

W. Jia (✉)
The First Affiliated Hospital of Xinjiang Medical University, Urumqi, China

H. Li et al. (eds.), *Radiology of Infectious and Inflammatory Diseases - Volume 1*,
https://doi.org/10.1007/978-981-99-0039-8_15

such as interleukin-1 due to the multiple biological activities of spirochete lipopolysaccharide as an endotoxin (IL-l), with mononuclear cell infiltration around the blood vessels of the brain parenchyma and in the brain nerves (especially the facial, oculogyric and adductor nerves). Stage III neuro-Lyme disease occurs as a result of the body's immune response to *Borrelia* spirochetes, with increased immune complexes in the patient's blood, low activity of suppressor T cells, and increased naïve responses against specific antigens and lymphocytes in the cerebrospinal fluid (CSF). There is lymphocytic infiltration around the vessels in the neuropathy, thickening of the vessel walls, demyelination of the nerves, and proliferation of collagen fibers. In this stage, proliferative erosive synovitis, synovial villous hypertrophy with vascularization, fibrin deposition, and mononuclear cell infiltration are seen at the joint. There were also varying degrees of erosive destruction of bone and cartilage, as well as skin depigmentation, atrophy, or thickened, closely aligned bundles of collagenous fibrous tissue, similar to scleroderma damage and atrophic acrodermatitis [3].

15.3 Imaging

15.3.1 CT Findings

Most lesions are not abnormal on CT. Multiple or fused cases appear on the surface of the brain or around deep vessels. Patchy cerebral white matter demyelinating lesions appear as multiple patchy or large hypodense lesions on CT, some of which may have abnormal enhancement on enhanced scans, and some cases may have abnormal meningeal enhancement.

15.3.2 MRI Findings

It shows intracerebral parenchymal changes mainly in the bilateral periventricular and/or subcortical multiple diameters 2–3 mm patchy lesion, lesion T_1WI with low signal or isosignal (Fig. 15.1a), T_2WI with high signal (Fig. 15.1b), FLAIR with high signal (Fig. 15.1c), mostly without occu-

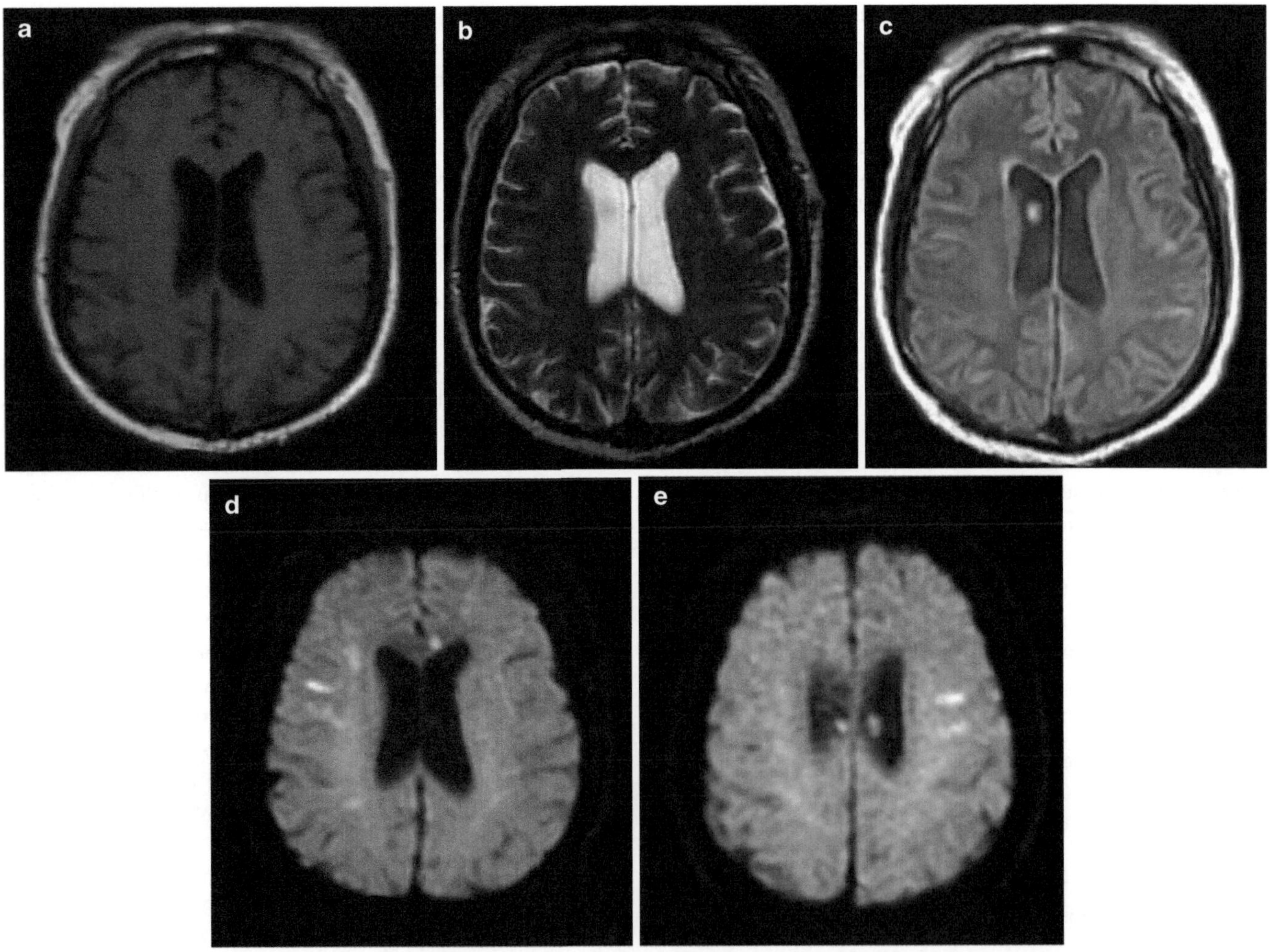

Fig. 15.1 Lyme disease. (**a**) T_1WI shows multiple patches of isosignal or slightly low signal around the lateral ventricles bilaterally; (**b**) T_2WI shows a slightly high signal; (**c**) FLAIR shows a high signal; (**d**, **e**) DWI shows a high signal, and the lesions are mostly vertically aligned with the ventricles. (Image courtesy of Wang Yan, People's Hospital of Xinjiang Uygur Autonomous Region)

pancy effect. Lesions are also seen in the basal ganglia and brainstem. In typical cases, the lesion is often located bilaterally next to the lateral ventricles and is aligned mostly perpendicular to the ventricles (Fig. 15.1d, e). There are often no signs of periventricular white matter involvement in the proximal ventricles. The lesions in the brain parenchyma show patchy enhancement on enhanced scans, and in some cases, there may be abnormal meningeal enhancement on enhancement. Enhancement of the nerve roots may suggest radiculitis and, in advanced stages, cerebral atrophy. MRV may show venous stenosis. Abnormal reinforcement of the meninges and nerve roots is important in the diagnosis of Lyme disease [4].

15.4 Diagnostic Key Points

1. Prevalent in young adults with a history of exposure to infected areas and a history of exposure or tick bites.
2. The presence of characteristic chronic wandering erythema in a patient with lesions larger than 10 cm in diameter is highly suggestive of the disease.
3. Typical cases often present as multiple round-like patchy lesions (diameter 2–3 mm) bilaterally adjacent to the lateral ventricles, aligned mostly perpendicular to the ventricles.
4. The lesions in the brain parenchyma showed patchy enhancement after an enhanced scan. Abnormal reinforcement of the meninges and nerve roots is important in the diagnosis of Lyme disease.
5. Detection of specific antibodies or *Borrelia* spirochetes from infected tissue or body fluids can confirm the diagnosis.

15.5 Differential Diagnosis

Lyme disease is a human-animal disease caused by *Borrelia* spirochetes. *Borrelia* spirochetes can cause damage to multiple systems and organs in humans, causing disability and even death in severe cases. Lyme disease needs to be differentiated from multiple sclerosis, progressive multifocal leukoencephalopathy, and acute disseminated encephalomyelitis.

1. **Multiple sclerosis (MS)** and Lyme disease can both manifest pathologically as demyelinating changes in the white matter of the brain. Multiple sclerosis is more common in young women, with no apparent precipitating factor, whereas Lyme disease is more common in young adult males, with a history of prior exposure to infected areas and a history of exposure or tick bites, and early visible wandering erythema of the skin. Multiple sclerosis is characterized by multiple round-like lesions in the paraventricular white matter with a perpendicular distribution to the ventricles, typically showing a "right-angle demyelination sign," whereas Lyme disease lesions are often located bilaterally next to the lateral ventricles, mostly vertically aligned with the ventricles, but less pronounced than in multiple sclerosis; multiple 2–3 mm patchy lesions of bilateral lateral ventricles and/or subcortical diameter, less large than in multiple sclerosis, with halo edema shadows visible around them, often without adjacent periventricular white matter involvement. Abnormal enhancement is seen in patchy lesions on enhanced scans. Multiple sclerosis is usually without abnormal enhancement of meninges and nerve roots, whereas Lyme disease may be accompanied by abnormal enhancement of meninges and may have characteristic abnormal enhancement of nerve roots, and it is not difficult to distinguish between the two.
2. **Progressive multifocal leukoencephalopathy**. Subacute demyelinating disease of the central nervous system in a hypoenergetic state is strongly associated with exposure to the JC virus, whereas Lyme disease has a history of exposure in an infected area and a history of exposure or tick bites, with early visible wandering erythema of the skin. Imaging manifestations. The lesions are found in the subcortical white matter of the parieto-occipital area, far from the periventricular area, with an asymmetric distribution, and there is a tendency for the lesions to gradually fuse and increase in size. Multiple small subcortical patchy lesions (diameter 2–3 mm), smaller lesions compared to PML, and patchy enhancement are seen on enhanced scans. There is generally no abnormal enhancement of meninges or nerve roots, whereas Lyme disease may be distinguished by abnormal enhancement of meninges, which may be accompanied by characteristic abnormal enhancement of nerve roots.
3. **Acute disseminated encephalomyelitis (ADEM)** is prevalent in children, often with a history of infection or vaccination prior to onset, while Lyme disease has a history of epidemic areas and exposure or tick bite, with visible wandering skin erythema in the early stage. ADEM is a diffuse multifocal CNS demyelinating disease with predominantly white matter invasion; imaging manifests as multiple patchy lesions with small peripheral edema and insignificant occupying effects, mild enhancement or circumferential enhancement on enhanced scans, or no significant abnormal enhancement, whereas intracerebral parenchymal changes in Lyme disease mainly manifest as bilateral lateral periventricular and/or subcortical Multiple 2–3 mm patchy lesions with halo edema shadows visible around them, often without adjacent periventricular white matter involvement. There are mostly manifestations of spinal cord involvement, whereas Lyme

disease can be associated with abnormal meningeal enhancement and can have characteristic abnormal nerve root enhancement, and the two manifestations are different and easily distinguished.

15.6 Status and Progress of Research

In recent years, with the rise of various new MRI techniques and the popularity of clinical use, the efficiency of MRI diagnosis and differential diagnosis has been greatly improved.

CT and MRI can be used for Lyme disease, but MRI is predominant. MRI has high soft tissue resolution, and its multisequence, multimodal examination can provide a wealth of useful information for localization, characterization, and even quantification of Lyme disease. MR perfusion imaging includes dynamic magnetic sensitive enhanced perfusion and dynamic contrast-enhanced perfusion, and the latter can provides information about hemodynamics and vascular permeability. MR Diffusion-related techniques (including diffusion-weighted imaging, diffusion tensor imaging, etc.) can provide information on the diffusion of water molecules within the lesion and the travel of white matter fiber tracts in the brain. SWI can provide calcification and hemorrhage within the lesion.

References

1. Fallon BA, Levin ES, Schweitzer PJ, et al. Inflammation and central nervous system Lyme disease. Neurobiol Dis. 2010;37(3):534–41.
2. Hildenbrand P. Lyme neuroborreliosis: manifestations of a rapidly emerging zoonosis. Am J Neuroradiol. 2009;30(6):1079–87.
3. Hongjun L. Practical infectious disease imaging. Beijing: People's Health Press; 2014.
4. Agarwal R, Sze G. Neuro-Lyme disease: MR imaging findings. Radiology. 2009;253(1):167–73.

Intracranial Rickettsial Infection

16

Fei Dong, Jiaying Tang, and Pingfeng Dai

16.1 Overview

Rickettsial infection of the brain is an infection resulting from the invasion of the central nervous system by Rickettsia. Rickettsia is a group of Gram-negative, strictly intracellular parasitic prokaryotic microorganisms that use arthropods (ticks, lice, fleas, mites, etc.) as vectors of transmission. There are more than 30 known species of Rickettsia, and the prevalence of rickettsial disease is distinctly regional and seasonal due to the different geographical distribution and activity times of the various arthropods that are vectors of Rickettsia. The more common rickettsial diseases in the country include epidemic typhus, endemic typhus, tsutsugamushi disease, and Q fever.

The clinical manifestations of Rickettsia infection include sudden onset of high fever, malaise, generalized pain, facial and conjunctival congestion, and other signs of generalized toxemia. About 90% of patients have hemorrhagic macules, 70%–100% of patients with scrub typhus may develop scab or ulcers, and most patients may develop splenomegaly, and a few have hepatomegaly. Also, 12%–28% of patients with rickettsial disease can develop neurologic infections, with the most common type of patient in this group being rickettsial infection (i.e., Rocky Mountain typhus), and approximately 80% of patients with neurologic rickettsial infections have a definite history of arthropod bites. Neurological infections mainly manifest as encephalitis and meningitis, the most prominent manifestation of which is persistent severe headache, in addition to dizziness, insomnia, tinnitus and hearing loss, and even unresponsiveness, delirium, mania, tremors, convulsions, opisthotonos, muscle rigidity and signs of meningeal irritation [1–8].

Currently, indirect fluorescent antibody testing is the method of choice for the diagnosis of rickettsial infection. However, there is still a lack of better laboratory methods for early diagnosis of the disease [2].

16.2 Pathological Manifestations

The direct damage to endothelial cells and the release of endotoxin by Rickettsia will cause systemic microcirculatory disorders and clinical signs of tissue and organ damage. Intracranial infections mainly involve the brain and meninges, with gross specimens showing brain edema, sometimes visible as subcortical hemorrhagic spots [2, 5, 9].

The basic lesion of rickettsial infection is small-vessel vasculitis, which can be seen microscopically as diffuse "typhus nodules" around small vessels, i.e., proliferative, thrombotic, necrotizing vasculitis and surrounding inflammatory cell infiltration resulting in rickettsial granulomas. There is severe degeneration of the vessels in the center of the lesion, with swelling of the endothelium, obstruction of the lumen, and small focal necrosis visible due to embolization of small arteries [2].

16.3 Imaging

16.3.1 CT Findings

Due to rickettsial infection followed by a major invasion of small vessel and capillary endothelial cells, the imaging presentation is a terminal arterial infarct-like lesion. When the lesion involves the brain parenchyma, cranial CT plain scan may be unremarkable in some cases, and poorly defined hypodense foci with/without diffuse brain swelling are seen when the lesion is significant, and the lesion has no obvious

F. Dong · P. Dai (✉)
The Second Affiliated Hospital of School of Medicine, Zhejiang University, Hangzhou, China
e-mail: dongfei@zju.edu.cn

J. Tang
The First Affiliated Hospital of Xinjiang Medical University, Urumqi, China

H. Li et al. (eds.), *Radiology of Infectious and Inflammatory Diseases - Volume 1*,
https://doi.org/10.1007/978-981-99-0039-8_16

occupying effect. When the lesion involves the meninges, swelling of the adjacent cerebral cortex may occur due to inflammatory stimulation; CT scan shows narrowing of the cerebral sulcus, cerebral fissure, and cerebral pool, and enhanced scan shows thickening of the meninges [5, 6, 9].

In rare patients with hypercoagulability due to inflammatory stimulation, intracranial venous thrombosis may occur. CT scan direct signs include striations and high-density triangles in the involved veins (sinuses); indirect signs include cerebral edema, ischemic infarcts, hemorrhagic infarcts, ventricular obstruction, or obstructive hydrocephalus in the corresponding venous/venous sinus drainage areas; CTV may show intraventricular sinus thrombus in the form of filling defect-like lesions, with characteristic empty triangle sign seen in superior sagittal sinus thrombosis.

16.3.2 MRI Findings

Lesions in brain parenchyma showed patchy iso or slightly hyperintense with unclear boundary on T1WI and slightly hyperintense or hyperintense on T2WI, which may involve the lobes, subcortical white matter, cerebellar peduncle, corpus callosum, and cerebral bridge [6]; after the enhanced scan, some lesions may have speckle/patch. The enhancement of some lesions may be patchy, suggesting the presence of vascular damage [5].

In combination with intracranial venous thrombosis, at the early stage, normal vascular flow void disappeared on T1WI, with iso T_1 and short T_2 vascular filling shadow; 1–2 weeks after increased methemoglobin, T_1WI and T_2WI is high signal; MRV examination reveals a filling defect in the involved venous/sinus.

16.3.3 Digital Subtraction Angiography

The essential lesion of Rickettsia infection is small vessel vasculitis, mainly involving small arteries, microscopic arteries, and capillaries, so angiography may be negative. When a patient has a combination of intracranial venous sinus thrombosis, DSA is the gold standard for confirming the diagnosis, but it is not advantageous for diagnosing simple cortical vein thrombosis, so DSA is usually used when the diagnosis cannot be confirmed after other tests are completed or when concurrent transcatheter drug therapy is required.

16.4 Diagnostic Key Points

1. Most have a clear history of arthropod bites in the infected area.
2. The lesions are found in the terminal arterial supply area, predominantly in the basal ganglia region.
3. Lesions may be single or multiple. The lesion manifest as hypodense on CT plain scan. MR plain scan shows iso/hypointensity on T_1WI and hyperintensity on T_2WI, and some lesions may have patchy like enhancement on the enhanced scan.
4. DWI sequence lesion shows a high signal.
5. On cerebrospinal fluid examination, lymphocytosis and mildly elevated cerebrospinal fluid protein levels are observed.
6. Indirect fluorescent antibody tests are of great value in the diagnosis of rickettsial infections.

16.5 Differential Diagnosis

Rickettsia infection in the brain is relatively rare, and the CT and MRI plain scan presentations lack specificity; its qualitative diagnosis mainly relies on history, physical signs, and laboratory tests of cerebrospinal fluid. Cerebral rickettsial infections need to be differentiated from vasculitis, multiple lacunar cerebral infarcts, and metastases.

1. **Vasculitis.** The vast majority of patients with cerebral vasculitis have neurological imaging abnormalities, the most common manifestation being extensive cortical and white matter damage, which may involve unilateral or bilateral hemispheres or may be disseminated, with soft meningeal enhancement on enhanced scans, wall enhancement of the involved vessels on high-resolution MR angiography, and positive findings on DSA in approximately 60% of patients, mainly manifesting as multiple alternating stenoses and dilatations of blood vessels. In contrast, vasculitis due to rickettsial infection mainly involves small arteries, microscopic arteries and capillaries, and therefore CT, MR angiography, or DSA examinations may be negative.
2. **Multiple lacunar cerebral infarction.** Most often, cases are seen in 50 years and older. Patients present with comorbid hyperlipidemia, atherosclerosis, hypertension, or diabetes. The lesions are caused by occlusion of deep cerebral penetrating branches, so the lesions are mostly located in the centrum semiovale, the white matter around the lateral ventricles, and the internal capsule of basal ganglia but can also occur in the brainstem. CT lesions are hypointense on the plain scan; small CT lesions are difficult to detect on the plain scan. Lesions show iso or hypointense on MR T1WI and hyperintense on T_2WI; recent lesions may have restricted diffusion on DWI and mild enhancement. The above imaging presentation is similar to that of rickettsial infection, but the latter usually has a history of exposure to the infected area or tick, lice, or mite bites, and the majority of patients present with fever and rash, which can be used to differentiate between the two.

3. **Intracranial metastases** are often multiple, varying in size, and prone to necrosis. CT scan is hypointense. MR examination shows that T_1WI lesion is equivocal/hyposignal, T_2WI is high signal, enhanced scan is mostly accompanied by enhancement, and the lesion with necrosis is circumferentially enhanced; however, intracranial metastasis tumors tend to occur in middle-aged and elderly people with a history of extracranial tumors. Intracranial lesions of rickettsial infection with necrosis are rare and show mild patchy enhancement on enhanced scans; since rickettsial infection usually presents with significant fever and rash, it is not difficult to differentiate the two with the history.

16.6 Status and Progress of Research

Currently, CT and MR examinations are commonly used for cerebral rickettsial infections. About 20% of patients have imaging abnormalities, and patients with normal MRI presentations usually have a better prognosis. Because of the good soft-tissue resolution of MRI, routine MR examination can be the examination of choice for the diagnosis and follow-up of this disease; although CT has less soft-tissue resolution than MR, it can be the examination of choice for the screening of intracranial disease. DSA is not the test of choice for this disease, but in combination with intracranial venous sinus thrombosis, DSA may provide some diagnostic information. The main aspects of advances in imaging research include the following.

1. **Magnetic resonance diffusion-weighted imaging (DWI)**. With intracranial infection in the early stage of the lesion, DWI shows a high signal and ADC shows a low signal; when the lesion involves the corpus callosum pressure, it may show the characteristic "boomerang sign"; If there is DWI high signal in the brain parenchyma in addition to the corpus callosum pressure, it is called "boomerang superimposed sign" [3].
2. **Magnetic resonance magnetic sensitivity imaging (SWI)**. It's less commonly used for intracranial rickettsial infection. On examination of Rickettsia infection, when subcortical hemorrhage is present, the corresponding areas are seen as speckled low signal on SWI due to iron-containing heme deposition, providing diagnostic information for microhemorrhages.

References

1. Miller JR, Jubelt B. Bacterial infections in Merritt's neurology. 10th ed. Philadelphia: Lippincott Williams & Wilkins; 2000.
2. Moy WL, Ooi ST. Case report: abducens nerve palsy and meningitis by Rickettsia typhi. Am J Trop Med Hyg. 2015;92(3):620–4.
3. Mathew T, Badachi S, Sarma GRK. Boomerang plus sign in Rickettsial encephalitis. Pediatr Neurol. 2016;56(88):89.
4. Huntington MK, Allison J, Nair D. Emerging vector-borne disease. Am Fam Physician. 2016;94(7):551–7.
5. Duque V, Ventura C, Seixas D, et al. Mediterranean spotted fever and encephalitis: a case report and review of the literature. J Infect Chemother. 2012;18(1):105–8.
6. Aliaga L, Sánchez-Blázquez P, Rodríguez-Granger J, et al. Mediterranean spotted fever and encephalitis. J Med Microbiol. 2009;58(Pt4):521–5.
7. Tzavella K, Hatzizisis IS, Vakali A, et al. Severe case of Mediterranean spotted fever in Greece with predominantly neurological features. J Med Microbiol. 2006;55(3):341–3.
8. Lindblom A, Severinson K, Nilsson K. Rickettsia felis infection in Sweden: report of two cases with subacute meningitis and review of the literature. Scand J Infect Dis. 2010;42(11/12):906–9.
9. Walker DH, Gear JH. Correlation of the distribution of Rickettsia conorii, microscopic lesions, and clinical features in South African tick bite fever. Am J Trop Med Hyg. 1985;34(2):361–71.

17 Other Types of Intracranial Infectious (Creutzfeldt–Jakob Disease)

Yongxiao You, Wenhuan Du, Jian Wang, and Yinhua Jin

17.1 Overview

Creutzfeldt–Jakob disease (CJD) is a progressive, fatal neurological disease caused by prion infection in humans, also known as cortico-striatal-spinal cord degeneration, and was reported by European neuropathologists Creutzfeldt and Jakob successively in 1920. CJD is the most common clinical type of protein particle disease, with a diverse clinical presentation, a rapidly progressive course, and a very poor prognosis. Definitive diagnosis of CJD requires pathological confirmation, but brain tissue biopsy may cause an iatrogenic infection and is generally not recommended.

CJD can be divided into sporadic (sCJD), familial (or genetic CJD, fCJD, or gCJD), iatrogenic (iCJD), and variant CJD (vCJD), most of which are sporadic in the clinic.

The age of onset of CJD is around 60 years, and the prominent clinical manifestation of early onset is abnormal mental behavior and rapidly progressive dementia, which may be related to the deposition of prions in the frontotemporal cortex, causing the involvement of higher cortical functions. It has an acute onset with blurred vision as the first symptom with unsteady gait and a subacute onset with memory loss with mental retardation as the first symptom [1], also with unsteady gait with slurred speech as the first symptom. As the disease progresses, patients exhibit increased word-finding difficulties, nominal aphasia, retelling dysfunction, alexia, and disorientation. About 20 days after onset, the patient may have language comprehension disorders, paraphasia, retelling dysfunction, logagraphia, fidgety, forced crying or laughter, and more delayed movements. At about 35 days, the patient may become reticent and can't recognize the relatives, develops comprehensive cognitive dysfunction, and walks to the right, recurrent facial and limb twitching, right upper extremity groping, strong grip syndrome, intermittent episodic myoclonus, and sucking reflexes and jaw reflexes can be elicited, and high muscle tone in the extremities is evident in the upper extremities bilaterally.

In general, patients with early CJD have a disintegration of the basic rhythm of the EEG with a high degree of rhythmical dysregulation or irregular slowing of the background brain waves; if there are periodic synchronous discharges (PSD) of medium to high amplitude on a slow wave background, this indicates CJD in an intermediate to late stage; the presence of typical periodic high amplitude sharp slow wave syndrome is then an important hint for the clinical diagnosis of CJD. Therefore, it is important to perform continuous dynamic EEG tracking in patients with suspected CJD. The presence of 14-3-3 protein in cerebrospinal fluid can also be used as an early detection marker for CJD and positive cerebrospinal fluid 14-3-3 protein has a high reference value for the diagnosis of this disease with a sensitivity and specificity of 92% or more [2].

Abnormal folding of prion protein into SC type prion protein (PrPsc), which cannot be digested by the protease K, causes large quantitative deposition of PrPsc in the brain tissue, and destroys its own nervous system, resulting in the apoptosis and loss of a wide range of nerve cells in the brain and the formation of spongiform encephalopathy. Immunohistochemistry can directly show the presence of PrPsc in brain and lymphoreticular tissue, which has a good confirmatory value.

Y. You
Beijing Shunyi Maternal and Child Health Hospital, Beijing, China

W. Du
People's Hospital of Gaochang District, Turpan, Turpan, China

J. Wang (✉)
Medical Imaging Center, First Affiliated Hospital of Xinjiang Medical University, Urumqi, China

Shanghai Universal Medical Imaging Diagnostic Center, Shanghai University, Shanghai, China

Y. Jin
Xiamen Fifth Hospital (Xiang'an Hospital of the First Affiliated Hospital of Xiamen University), Xiamen, China

H. Li et al. (eds.), *Radiology of Infectious and Inflammatory Diseases - Volume 1*,
https://doi.org/10.1007/978-981-99-0039-8_17

17.2 Pathological Manifestations

Pathological histological features of CJD: spongiform degeneration of brain tissue (including spongy changes and spongy states), atypical neuronal degeneration and deletion with astrocytic proliferation, and additional amyloid plaques. The spongiotic changes in brain tissue may be focal, with lesions often invading the cerebral cortex, striatum, parts of the thalamus, substantia nigra, cerebellum, medulla oblongata, and anterior horn of the spinal cord, often in a laminar distribution within the cortex. The lesions are bilaterally asymmetric, with the cerebral cortex and striatum being the most severe. The spongiform degeneration of CJD is not limited to superficial cells (layers I and II), but rather the underlying cells undergo changes, and the lower hippocampal gyrus and parahippocampal gyrus often lack such changes, and this feature can help in the differential diagnosis of the clinical disease. The vacuolar changes in the upper cerebral cortex are generally caused by hypoxia and metabolic disturbances. Routine tests that negate any other diagnoses can prompt diagnosis.

Light microscopy after myelin staining showed no demyelinating changes and no inflammatory cell infiltration. The cortical nerves showed macular vacuolation, a marked reduction in the number of neuronal cells, especially pyramidal cells, a high presence of lipofuscin in the cytoplasm of the remaining neuronal cells, and mild to moderate proliferation of glial cells.

Electron microscopy results showed no viral particles. There are many inflatable membrane vesicles in the nerve sensation, and some of which are visible as convoluted membrane fragments. Glial cells proliferated significantly (mainly oligodendrocytes and astrocytes). The rough endoplasmic reticulum is highly dilated and some cells contain lipofuscin. Some myelinated axons were cavitated and swollen, with partial narrowing of the capillaries.

17.3 Imaging

17.3.1 CT Findings

CT is usually unremarkable and may show progressive brain atrophy and ventricular dilatation.

17.3.2 MRI Findings

In early-stage CJD, T_2WI and FLAIR are normal. On T_2WI, CJD is mainly characterized by abnormal hyperintense in the cerebral cortex and basal ganglia and rapidly developing brain atrophy. DWI is more sensitive than T_2WI and FLAIR, and its typical MRI features are the “drifting band sign” of DWI sequence along the cortex and hyperintense in bilateral basal ganglia area. This manifestation is earlier and more sensitive than the periodic synchronous discharge of EEG, and even than the clinical signs of myoclonus and symptoms of dementia. The DWI can suggest the diagnosis of CJD before the onset of brain atrophy or abnormal T_2WI signal.

With the in-depth study of CJD, no significant differences were found between sCJD, fCJD, and iCJD in terms of imaging presentation, while sCJD and vCJD differed significantly, especially in DWI sequences. Patients with vCJD usually show a symmetrical distribution of hyperintense in the bilateral thalamic occipital nuclei on T_2WI, FLAIR, and DWI sequences, and this characteristic manifestation called the “occipital sign” [3], and hyperintensity in the dorsomedial nucleus of thalamus is called “hockey stick sign” (Fig. 17.1). While sCJD often shows symmetrical or asymmetrical hyperintense in the striatum and cerebral cortex, occipital nucleus of the thalamus also shows hyperintense, but its signal is usually lower than that of the

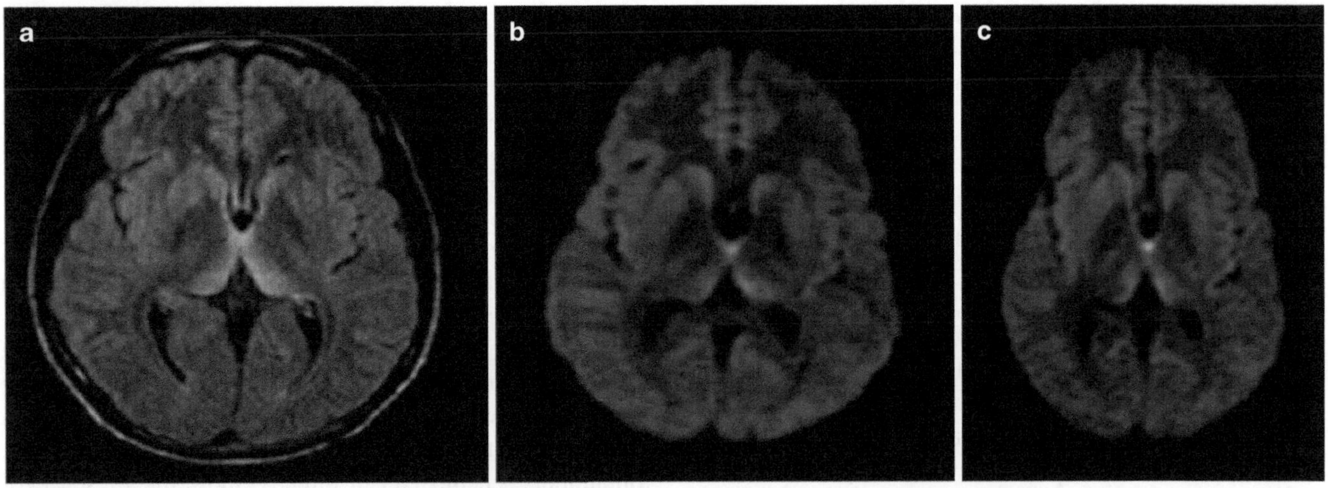

Fig. 17.1 Variant Creutzfeldt–Jakob disease. (**a**) FLAIR sequence shows hyperintense in bilateral dorsomedial thalamic nuclei and occipital nuclei of the thalamus, i.e., “hockey stick sign” and “occipital sign”; (**b**) DWI shows that the above lesions still manifest hyperintensity, with lower signal intensity than FLAIR sequence; (**c**) A review 1 months later, DWI shows abnormally hyperintense in the thalamus bilaterally and further elevated signal in the occipital nucleus of the thalamus

striatum. The early stage of sCJD is characterized by a band-like hyperintensity along the cortical sulcus ("drifting band sign") and abnormal hyperintensity in the bilateral basal ganglia on DWI. The lesions in the basal ganglia often involve caudate nucleus and putamen, rarely involving globus pallidus, often accompanied by brain atrophy, and generally have no enhancement on enhanced scanning (Figs. 17.2 and 17.3).

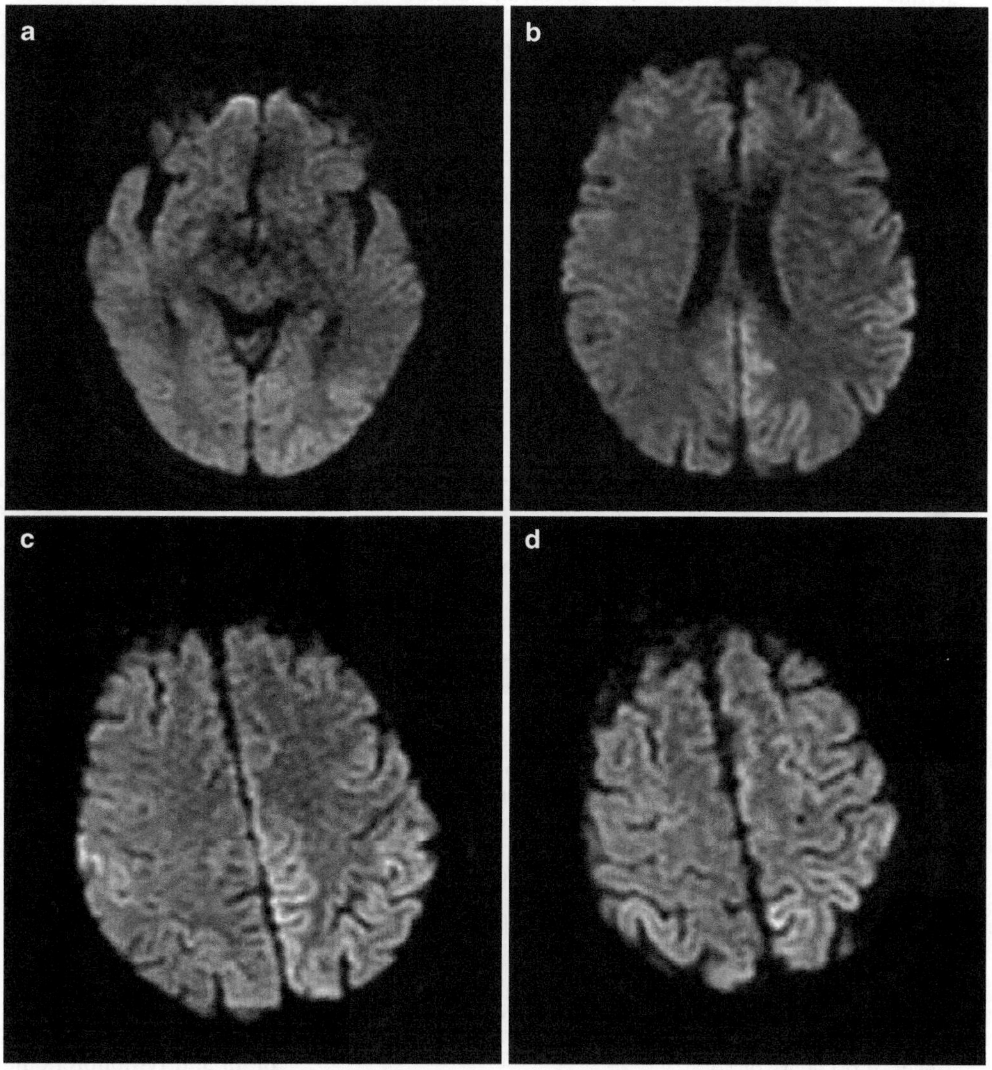

Fig. 17.2 Cerebral Creutzfeldt–Jakob disease. (**a**–**d**) DWI showed abnormal increase of cerebral cortical signal and a widening and deepening of the sulcus, manifested as a "drifting band sign" along the cortex (CD)

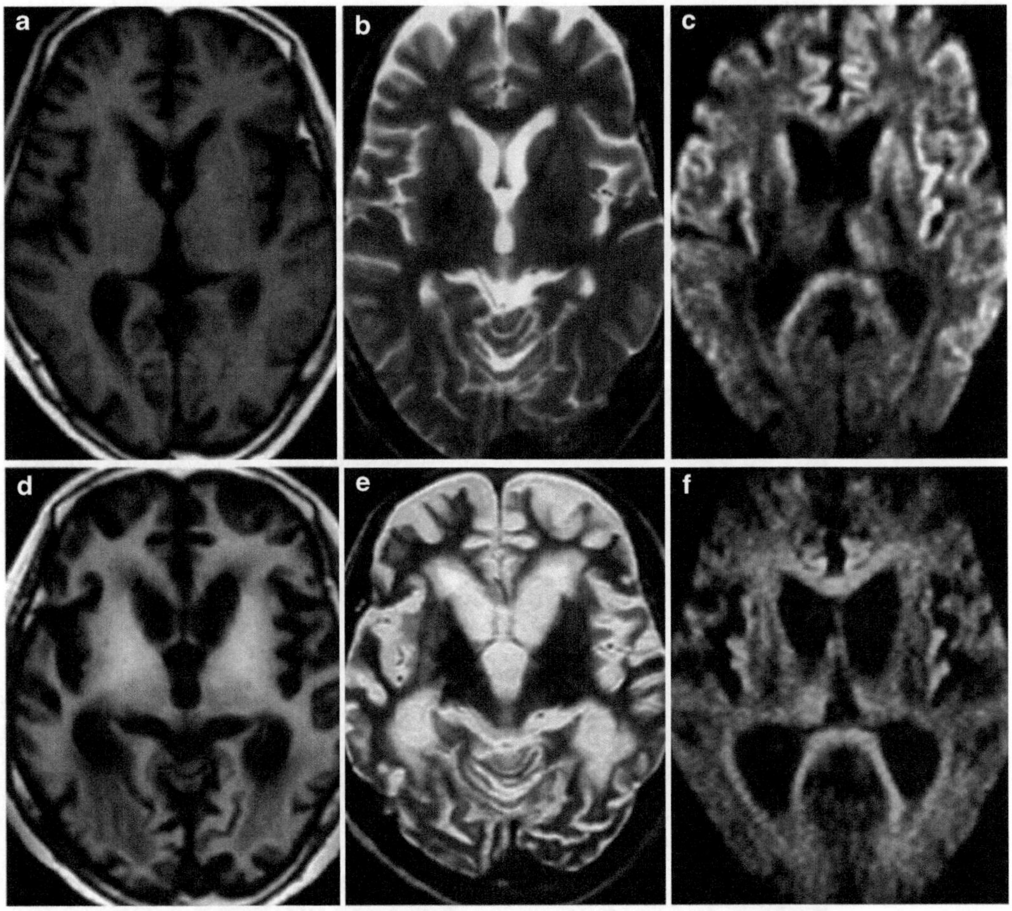

Fig. 17.3 Sporadic Creutzfeldt–Jakob disease. The case was negative for cerebrospinal fluid 14-3-3 protein 7 weeks after the onset of dementia and 2 weeks before the onset of periodic abnormalities in the EEG. (**a**) MRI T_1WI shows no significant intracranial abnormalities; (**b**, **c**) DWI shows symmetrical hyperintense in the bilateral frontotemporal cortex, caudate nucleus, and shell nucleus, and is reexamined 27 weeks after the onset of clinical symptoms; (**d**) T_1WI shows significant brain atrophy; (**e**) T_2WI shows increased white matter signal around the ventricles, atrophy in the caudate nucleus, and asymmetrical hyperintense in the bilateral basal ganglia; (**f**) DWI shows loss of hyperintensity in the bilateral basal ganglia. (Image courtesy of Li Hongjun, Beijing You'an Hospital, Capital Medical University)

17.4 Diagnostic Key Points

1. A clear history of prion infection, with a mean age of onset of 60 years or so.
2. The MRI main findings are abnormal hyperintensity in the cerebral cortex, basal ganglia region, and rapidly developing brain atrophy.
3. The DWI sequence of vCJD is characterized by the "occipital sign" and "hockey stick sign" and typically shows a band of hyperintensity along the cortical sulcus ("drifting band sign") and abnormal hyperintensity in the bilateral basal ganglia region, often accompanied by extensive mild brain atrophy.
4. Periodic synchronous EEG discharges can suggest CJD, and the presence of a typical periodic high-amplitude spike and slow wave syndrome is an important indicator for the clinical diagnosis of CJD.
5. A positive cerebrospinal fluid 14-3-3 protein is highly informative for the diagnosis of this disease.
6. Immunohistochemistry showed the presence of PrPsc in brain and lymphoreticular tissue, which has a good confirmatory value.
7. Definitive diagnosis requires pathological confirmation, and routine examination negates any other diagnosis that could suggest the diagnosis.

17.5 Differential Diagnosis

The clinical manifestations of CJD are varied, with a rapidly progressive course and an extremely poor prognosis. Confirmation of the disease requires pathological confirmation, but brain tissue biopsies can cause iatrogenic infections, so they are difficult to perform. The clinical manifestations of CJD are typical rapid progressive dementia, focal neurological signs, and myoclonus. CJD needs to be differentiated from Alzheimer's disease, mitochondrial encephalopathy, osmotic demyelination syndrome, and Wilson's disease.

1. Alzheimer's disease and CJD both with progressive dementia as the main clinical manifestations. Alzheimer's disease is mainly characterized by widening of the gyrus and sulcus, enlargement of the ventricles, especially in the hippocampus and medial temporal lobe, and an average reduction in hippocampal volume of 20% to 25%. CJD may show symmetrical involvement of the basal ganglia with characteristic "occipital," "hockey stick," and "drifting band" signs, often accompanied by extensive brain atrophy. The two behave differently for identification purposes.
2. Mitochondrial encephalopathy has a diversity of brain imaging manifestations. Most show abnormal signal in the deep nuclei and surrounding white matter, and an elevated lactate peak in the magnetic resonance spectrum can suggest the disease. In the brain, it presents as a multicortical lesion across blood supply regions and is prone to involve the parieto-occipital lobe. CJD may show symmetrical involvement of the basal ganglia with characteristic "occipital," "hockey stick," and "drifting band" signs, often accompanied by extensive atrophy, and easy to differentiate.
3. Infiltrative demyelination syndrome. MRI may show a lamellar abnormal signal with symmetrical distribution in bilateral thalamus, slightly hypointense on T_1WI, slightly hyperintense on T_2WI and hyperintense on FLAIR, and the lesion is enhanced distinctly on enhanced scan. CJD may show symmetrical involvement of the dorsomedial nucleus of thalamus with characteristic "hockey stick" sign, and no enhancement on enhanced scan. It is not difficult to differentiate the two disease.
4. Wilson's disease. It mainly involves basal ganglia and midbrain, and the typical presentation is hyperintense in the nucleus accumbens, pallidum, caudate nucleus, and thalamus on FLAIR sequence. The thalamic lesions are often confined to the ventral lateral nucleus with rare cortex involvement. CJD is characterized by hyperintense in the dorsomedial nucleus of thalamus, which is symmetrically distributed and resembles a "hockey stick" and is the characteristic performance of CJD. It often associated with widespread brain atrophy. The two diseases can be differentiated.

17.6 Status and Progress of Research

1. *Magnetic Resonance Diffusion Weighted Imaging (DWI).* In recent years, MRI examinations (especially DWI and FLAIR sequences) are of increasing interest in the early diagnosis of CJD. sCJD shows hyperintense in at least two cortical areas in the frontal, parietal, and occipital lobes on DWI sequences or FLAIR, or symmetrical hyperintense in the caudate and shell nuclei, while vCJD shows characteristic posterior thalamic hyperintensity (i.e., thalamic "occipital sign") [3]. DWI is more sensitive and specific in early diagnosis compared to FLAIR. but DWI also has several shortcomings for CJD detection: (a) the abnormal brain signal is not consistent with the severity of the disease, but disappears in the late stage of the disease; (b) the abnormal brain signal is not unique to CJD and is occasionally seen in mitochondrial encephalomyopathy, carbon monoxide poisoning, cryptococcal meningitis, viral encephalitis, etc.; (c) in very few patients with CJD, DWI may also have no abnormal changes. DWI images may show hyperintense damage to cortical and basal ganglia areas, and in cases where only cortical areas are hyperintense on DWI images, they need to be differentiated from diseases that cause progressive exacerbation of cognitive dysfunction (chronic herpetic encephalitis, lactic acidosis, mitochondrial encephalomyopathy, etc.). Diagnosis in the current anatomical structural sense has been extended from cortical–basal ganglia–thalamic regions to the ocular, frontal, parietal, temporal, limbic system and hippocampal cortices. The hyperintense areas on DWI images are associated with clinical symptoms and disease progression; e.g., DWI shows hyperintense in the basal ganglia region, patients have a shorter survival time and a higher incidence of myoclonus, and DWI hyperintense in the occipital cortical region is associated with time from onset to the onset of inactivity mutism. The preferred method of early imaging in CJD is DWI, as the disease progresses, the abnormal hyperintensity shown by DWI is instead reduced, so the DWI presentation needs to be followed.
2. *Magnetic resonance hydrogen proton spectrum (^{1}H-MRS).* In 2008, Sarac et al. [4] used ^{1}H-MRS for the early diagnosis of CJD, suggesting for the first time that functional MRI and ^{1}H-MRS are valuable for the early diagnosis of CJD, but further studies are needed on the role of ^{1}H-MRS in the assessment of CJD outcomes.

It has been suggested that serial magnetic resonance imaging, MRS studies, and measurement of cerebrospinal fluid phosphorylated tau protein to total tau protein ratio may improve the early diagnosis of sCJD. It was found that thalamic NAA levels were reduced in monosomal ^{1}H-MRS, consistent with changes in neurodegenerative disease. The NAA/Cr correlated with disease duration and was lower in short disease duration [5]. However, in the early stages of the disease, there is no significant decrease in NAA, suggesting a predominance of spongiform degeneration in the early stages of sCJD and mainly neurodegenerative lesions in the late stages [6].

CT and MRI can be used for the examination of CJD, but MRI is the main method, which has high soft tissue resolution and provides a lot of valuable information for the localization, characterization, and even quantification of CJD with multi-series and multi-modality examination. In recent years, with the emergence of new magnetic resonance techniques and the popularization of clinical use, the clinical application of MRI for diagnosis, differential diagnosis, and post-treatment follow-up has been greatly enhanced. MRS can provide metabolic information of lesions, and MRI diffusion related techniques (including diffusion weighted imaging and diffusion tensor imaging, etc.) can provide information on diffusion of water molecules and orientation of cerebral white matter fiber tracts. CT is widely used in the screening of intracranial lesions because of its fast scanning speed and low cost, and it is also advantageous in showing microcalcifications and cortical disruption. CT-enhanced scans can show blood–brain barrier disruption, and MRA, CTA, and DSA can provide vascular information.

References

1. Kim MO, Geschwind MD. Clinical update of Jakob-Creutzfeldt disease. Curr Opin Neurol. 2015;28(3):302–10.
2. Muayqil T, Gronseth G, Camicioli R. Evidence based guideline: diagnostic accuracy of CSF 14-3-3 protein in sporadic Creutzfeldt-Jakob disease. Neurology. 2012;79(14):1499–506.
3. Collie DA, Summers DM, Sellar J, et al. Diagnosing variant Creutzfeldt-Jakob disease with the pulvinar sign: MR imaging findings in 86 neuropathologically confirmed cases. Am J Neuroradiol. 2003;24(8):1560–9.
4. Sarac H, Hajnsek S, Basi S, et al. Magnetic resonance spectroscopy and measurement of tau epitopes of autopsy proven sporadic Creutzfeldt-Jakob disease in a patient with non-specific initial EEG, MRI and negative 14-3-3 immunoblot. Coll Antropol. 2008;32(1):199–204.
5. La Morgia C, Parchi P, Capellari S, et al. "Agrypnia excitata" in a case of sporadic Creutzfeldt-Jakob disease VV2. J Neurol Neurosurg Psychiatry. 2009;80(2):244–6.
6. Kim JH, Choi BS, Jung C, et al. Diffusion-weighted imaging and magnetic resonance spectroscopy of sporadic Creutzfeldt-Jakob disease: correlation with clinical course. Neuroradiology. 2011;53(12):939–45.

18 Specific Types of Intracranial Inflammatory Diseases

Jingjing Xu, Xin Gao, Pingfeng Dai, Hong Li, Hui Tian, Chao Wang, and Jundi Liu

18.1 Acute Disseminated Encephalomyelitis

Jingjing Xu, Xin Gao, and Pingfeng Dai

18.1.1 Overview

Acute disseminated encephalomyelitis (ADEM), also known as post-infectious encephalomyelitis, is an immune-mediated acute, subacute, or hyperacute inflammatory disease of the central nervous system [1–3]. ADEM is characterized by demyelination of the brain and spinal cord, which in some cases can involve the optic nerve, with a mostly transient, multifocal, and unidirectional course [4]. In pediatrics, ADEM has corresponding diagnostic criteria [5], but adults lack a widely accepted diagnostic consensus. Therefore, to make an accurate clinical diagnosis of ADEM, the clinical features, imaging findings, and cerebrospinal fluid findings must be combined with other neurological infections and inflammatory conditions, and other central nervous system infections and inflammations and systemic diseases such as multiple sclerosis should be ruled out. At the same time, ADEM clinical differential diagnosis is challenging because brain tissue biopsy is more limited in clinical application as the gold standard [1–4].

ADEM is a rare condition that can occur at any age, commonly in children, mostly in children under 10 years old [2, 3]. The annual childhood incidence has been reported to be 0.07 to 0.64 per 100 thousand, and incidence in the adult stage has not been reported. ADEM is more common in males, with a male-to-female ratio of about 1.3:1, and is more frequent in spring and winter. Also, 50% to 75% of ADEM patients have a preexisting history of infection or vaccination, most cases secondary to viral or bacterial infection [4–7]. It is important to note that while vaccination is frequently reported to trigger ADEM, it only accounts for a small proportion of patients with ADEM, and upper respiratory tract infection is still the most common precursor event [1–4]. The lag time of ADEM can be as long as 60 days (mean 26 days), often with acute onset and rapid progression, characterized by multiple neurological symptoms, requiring early admission to the hospital [4–7].

ADEM atypical symptoms include fever, headache, malaise, nausea, and vomiting. Furthermore, 20% to 52% of adult cases may develop psychiatric symptoms, including irritability, confusion, drowsiness, and even coma. Some patients may also present with motor and sensory symptoms, such as paresis of lower limb or extremities; brainstem dysfunction (e.g., dysarthria, abnormalities in motor-eye function) or other neurological symptoms (such as epilepsy, meningeal irritation signs, ataxia, aphasia, nystagmus, optic neuritis, increased intracranial pressure, or extrapyramidal symptoms) may also be present. Some adults with ADEM may also develop peripheral nervous system involvement with EMG abnormalities, sensory abnormalities in the extremities, sensory deficits, or muscular atrophy. Peripheral nervous system involvement often predicts a poorer prognosis for patients and predisposition to recurrence [1–7].

Acute hemorrhagic encephalomyelitis (AHEM) is a hyperacute variant of ADEM that presents with acute progression, coma, and even life-threatening [1–4]. AHEM is similar to ADEM and is often triggered by infectious agents or vaccines, with symptoms including asymmetric multifocal neurological symptoms, meningitis symptoms, headaches, and convulsions. Cranial CT or MRI may reveal intracranial focal hemorrhage, edema, punctate or paravalvular hemorrhage, vascular disruption, fibrous deposits, and neutrophil infiltration [1–7].

J. Xu · P. Dai (✉) · H. Li · C. Wang
The Second Affiliated Hospital of School of Medicine, Zhejiang University, Hangzhou, China

X. Gao · H. Tian · J. Liu
The First Affiliated Hospital of Xinjiang Medical University, Urumqi, China

H. Li et al. (eds.), *Radiology of Infectious and Inflammatory Diseases - Volume 1*,
https://doi.org/10.1007/978-981-99-0039-8_18

ADEM patients with signs of meningeal irritation, fever, acute encephalopathy, and signs of inflammation on blood or cerebrospinal fluid examination should be started on empirical acyclovir treatment [4–7]. The primary treatment should be immunosuppressive therapy, i.e., high-dose intravenous glucocorticoids, which should be started at the same time as acyclovir or antibiotic therapy. If patients' symptoms do not improve or if glucocorticoid therapy does not respond well, try immunoglobulin IV, plasma exchange, or cyclophosphamide [4–7]. ADEM has a good long-term prognosis, with full recovery mostly after 1 to 6 months. Some patients may have sequelae, including motor impairment, visual impairment, and convulsions. Some ADEM patients also develop attention, executive ability, and behavior-related neurocognitive deficits years after the disease [2–6].

ADEM diagnosis based on clinical presentation requires MRI imaging evidence to support [3–6]. ADEM has a diverse clinical presentation and lacks specific biomarkers. The main aim of differential diagnosis is to exclude other pathologies, the primary exclusion is central nervous system infection, but clinical application of cerebrospinal fluid examination, serum and cerebrospinal fluid oligoclonal IgG, and other serum laboratory tests (routine blood, erythrocyte sedimentation rate, C reactive protein, anti-neutrophil cytoplasmic antibodies, etc.) may be carried out to differentiate. The most important disease to be distinguished on imaging from ADEM is multiple sclerosis, as the prognosis and treatment of the two are completely different [1, 2].

18.1.2 Pathological Manifestations

Biopsy of intracerebral lesions is the gold standard for ADEM diagnosis [1–3]. ADEM pathological features: microscopic manifestations include perivascular demyelinating changes and perivascular inflammation in the brain or spinal cord. AHEM may present perivascular demyelination, acute inflammation, vascular fiber necrosis, and punctate hemorrhage. Although perivascular inflammation is also a feature of multiple sclerosis pathology, the pattern of ADEM demyelination is different from that of multiple sclerosis. There will also be a mixture of macrophage infiltration and reactive astrocyte proliferation in areas of complete demyelination in ADEM [2–6].

The precise pathogenic mechanism of ADEM is not fully proven, but ADEM has long been considered an inflammatory response triggered by external environmental stimuli in genetically susceptible individuals, a central nervous system autoimmune disease, an environmentally triggered cell-mediated or antibody-triggered cross-reaction to myelin autoantigens, with demyelination as a feature [1–3]. Another possible mechanism is that after vaccination or infection, the inflammatory response and the presence of immune complexes in the blood allow for increased CNS vascular permeability and CNS vascular mononuclear cell infiltration, causing perivascular gap edema and hemorrhage, leading to destruction of adjacent nerve cells, pathological changes such as demyelination, necrosis, gliosis, and eventually clinical symptoms. ADEM-associated inflammation and increased vascular permeability may also disrupt the blood–brain barrier, producing CNS antigen and inflammatory cell infiltration with associated cell-mediated immune responses [6, 7].

18.1.3 Imaging

MRI is used for the clinical assessment of ADEM [1–7]. Lesions manifest as hyperintense on T_2WI and FLAIR sequences. T_1WI cannot find lesions easily, and the larger ones may display hypointense. ADEM lesions can be single or multiple lesions of variable size, partially fusible. Sites of occurrence can be the whole brain white matter (e.g., paraventricular or subcortical) and gray matter (e.g., basal ganglia, thalamus, and cortex). White matter lesions are typically multiple and asymmetrical, whereas gray matter lesions are more symmetrical and involve the thalamus and basal ganglia regions. Multiple foci are mostly in the same period [1–7]. Typical MRI findings of ADEM: asymmetric patchy abnormal signal on both sides with blurred borders and variable size, some lesions may be associated with perifocal edema (Fig. 18.1). Typical ADEM often involves the subcortex and white matter, cortico-white matter junction, thalamus, basal ganglia, cerebellum, and brainstem. Lesions occurring alone in the subscripts are rare [2–4]. On imaging, the borders of ADEM are blurred, and that helps distinguish it from multiple sclerotic lesions, which have clear borders (Fig. 18.2). One-third of patients may have spinal cord involvement, manifesting as a larger multisegmental fusion lesion, which may be accompanied by spinal cord edema, and some lesions may be enhanced on enhanced scan [3–7]. MRI signal intensity, distribution, and mode of enhancement of the lesion do not correlate with prognosis [1–6].

It is worth noting that MRI of ADEM patients may show normal; i.e., MRI reveals no abnormal lesions or even negative results on multiple examinations [1–3]. This is because ADEM lesions are not revealed by MRI until a few weeks after the patient becomes symptomatic, and most MRI findings resolve within 18 weeks, so a review of MRI is necessary. The current review protocol is usually 3 months and 9 to 12 months after the onset of the disease to exclude other active progressive diseases [3–6]. However, repeat examinations must take into account the age and clinical features of the patient and should be considered in the case of children who require sedation [6].

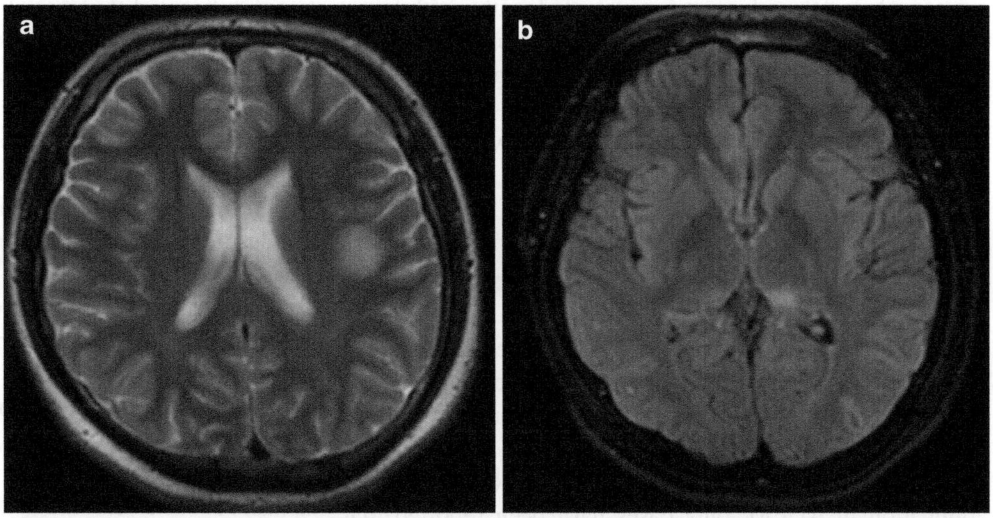

Fig. 18.1 ADEM intracerebral lesion (1). (**a**) Patchy slightly hyperintense visible in the left temporal lobe on T_2WI; (**b**) FLAIR shows slightly hyperintense in the left thalamus

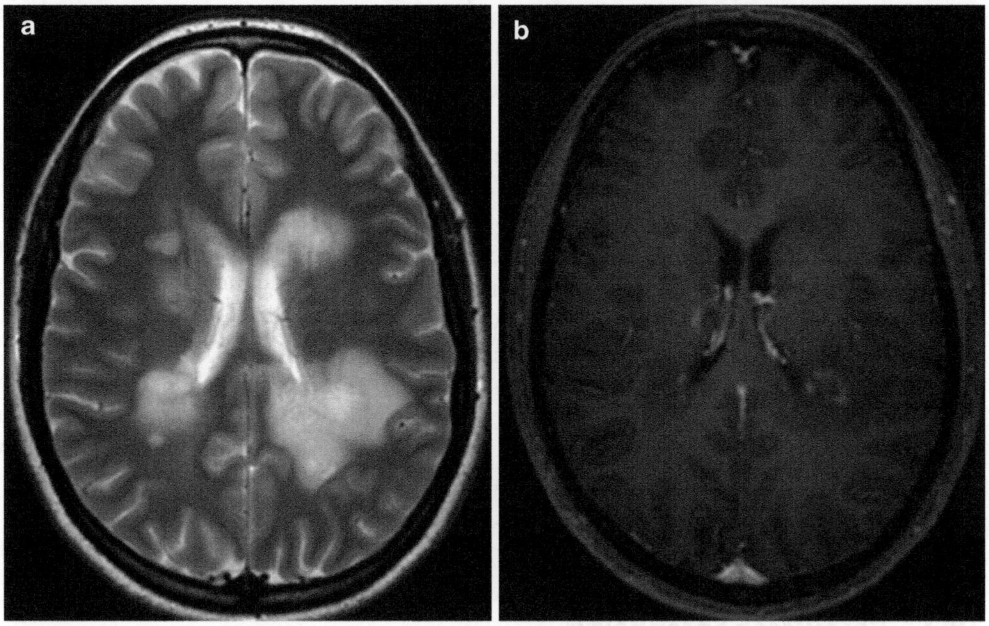

Fig. 18.2 ADEM intracerebral lesions (2). (**a**) T_2WI shows multiple patchy hyperintense next to the ventricles on both sides; (**b**) Enhancement is seen in some lesions on enhanced scan

18.1.4 Diagnostic Key Points

1. Most of them have a history of precursor infection or vaccination.
2. The patient presented with symptoms of multiple neurological deficits and no previous history of neurological abnormalities.
3. MRI findings: T_2WI or FLAIR sequences show asymmetric patchy hyperintense on both sides with blurred borders and variable size, which may involve all gray matter, white matter, subtentorial structures, and the spinal cord, and some lesions may show enhancement.
4. The MRI follow-up during the course of the disease is important.
5. Cerebrospinal fluid examination: abnormal increase in lymphocytes.

18.1.5 Differential Diagnosis

Children with ADEM have a younger age of onset than multiple sclerosis and often have systemic symptoms such as fever, vomiting, meningeal irritation, and headache. Intrathecal oligoclonal IgG synthesis is a characteristic manifestation of childhood multiple sclerosis and is rare in ADEM. In adult patients, ADEM is difficult to distinguish from first-onset multiple sclerosis based on clinical symptoms or imaging evidence alone. But an accurate diagnosis is crucial to choosing a treatment plan. Although multiple sclerosis characteristically presents with recurrent neurological symptoms and is temporally and spatially variable, there is much overlap in the CNS symptoms and imaging manifestations of ADEM and multiple sclerosis. ADEM patients are more likely to have prodromal infection symptoms, such as those of infectious encephalopathy with fever, sniff neck, ataxia, and confusion, while patients with multiple sclerosis are less likely to have these symptoms. In addition, multiple sclerosis more often presents with a single symptom, such as optic neuritis alone, and with a chronic recurrent course [1–6].

18.1.6 Status and Progress of Research

Reports of the signal intensity of ADEM lesions in DWI sequences vary from increased signal to decreased signal. However, in a summary of pediatric cases, the results showed an increase in ADC values in 70% of the lesions, which is consistent with vasogenic edema [1, 2]. MRS has limited application in ADEM; only cases have been reported that NAA can be reduced [3–6]. MTI and DTI help reflect the involvement of brain parenchymal that manifests as normal on conventional sequences. There are reports of MTI and DTI showing no significant difference between brain tissue that manifest as normal in signal in ADEM cases and the healthy controls, suggesting that brain tissue showing normal signal during ADEM pathology in conventional sequences was not involved pathologically [4, 6]. DTI can differentiate ADEM and multiple sclerosis lesions. In age-matched ADEM and multiple sclerosis patients, DTI baseline scan analysis of the region of interest showed differences in the final diagnosis between the two groups, with patients with multiple sclerosis showing a lower rate of anisotropy and higher radial diffusion rates compared to ADEM patients. Anisotropic fraction and radial diffusivity measurements may have potential as biomarkers to differentiate between ADEM and the onset of multiple sclerosis [2–6].

18.2 Rasmussen Encephalitis

Hong Li, Hui Tian, and Pingfeng Dai

18.2.1 Overview

Rasmussen encephalitis, also known as Rasmussen syndrome, is a rare, acquired, progressive, chronic inflammatory disease involving the unilateral brain, manifested by refractory focal epilepsy, progressive hemiparesis, and cognitive decline, named for first reported by Rasmussen of the Montreal Neurological Institute, Canada, in 1958. Rasmussen encephalitis occurs mainly in children, with an average age of onset of about 6 years, from infancy to adolescence, and is predominantly disseminated. The disease affects approximately 18 of every ten million people in the population, with no significant differences by gender, race, or geographic location. The pathogenesis of the disease is unclear, but it is currently thought to be related to an immune response and is a localized autoimmune encephalitis [8].

Studies in the twentieth century divided the natural clinical course of Rasmussen encephalitis into three stages. (1) Prodromal phase: the clinical presentation is nonspecific and can last for several years, presenting only with mild hemiparesis or occasional seizures. (2) Acute phase: patients have frequent seizures, often accompanied by partial persistent epilepsy (about 50%) and are difficult to control with antiepileptic drugs; the presence of a diversity of seizure symptoms may suggest recent involvement of the hemispheric cortex; if left untreated at this stage, patients develop progressive hemiparesis, hemianopia, cognitive decline, and aphasia about 1 year later (when the dominant hemisphere is affected). (3) Sequelae phase: patients with relatively uneventful disease course, with residual severe neurological deficits, motor and cognitive problems, and refractory recurrent seizures.

Some patients with Rasmussen encephalitis have a different clinical presentation. Approximately 10% of Rasmussen encephalitis starts in adolescents or adults, usually with a slow clinical course and ultimately less severe functional impairment than in those with childhood onset, with seizure symptoms more consistent with temporal lobe epilepsy, and with unilateral movement disorders manifesting as lateralized athetosis and lateralized dystonia. Very few cases present with bilateral hemispheric involvement, and no cases have been reported in which surgical treatment causes contralateral hemispheric involvement.

18.2.2 Pathological Manifestations

Rasmussen brain specimens from children with encephalitis showed mainly diffuse brain tissue atrophy, arachnoid thickening, and widening of the subarachnoid space. Pathological changes are mainly cortical damage, with the best sites being the frontal-insular cortex, with lesser involvement of the occipital cortex, and the basal nucleus, brainstem, and cerebellum can also be involved. The pathological features are mainly gliosis, microglial nodules, lymphocytic infiltration forming perivascular sleeves, neuronal necrosis, and neutrophilic cells. Some scholars have divided the disease into four periods according to the cortical pathological changes [9]: (1) early stage. cerebral cortex with only mild limited inflammation and glial cell hyperplasia, little and limited neuronal loss, mild to moderate microglial cell hyperplasia, mild to moderate infiltration of T lymphocytes, a few formation of cell clusters and perivascular cuff; (2) medium stage: inflammation and gliosis in all layers of the cerebral cortex, with multifocal moderate and severe neuronal loss, microglia activation and marked infiltration of T lymphocytes in all layers, forming perivascular sleeves; (3) late stage: degeneration and glial cell proliferation in all layers of the cerebral cortex, with severe neuronal loss and large round cell-forming astrocytes in all layers; (4) terminal stage: cystic changes and glial cell hyperplasia were seen in all layers of the cerebral cortex, while neurons were rare. It was found that the T lymphocytes that infiltrate the perivascular infiltration in Rasmussen encephalitis are mainly $CD8^+$ T lymphocytes, while $CD79^+$, $CD20^+$, and $CD10^+$ B lymphocytes were rare, and there were no viral inclusion bodies.

18.2.3 Imaging

18.2.3.1 CT Findings

Early CT scans in the prodromal phase of Rasmussen encephalitis tend to be normal, with no obvious signs of cortical atrophy. Focal cerebral cortical edema may occur in patients with Rasmussen encephalitis in the presence of persistent epilepsy. This is followed by signs of progressive, multifocal cortical atrophy and widening of the cerebral sulcus in the cerebral hemisphere, varying degrees of enlargement of the lateral ventricles ipsilateral to the atrophied cerebral hemisphere, and widening of the subarachnoid space.

18.2.3.2 MRI Findings

Due to the Rasmussen encephalitis patient condition, the rate of progression varies, the disease is complex and variable, and the imaging presentation varies from case to case. Signal abnormalities in the cortical and deep gray matter nuclei of Rasmussen encephalitis can change as the lesion evolves, manifesting as decreased and increased signal, the appearance of new lesions, or involvement of new sites [10]. The imaging features that determine Rasmussen encephalitis should emphasize the abnormal signal changes in the area of the lesion with brain atrophy and progressive changes. Bien et al. [11] followed up ten patients with this disease and compared the MRI and histopathological features in different periods, and classified them into four phases according to the T_2WI signal alterations in cortical, i.e., hyperintense cortical with swelling, hyperintense cortical with normal volume, hyperintense cortical with atrophy, and normal-signal cortical with progressive atrophy.

1. Phase of hyperintense cortical with swelling: in most patients, cortical involvement occurs mainly in the frontal, temporal, and insular cortices, with focal cortical swelling and hyperintense on T_2WI/FLAIR in one cerebral hemisphere and hypointense on T_1WI. The cerebral edema may be caused by the large numbers of T lymphocyte infiltration during the onset of infection [12]. Hyperintensity on T_2WI and FLAIR can better show neuronal damage or glial cell proliferation, especially FLAIR, which is sensitive to the progressive development of epileptic lesions later on [13].
2. Phase of hyperintense cortical with normal volume: T_1WI shows hypointense and T_2WI/FLAIR shows only focal cortical hyperintense on one side of the cerebral hemisphere, and cortical swelling begins to subside at this stage, possibly associated with the decrease in the number of T lymphocytes and the proliferation of reactive astrocytes. Adjacent white matter and deep gray matter nuclei can be found in some cases of a cluster and appear to have a similar signal change.
3. Phase of hyperintense cortical with atrophy. The cortical extent that involved by lesion may progressively increase and the cortical manifests as hyperintense on T_2WI/FLAIR and hypointense on T_1WI with atrophy, and may be accompanied by ipsilateral lateral ventricular enlargement and widening of temporal horn and lateral fissure pool. The involvement of adjacent white matter is more pronounced and may be related to demyelination of white matter fibers. The atrophy of the affected deep gray matter nuclei is not secondary to the lesion, but is the result of direct involvement. The shell nucleus is often more distinctly atrophied than the caudate nucleus (Figs. 18.3 and 18.4).
4. Normal signal cortical with progressive atrophy phase: diffuse cortical atrophy in one hemisphere of the brain is significant, but the signal on T_2WI tends to be normal, and in some cases, the signal on T_1WI may be increased. The lateral ventricles and sulci are enlarged and the subarachnoid space is widened. The affected white matter is extensively involved, with hypointense on T_1WI and hyperintense on T_2WI.

MRI enhanced scan revealed Rasmussen with no significant enhancement in the area of the encephalitis lesion. In addition, atrophy of the healthy hemisphere also occurs in patients with Rasmussen encephalitis, but the atrophy is relatively slow and may be affected by Wallerian degeneration of the combined fibers of the right and left hemispheres, prolonged seizures, or medication, or it may be a rare bilateral hemispheric involvement.

18.2.4 Diagnostic Key Points

1. The clinical presentation is mostly refractory partial epilepsy, progressive hemiparesis, and cognitive decline.
2. The lesions are found in the frontal, temporal, and insular cortices and are progressive, multifocal cortical atrophy.

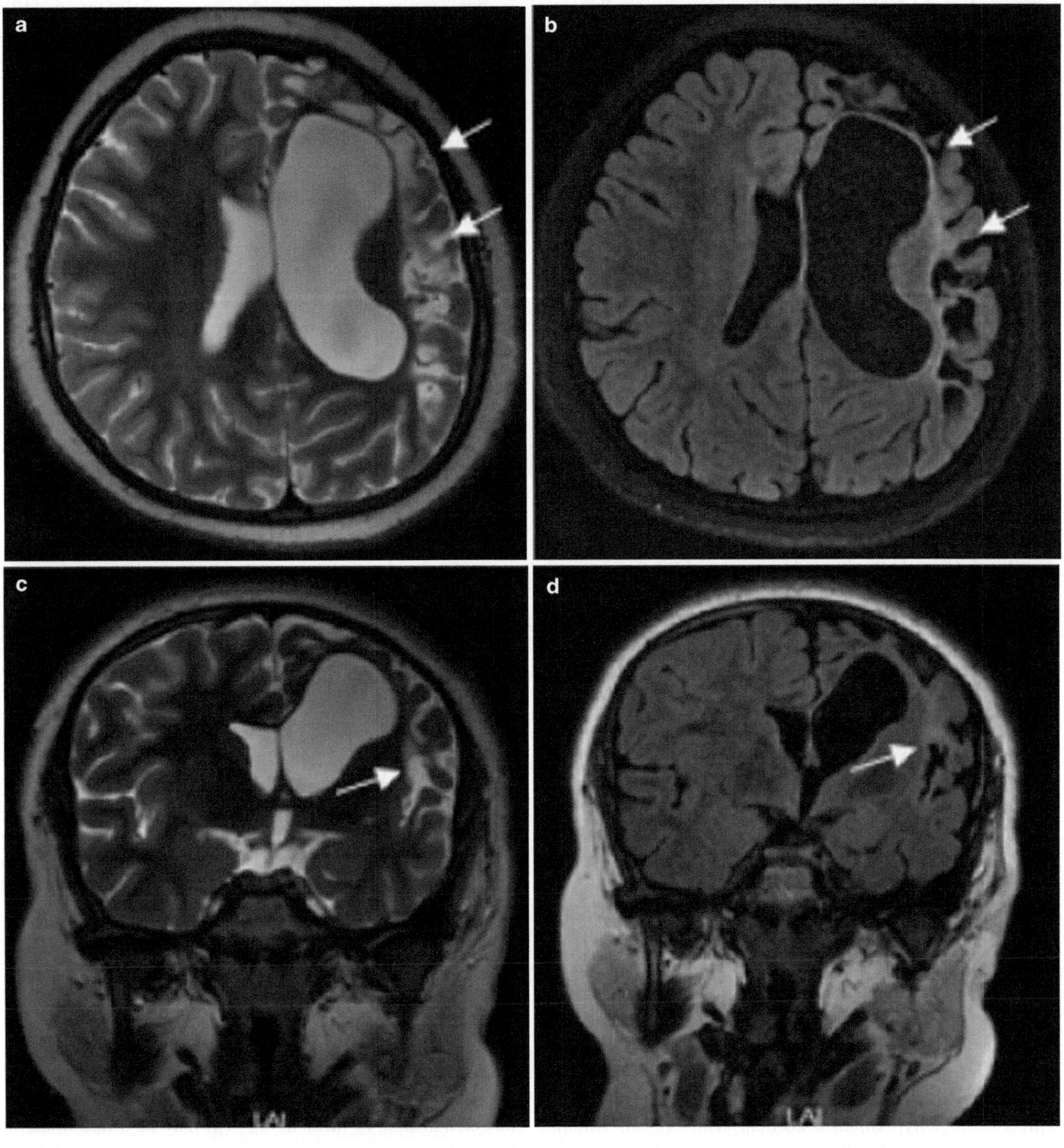

Fig. 18.3 Rasmussen encephalitis hyperintense cortical with atrophy phase (1). Multiple cortical atrophy in the left cerebral hemisphere with enlarged and widened ipsilateral ventricles and corresponding sulci. (**a**, **c**) T_2WI shows hyperintense in the involved cortex (axial, coronal). (**b**, **d**) FLAIR sequence shows hypointense in the involved cortex, with patches of slightly hyperintense visible in the periphery (axial, coronal)

3. MRI Findings: progressive atrophy of the cortical and deep gray matter nuclei of one cerebral hemisphere, with changes in cortical signal with the evolution of the disease, varying degrees of enlargement of the ipsilateral lateral ventricles, and widening of the subarachnoid space.
4. Unilateral EEG hemispheric slow activity with or without epileptiform discharges and unilateral seizures.
5. Histopathological manifestations of the brain: T lymphocyte-dominated encephalitis with microglia hyperplasia and reactive glial cell hyperplasia.

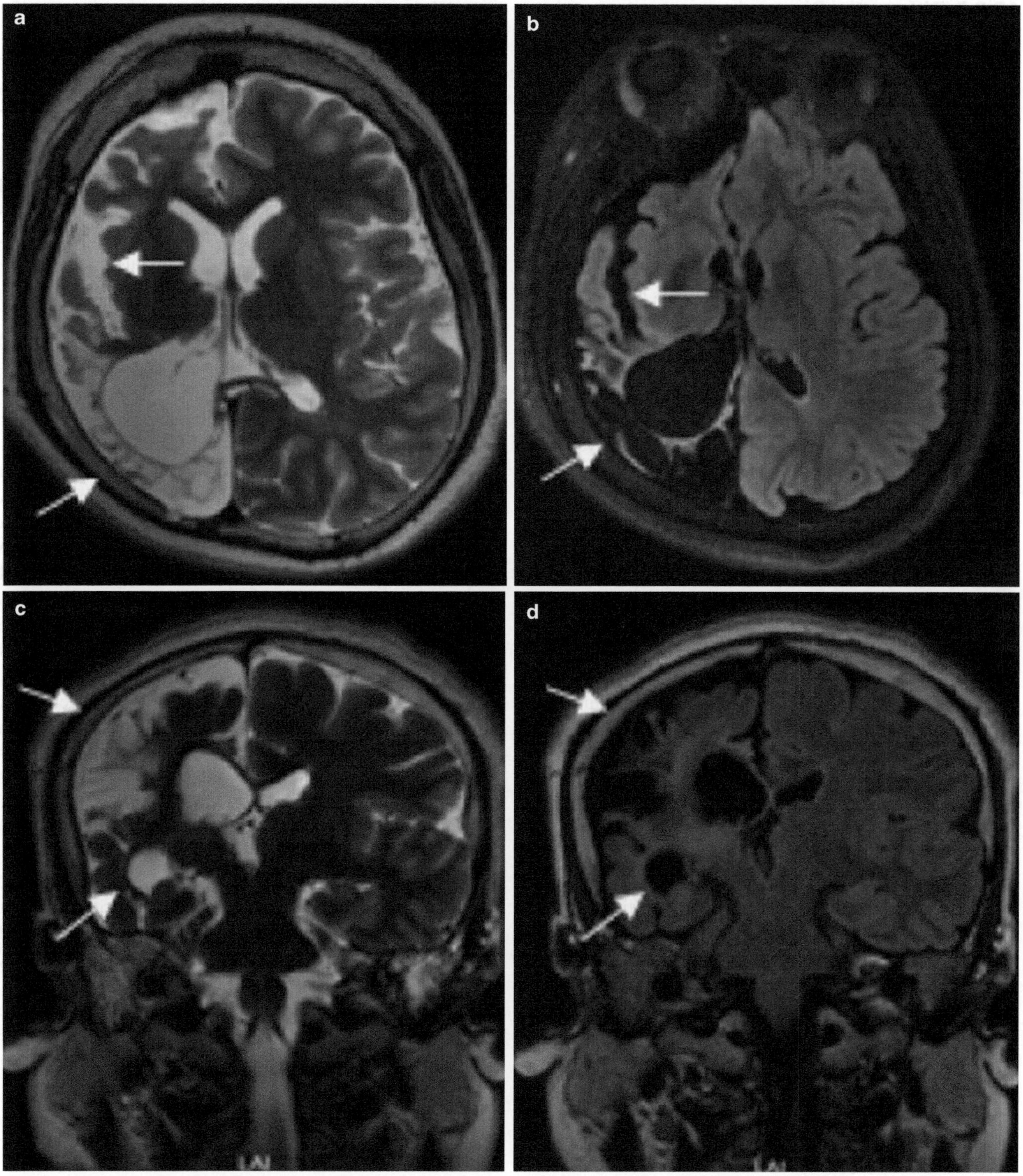

Fig. 18.4 Rasmussen encephalitis hyperintense cortical with atrophy phase (2). Multiple cortical atrophy in the right hemisphere with enlargement and widening of the ipsilateral ventricles, temporal horn, and corresponding sulci. (**a**, **c**) T_2WI shows hyperintense in the involved cortex (axial, coronal). (**b**, **d**) FLAIR sequence with predominantly hypointense in the involved cortex, with patches of slightly hyperintense visible in the periphery (axial, coronal)

18.2.5 Differential Diagnosis

18.2.5.1 Mitochondrial Encephalopathy

It is prevalent in adolescents and young adults who may be older than patients with Rasmussen encephalitis, the lesions are migratory, and most of the hemispheres are involved bilaterally, usually without atrophic changes such as unilateral widening of the lateral fissure and enlargement of the ventricles.

18.2.5.2 Cortical Dysplasia

Imaging shows localized cortical thickening, indistinct gray-white matter demarcation, reduced white matter, localized enlargement of the cerebral gyrus, and widening of the sulcus. MRI shows subcortical linear, radiolucent, and funnel-like abnormal signals, which display hypointense on T_1WI and hyperintense on T_2WI and can range from the gray-white matter junction area to the lateral margin of lateral ventricular. Patients with Rasmussen encephalitis show limited, progressive atrophy of the diseased cortex and the phenomenon progressively worsens as the disease progresses, whereas cortical dysplasia is generally less markedly changed.

18.2.5.3 Sturge–Weber Syndrome

The lesion site of the patient's brain may occur cortical atrophy, and signal changes, often with calcification, and enhanced scans reveal varying degrees of meningeal enhancement and the presence of thickened and increased abnormal venous vessels in the brain parenchyma. In contrast, patients with Rasmussen encephalitis rarely present with cortical calcification, and Sturge–Weber syndrome also presents with typical facial hemangiomas.

18.2.5.4 Cerebral Vasculitis

Vasculitis presents often with diverse imaging manifestations and lack of characteristics; some vasculitis is difficult to differentiate from Rasmussen encephalitis without brain tissue biopsy, and MRI and CT enhancement examinations may reveal leptomeningeal enhancement involving part of the cerebral cortex or diffuse parenchymal vascular enhancement in the patient's brain.

18.2.6 Status and Progress of Research

Brain tissue biopsy, although definitive in diagnosis, is severely limited as an invasive test. The development of neuroimaging has greatly assisted in the clinical diagnosis of Rasmussen encephalitis. CT and MRI can be applied to Rasmussen encephalitis diagnosis, and MRI is the predominant test [12].

CT, although not the preferred means of examination, is particularly suitable in this disease for patients with persistent status epilepticus or epilepsy that is difficult to control with medication because of its fast scanning speed and low price and helps to clarify the morphology, structure and density of intracranial tissues and serves as a preliminary screen, but it is less sensitive than MRI. In recent years, the widespread use of MRI has provided a wealth of information for the localization, characterization, and even quantitative diagnosis of the disease. With the development of multimodal sequences, MRI provides important information for the diagnosis, differential diagnosis, and treatment of the disease. MRS helps diagnose this disease and monitor disease progression and metabolic changes. MRA may reflect the presence or absence of alterations in the affected vessels.

18.2.6.1 Hydrogen Proton Spectrum Imaging (^{1}H-MRS)

It can be used as an important complementary diagnostic method to conventional MRI, capable of reflecting biochemical changes that occur prior to morphological structural changes. The affected area will show a decrease in the NAA peak and an increase in the Cho and mI peaks. The NAA peak decrease represents progressive neuronal destruction and loss, the Cho peak increase reflects the degree of cell membrane disruption, and the mI is a marker of glial cells and is involved in the regulation of osmotic pressure. Some studies have found elevated Glu/Gln peaks in the affected region or even the corresponding region contralaterally, which may suggest a potential mechanism of action of abnormal excitatory neurotransmitters in the disease [14]. In addition, large metabolite peaks (0.8 ppm, 1.3 ppm) are significantly elevated in the affected and contralateral regions, respectively, representing an active demyelination process.

18.2.6.2 Magnetic Resonance Angiography (MRA)

It is able to reflect the presence or absence of significant changes in each major artery and its branches, combined with the imaging features of MRI conventional imaging, which helped to diagnose Rasmussen encephalitis [15]. Some patients with Rasmussen encephalitis will have reduced arterial vessels on the affected side compared to the opposite side, notably in the middle cerebral artery.

18.2.6.3 Task-State Functional MRI (fMRI)

Surgical intervention is the only method of preventing continued seizures, but clinical attention should be paid to speech function in functional hemisphere resection to prevent the occurrence of postoperative aphasia. Functional MRI with the language task state has the advantage of simultaneous preoperative acquisition of functional and anatomical images and is easy to perform, reproducible, noninvasive, and inexpensive as a routine clinical scan to predict and reduce the likelihood of postoperative language deficits in patients with Rasmussen encephalitis requiring surgical treatment and to guide clinical surgical decisions.

18.3 Autoimmune Encephalitis

Chao Wang, Jundi Liu, and Pingfeng Dai

18.3.1 Overview

Encephalitis is a serious inflammatory lesion of the brain parenchyma with many possible causes, the most common cause of encephalitis being infection. However, over the past 10 years, there has been an increasing number of patients with noninfectious encephalitis, which includes autoimmune encephalitis. The first description of autoimmune encephalitis dates back to 1888 when Hermann Oppenheim first described a patient with neurological symptoms but no underlying brain pathology [16]. In the twentieth century, brain sections from some patients with subacute encephalitis with emotional and behavioral abnormalities showed that inflammatory lesions in the brain occurred mainly in limbic structures such as the hippocampus and amygdala, leading to the term limbic encephalitis [16]. It was not until 2007 that autoantibodies against N-methyl-D-aspartate receptors (NMDAR) and many other anti-neuronal cell surface or synaptic proteins continued to be discovered. Anti-NMDAR encephalitis is by far the most common autoimmune encephalitis, accounting for 80% of autoimmune encephalitis. The first case of anti-NMDAR encephalitis was reported in China in 2010. Since then, other types of cases have been reported, including leucine-rich glioma inactivated 1 antibody (LGI 1), γ-aminobutyric acid B type receptor (GABABR) antibody, alpha amino-3-hydroxy-5-methyl-4-isoazole propionic acid receptor (AMPAR) antibody-related encephalitis, and anti-contact protein-associated protein 2(CASPR2) antibody-associated Morvang syndrome [17]. This broad class of novel autoimmune encephalitis differs markedly from classical paraneoplastic limbic encephalitis in that its immunotherapy is more effective because the target antigens in this type of autoimmune encephalitis are located on the surface of neuronal cells and they cause relatively reversible neuronal damage primarily by mediating humoral immune responses; however, in classical paraneoplastic limbic encephalitis, the target antigens are located within neuronal cells and they cause relatively reversible neuronal damage primarily by cellular immune mechanisms and the neuronal damage caused by the system is often irreversible [17]. The diagnosis of autoimmune encephalitis requires a combination of clinical manifestations, neuroimaging, cerebrospinal fluid examination, and electroencephalography, followed by the selection and testing of antibodies associated with autoimmune encephalitis. The clinical manifestations are mainly of acute or subacute onset (3 months) with symptoms of the limbic system, encephalitis syndrome, clinical manifestations of basal ganglia and/or mesencephalic/hypothalamic involvement, and psychiatric disorders and neurological and psychiatric symptoms not compatible with nonorganic disease in the opinion of psychiatric specialists, and one or more of the above four clinical syndromes should be matched. Cerebrospinal fluid examination shows that cerebrospinal fluid leukocytes may be mildly increased, cerebrospinal fluid cytology is mostly lymphocytic inflammation, and oligoclonal zone bands may be positive. For anti-neuronal antibodies, both cerebrospinal fluid and serum are recommended. Positive autoantibodies to anti-neuronal surface antigens are the basis for confirming the diagnosis of autoimmune encephalitis [17, 18].

18.3.2 Pathological Manifestations

Autoimmune encephalitis is a group of encephalitis mediated by autoimmune mechanisms, and the diagnosis is confirmed by positive autoantibodies to anti-neuronal surface antigens. The Chinese Consensus on Expert Diagnosis and Treatment of Autoimmune Encephalitis states that the criteria for confirming the diagnosis of anti-NMDAR encephalitis require both clinical manifestations and cerebrospinal fluid anti-NMDAR while other types of autoimmune encephalitis require clinical manifestations, ancillary tests, and serum and cerebrospinal fluid antibody tests as necessary to confirm the diagnosis [17, 18].

18.3.3 Imaging

The current imaging diagnosis of autoimmune encephalitis is mostly based on conventional MRI. However, only some cases of cranial MRI showed positive [16–19]. The involvement was predominantly in the brain parenchyma, with the occipital lobe, bilateral hippocampus, temporal lobe, frontal lobe, parietal lobe, cerebellum, insula, thalamus, and caudate nucleus head [19] in that order. Involvement of the hippocampus often appears as a diffuse lesion, while the involvement of other areas often appears as a patchy or "gyrus-like" lesion. T_1WI shows a low signal, T_2WI and FLAIR show a high signal, and the FLAIR sequence shows the most obvious lesion [16, 19]. Some cases may present with meningeal abnormalities as linear enhancement of the meninges and increased vascular shadowing. The morphology of hippocampal lesions is often a symmetrical diffuse change in the hippocampus. Lobar lesions are gyrus-like or patchy, and thalamic lesions are patchy with abnormal signals [16, 19]. The

DWI signal varies, depending on the course of the disease, with cytotoxic edema in the early stage of the disease, which is characterized by DWI high signal, and vasogenic edema in the late stage of the disease, which is characterized by reduced DWI signal. Usually, DWI high signal and ADC value reduction [16, 19] are seen in patients with MRI performed at the beginning of the onset (within 1 week).

Anti-NMDAR encephalitis is the most common type of autoimmune encephalitis (Fig. 18.5). Most patients with anti-NMDAR encephalitis have normal cranial MRI examinations, and only 23%–50% have abnormalities findings without specific changes, mostly nonspecific gray and white matter changes, mainly small patchy frontal, temporal, thalamic, cerebellar, and brainstem lesions, with rare lesions in the basal ganglia region, of which about 1/4 patients have enhancement on enhanced scans [16, 19] (Fig. 18.5). Anti-NMDAR lesions in the brainstem, basal ganglia, and cerebellum are relatively rare in patients with encephalitis, and their imaging manifestations do not change with disease progression or are only slightly altered [16, 19].

18.3.4 Diagnostic Key Points

1. The course of the disease is acute or subacute and presents with one or more neurological and psychiatric symptoms or clinical syndromes.
2. MRI Findings: Involvement is predominantly parenchymal, with involvement of the hippocampus often showing diffuse lesions, and involvement of other sites often showing patchy or "gyral-like" lesions. T_1WI shows a low signal, T_2WI and FLAIR show a high signal, and enhancement can be seen on enhancement scans.
3. Positive autoantibodies to cerebrospinal fluid and/or serum anti-neuronal surface antigen.

18.3.5 Differential Diagnosis

Confirmation of autoimmune encephalitis requires a combination of clinical manifestations, neuroimaging, cerebrospinal fluid examination, and electroencephalography followed by selection and testing of autoimmune encephalitis-related antibodies, the main basis for confirmation of diagnosis

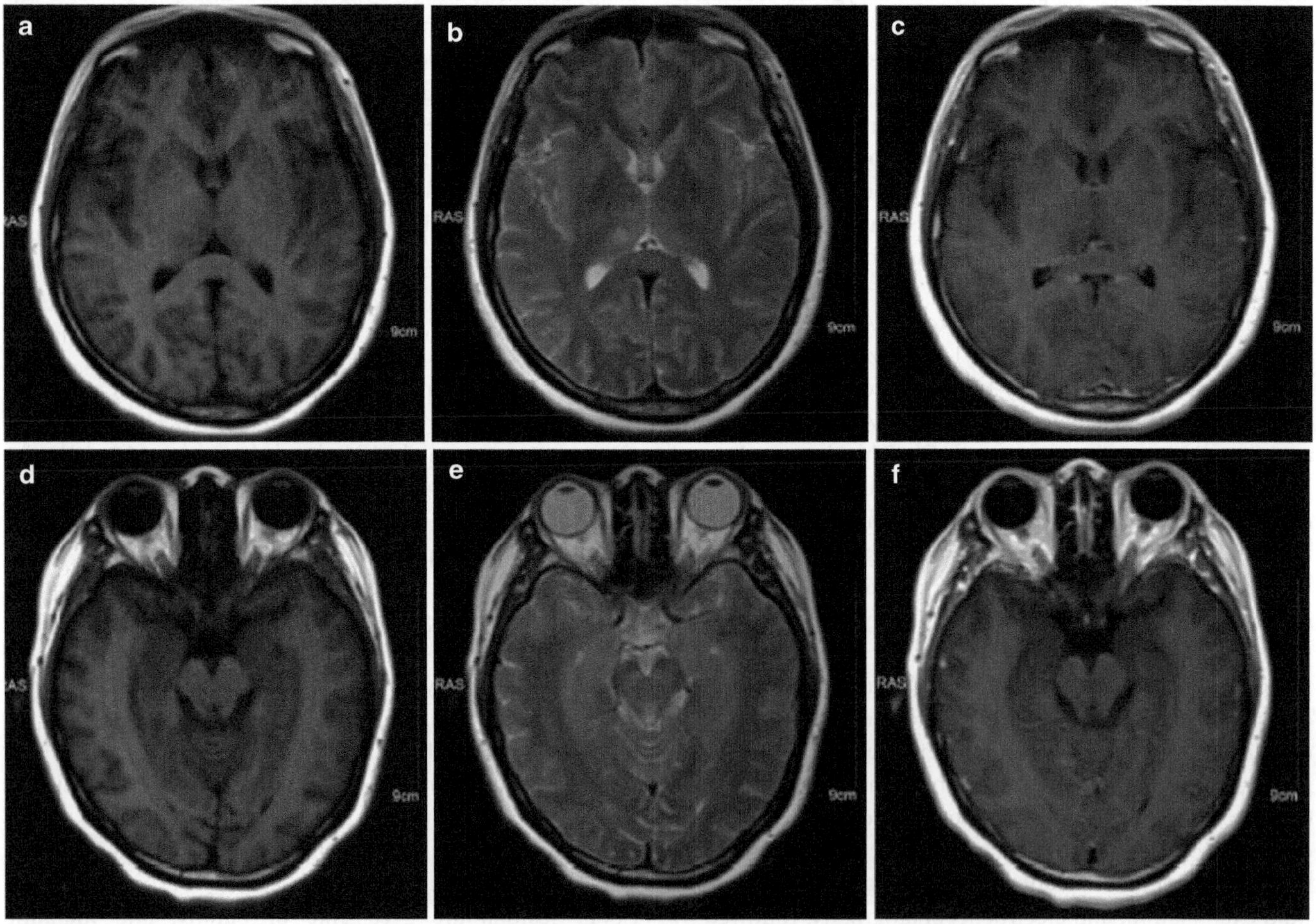

Fig. 18.5 Anti-NMDAR encephalitis. (**a**, **d**) T_1WI slightly low signal is seen in the bilateral dorsal thalamus and medial temporal lobe; (**b**, **e**) T_2WI slightly high signal is seen in the bilateral dorsal thalamus and medial temporal lobe; (**c**, **f**) No significant enhancement is seen after enhancement

being positive anti-neuronal antibodies. Its needs to be differentiated from herpes simplex virus encephalitis and hippocampal sclerosis.

1. Herpes simplex virus encephalitis: Bilateral temporal lobe involvement is its characteristic presentation, often asymmetrical. Moreover, a large patch of abnormal signal in the temporal, insular, or frontal lobes of the cerebral hemisphere, mostly involving cortical and subcortical white matter, is often seen, and the lesions are often associated with hemorrhage. The lesion starts in the medial temporal lobe region and gradually expands progressively to the frontal lobe and the limbic system such as the hippocampus [20].
2. Hippocampal sclerosis: Autoimmune encephalitis manifesting as symmetrical diffuse hippocampal changes also needs to be differentiated from hippocampal sclerosis, which, in addition to abnormally high hippocampal T_2WI signals, can also be seen as a reduction in hippocampal volume, with unilateral atrophic changes most likely to be found when comparing the size of the hippocampus on both sides in coronal view, with enlargement of the temporal horn of the affected ventricle [21].

18.3.6 Status and Progress of Research

1. Arterial spin labeling (ASL): ASL is a noninvasive magnetic resonance functional imaging technique that allows for the quantitative measurement of cerebral tissue perfusion using endogenous tracers. Autoimmune encephalitis is mainly mediated through autoimmune mechanisms and can cause the aggregation of inflammatory cells such as phagocytes and inflammatory factors, which leads to inflammatory vasodilation and increased blood flow, resulting in increased blood flow to the brain tissue and a manifestation of ASL hyperperfusion.
2. Magnetic resonance spectroscopy (MRS): MRS is a magnetic resonance detection method that uses chemical shift phenomena to determine the molecular composition of a substance. Cr peaks may be normal or slightly decreased in autoimmune encephalitis, Cho peaks may be normal or slightly increased, and NAA peaks may be decreased to varying degrees. The Cho peaks may not be significantly altered due to insignificant neuronal cell necrosis in the early stages of autoimmune encephalitis, but early neuronal cell and axonal damage may occur, which may lead to a decrease in the NAA peaks.
3. Positron emission tomography (PET): PET is useful in the diagnosis of limbic lobe encephalitis, and some patients with negative MRI findings of limbic lobe encephalitis show hypermetabolism in the medial temporal lobe on PET. It has also been found that patients with anti-NMDAR encephalitis have increased metabolism in the frontal and temporal lobes with decreased metabolism in the occipital lobe, that the degree of alteration of this metabolic gradient is positively correlated with disease severity, and that cortical metabolism returns to normal in these patients after clinical cure.

References

1. Koelman DL, Mateen FJ. Acute disseminated encephalomyelitis: current controversies in diagnosis and outcome. J Neurol. 2015;262(9):2013–24.
2. Young NP, Weinshenker BG, Lucchinetti CF. Acute disseminated encephalomyelitis: current understanding and controversies. Semin Neurol. 2008;28(1):84–94.
3. Pohl D, Alper G, van Haren K, et al. Acute disseminated encephalomyelitis: updates on an inflammatory CNS syndrome. Neurology. 2016;87(9 Suppl 2):S38–45.
4. Steiner I, Kennedy PG. Acute disseminated encephalomyelitis: current knowledge and open questions. J Neurovirol. 2015;21(5):473–9.
5. Krupp LB, Banwell B,Tenembaum S, et al. Consensus definitions proposed for pediatric multiplesclerosis and related disorders. Neurology, 2007;68:S7–12.
6. Burton KLO, Williams TA, Catchpoole SE, et al. Long-term neuropsychological outcomes of childhood onset acute disseminated encephalomyelitis (ADEM): a Meta-analysis. Neuropsychol Rev. 2017;27(2):124–33.
7. Bookstaver PB, Mohorn PL, Shah A, et al. Management of viral central nervous system infections: a primer for clinicians. J Cent Nerv Syst Dis. 2017;9:1179573517703342.
8. Varadkar S, Bien CG, Kruse CA, et al. Rasmussen's encephalitis: clinical features, pathobiology, and treatment advances. Lancet Neurol. 2014;13(2):195–205.
9. Pardo C, Vining E, Guo L, et al. The pathology of Rasmussen syndrome: stages of cortical involvement and neuropathological studies in 45 hemispherectomies. Epilepsia. 2004;45(5):516–26.
10. Yacubian E, Marie S, Valério R, et al. Neuroimaging findings in Rasmussen's syndrome. J Neuroimaging. 1997;7(1):16–22.
11. Bien CG, Urbach H, Deckert M, et al. Diagnosis and staging of Rasmussen's encephalitis by serial MRI and histopathology. Neurology. 2002;58(2):250–7.
12. Tien R, Ashdown B, Lewis DJ, et al. Rasmussen's encephalitis: neuroimaging findings in four patients. Am J Roentgenol. 1992;158:1329–32.
13. Chiapparini L, Granata T, Farina L, et al. Diagnostic imaging in 13 cases of Rasmussen's encephalitis. Neuroradiology. 2003;45(3):171–83.
14. Geller E, Faerber E, Legido A, et al. Rasmussen encephalitis: complementary role of multi technique neuroimaging. Am J Neuroradiol. 1998;19(3):445–9.
15. Wagner J, Schoene-Bake JC, Bien CG, et al. Automated 3D MRI volumetry reveals regional atrophy differences in Rasmussen encephalitis. Epilepsia. 2012;53(4):613–21.
16. Heine J, Prüss H, Bartsch T, et al. Imaging of autoimmune encephalitis-relevance for clinical practice and hippocampal function. Neuroscience. 2015;309:68–83.
17. Chinese Medical Association, Neurology Branch. Expert consensus on the diagnosis and treatment of autoimmune encephalitis. Chin J Neurol. 2017;50(2):91–8.
18. Graus F, Titulaer MJ, Balu R, et al. A clinical approach to diagnosis of autoimmune encephalitis. Lancet Neurol. 2016;15(4):391.
19. Du C, Zhang L, Guo X, et al. Clinical presentation and MRI characterization of autoimmune encephalitis. Chin J Neuropsychiatr Disord. 2017;43(6):341–5.
20. Zhang Y, Li Y, Wang X, et al. Herpes simplex virus encephalitis CT and MRI manifestations. Radiol Pract. 2014;29(3):276–8.
21. Zhang L, Feng Y, Chen X, et al. Diagnostic value of MRI and 18 F-FDG PET/CT for hippocampal sclerosis. J Jinan Univ (Med Ed). 2013;34(2):216–20.

19 Cerebral Vasculitis

Yuehua Li, Kai Shang, Xiaoqing Cheng, and Zhiqiang Zhang

Vasculitis is a group of vascular inflammatory diseases characterized by inflammatory and fibrinoid necrosis of the vessel wall as the main pathological feature, which can involve vessels of any size. In recent years, with the increase in the number of clinical tissue biopsy cases, there has been an increase in the number of affected vessels, tissues, types of infiltrating cells in the tissues, detectable autoantibodies in the serum, and vasculitis. The understanding of other relevant factors causing vasculitis has led to a continuous expansion and updating of the clinical classification of vasculitis. The 2012 Chapel Hill Conference further refined the understanding of vasculitis and updated the classification of vasculitis, which is currently the most widely used classification. In this classification, vasculitis has been classified into seven main categories, known as large vessel vasculitis (LVV) (includes Takayasu arteritis (TAK) and giant cell arteritis (GCA)), medium vessel vasculitis (MVV) (includes polyarteritis nodosa (PAN) and Kawasaki disease (KD)), small vessel vasculitis (SVV) (includes antineutrophil cytoplasmic antibody (ANCA)-associated vasculitis microscopic polyangiitis (MPA), granulomatous polyangiitis (GPA)/Wegener's granulomatosis (WG), eosinophilic granulomatous polyangiitis (EGPA)/Churg–Strauss syndrome (CSS), immune complex small vessel vasculitis, anti-glomerular basement membrane disease, cryoglobulinemic vasculitis (CV), IgA vasculitis (IgAV), and hypocomplementemic urticarial vasculitis (HUV)/anti-C1q vasculitis), variant vasculitis (VVV) (includes Behcet's disease (BD), Cogan's syndrome (CS)), single organ vasculitis (SOV) (cutaneous leukocytoclastic vasculitis, cutaneous arteritis, primary central nervous system vasculitis, isolated aortitis), vasculitis associated with systemic diseases (includes lupus vasculitis, rheumatoid vasculitis, and sarcoidosis vasculitis), and vasculitis associated with possible causes (includes hepatitis C virus-associated cryoglobulinemic vasculitis, hepatitis B virus-associated vasculitis, syphilis-associated aortitis, drug-associated immune complex vasculitis, drug-associated ANCA associated vasculitis, tumor-associated vasculitis, and other).

Central nervous system (CNS) vasculitis has also been classified in various ways and can be divided etiologically into primary angiitis of the central nervous system (PACNS) and secondary CNS vasculitis. PACNS means that the vasculitis is confined to the central nervous system (including the brain, meninges, and spinal cord) and does not involve other systems; vasculitis is secondary if it is secondary to a systemic or systemic disease, including mainly infectious diseases, connective tissue diseases, systemic vasculitis, and chronic inflammatory diseases. By pathology CNS vasculitis can be classified as granulomatous, lymphocytic, and necrotizing vasculitis. According to the size of the involved vessels, CNS vasculitis can be divided into large, medium, and small vasculitis.

19.1 Infectious Vasculitis

Yuehua Li, Kai Shang, and Xiaoqing Cheng

19.1.1 Overview

Infectious vasculitis of the central nervous system can be caused by a variety of pathogens, including bacteria, fungi, viruses, and spirochetes, such as those caused by acute septic meningitis, *Mycobacterium tuberculosis*, neurosyphilis, varicella-zoster, and fungi (*Mucor*, *Aspergillus*).

Y. Li (✉)
The Sixth People's Hospital of Shanghai Jiao Tong University, Shanghai, China

K. Shang
Shanghai Sixth People's Hospital, Shanghai, China

X. Cheng
Eastern War Zone General Hospital, Nanjing, China

Z. Zhang
General Hospital of Eastern Theater Command, Nanjing, China

H. Li et al. (eds.), *Radiology of Infectious and Inflammatory Diseases - Volume 1*,
https://doi.org/10.1007/978-981-99-0039-8_19

Acute septic meningitis can be caused by a variety of bacteria and can cause cerebral vasculitis and cerebral infarction in 5% to 15% of adults [1]. The patient had a significant elevation in serum C reactive protein (CRP), a common elevated white blood cell count on cerebrospinal fluid examination, a decreased cerebrospinal fluid glucose to serum glucose ratio, and a positive Pan's test.

Cerebral vasculitis due to *Mycobacterium tuberculosis* infection may be seen in 30% to 40% cases of tuberculous meningitis, most often involving the basilar vessels. It is mainly due to the rupture of the tuberculous nodules and the spread of *Mycobacterium tuberculosis* along the subarachnoid space involving the meninges, producing inflammatory exudates that then spread along the cerebral sulci and pools to the base of the brain, especially the lateral fissure pools of the brain, leading to vasculitis in the vessels traveling within them. Inflammatory exudates can also impede cerebrospinal fluid circulation and absorption, leading to obstructive or traffic hydrocephalus. Cerebrospinal fluid examination shows elevated protein levels and decreased chloride and sugar levels. In addition, cerebrospinal fluid adenosine deaminase (ADA), cerebrospinal fluid *Mycobacterium tuberculosis* (TB)-DNA test, plasma T cell spot test (T-SPOT), and other indicators are important indicators for the diagnosis.

Vasculitis due to neurosyphilis is generally thought to be the result of direct attack by syphilis spirochetes on vascular endothelial cells, causing necrosis of the endothelium and epithelium, followed by thrombosis, resulting in local cerebral tissue ischemia and infarction, which may have a subacute or chronic onset with progressive exacerbation. Lesions have a long latency period and can become symptomatic months to 12 years after infection. The characteristic presentation is usually headache and local neurological dysfunction associated with vascular lesions, which may be accompanied by abnormal changes in the central nervous system. The middle cerebral artery is most frequently involved, followed by the basilar artery. Currently, commonly used cerebrospinal fluid tests in neurosyphilis include routine cerebrospinal fluid, biochemical cerebrospinal fluid tests and specific and nonspecific detection tests for syphilis spirochetes, of which the Cerebrospinal Fluid Venereal Disease Research Laboratory (VDRL) examination is highly specific, and a positive result after excluding blood contamination is diagnostic of neurosyphilis, but is less sensitive.

Varicella-herpes zoster-associated vasculitis tends to involve the middle and anterior cerebral arteries, leading to secondary changes such as ischemic infarction, cerebral hemorrhage, and aneurysm formation, but bilateral infarcts in the basal ganglia region are less common. Virus-specific IgG or IgM antibodies in the serum or cerebrospinal fluid are important for virus detection.

Aspergillus, *Candida*, *Cyclospora*, and *Mucor* are the four most common CNS pathogens and can be chronic complications of acute or subacute CNS infections. These fungi can directly invade blood vessels leading to vasculitis and are more susceptible in people with sepsis, leukopenia, and immunosuppression, with *Candida albicans* being the most common and hematogenous infection being its primary route of infection. The formed mycelial colonies can invade and block large, medium, and small cerebral arteries, leading to cerebral infarction and encephalitis. Patients tend to have increased intracranial pressure, increased cerebrospinal fluid cell count and protein content, and normal or slightly low glucose and chloride. However, it is not specific, and sometimes cerebrospinal fluid tests can be abnormal in patients with *Aspergillus* infection. In addition, antigen and antibody tests in serum and blood fungal smears and cultures are also valuable in the diagnosis of fungal infections of the central nervous system.

Therefore, the diagnosis of CNS infectious vasculitis needs to be considered in the context of the patient's clinical presentation, imaging manifestations, laboratory tests, and pathological changes, and the possibility of the disease should be considered for unexplained headaches, behavioral cognitive abnormalities, and stroke in young people. CT and MRI are helpful as noninvasive tests for the diagnosis of vasculitis but lack specific changes and the gold standard for diagnosis remains brain pathology.

19.1.2 Pathological Manifestations

Vasculitis is characterized by non-atherosclerotic inflammation and necrosis of the vessel wall, and both arteries and veins can be involved. The diagnosis of infectious vasculitis must be confirmed by finding direct or indirect evidence of microbial infection [2].

Cerebral vasculitis due to *Mycobacterium tuberculosis* is mainly caused by direct invasion of the vessel wall by *Mycobacterium tuberculosis* or by surrounding inflammation. The adventitia was first involved, producing a strong polymorphonuclear reaction, followed by infiltration of lymphocytes, plasma cells, and macrophages. After the destruction of the outer membrane and elastic fibers, the inflammation gradually spreads to the inner membrane. Eventually, fibrin-like degeneration of small arteries and veins occurs, leading to thrombosis, focal hemorrhage, and occlusive vasculitis. Microscopically, the lesion shows a large accumulation of epithelioid cells and monocytes, as well as a typical nodule of tuberculosis consisting of giant cells from Langhans with a central caseous necrosis.

The typical pathological features of neurosyphilis-associated vasculitis are occlusive vasculitis and chronic inflammatory cell infiltration of the gray and white matter and soft meningeal vessels, with a central ischemic necrotic area visible in the lesion, surrounded by granulation tissue hyperplasia, and a reactive proliferating neuroglial tissue in the outer layer, and a large number of plasma cell infiltrates are its characteristic manifestations, but this manifestation is not specific, and the sensitivity of brain biopsy is low. So, the diagnosis can be made without relying on brain tissue biopsy if there is a clear history of syphilis infection or if the cerebrospinal fluid and serum syphilis tests are positive and there is improvement with syphilis repellent treatment.

19.1.3 Imaging

19.1.3.1 Angiography

The general presentation of routine angiography in infectious vasculitis is as follows: (1) alternating stenosis and dilatation of the affected vessels; (2) localized stenosis and occlusion of the vessels; (3) stenosis and pseudoaneurysm of long segments, etc. Different types of infections involve slightly different sites and patterns of blood vessels.

Tuberculous meningitis most often involves the arteries at the base of the skull resulting in vasculitis, especially the superior aspect of the internal carotid bed and the middle cerebral artery M1 segments, causing lumen occlusion and stenosis. The outer and middle membranes of the vessel are the first to be involved, and the inner membrane is the last to be involved; the angiogram may show short-segment stenosis, long-segment uniform stenosis, bead-like irregular stenosis, or complete occlusion.

Cerebral vasculitis due to neurosyphilis involves arteries with segmental irregular narrowing, dilatation, or "salami"-like changes, often asymmetrical bilaterally, and more pronounced in the proximal segments, with the supratentorial segment of the internal carotid artery, the horizontal segment of the internal carotid artery, the middle cerebral artery, and the beginning segment of the anterior cerebral artery being more common. Large vessel lesions present as concentric or asymmetric stenosis, and small vessels may be associated with aneurysmal dilatation.

Varicella-herpes zoster-associated vasculitis may be associated with aneurysms and localized vascular entrapment of the middle and anterior cerebral arteries, etc. DSA/MRA may show segmental stenosis, thrombosis, and bead-like changes in the anterior and proximal branches of the middle cerebral artery, mostly unilateral [3].

Fungal vasculitis angiography may show the narrowing of the basal or cortical vessels of the brain. Among these, vasculitis and secondary thrombosis resulting from invasion of the orbit and skull by *Trichoderma* infection can cause narrowing and occlusion of the superior ophthalmic vein, ophthalmic artery, or internal carotid artery, but complete occlusion of the unilateral internal carotid artery is less common (Fig. 19.1).

19.1.3.2 CT Finding

CT plain scan is relatively insensitive and may appear normal or may show corresponding secondary signs, such as ischemic/infarction, which appears as multiple hypointense shadows in the basal ganglia area, subcortical, and sometimes visible hemorrhage. Enhanced CT shows lesion display patchy enhancement, and if the meninges are involved, the adjacent meninges may also be enhanced. The foci of cerebral infarction due to syphilitic vasculitis are characteristic and usually present as of varying size multiple hypodense foci, often involving the cortex and subcortex, in a triangular or scalloped shape with the bottom edge outward.

19.1.3.3 MRI Findings

1. Bacterial vasculitis. Bacterial involvement of blood vessels can lead to the development of vasculitis, and the irritation of blood vessels by inflammatory exudates causes vasospasm and (or) thrombosis, resulting in arterial or venous infarction, which is the most common complication in adults. Of these, occlusion of small penetrating

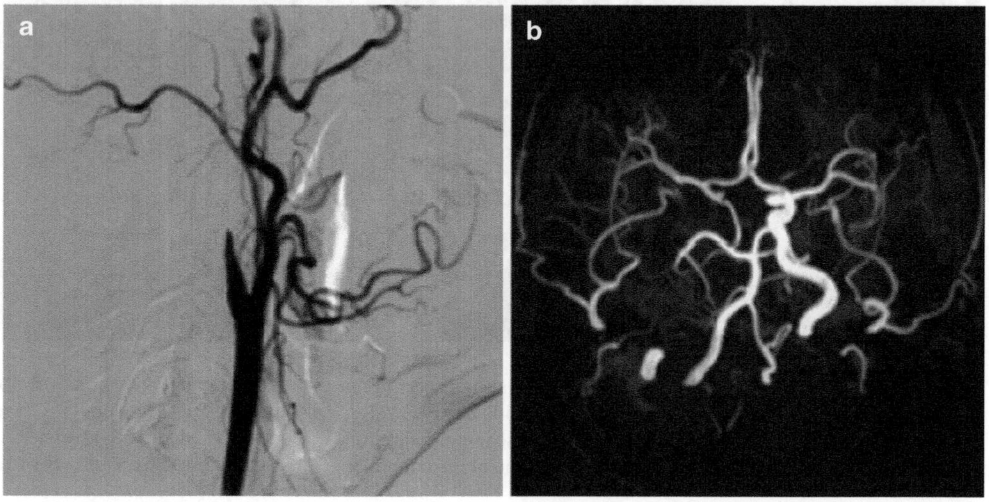

Fig. 19.1 *Mucor* infection-associated vasculitis. Right internal carotid artery lesion. (**a**) DSA showing complete occlusion of the right internal carotid artery after bifurcation of the common carotid artery; (**b**) 3D TOF-MRA showing complete occlusion of the right internal carotid artery. (Image courtesy of Eui Jong Kim, Kyung Hee University Hospital, Gangdong, Korea)

arteries may cause focal infarction of the basal ganglia, and spasm of the anterior and middle cerebral arteries may lead to large cerebral infarction. MR DWI sequence confirms an acute cerebral infarct lesion, which shows significant hyperintense. Hemorrhagic cerebral infarction may have characteristic changes depending on the time of infarction and the extent of hemorrhage, showing hypointense in the acute phase on T_2WI, and hyperintense in the subacute phase. During the evolution of hemorrhage from acute to subacute phase, cerebral cortical vein occlusion with or without thrombosis of the dural venous sinuses can result in hyperintense submoccipital cortex and subcortical cerebral white matter that does not correspond to the arterial distribution area. MR also has advantages for the demonstration of extravascular lesions of meningitis, such as subdural abscesses and meningeal and ventricular canal involvement.

2. Tuberculous vasculitis. Tuberculous exudate can involve the vessels through which it flows leading to vasculitis, with the pulsatile and middle cerebral arteries being the most susceptible, leading to narrowing or occlusion of the vessels [4]. Thus, ischemic cerebral infarction is a common complication of tuberculous vasculitis (Fig. 19.2), with common regions being the thalamus, basal ganglia region, and internal capsule, showing multiple small patchy hypointense on T_1WI and hyperintense on T_2WI and DWI with no enhancement on the enhanced scan. DWI shows an infarct area that is often larger than T_2WI, which can detect early cerebral infarction and is not significantly different from the presentation of infarct foci due to cerebrovascular lesions.
3. Syphilitic vasculitis. Multiple asymmetric hemispheric (including white and gray matter) infarct foci are common, showing hypointense on T_1WI and hyperintense on T_2WI and DWI, and the lesions are scattered and do not fully conform to the vascular distribution, located mainly in the subcortical and deep cerebral white matter, including the corpus callosum and internal capsule. Lesions are often with migration, with recurrence-remission, and new lesions may appear during follow-up, while old lesions may be significantly reduced. This feature is an important basis for differentiation from other lesions such as cerebrovascular disease and tumors. The signal after encephalomalacia is the same as in cerebrospinal fluid, displaying hypointense on T_1WI and hyperintense on T_2WI.
4. Viral vasculitis. Most viruses mainly affect the brain substantially; a few viruses can infect the cerebral vessels and cause cerebral vasculitis. The possibility of varicella-zoster vasculitis needs to be considered in pediatric patients presenting with unilateral basal ganglia infarcts, and infarcts in the bilateral basal ganglia region of this disease are rarely seen [1].
5. Fungal vasculitis. MR shows various secondary manifestations of fungal infections of the central nervous system, is superior to CT in the evaluation of skull base lesions and cerebrovascular occlusions, and is the imaging method of choice for demonstrating fungal infections. *Aspergillus* and *Mucor* can cause infection of the central nervous system by directly infection via the nasal cavity or sinuses or hematogenous dissemination. Among them, *Aspergillus* is mostly hematogenously disseminated, and direct infection often occurs with vascular involvement, mainly involving the cavernous sinus and the Willis ring, leading to vasculitis, thrombosis, and cerebral infarction; mycelial embolism can cause cerebrovascular occlusion and hemorrhagic cerebral infarction, and the lesion is usually far from the location of the primary focus, which can then progress to septic cerebral infarction, manifest-

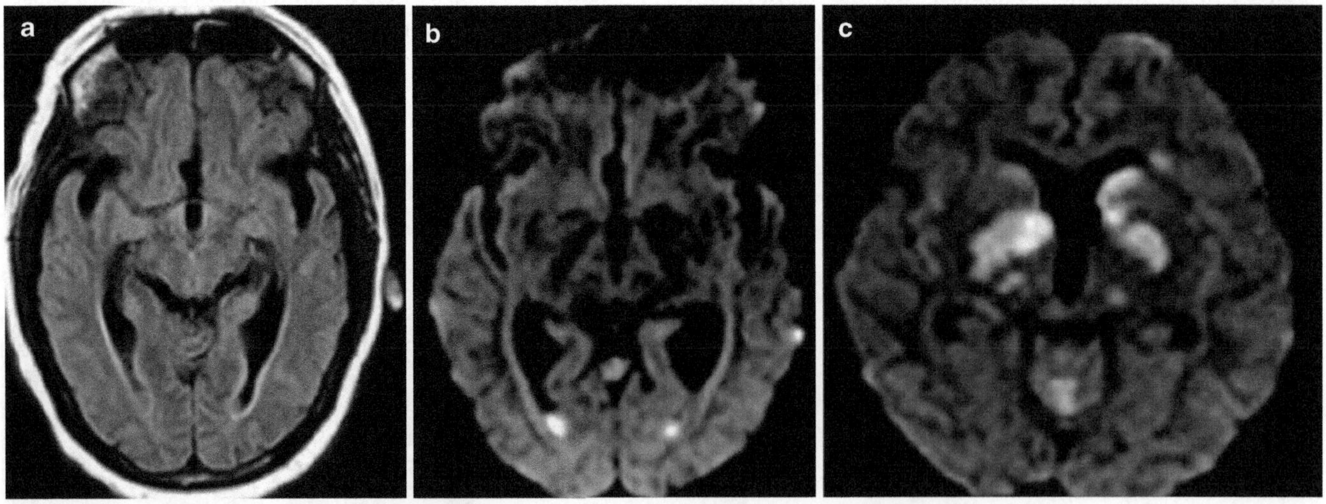

Fig. 19.2 Tuberculous vasculitis. (**a**) FLAIR shows the lesion is not obvious; (**b**, **c**) DWI shows that tuberculous vasculitis easily involves the penetrating branches and subcortex leading to ischemic infarction, and multiple foci of cerebral infarction are seen in the brainstem, bilateral basal ganglia area and the posterior horn of the lateral ventricle in this patient, showing obvious hyperintense on DWI. (Image courtesy of Chongqing Medical University Affiliated First Hospital of Chongqing Medical University, courtesy of Li Yongmei)

ing as hypointense on T_1WI and hyperintense on T_2WI with ring-like enhancement, or poorly defined borders, and may be associated with occupying effects. CNS infections caused by Coccidioides are primarily the result of hematogenous dissemination of spores from foci of pulmonary infection, characterized by meningeal infections with pus and caseous granulomas, preferably at the base of the brain, and vasculitis with vascular involvement, but occlusive vasculitis is less common. Candidiasis albicans occurs in young infants. Approximately 50% of deaths from invasive candidiasis have central nervous system involvement, with thrombosis, secondary infarction, and hemorrhage, followed by encephalomalacia and necrosis in the presence of intracranial vascular involvement, and venous sinus embolism and brain atrophy-like changes later in the disease [2].

19.1.4 Diagnostic Key Points

1. For unexplained headaches, behavioral-cognitive abnormalities, and strokes in youth, possibility of vasculitis should be considered.
2. CT and MRI examinations may show secondary infarction and abscess formation.
3. Cerebral angiography may show multiple irregular stenoses and dilatations alternating with the involvement of any intracranial vessels of varying size. The distribution characteristics of the lesions are not consistent with typical atherosclerotic changes.
4. The pathological manifestations are mainly inflammation and necrosis of the vessel wall, common in vasculitis. The diagnosis of infectious vasculitis requires direct and indirect evidence of microbial infection.

19.1.5 Differential Diagnosis

The diagnosis of infectious vasculitis is usually based on a combination of the patient's clinical presentation, brain MRI, and cerebral angiography findings. Vascular changes are usually localized stenosis, dilatation, and occlusion of vessels, and MR may show secondary manifestations following the involvement of vessels by various infections, mostly nonspecific. The specific manifestations of some pathogenic infections are suggestive of clinical significance. This disease needs to be differentiated from noninfectious vascular lesions.

19.1.5.1 Primary Central Nervous System Vasculitis

It is an etiology potentially serious inflammatory disease of unknown origin, which has no any obvious systemic vasculitis or possible etiology, diagnosed clinically primarily by exclusion. The clinical and imaging manifestations of the disease are varied, with the diseased vessels often showing alternating stenosis and dilatation and, rarely, long-segment stenosis, occlusion, and acute aneurysm formation, usually involving secondary and tertiary branch vessels more frequently. The classical change of intracerebral lesions is multiple, morphologically diverse, old and new, morphologically atypical, and not conforming to the cerebrovascular distribution of punctate or gyrus-like infarct lesions in the brain involving both the cortex and subcortex, unilaterally or bilaterally. Laboratory tests are nonspecific, and a brain biopsy is ultimately required to confirm the diagnosis.

19.1.5.2 Intracranial Atherosclerosis

See Sect. 19.2 of this chapter for details of identification.

19.1.5.3 Reversible Cerebral Vasoconstriction Syndrome

See Sect. 19.2 of this chapter for details of the differential diagnosis.

19.1.6 Status and Progress of Research

19.1.6.1 Angiography

DSA is the gold standard for the diagnosis of this disease. If the laboratory test is positive and the MR/MRA test is negative, a DSA test is required. DSA shows multiple luminal stenoses with smooth or mildly irregular walls alternating with segmental dilatation; any intracranial vessel of variable size may be involved; lesion characteristics and distribution are not consistent with typical atherosclerotic changes. CTA/MRA may aid in the diagnosis of cerebral vasculitis. CTA is mainly used to evaluate the vessel wall and lumen condition, and its spatial resolution is higher than MRA, and it is more reliable in the determination of intracranial and extracranial arterial stenosis, and it has a very high sensitivity (95% or more) and specificity (near 100% or more) in the diagnosis of asymptomatic vascular anomalies. MRA has the advantage of being noninvasive and easy to perform. But the most widely used 1.5T and 3.0T MRA only show alterations in above moderate vessels and have low temporal resolution, providing relatively little hemodynamic information. If the vascular abnormalities showed in MRA are inconsistent with the extent of the lesion, it may be an ischemic change due to a hypoperfusion state and chronic compensation, rather than a true infarct.

19.1.6.2 Three-Dimensional Volumetric Isotropic Fast Spin-Echo Technique (3D-VISTA)

It is a type of high-resolution fast spin-echo sequence with variable flip angle and refocusing pulses, which can effectively suppress blood flow effects and have a higher signal-to-noise ratio compared to ordinary high-resolution MR sequences. This technique allows reconstruction of the target vessel in any plane with the aid of multiplanar reconstruction (MPR), minimizes the misestimation of wall thickness due to vessel distortion, reduces the bias of stenosis measurement, clearly shows the morphology, signal, surface condition, and degree of enhancement of the vessel wall, shows the wall and lumen in all aspects, and helps to identify the cause of intracranial artery.

19.1.6.3 Magnetic Resonance High-Resolution Vascular Wall Imaging (HR-VWI)

For details, see the status and progress of research in Sect. 19.2 of this chapter.

19.1.6.4 Magnetic Resonance Arterial Spin Labeling (ASL)

It is a contrast-free MR perfusion method that uses blood in the artery as an endogenous marker, suppresses the arterial blood flowing into the imaging area by saturating the pulse, then marks the inflowing arterial blood using the inversion pulse, and finally subtracts the marked image from the unmarked image to obtain perfusion information by detecting the signal intensity change in the tissue. CBF can perform an early detection of altered cerebral perfusion status in patients with neurosyphilis and can provide an important basis for early diagnosis and treatment of neurosyphilis. Elevated CBF values indicate that acute syphilis attacks or disease in active phase and decreased CBF values indicate reduced inflammation, which indirectly reflects the effect of treatment, so CBF can be used as a reference to evaluate the effect of treatment for neurosyphilis.

19.2 Noninfectious Vasculitis

Yuehua Li, Kai Shang, and Zhiqiang Zhang

19.2.1 Primary Angiitis of the Central Nervous System

19.2.1.1 Overview

Primary angiitis of the central nervous system (PACNS), also known as primary cerebral vasculitis, is a rare and severe immunoinflammatory disease of small and medium-sized vessels mainly confined to the brain parenchyma, spinal cord, and leptomeninges. It can involve both arteries and veins, but is predominantly arterial. The etiology is unclear and may be related to immune abnormalities.

PACNS can occur at any age, with 40 to 60 years of age, and is the most common and occasionally seen in children. Most have a slow onset, a few have an acute onset, and the course of the disease may alternate between relapses and remissions or be progressively worse. The clinical signs and symptoms are nonspecific, mainly presenting as headache, cognitive impairment, persistent neurological deficits, and stroke. Epilepsy is most often seen in pediatric patients, and hemiparesis can occur with the involvement of larger blood vessels. Symptoms of systemic vasculitis such as fever, peripheral neuropathy, weight loss, and joint and muscle aches are less common. Early diagnosis and early treatment (including hormonal therapy and immunosuppressive therapy) of PACNS can significantly improve prognosis.

In recent years, there has been a clinical tendency to consider PACNS as a spectrum of disease with multiple clinical and pathological subtypes, with new subtypes such as PACNS with amyloidosis, meningeal small-vessel vasculitis, tumor-like lesions, angiographically negative PACNS, and progressive forms. The gold standard for the diagnosis of PACNS is still brain biopsy, and the most widely used clinical diagnostic criteria are those developed by Calabrese and Mallek in 1998. The details are as follows. (1) Clinical criteria, patient's history or clinical findings suggesting neurological deficits that cannot be explained by other lesions; (2) imaging and histological criteria, imaging and/or pathologically confirmed vascular inflammatory process in the CNS; (3) exclusion criteria, no evidence of systemic vasculitis or any evidence that the vasculitis is secondary, such as syphilis-associated vasculitis. The diagnosis of PACNS should meet all the above criteria, while the childhood-type PACNS requires an age of onset of 1 month to 18 years.

There are no clear laboratory indicators to diagnose or rule out PACNS, and the purpose of laboratory tests is mainly to rule out other diseases similar to its presentation. Elevated erythrocyte sedimentation rate (ECR) and C reactive protein (CRP) are seen in a small number of patients with PACNS. If the former is significantly elevated, along with anti-neutrophil cytoplasmic antibodies (ANCA), anticardiolipin antibodies (ACLA), serum complement, lupus anticoagulant, cold precipitated globulin, and other acute phase reactants were significantly elevated, secondary CNS vasculitis such as infection or inflammatory response process involving the whole body, associated connective tissue disease should be considered. Cerebrospinal fluid abnormalities are not specific for PACNS, mostly presenting as aseptic meningitis; protein levels and lymphocyte counts in the cerebrospinal fluid may be mildly to moderately elevated, with occasional positive oligoclonal bands and increased rates of IgG intrathecal synthesis.

19.2.1.2 Pathological Manifestations

The typical pathological changes in PACNS are vascular permeability damage and vascular destructive inflammatory responses, with the brain most frequently involved (95%), followed by the pons and medulla oblongata (32%), cerebellum (18%), and spinal cord (16%). Major histopathologic subtypes include granulomatous vasculitis, lymphocytic vasculitis, necrotizing vasculitis, and beta amyloid-associated cerebral vasculitis (ABRA). Granulomatous vasculitis is most common and presents as a vascular-centered mononuclear cell infiltrate with granuloma formation; granulomas are seen throughout the canal wall. Lymphocytic vasculitis presents with a large perivascular infiltrate of lymphocytes and a small number of plasma cells, with an unremarkable inflammatory response in the brain parenchyma. Necrotizing vasculitis primarily involves small muscular arteries and manifests as an acute inflammatory response in the vessel wall, destruction of the internal elastic lamina, and transmural-like avascular necrosis, often accompanied by subarachnoid hemorrhage. This type progresses rapidly and has a poor prognosis. ABRA often manifests as a giant cell, lymphocytic infiltrative inflammatory reaction and amyloid deposition around the leptomeninges and small cortical vessels with granuloma formation, and fibrinoid necrosis, focal hemorrhage, embolization, and recanalization are also seen.

The pathological diagnostic criteria of the University of Michigan Hospital and Health Center for PACNS are as follows: lymphocytic infiltration of at least two layers or more in the wall or perivascular canal of cerebral parenchymal vessels or meningeal vessels; necrosis or suspected necrosis of structures in the canal wall of the involved vessels; pinkish cytoplasm or nuclear condensation of neurons with or without astrocyte condensation or gliosis; neurophilic manifestations; brain parenchymal edema; exclusion of other pathologic diagnoses.

19.2.1.3 Imaging

Angiographic Manifestation

Angiography is not very sensitive to the diagnosis of PACNS, and a positive result can be used as evidence for the suspected diagnosis of PACNS. The diagnosis of PACNS requires the combination of appropriate clinical data and laboratory tests and the exclusion of other causes of similar cerebrovascular morphological changes.

According to the morphological changes and characteristics of the lumen, there are mainly three manifestations.

(1) Vascular stenosis: There are various types of stenosis, among which bead-like stenosis and multiple focal stenoses are the most common, usually bilateral, and are characterized by alternating luminal narrowing and dilatation of the lesioned vessel, mutual migration of the lesioned lumen and the normal lumen, and wall irregularities. In segmental stenosis, the degree of stenosis varies, the length of the lesion varies, and the wall is often not smooth. Single focal stenosis is the least common and is characterized by a localized narrowing of the lesion lumen, which is centripetal in nature and has a smooth wall. (2) Focal vascular occlusion: the occluded vessel is completely unremarkable, with an abrupt truncation sign or a ratty appearance, and the lesion may be surrounded with or without collateral circulation. (3) Aneurysm formation or aneurysmal dilatation: the lesioned vessel is cystically dilated, with localized dilatation centered on the lesioned vessel (Fig. 19.3). Cerebral angiography is often negative when the diameter of the involved vessels is less than 0.2 mm. In contrast, long segmental stenoses, microaneurysms, and complete occlusion of vessels are rare [5, 6].

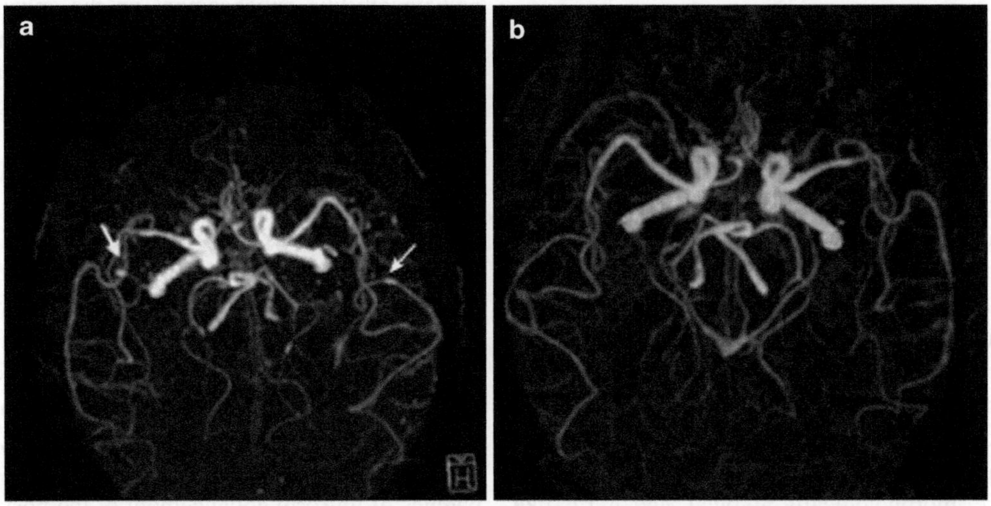

Fig. 19.3 Comparison of PACNS before and after treatment. Changes in the bilateral middle cerebral artery and its branching microangiomas during the course of the disease. (**a**) CT angiography-maximum intensity projection (CTA-MIP) before treatment showing multiple aneurysmal-like changes in bilateral anterior cerebral arteries, bilateral middle cerebral arteries, and bilateral posterior cerebral arteries (arrows); (**b**) CTA-MIP review after treatment showing the disappearance of aneurysms and essentially normal vascular morphology and structure. (Image courtesy of Chen Hongyan, Beijing Tiantan Hospital, Capital Medical University)

MRA and CTA are more effective in evaluating proximal cerebral arteries with larger diameters (including internal carotid artery, basilar artery, intracranial segment of vertebral artery, middle cerebral artery M1 segment, anterior cerebral artery A1 segment and posterior cerebral artery P1 segment, etc.), while PACNS usually affects small and medium-sized vessels of the CNS, so MRA and CTA are slightly less sensitive to PACNS. However, even DSA lacks the spatial resolution to evaluate the smallest vessels (<0.2 mm), so its sensitivity to PACNS is 60% to 70%. The specificity of DSA for the diagnosis of PACNS is also low (about 30%), partly because DSA cannot distinguish between vascular lesions and vasculitis. If manifestations such as large artery stenosis are present on MRA or CTA, other pathologies such as reversible cerebral vasoconstriction syndrome, atherosclerosis, arterial dissection, fibromuscular dysplasia, and Moyamoya disease should also be considered.

CT Findings

CT scan is relatively insensitive and usually normal, but some secondary changes, such as ischemia or infarction, are seen as multiple hypodense foci, particularly in the basal ganglia and subcortical white matter.

About 12% of PACNS patients with intracranial hemorrhage, mostly in women, have a subacute onset and may present with hyperdense shadow in the brain parenchyma, subarachnoid space, and intracerebroventricular space. Cerebral parenchymal hemorrhage is more common than subarachnoid hemorrhage, deep cerebral white matter hematomas are mostly caused by ruptured vessels, and hemorrhagic cortical infarction is mostly associated with reperfusion injury. Deep white matter calcification may also be present.

MRI Findings

MRI is the most sensitive imaging method and 90% to 100% of patients may have positive findings. Conventional MRI presentation may resemble infarction, demyelinating-like lesions, hemorrhage, or tumor-like lesions, with new lesions constantly appearing as the disease progresses, while old lesions may shrink or disappear, or malacic foci may remain, with lesions varying in age (Fig. 19.4). PACNS ischemic lesion mainly involving large and medium vessels have a higher incidence of vascular wall enhancement and PACNS mainly involving small vessels have a higher incidence of hemorrhage and MR enhancing lesions [7].

The classical changes in PACNS are multiple, morphologically diverse, morphologically atypical, and gyrus-like infarct lesions in unilateral or bilateral brains involving both the cortex and subcortex, with common sites being subcortical white matter, deep gray matter, deep white matter, and cortical in that order [2]. MRI T_1WI shows hypointense and T_2WI and FLAIR show hyperintense and the pathological basis of these signal changes is the narrowing and occlusion of the lumen caused by thrombus formation in the affected micro arteries in the lesion area, resulting in focal or diffuse ischemia of the brain tissue, producing cytotoxic cerebral edema or angiogenic cerebral edema. DWI hyperintense helps in the early detection of lesions, commonly in the acute phase of PACNS with concomitantly reduced ADC values, whose main pathological basis is cytotoxic brain edema. Elevated ADC values of lesions in the subacute and chronic phase can be seen as the disease progresses. Therefore, at follow-up review, DWI and ADC maps can be used to observe the dynamic changes of PACNS old and new alternating lesions and help to assess whether PACNS is in the active phase.

Other manifestations of PACNS: (1) Small and large hematomas in the brain parenchyma, vascular rupture due to permeable inflammatory infiltration of the involved vessels, and reperfusion injury in the infarcted area may be the cause of the PACNS intra-focal hemorrhage. The probability of brain parenchymal hemorrhage reported in the current literature regarding PACNS varies widely from 8% to 55%. Signal is heterogeneous in the case of intrafocal hemorrhage and may display hyperintense on T_1WI or hypointense on T_2WI, depending on the period of hemorrhage. Partial PACNS lesion presents only as a hemorrhagic cerebral infarction with diffusely distributed punctate and patchy hemorrhage seen around the lesion vessels. (2) Progressive fusion of white matter lesions, which can be solitary or multiple, can be easily misdiagnosed as demyelinating disease. When PACNS lesions are extensive and perifocal edema is evident, there can be an occupying effect, and there can be mass-like and wreath-like enhancement on the enhanced scan. This presentation is difficult to differentiate from brain tumors. (3) Enlargement of the perivascular space with enhancement and foci of enhancement in the leptomeninges. (4) Normal manifestation, seen in a few early PACNS. Magnetic resonance perfusion imaging can early detect abnormal perfusion areas, suggesting lesion location.

Spinal cord types account for about 5% of PACNS. Spinal cord involvement is not clearly sequential with brain involvement and may occur before, after, or simultaneously with it; involvement of the spinal cord alone is rare. The involvement of the thoracic segment of the spinal cord is commonly seen on MRI the examination. Multiple small patches of abnormal enhancement are seen on enhancement, which is more uniform and best observed in the sagittal view, and small patches of uniform enhancement of the posterior part of the spinal cord and soft spinal membranes are seen on the axial view. Patients who present with spinal cord lesions often have a poor prognosis.

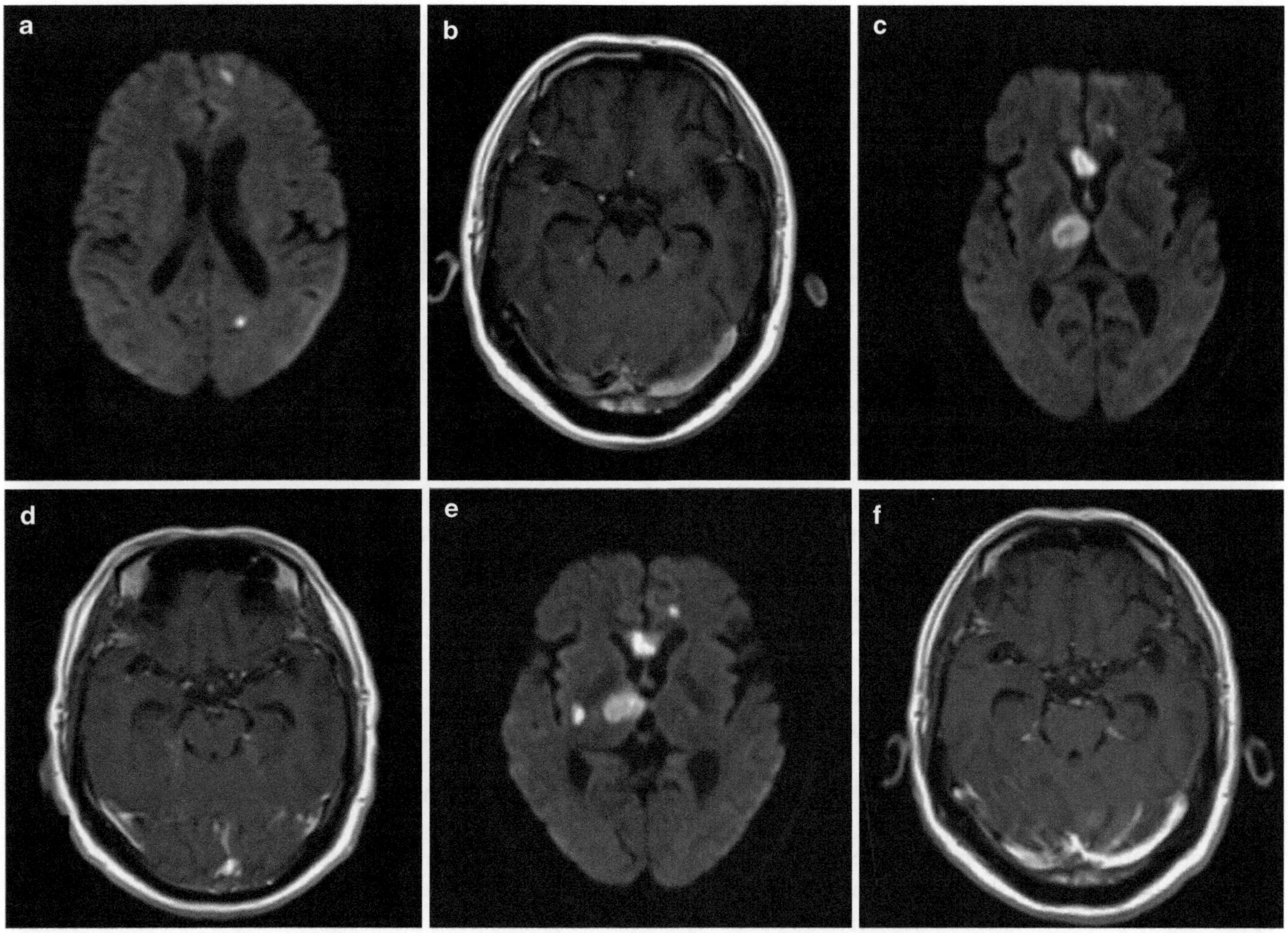

Fig. 19.4 Follow-up dynamic change of PACNS. The patient, female, 59 years old, was admitted to the hospital with recurrent dizziness for more than 5 months and was diagnosed with PACNS. **a**, **b** examined on November 2, 2016, **c**, **d** examined on December 1, 2016. The examination of **e**, **f** took place on March 1, 2017, and the site and size of the lesions and meninges of the patient's bilateral cerebral hemispheres changed dynamically during the follow-up. (**a**) DWI showing multiple acute cerebral infarcts in the left frontal, parietal, and occipital lobes. (**b**) T_1WI enhancement shows localized nodular enhancement of the meninges; (**c**) DWI shows multiple foci in the brainstem, right dorsal thalamus, basal ganglia area and genu of corpus callosum, deep white matter areas of both frontal lobes, and cerebellum (some foci disappear, some foci are new with migration, and with significant signal changes); (**d**) T_1WI enhancement shows localized thickening of the meninges with multiple nodular enhancement and multiple nodules in the vascular travel area; (**e**) DWI shows multiple foci in the genu of the corpus callosum, right thalamus, and right paraventricular and right cerebellar hemisphere; F. T_1WI enhancement shows meningeal enhancement which is similar to the previous. (Image courtesy of Chen Hongyan, Beijing Tiantan Hospital, Capital Medical University)

19.2.1.4 Diagnostic Key Points

1. PACNS has a wide range of age involvement (childhood to adulthood, with a mean age of 42 years).
2. CT and MR may show secondary manifestations of vasculitis (ischemia, infarction), commonly in the basal ganglia area and subcortical white matter.
3. DSA is the gold standard, with common presentations of bead-like stenosis, long segmental stenosis, vascular occlusion, and microaneurysms are rare, and small and medium-sized vessels are more frequently involved.
4. Typical pathological changes in PACNS are characterized by vascular permeability damage and vascular destructive inflammatory response; lesions may involve small and medium-sized vessels in the brain parenchyma, spinal cord, and leptomeninges, with nonspecific clinical presentation. There are no clear laboratory test indicators to diagnose or exclude PACNS.

19.2.1.5 Differential Diagnosis

The diagnosis of PACNS relies primarily on the patient's clinical presentation, imaging findings, and pathological change characteristics of the disease, which should be considered for unexplained headaches, chronic vasculitis, and strokes presenting in young adults. Although imaging is important, the gold standard for diagnosis remains pathology.

Cerebrovascular changes in PACNS need to be differentiated mainly from the following diseases.

Reversible Cerebral Vasoconstriction Syndromes (RCVS)

It is most often seen in young women aged 20 to 40 with reversible, multiple cerebral artery constriction. Patients may have severe, flash-like headaches, with or without focal neurological deficits, and the onset is most often triggered by stimulated vasospasm, such as postpartum, physiological stimuli, and drugs. DSA is essential for its diagnosis (sensitivity 100%); RCVS often involves large and middle arteries, with diffuse, multiple, segmental stenoses, mostly centripetal, sometimes with a "bead-like" or "salami-like" appearance. Intermittent DSA examination may show rapid improvement after administration of vasodilator medication. CT plain scan is often negative, and about 20% of patients may have a small amount of subarachnoid hemorrhage with or without parenchymal hemorrhage. CTA/MRA may show diffuse and segmental arterial stenosis and may appear normal (10%) if changes are mild. MRI commonly shows vascular-derived cerebral edema and watershed infarction, and high resolution (HR)-MRI mostly has no vessel wall enhancement.

Moyamoya Disease

It is an angiographically nonspecific disease, which can be acquired or inherited. Any slow progressive occlusion of the superior aspect of the internal carotid artery bed can develop into a manifestation of moyamoya disease. In the early stages of angiography, stenosis of the internal carotid artery and proximal segment of the circle of Willis is seen. In the middle stages, cloudy nucleus striatum arteries and collateral circulation of the thalamus penetrating arteries are seen, and in the late stages, collateral circulation of the external–internal carotid artery and transdural and transosseous collaterals is seen.

Intracranial Atherosclerosis

It is a major cause of ischemic stroke in older patients with eccentric, irregularly narrowed vessels that may be associated with ulceration and calcification. Enhanced scans may show heterogeneous mild to moderate enhancement of vascular wall or ring-like enhancement of vascular wall resembling vasculitis; dilated tortuous vessels are rare. The terminal basilar artery or the cavernous sinus/supraclinoid segment of the internal carotid artery is the most common site, while the circle of Willis and the middle cerebral artery are rare (about 2%). T_1WI and T_2WI exhibit diminished or absence of vascular flow void signal; FLAIR may show hyperintense due to slow blood flow or lumen occlusion, most commonly occurs in the proximal segment or bifurcations of arterial branches, which may be enhanced after enhancement and may be associated with an inflammatory response or neovascularization.

Intracerebral lesions in PACNS are primarily identified with cranial MRI-positive disease, where multiple foci of punctate or gyral-like infarction need to be differentiated from autosomal dominant hereditary cerebral arteriopathy with subcortical infarction and white matter encephalopathy, the latter mostly with a family history and positive genetic screening for notch3 gene mutation. Solitary tumor-like white matter lesions with occupying effects need to be differentiated from brain tumors (e.g., gliomas, lymphomas, etc.) and tumor-like demyelinating diseases; multiple white matter lesions need to be differentiated from inflammatory demyelinating diseases such as multiple sclerosis and progressive multifocal leukoencephalopathy, which have overlapping in imaging manifestations and no obvious specificity, and are difficult to differentiate on imaging, and need to be differentiated based on pathology.

Other diseases that need to be identified include infectious vasculitis, systemic vasculitis, and cardiogenic multiple cerebral infarctions.

19.2.1.6 Status and Progress of Research

Magnetic Resonance High-Resolution Vessel Wall Imaging (HR-VWI)

The use of intracranial three-dimensional (3D) vessel wall imaging has become increasingly widespread in recent years. 3D acquisition can reconstruct isotropic volume acquisition in any plane by isotropic scanning and the use of increased brain coverage area, showing the tortuous intracranial vessels with resolutions up to 0.4 mm. The "black blood technique" makes the canal wall more visible by suppressing intracranial blood flow signals and perivascular cerebrospinal fluid signals (Fig. 19.5). The typical presentation of involved vessels in PACNS is smooth, homogeneous marked centripetal enhancement, but with low specificity, mostly in large/medium vessels, which may show secondary ischemic signs [8]. Some patients with biopsy pathologically confirmed PACNS did not show wall enhancement, which may be related to inflammation involving small diameter vessels beyond the resolving power of wall imaging.

Magnetic Resonance Magnetic Sensitivity Weighted Imaging (SWI)

It is a technique for imaging magnetic sensitivity differences between different tissues using deviations in magnetization rates dependent on oxygen saturation. SWI is less disturbed by blood flow velocity, has a significant imaging advantage for small vessels around vasculitis, and is a superior sequence for diagnosing PACNS, which can show compensatory thickened vessels around vasculitis. It is also sensitive to trivalent iron and can show microhemorrhagic foci and hemosiderin

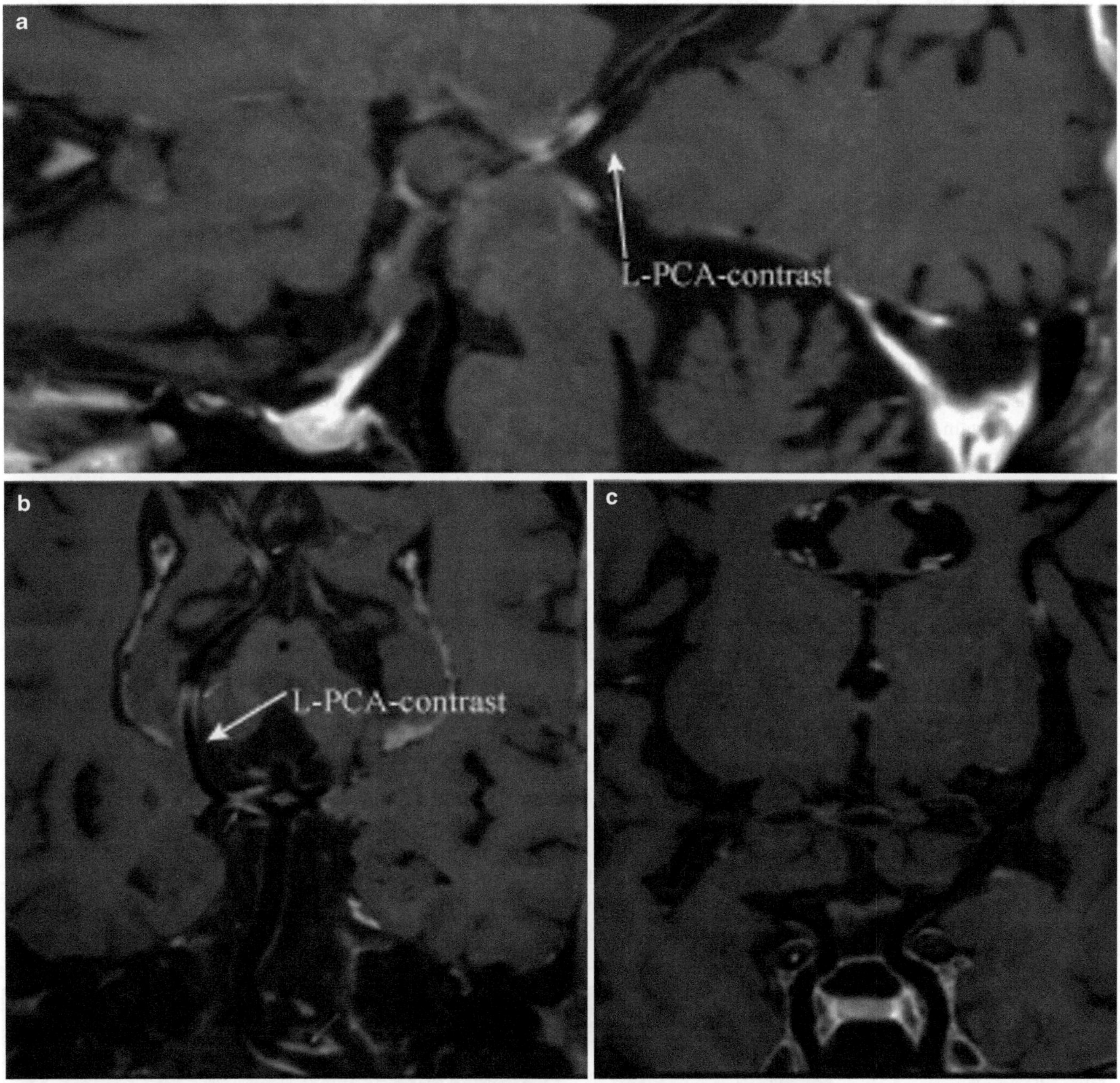

Fig. 19.5 Cerebrovascular changes of PACNS. The patient, male, 49 years old, was admitted to the hospital with "impaired right side limb movement with adverse speech for more than 3 months." The imaging study shows significant enhancement of the cerebral vessel wall. (**a**, **b**) HR-VWI shows localized wall thickening and marked enhancement of the P2 segment of the left posterior cerebral artery; (**c**) HR-VWI shows segmental centripetal enhancement of the M2 segment of the left middle cerebral artery. (Image courtesy of Xia Shuang, Tianjin First Central Hospital)

deposition. The microhemorrhagic foci show a significant signal intensity loss in multiple spots on SWI, which is caused by increased permeability of the vessel wall after infiltration by inflammatory cells causing blood leakage, which is also highly suggestive of the small vessel damage characteristic of PACNS. The possibility of PACNS should be highly suspected in extensive hemorrhage, primarily cortical-subcortical, especially in the presence of chronic, quiescent punctate hemorrhage combined with multifocal ischemic lesions.

Magnetic Resonance Diffusion-Weighted Imaging (DWI)

PACNS patients with diffuse changes in brain tissue may show diffusion restriction throughout the corona radiata and centrum semiovale, the thalamus, and the posterior part of the internal capsule. Combined ADC analysis helps to elucidate the extent of vascular abnormalities in the central nervous system. CNS vasculitis is often combined with cytotoxic cerebral edema, showing hyperintense on DWI and hypointense on ADC. DWI combined with ADC can indicate the stage of vasculitis. DWI is more sensitive to early lesions and small lesions and can show the superposition of lesions from different periods [9].

Magnetic Resonance Perfusion Imaging (PWI)

Currently, there are two different PWI imaging methods: dynamic contrast-enhanced magnetic resonance imaging and arterial spin labeling. The former method requires the injection of a contrast agent and rapid acquisition of continuous images at a given location. Several physiological maps can be obtained from the first-pass curve, including cerebral blood volume, cerebral blood flow, peak time, and mean time to pass. The latter method does not require a contrast agent [1]. The distinguishing feature of PACNS is a state of hypoperfusion in certain areas due to vasculitis, and abnormalities in different parameters may show local microcirculatory alterations suggestive of microangiopathy.

19.2.2 Various Other Vasculitis

19.2.2.1 Large Vessel Vasculitis

1. Aortitis. It is a chronic, nonspecific inflammatory disease affecting the aorta and its major branches, of unknown etiology, occurring in people between 20 and 30 years of age. Vascular involvement manifests as vessel wall thickening, lumen narrowing, occlusion, dilatation, and aneurysm formation (Fig. 19.6). CT plain scan of the early stage of the lesion shows vessel wall hyperdensity with calcification, and vessel wall enhancement is seen on enhanced scan; T_2WI sequence shows vessel wall thickening with hyperintense shadow in the lumen and around the vessel. The chronic phase presents with segmental stenosis and marked dilatation of the common carotid and subclavian arteries, and a large number of accompanying collateral branches of the bypass may be present in the event of complete occlusion at the beginning of the vessel. The disease can be diagnosed when the lesion is shown to involve the aorta or at least two medium vessels on DSA.
2. Giant cell arteritis. It is a chronic granulomatous vasculitis, involving mainly the superficial temporal artery, but also the occipital artery, with an age of onset mostly above 55 years. The main manifestation is wall thickening, T_2WI sequence may show wall edema, and enhancement of the wall may occur.

19.2.2.2 Medium Vessel Vasculitis

1. Arteritis nodosa. It is a necrotizing inflammatory disease affecting the middle arteries involving the entire lamina, with characteristic pathologic changes of multiple aneurysm formation, with imaging primarily showing luminal narrowing or occlusion and aneurysm formation (Fig. 19.7).
2. Kawasaki disease. It is most commonly seen in children and is associated with sudden high fever, oral mucositis, rash, bilateral conjunctival congestion, and enlarged cervical lymph nodes, and may be associated with nonspecific cerebral infarction, cerebral atrophy, recurrent T_2WI hyperintense foci, and subcortical lesions with subdural exudates.

19.2.2.3 Small Vessel Vasculitis

1. IgA vasculitis: It is a vasculitis caused by the deposition of IgA immune complexes in the walls of blood vessels, commonly in children aged 4 to 7 years. Involvement of the central nervous system is rare, sometimes with hyper-

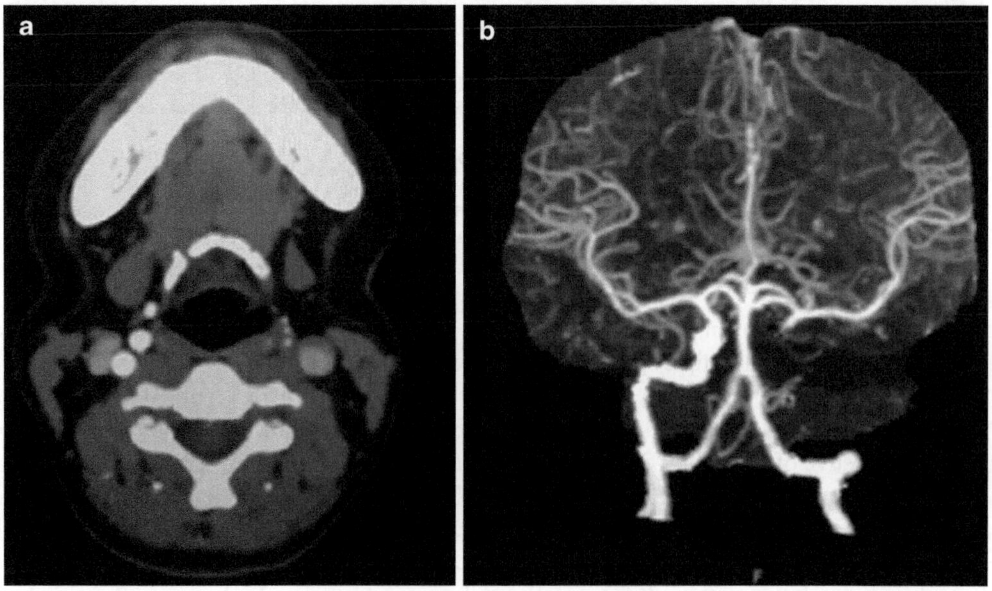

Fig. 19.6 Takayasu arteritis. Left internal carotid artery lesion. (**a**) CT-enhanced scan showing ring-like thickening of the wall of the left common carotid artery with luminal narrowing; (**b**) CTA-MIP showing occlusion of the entire left internal carotid artery

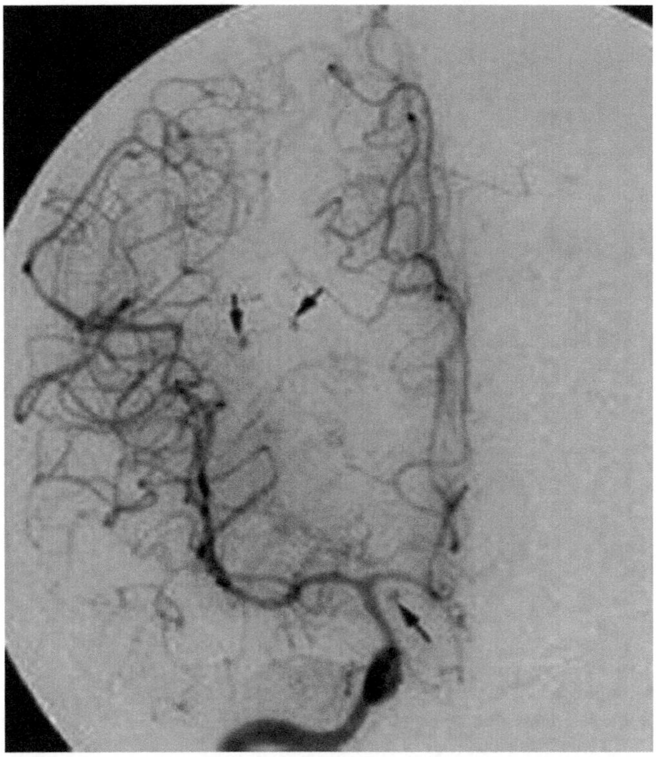

Fig. 19.7 Nodular arteritis. DSA showing multiple microaneurysms of the right middle cerebral artery branches (arrow). (Image courtesy of Li Yongmei, The First Hospital of Chongqing Medical University)

tensive encephalopathy and localized ischemic and hemorrhagic lesions.

2. Granulomatous polyangiitis. It is a vasculitis affecting small vessels and positive for anti-neutrophil cytoplasmic antibodies, involving the central nervous system in more than 35% of patients, showing enhancement of leptomeninges and intracerebral and intraspinal lesions. Necrotizing cerebral vasculitis often occurs in conjunction with sinusitis, otitis, or pulmonary disease. CT scan shows granuloma with soft tissue density in the nasal cavity and hypointense on T_1WI and T_2WI. CT and MR enhancement shows varying degrees of enhancement.

19.2.2.4 Vasculitis Associated with Systemic Disease

1. Systemic lupus erythematosus. T_2WI shows the main four types of CNS involvement, namely focal gray matter hyperintense, multiple T_2WI hyperintense (microinfarcts), new infarcts, and extensive, reversible white matter lesions (cerebral edema). Brain atrophy may occur in a small percentage of patients, and intracranial hemorrhage is rare (3%).
2. Dry syndrome. Around 25% to 30% of patients with dry syndrome involve the central nervous system with trigeminal neuropathy, recurrent aseptic encephalitis encephalopathy, extensive white matter, intra-gray matter lesions and microhemorrhagic foci, and hypertrophy of the lacrimal and salivary glands.
3. Rheumatoid arthritis. Dural meningitis with enhancement of the leptomeninges, as well as dural nodules, and cerebral vasculitis is rarer.
4. Antiphospholipid antibody syndrome. The main symptoms are arterial and venous thrombosis, thrombocytopenia, and habitual abortion, and the DWI and SWI sequences show a significant advantage for secondary changes such as cerebral infarction and microhemorrhage.
5. Scleroderma. It is a progressive disease that results in hardening of the skin and its connecting tissues with MR manifestations that are nonspecific and include nonspecific infarcts, massive or small amounts of hemorrhage, and extensive calcifications.

19.2.2.5 Vasculitis Due to Drug Abuse

Drugs including amphetamines, cocaine, heroin, phenylpropanolamine, and ergot can directly or indirectly (usually as a hypersensitivity reaction to contaminants) damage blood vessels. Cocaine can cause vasculitis, vasospasm, platelet aggregation, and eventually cerebral infarction, cerebral leukomalacia, and cerebral hemorrhage, and smoldering revascularization in chronic dependence. Heroin abusers present more commonly with spongiform white matter lesions [2].

19.2.2.6 Radiation Injury

Acute arteritis can cause transient white mass edema, with more severe chronic changes, and is often associated with vascular occlusion and ischemic necrosis of brain tissue, leukomalacia, mineralized microangiopathy, and cerebral atrophy, with thickening of the walls of the affected large vessels and permanent enhancement of the walls.

19.3 Sarcoidosis

Yuehua Li, Kai Shang, and Zhiqiang Zhang

19.3.1 Overview

Sarcoidosis is a multisystem inflammatory disease of unknown etiology, typically characterized by the formation of non-caseating granulomas, most often involving the lungs, but also the eyes, skin, liver, spleen, and nervous system. The incidence of sarcoidosis is 10–65/100 thousand, with neurological involvement of 5%–15% and a mean age of onset of 33–41 years, which is later than other types of sarcoidosis. Neurosarcoidosis (NS) has a tendency to spread perivascularly and can also lead to disease of parenchymal, leptomeninges, or dural mater and can result in granulomatous vasculitis. Isolated neurological sarcoidosis is very rare.

The clinical presentation of neurological sarcoidosis is varied and is primarily related to the location and size of the granuloma. The cerebral nerves (especially the facial nerve) are most frequently involved, mainly in the form of multiple cerebral nerve palsy, and bilateral peripheral facial palsy is considered to be the characteristic clinical manifestation of neurological sarcoidosis, followed by spinal cord lesions, parenchymal lesions, meningeal lesions, and peripheral neuropathies. Common nonspecific symptoms include headache, fatigue, nausea, vomiting, depression, ataxia, and tremor. Cerebrovascular events due to neurological sarcoidosis include mainly transient cerebral ischemia, cerebral infarction, cerebral hemorrhage, and central venous thrombosis and are mainly associated with granuloma invasion of the vessel wall and compression of larger vessels by the granuloma. Hypothalamic and pituitary involvement can lead to endocrine abnormalities, which can manifest as uremia, hyperprolactinemia, and autonomic dysfunction. About 40% of patients may present with acute or chronic meningitis.

Routine serological tests for neurological sarcoidosis are usually unremarkable; some patients may present with serum angiotensin-converting enzyme (ACE), which is elevated but not specific. Elevation of total protein on cerebrospinal fluid examination was most common (63% to 69%), followed by lymphocytosis (47% to 58%), with a lower incidence of low glucose (about 14%). Cerebrospinal fluid ACE is not sensitive for neurological nodal disease but has a high specificity (up to 94% to 95%) and can be used to monitor disease activity and treatment efficacy. Elevated soluble interleukin 2 receptor (sIL2R), a marker reflecting the degree of lymphocyte activation, is also suggestive, but not specific, and can be seen in patients with intracranial infections or malignancies.

There are two main types of neurological sarcoidosis. (1) Involvement of the meninges or ependyma, most commonly present as granulomatous meningitis. The lesions are usually distributed at the base of the brain, with the saddle most susceptible (including the optic cross, pituitary, and hypothalamic regions), and are diffuse or confined. This type is more common. (2) Brain parenchymal involvement, including non-caseating necrotizing granulomas of the brain parenchyma and brain tumor-like solitary giant masses. This type is less common.

19.3.2 Pathological Manifestations

Histological biopsy of the lesion site is the gold standard for the diagnosis of sarcoidosis. The characteristic pathologic manifestation of sarcoidosis is a noncaseating epithelioid cell granuloma (Fig. 19.8), consisting primarily of highly activated mononuclear phagocytes and lymphocytes. Two relatively specific types of inclusion bodies are seen in the cytoplasm of multinucleated giant cells in about 60% of patients with sarcoidosis, one of which is radial astral vesicles that are strongly eosinophilic, and the other is lamellar vesicles formed by iron- and calcium-containing proteins. However, non-caseating granulomas are not a specific change in sarcoidosis, and tuberculosis, fungal infections, and beryllium granulomas should also be excluded in the diagnosis of the disease.

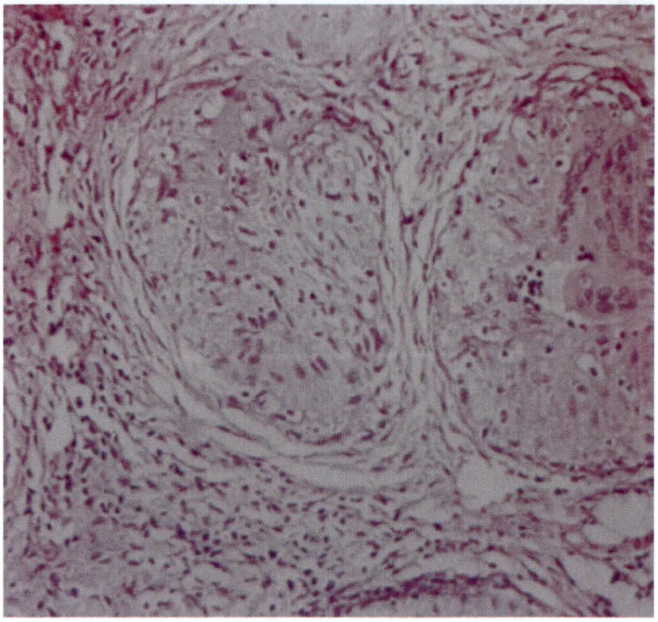

Fig. 19.8 Sarcoidosis. Pathological sections showed epithelioid cells, lymphocytes, and multinucleated giant cells forming multiple nodules in the lesion, with no caseous necrosis in the nodules

19.3.3 Imaging

19.3.3.1 Angiographic Findings

Intracerebral granulomas mainly in the middle and small perivascular vessels (tube size such as penetrating arteries), most likely to involve the outer membrane, with less involvement of the middle and inner membranes [10], so cerebral angiography such as DSA and MRA usually show negative results. Involvement of large vessels is rare and may be due to compression by granulomas or masses.

19.3.3.2 CT Findings

1. Brain parenchyma. Nodular granulomas or masses in the brain are manifest as slightly hyperdense on CT plain scan with relatively well-defined borders and may or may not with enhancement on the enhanced scan.
2. Meninges. Leptomeninges involvement is most common, with good skull base meningeal involvement. CT plain

scan does not easily reveal positive changes, and enhancement may show meningeal thickening with nodular or linear enhancement along the brain contour, which may extend to the sulcus, and the distribution of lesions may be diffuse, focal, or multiple.

3. CT plain scan may also show indirect signs such as hydrocephalus and intracranial calcifications. Also, 5% to 12% of neurological sarcoidosis may present with hydrocephalus and the main reason is that obstructed cerebrospinal fluid absorption leads to traffic hydrocephalus and obstructive hydrocephalus due to adhesions or separation of the ventricular system by meningeal involvement.

19.3.3.3 MRI Findings

1. Brain parenchymal changes. Sarcoidosis involving the brain parenchyma has mainly two types of changes. The first type presents with multiple periventricular or small subcortical white matter hyperintense on T_2WI without enhancement, usually without the Dawson finger sign, without leptomeninges or parenchymal enhancing lesions, and without correlation between clinical symptoms and imaging presentation; the second type is a multiple tumor-like lesion, often involving the adjacent leptomeninges (Fig. 19.9a), probably due to the spread of lymphocytes along the leptomeninges in the perivascular space. The lesion may also involve the meninges at the base of the skull and adjacent blood vessels, disrupting the blood–brain barrier, so enhanced lesions may appear after enhancement, and should be distinguished from brain abscesses and metastases. The clinical manifestations of this group of patients are related to the radiological manifestations and improve when the radiological manifestations subside. Pituitary involvement is uncommon, and when involved, the normal hyperintense of T_1WI of the posterior pituitary lobe is lost due to the absence of intracellular neurosecretory granules. Pituitary sarcoidosis may also present as a cystic, thick-walled mass in the saddle and suprasellar regions, encircling the optic cross and extending into the funnel and hypothalamus, which may be enhanced upon enhancement [11]. Ischemic/hemorrhagic stroke and other vascular manifestations are rare, and hemorrhage in the brain parenchyma usually presents as multiple small blebs in atypical sites of supratentorial [12].
2. Meningeal changes. Leptomeninges involvement is the most common manifestation of neurological sarcoidosis. T_1WI contrast enhancement shows the leptomeninges involvement best and manifested by leptomeninges thickening and marked diffuse or nodular enhancement, which can occur in any part of the meninges, mostly concentrated in the deep cerebral sulcus, preferably in the meninges at the base of the brain, especially in the saddle and frontal region (Fig. 19.9b). Some may form mass-like lesions, especially in the optic cross, the base of the third ventricle, and the pituitary stalk. Because sarcoidosis spreads mainly along the perivascular space with late involvement of the brain parenchyma, the presence of only leptomeninges involvement on imaging with little or no involvement of the brain parenchyma is usually indicative of early-stage disease. Dural mater involvement is mainly manifested by dural mater thickening, T_1WI with hypo to isointense which is similar to gray matter, and T_2WI with hypointense (probably related to fibrillar collagen accumulation); the lesion can be limited or diffusely distributed, and homogeneous enhancement is seen on enhanced T_1WI scan. Simultaneous involvement of dura mater and leptomeninges in the same location is rare and is related to the barrier cells of the arachnoid, which have no extracellular gaps, with a large number of cell junctions, and a basement membrane that separates them from the subarachnoid space and thus prevents lymphocyte infiltration.
3. Cerebral nerves. All brain nerves can be involved. Clinically, the involvement of the facial nerve is most common (Fig. 19.9c). The optic nerve is most frequently involved on imaging, with unilateral (69%) or bilateral (31%) onset, either in the optic cross or intraorbital segment. The imaging presentation of optic nerve dural sheath involvement is similar to that of optic nerve sheath meningioma, showing thickening of the involved optic nerve with abnormal enhancement. Other cerebral nerve involvement presented similarly, all showing nerve thickening and abnormal enhancement.
4. Spinal cord. Intramedullary lesions are rare, occurring in less than 1%, and can occur anywhere in the spinal cord but are common in the cervical and thoracic medulla. The imaging manifestation is spindle enlargement of the spinal cord, which displays hypointense on T_1WI and hyperintense on T_2WI, and the lesion is more clearly shown on the proton density-weighted image (PDW) and manifest as patchy abnormal enhancement on enhanced T_1WI scan (Fig. 19.9d). The presence of enhancing nodules and spinal pia mater involvement suggests a diagnosis. These imaging manifestations are often more severe than the clinical presentation, and a mismatch between imaging and clinical findings may be a clue suggestive of the disease.

19.3.4 Diagnostic Key Points

1. The signs or symptoms of neurological sarcoidosis depend on the location of the lesion, with cerebral nerve involvement being the most common.
2. The lesion usually spreads along the perivascular space and extends into the brain parenchyma to form a lesion.

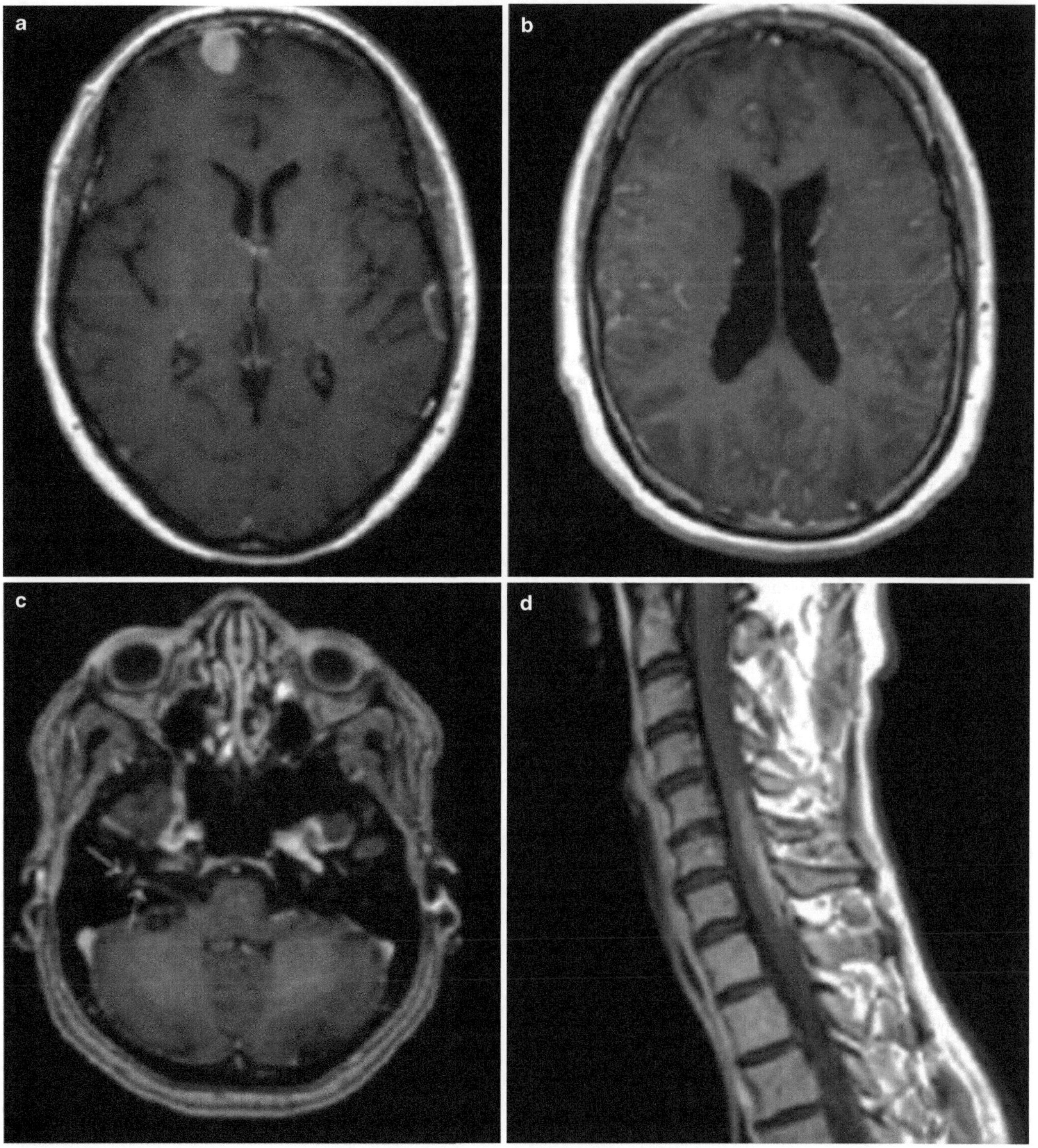

Fig. 19.9 Sarcoidosis of the nervous system. Intracerebral involvement, meningeal changes, cerebral nerve changes, and spinal cord involvement in neurological sarcoidosis. (**a**) T_1WI enhanced scan shows a right frontal lobe enhancing nodule with adjacent soft meningeal enhancement, suggesting soft meningeal involvement. (**b**) T_1WI enhanced scans shows abnormal leptomeninges enhancement; (**c**) T_1WI enhanced scan shows right facial nerve enhancement; (**d**) T_1WI enhanced scan shows lamellar abnormal enhancement foci in the spinal cord (sagittal position of the cervical spine). (Images courtesy of Huang Guang, Fuxing Hospital, Capital Medical University)

3. The typical presentation is leptomeningitis of cranial base or diffuse granulomatous leptomeningitis. CT and MR may show leptomeninges thickening and marked diffuse or nodular enhancement with secondary changes in the optic chiasm, hypothalamus, base of the third ventricle, and pituitary gland.
4. The typical pathology of sarcoidosis is a non-caseating granuloma with aggregates of multinucleated macrophages and epithelioid cells in the center of the lesion surrounded by peripheral lymphocytes. Laboratory tests may show inflammatory changes in the central nervous system such as increased protein content or increased cell count in the cerebrospinal fluid and positive oligoclonal bands.

19.3.5 Differential Diagnosis

Meningitis and vasculitis are more common in neurological sarcoidosis than in parenchymal brain lesions, usually spreading along the perivascular space and involving the vessels at the base of the brain. Typical presentation is cranial base or diffuse granulomatous leptomeningitis with secondary changes in the optic chiasm, hypothalamus, base of the third ventricle, and pituitary gland; multilevel T_1WI enhanced scan clearly shows the above lesions. Cerebral ischemia or cerebral infarction due to vasculitis is demonstrated on T_2WI as hyperintense in cerebral white matter and basal ganglia on DWI to confirm acute cerebral infarction. Its needs to be differentiated from the following diseases.

19.3.5.1 Multiple Sclerosis

It is the most common inflammatory demyelinating lesion of the central nervous system that occurs in young and middle-aged people but can also occur in older adults. According to the diagnostic criteria of McDonald, the diagnosis requires objective evidence of spatial and temporal dissemination of the lesion. Thus, MRI plays an important role in the diagnosis of multiple sclerosis, not only by showing multiple foci (spatial spread) but also by detecting new foci (temporal spread) by tracking patients with clinically occult onset. Multiple sclerosis has a typical site of onset in the white matter area. This includes the corpus callosum region, subcortical fibers, brainstem, cerebellum, and spinal cord. On MRI, multiple sclerosis usually shows hyperintense on T_2WI and hypointense on T_1WI. After intravenous gadolinium administration, some lesions may show enhancement, while others may not.

19.3.5.2 Primary CNS Vasculitis

See the differential diagnosis in Sect. 19.1 of this chapter for details.

19.3.5.3 Infectious Lesions

Differential diagnosis is also required for tuberculosis and fungal infections (e.g., *Candida* infection, coccidioidomycosis, etc.), all of which can manifest as intracerebral miliary nodules that enhance on enhanced scan, and it should be evaluated in conjunction with a combination of clinical and laboratory tests.

19.3.6 Status and Progress of Research

1. MRI is of great value in the diagnosis of neurological sarcoidosis, and although MRI does not directly show small vessels, it is sensitive to small infarct foci and small hemorrhagic foci, which can suggest the presence of vasculitis and is far superior to CT. Typically, noninvasive angiography including CTA/CTV and MRA/MRV provides sufficient vascular picture without the need for invasive cerebral angiography. Because of the rarity of neurologic sarcoidosis involving blood vessels and the risks associated with invasive imaging, enhancement MR and MRA are usually the preferred options.
2. *Magnetic Resonance Magnetic Sensitivity Weighted Imaging (SWI).* It uses the difference of magnetic sensitivity between tissues and bold effect imaging; that is, use deoxyhemoglobin in blood vessels as an endogenous contrast agent. It is safe, noninvasive, sensitive to veins and blood metabolites, and can show low-flow arteries and veins, including increased, thickened fine veins (1 mm diameter) and tortuous thickened draining veins, independent of blood flow velocity and direction. The normal diameter of the deep medullary cerebral vein is 0.1–0.3 mm, and its length does not exceed 1.0–1.5 cm. Deep medullary vein engorgement (DMVE) sign is an increase in the diameter of the deep medullary vein perpendicular to the lateral ventricles or dilatation compared to the same mirror area and is a common manifestation of neurological sarcoidosis, probably caused by increased resistance to venous blood flow due to venous and peripheral inflammation, not secondary to venous thrombosis. DMVE is seen in approximately 1/3 of patients and is associated with an increased incidence of microhemorrhage and cerebral edema, suggestive of the diagnosis of neurological sarcoidosis. But the sign is not specific and can also be seen in patients with primary CNS vasculitis and acute stroke [13].
3. Gallium scanning and ^{18}F-FDG PET examinations can detect foci of radio-concentrated neurological sarcoidosis and help to identify biopsy sites and assess the activity of sarcoidosis.

4. Imaging can be used not only to detect lesions, but also to guide the clinical treatment process, rational drug use, and follow-up. Of these, MRI is the most useful follow-up, and enhanced T_1WI is necessary for follow-up and can be used to observe blood–brain barrier permeability. Because inflammatory lesions are a major factor affecting the integrity of the blood–brain barrier, treatment with corticosteroids inhibits the inflammatory response and decreases blood–brain barrier permeability, and thus disease activity can be determined by enhanced T_1WI observations. In addition, the use of MRI allows for follow-up observation of mass lesions and their surrounding edematous changes.

References

1. Abdel Razek AA, Alvarez H, Bagg S, et al. Imaging spectrum of CNS vasculitis. Radiographics. 2014;34(4):873–94.
2. Osborn AG. In: Wu W, Huang XS, Zhang XW, et al., editors. Diagnostic brain imaging. Section 2 version. Beijing: People's Medical Publishing House; 2013.
3. Bae MS, Kim EJ, Lee KM, et al. Rapidly progressive rhino-orbi- to-cerebral mucor mycosis complicated with unilateral internal carotid artery occlusion: a case report. Neurointervention. 2012;7(1):45–9.
4. Carod Artal FJ. Clinical management of infectious cerebral vasculitides. Expert Rev Neurother. 2016;16(2):205–21.
5. Mandal J, Chung SA. primary angiitis of the central nervous system. Rheum Dis Clin North Am. 2017;43(4):503–18.
6. Beuker C, Schmidt A, Strunk D, et al. Primary angiitis of the central nervous system: diagnosis and treatment. Ther Adv Neurol Disord. 2018;11:1756286418785071.
7. Thaler C, Kaufmann-Bühler AK, Gansukh T, et al. Neuroradiologic characteristics of primary angiitis of the central nervous system according to the affected vessel size. Clin Neuroradiol. 2019;29(1):37–44.
8. Ting CS, Shuang X. Imaging features and research progress in vasculitis of the central nervous system. Int J Med Radiol. 2019;42(1):54–8.
9. Hu JX, Wang LN, Zhang XF, et al. Primary CNS vasculitis in MRI feature. Chin Med Imaging Technol. 2019;35(2):191–4.
10. Jachiet V, Lhote R, Rufat P, et al. Clinical imaging and histological presentations and outcomes of stroke related to sarcoidosis. J Neurol. 2018;265(10):2333–41.
11. Longjiang Z, Ji Q. Imaging of central nervous system sarcoidosis. Foreign Med Vol Clin Radiol. 2007;30(2):73–6.
12. Bathla G, Singh AK, Policeni B, et al. Imaging of neurosarcoidosis: common uncommon and rare. Clin Radiol. 2016;71(1):96–106.
13. Zamora C, Hung SC, Tomingas C, et al. Engorgement of deep medullary veins in neurosarcoidosis: a common-yet-underrecognized cerebrovascular finding on SWI. AJNR Am J Neuroradiol. 2018;39(11):2045–50.

Spinal Cord and Spinal Canal Infections and Inflammatory Diseases

20

Guihua Jiang, Jianping Zhang, Xiaoping Yin, Zongjun Zhang, Qiang Liu, Hui Xing, Zhiqiang Xu, Yuanyuan Fang, Dan Zhang, Yulin He, Jian Wang, Fei Wang, Luolin Yin, Rui Huang, Jianhua Ma, Cong Huang, Ning Xu, and Hongyan Chen

20.1 Viral Infection of Spinal Cord and Spinal Canal

20.1.1 AIDS-Related Spinal Cord Infection

Guihua Jiang, Jianping Zhang, and Xiaoping Yin

AIDS-related spinal cord infection refers to human immunodeficiency virus (HIV) that invades the spinal cord or causes opportunistic infections of the human spinal cord, leading to inflammatory changes in the spinal cord. HIV is a member of the human lentivirus group of the retrovirus family and can invade the nervous system, including the brain, spinal cord, and peripheral nerve cells. The main pathogens of common AIDS-related opportunistic spinal cord infections include protozoa, viruses, fungi, and bacteria, which are more common in the late stages of AIDS.

20.1.1.1 AIDS-Related Toxoplasma Spinal Cord Infection

Overview

AIDS patients have a high probability of infecting toxoplasma during the incubation period, which can be complicated by widespread dissemination and fatal infection, and can develop toxoplasmosis of the spinal cord. Toxoplasma is an intracellular parasite that enters the human body mainly through the digestive tract. Toxoplasma has an affinity for the nervous system, infections of organs outside the brain are rare, and toxoplasma infections of the spinal cord are even rarer. The incidence of toxoplasmosis of the nervous system in AIDS patients is 26%. Toxoplasmosis of the spinal cord is clinically subacute. The clinical manifestations include headache, hemi-limb sensory disturbance, focal neurological abnormalities, convulsions, disturbance of consciousness,

G. Jiang
Guangdong Second People's Hospital, Guangzhou, China

J. Zhang
Tianshui Xin Tiantan Trauma and Orthopaedic Hospital, Tianshui, China

X. Yin
The Affiliated Hospital of Hebei University, Baoding, China

Z. Zhang
Jiangsu Provincial Hospital of Integrated Traditional Chinese and Western Medicine, Nanjing, China

Q. Liu
Shandong Provincial Hospital, Jinan, China

H. Xing · Y. Fang · D. Zhang · F. Wang · J. Ma
The First Affiliated Hospital of Xinjiang Medical University, Urumqi, China

Z. Xu
Zhengzhou Central Hospital, Zhengzhou, China

Y. He
The First Affiliated Hospital of Nanchang University, Nanchang, China

J. Wang (✉)
Medical Imaging Center, First Affiliated Hospital of Xinjiang Medical University, Urumqi, China

Shanghai Universal Medical Imaging Diagnostic Center, Shanghai University, Shanghai, China

L. Yin
Beijing You'an Hospital, Capital Medical University, Beijing, China

R. Huang
Department of Radiology, Xijing Hospital, Air Force Military Medical University, Xi'an, China

C. Huang
The 926th Hospital of the Chinese People's Liberation Army Joint Logistics and Security Forces, Kaiyuan, China

N. Xu
Jinan first people's Hospital, Jinan, China

H. Chen
Beijing Tiantan Hospital, Capital Medical University, Beijing, China

H. Li et al. (eds.), *Radiology of Infectious and Inflammatory Diseases - Volume 1*,
https://doi.org/10.1007/978-981-99-0039-8_20

and fever. The clinical diagnosis is mainly based on histopathological section or cerebrospinal fluid examination showing toxoplasma, and serum toxoplasma antibodies (IgA, IgG) are positive.

Pathological Manifestations

Pathology is mainly manifested by liquefaction and necrosis of spinal cord tissue with a small amount of inflammatory cell infiltration. Cystic toxoplasma proliferators can be seen in the necrotic foci, which are granular with uneven sizes. Inflammatory reactions usually occur with necrotic foci, which are more obvious around necrotic foci, and are a direct manifestation of tissue necrosis. Necrotic substances can cause vasculitis.

Imaging

CT shows localized swelling and thickening of the spinal cord, and the lesion is isointense or hypointense on flat scan, which can be combined with calcification and appear as high density. Peripheral edema is banded hypodensity, and enhancement is seen as a ring or target enhancement. Studies have reported that toxoplasma infection can cause severe thoracic spinal cord atrophy and cause chronic arachnoid adhesion and even calcification, which may be the imaging manifestations of the chronic phase or cure of toxoplasma infection [1].

MR plain scan shows edema and thickening of local spinal cord tissues. In the spinal cord, there are patches of T_1WI low signal and T_2WI high signal. Lesion margin expresses with low T_1WI signal, equal or slightly high T_2WI signal ring, enhanced with a single ring-like, target-like, and node-like enhancement (Fig. 20.1).

Diagnostic Key Points

1. The patient has a history of HIV infection, with subacute onset and symptoms of transverse myelitis.
2. The imaging findings showed that the spinal cord was swollen and thickened, and the CT scan showed isodensity or hypodensity lesions. MR showed that the edge of the lesion manifests hypointense on T_1WI or slightly hyperintense on T_2WI and showed a single ring, target-like and nodular-like enhancement.
3. The white blood cell count in the cerebrospinal fluid increased slightly, and the protein content increased; the serum toxoplasma antibody (IgA, IgG) was positive, and the pathogen was confirmed by examination.

Differential Diagnosis

1. Bacterial abscess of the spinal cord is rare, mainly in patients with localized post-infection bacteraemia; most of the pathogenic bacteria are staphylococcus and streptococcus, with acute onset, short course of disease, and symptoms of fever and spinal cord damage. MRI examination showed that the lesions extending along the long axis of the spinal cord are characteristic and differentiated from Toxoplasma spinal cord. The capsule of bacterial abscess of the spinal cord shows a low signal on T_1WI and T_2WI, and the internal pus has a low signal on T_1WI and a high signal on T_2WI. MR-enhanced T_1WI shows that the abscess wall is ring-shaped and strengthened. The identification of AIDS-related toxoplasma spinal cord infection mainly depends on the patient's history of HIV infection and the positive test of serum toxoplasma antibody (IgA, IgG). The diagnostic criteria rely on histopathological biopsy.
2. AIDS-related tuberculosis abscess of spinal cord tuberculosis abscess with active tuberculosis in other adjacent organs or tissues, and MRI shows localized thickening of the spinal membrane and narrowing and occlusion of the subarachnoid space. Enhanced MRI shows typical tubular enhancement in the sagittal plane and circumferential enhancement in the transverse plane. AIDS-associated spinal cord toxoplasma infection MRI enhancement is

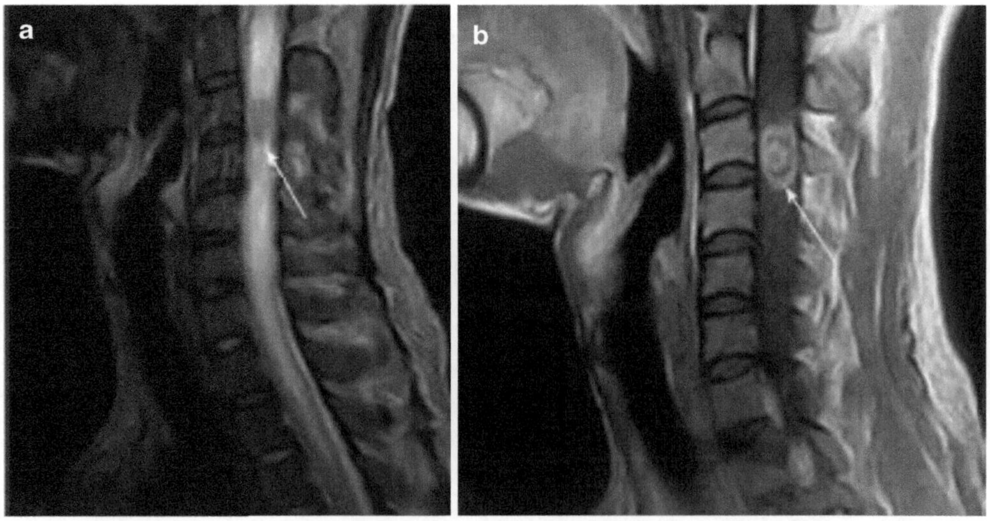

Fig. 20.1 AIDS-related toxoplasma spinal cord infection. (**a**) T_2WI showed that the cervical spinal cord was slightly thickened; the spinal cord at the level of the third cervical vertebra body showed a long band of hypointense (arrow); (**b**) enhanced scan showed that the intramedullary lesions showed a target-like or circular enhancement (arrow). (Image courtesy of Professor Li Hongjun, Beijing You'an Hospital Affiliated to Medical University)

often enhanced and can be differentiated from spinal tuberculosis abscess, less often spinal nodules. Sagittal scans of the spinal cord tend to show ring-like, spiral, or nodular heteronuclei extending along the long axis of the spine in a "flow-through" fashion [1].

Research Status and Progress

The diagnosis of AIDS-related toxoplasma spinal cord infection is mainly based on pathogenic examinations. At present, pathogenic examinations mainly include smear staining and isolation and culture to detect toxoplasma; immunological tests that can be applied when the pathogen is difficult to detect directly include staining tests. Indirect hemagglutination test and enzyme-linked immunosorbent test, both of which have good sensitivity and specificity, are mainly suitable for patients with normal immunity; organ transplantation and AIDS patients with limited immune function mainly apply molecular biological tests; for example, PCR detection can detect the DNA level of a single toxoplasma. Quantitative PCR is mainly used for the analysis of large samples to improve detection efficiency. The current nucleic acid molecular hybridization DNA chip technology has higher specificity, sensitivity, and faster detection speed and will play a major role in toxoplasma genetic diagnosis. Imaging examination can provide a certain reference, but the specificity is not high. It needs to be considered in combination with clinical manifestations and laboratory examinations.

20.1.1.2 AIDS-Related Spinal Herpes Simplex Virus Infection

Overview

Herpes simplex virus (HSV) is a double-stranded neurotrophic DNA virus, belonging to the human herpesvirus alpha subfamily. It is an enveloped virus that can cause lifelong infections. There are about 100 species that can infect humans and animals. The virus mainly causes the corresponding pathological changes after infection through the skin, mucous membranes, and nerve tissues. Immunocompromised patients with AIDS can trigger the activation of latent viruses, which are latent in ganglion nerve cells. The virus is activated in the ganglion nerve cells. Herpes simplex viral myelitis is an acute transverse spinal cord inflammatory lesion caused by allergy after infection with the herpes simplex virus. HSV is divided into two serotypes, HSV-1 and HSV-2. The infection methods and clinical manifestations of the two are different. HSV can cause primary infection, latent infection, and re-infection. The latent parts of HSV-1 in the human body are the trigeminal nerve and superior cervical ganglion, which are mainly transmitted through breathing, saliva, or sexual contact. The primary infections mainly cause oropharyngeal herpes, herpetic keratoconjunctivitis, and skin herpetic eczema. HSV-2 is mainly transmitted through sexual contact. The latent site is the sacral ganglia. Genital herpes is caused by infection of damaged skin and mucous membranes. The long-term latent herpes simplex virus can be activated when human cellular immune deficiency becomes a recurrent proliferative infection. After the infection is activated at the latent site, the infected virus descends along the sensory nerve fibers and returns to the end, and proliferates in the epithelial cells on the skin surface, causing local recurrence of herpes. The clinical manifestations of AIDS-related spinal herpes simplex virus infection are dyskinesia, sensory disturbance, and autonomic dysfunction.

Laboratory examination methods for herpes simplex virus infection: immunofluorescence, virus culture, PCR, and serological examination. If HSV-DNA is positive in the cerebrospinal fluid, HSV infection can be determined early.

Pathological Manifestations

The pathological changes of AIDS-related spinal herpes simplex virus infection are mainly manifested as acute inflammatory demyelination and necrosis of the spinal cord, which are often confined to several segments. The spinal cord is swollen, soft in texture, hyperemic, or inflammatory in the spinal cord. Exudate, the cut surface shows spinal cord softening and irregular edges, unclear boundaries of gray and white matter. Under the microscope, blood vessels in the spinal cord were dilated and congested, peripheral lymphocytes and plasma cells were infiltrated, and nerve cells were swollen and fragmented. Nucleus inclusion bodies could be found in infected cells, which eventually led to spinal cord softening, necrosis, atrophy, and scar formation.

Imaging Findings

MRI showed local swelling and swelling of the spinal cord in the diseased segment, scattered irregular T_1WI with low signal in the spinal cord, and high T_2WI signal (Fig. 20.2). The lesions are prone to hemorrhage. MRI-enhanced lesions generally do not enhance. In the chronic phase, the spinal cord is atrophy, the central canal of the spinal cord can be expanded, and the MRI findings are not specific.

Diagnostic Key Points

1. The patient has a history of HIV infection and clinical manifestations such as limb dysfunction, sensory disturbance, and quadriplegia.
2. MRI showed swelling of the spinal cord in the diseased segment, with low signal intensity on T_1WI and high signal intensity on T_2WI in the spinal cord. The lesions are prone to hemorrhage, and the enhanced lesions are generally not enhanced.
3. Cerebrospinal fluid examination is positive for HSV-DNA to confirm the diagnosis.

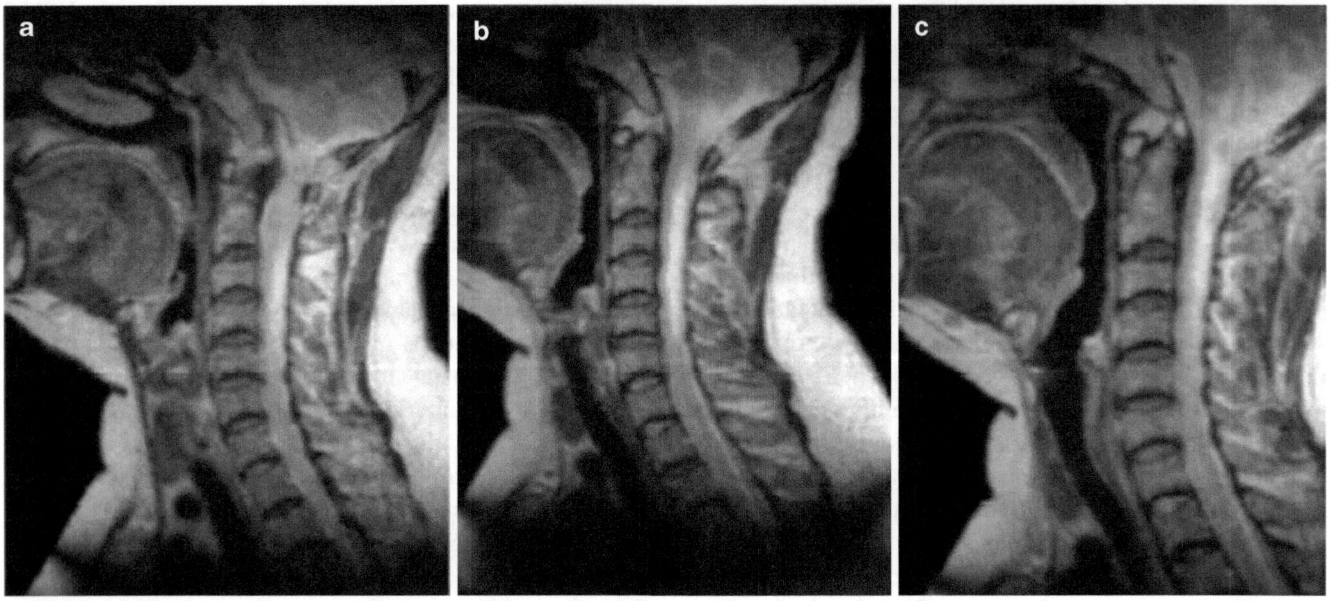

Fig. 20.2 AIDS-related spinal herpes simplex virus infection. (**a**–**c**) MRI shows localized swelling of the spinal cord at the level of the second to fifth cervical vertebrae, with striped T_2WI hyperintense. (Image courtesy of Prof. Li Hongjun, Beijing Youan Hospital, Capital Medical University)

Differential Diagnosis

1. **AIDS-related multiple sclerosis of the spinal cord.** HIV infection-related, acute or subacute onset, clinical symptoms are mostly unilateral or bilateral visual disturbances. Plain CT scans are mostly normal, but the acute phase of enhanced scan shows irregular ring enhancement, with low specificity. MR manifests as T_1WI and other signals in the spinal cord in the acute phase. T_2WI has a slightly high signal, with enhanced visible ring enhancement. The acute phase of multiple sclerosis is similar to the disease. The identification requires a comprehensive analysis of clinical manifestations and laboratory examination results.
2. **Spinal cord infarction.** It is rare due to the abundant blood supply of the spinal cord. The blood vessels are anastomosed into a net, and the arteries of the spinal cord are supplied from the anterior spinal artery, posterior spinal artery, and root artery of the vertebral artery. The anterior spinal artery supplies the anterior 2/3 area of the spinal cord, including the anterior horn of the spinal cord, the lateral horn, the anterior commissure of gray matter, the base of the posterior horn, the anterior cord, and the anterior part of the lateral cord. Arterial infarction is common with occlusion of the anterior spinal artery, which usually occurs in the deep perforating artery, so the gray matter of the spinal cord is the first to be affected, and finally the entire spinal cord is affected. In spinal cord vein thrombotic infarction, the symptoms are insidious, the course of the disease progresses slowly, and the lesion starts in the central area of the spinal cord and expands concentrically. Spinal arterial infarction has a rapid onset, a stroke-like process, and most of them have basic arteriosclerotic lesions. They are common in the thoracic and cervical spinal cord. The symptoms are acute pain at the lesion level, numbness of the limbs, and flaccid paralysis of the corresponding segment in a short time. The first choice for spinal cord infarction is MR examination. In the acute phase of MR, T_2 has its characteristic bilateral high signal, which is a typical manifestation of anterior spinal artery infarction, which is called "owl eye sign." The manifestation of spinal cord infarction on MR is similar to myelitis. It progresses rapidly within 1–2 days, and myelitis progresses rapidly. The early stage needs to be combined with clinical manifestations and the diagnosis of the disease.

Research Status and Progress

1H nuclear magnetic resonance (1H-NMR): The detection of HSV-1-infected human oligodendrocytes as an emerging metabolomics technique suggests that HSV-1 infection alters the metabolism of amino acids in human oligodendrocytes, providing a direction for the study of HSV-1 pathogenesis [2].

20.1.1.3 AIDS-Related Spinal Cytomegalovirus Infection

Overview

AIDS with cytomegalovirus myelitis: CMV infection is the most common viral opportunistic infection in AIDS patients. CMV is a double-stranded DNA virus, belonging to the herpesvirus β subfamily. It is named because it causes the infected cells to swell and enlarge the nucleus to form megakaryocytes. It has the biological characteristics of latent activation. CMV infected by humans is called human cytomegalovirus (HCMV). The host range of HCMV infection is narrow. Humans are the only host. It is human herpes virus type 5. CMV infection in the central nervous system is common in patients with AIDS or bone marrow transplantation and organ transplantation. Confirmation of CMV infection requires finding inclusion bodies in biopsy or isolating the virus [3].

A fourfold or greater increase in serum or plasma IgG antibodies in the early stages of primary CMV infection is confirmatory of the disease. The gold standard for active HCMV infection is the isolation of positive CMV IgM in cerebrospinal fluid cells, but the sensitivity is low and the specificity is high. IgM antibodies are early antibodies produced after antigenic stimulation of the body and are therefore an important indicator of early infection. The combination of HCMV IgM and IgG antibodies can improve the sensitivity and accuracy of the test, as IgG antibodies are important indicators of primary infection.

Pathological Manifestations

Pathological changes are mainly manifested as spinal cord congestion, edema, and spinal nerve demyelination. The lesions are initially located around blood vessels and then merge into large pieces and even form spinal cord softening and syringomyelia. The blood vessels around the lesion were dilated, and the surrounding inflammatory cells and glial cells were infiltrated. The spinal cord is atrophy in the late lesions, accompanied by the proliferation of glial cells, and scars can be formed in the softened area.

Imaging

1. CT findings: AIDS-infected patients with cytomegalovirus myelitis in AIDS-infected patients are most common in the cervical and lumbar segments of the spinal cord. CT scans show mild thickening of the spinal cord and uneven spinal cord density.
2. MRI findings: One or more segments of the spinal cord are thickened, with irregular strips of slightly hypointense on T_1WI and hyperintense on T_2WI and DWI (Fig. 20.3). No enhancement is seen on MRI-enhanced scans.

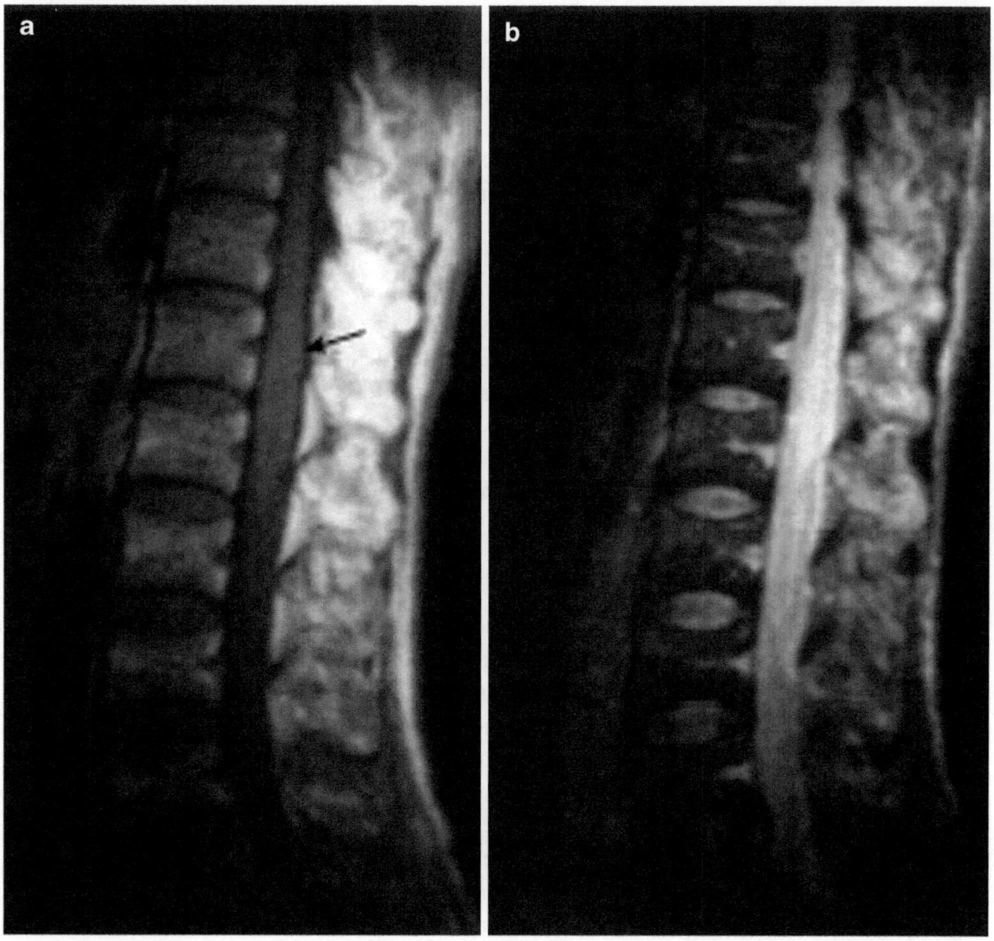

Fig. 20.3 AIDS-related spinal cytomegalovirus infection. (**a**, **b**) MR shows thickening of the thoracolumbar spinal cord with a low signal in T_1WI and a slightly high signal in T_2WI. (Image courtesy of Prof. Li Hongjun, Beijing Youan Hospital, Capital Medical University)

Diagnostic Key Points

1. With a clear history of HIV infection and clinical manifestations of HCMV-related diseases, AIDS combined with HCMV myelitis should be considered.
2. Imaging findings: CT shows localized thickening of the spinal cord and uneven spinal cord density; MR shows irregular strips of T_1WI low signal and T_2WI high signal in the spinal cord. Enhancement of the lesion is generally non-enhancing.
3. Laboratory examination: CMV IgM positive can be detected in cerebrospinal fluid cells. Isolation and culture is the gold standard for HCMV active infection, but it has low sensitivity and high specificity. Serological examinations are currently widely used.

Differential Diagnosis

Cytomegalovirus myelitis needs to be differentiated from slow-progressing spinal cord tumors. The tumor site is often accompanied by hemorrhagic necrosis, and enhanced scans show uneven enhancement. Cytomegalovirus myelitis is an acute disease with no enhancement or uniform enhancement.

Research Status and Progress

CMV has a wide range of susceptibility to humans and can be infected in a variety of ways. It is one of the more common opportunistic infections in AIDS patients. The imaging features of AIDS-related cytomegalovirus myelitis are few, and the diagnosis mainly depends on pathogenic examination. The specificity and sensitivity of fluorescence quantitative PCR in cerebrospinal fluid are relatively high. The immunity of AIDS patients is low, the CMV-IgM antibody produced is less, some are negative, and the specificity of imaging examination is low. It needs to be considered in combination with clinical manifestations, imaging manifestations, and laboratory examinations.

20.1.1.4 AIDS-Related *Staphylococcus aureus* Infection of the Spinal Cord

Overview

Most spinal cord *S. aureus* infections are caused by acute epidural abscesses, subdural abscesses, or direct bacterial infections within the spinal cord. AIDS patients have low immunity and have multiple infections throughout the body. Among them, purulent lung infections and adjacent soft tissue infections are the main ones. Before the symptoms of the spinal cord appear, it is mostly caused by septic bacteria that enter the spinal cord and meninges through the blood circulation [4]. Pain and banding sensation are common in the lesion. The thoracic spinal cord is more common, followed by the lumbar segment. Complete or incomplete paraplegia may occur.

Pathological Manifestations

Pathological changes are related to the way bacteria enter. In local infections, most of the spinal cord damage is located within several spinal cord segments; those with menstrual blood infections often have multiple or chronic lesions and are common in the thoracic and lumbar segments. Spinal cord swelling, congestion, edema, purulent secretions, thickening of the meninges, inflammatory exudate, and granulomas can be seen. Under the microscope, blood vessels in the meninges were congested, neurons in the spinal cord were degenerated or disappeared, neuronal axons were dissolved and demyelinated, and diffuse infiltration of inflammatory cells and proliferation of macrophages and glial cells were seen. Multiple small abscesses in the spinal cord can fuse with each other to form a larger spinal abscess. Suppurative myelitis with secondary spinal epidural abscess and spinal epidural abscess mainly changes with thickening of the spinal membrane, adhesions, and vascular obstruction.

Imaging

The imaging findings of AIDS-related spinal cord infection with *Staphylococcus aureus* are nonspecific, similar to other noninfectious inflammations and spinal cord demyelination changes. CT showed that the spinal cord was thickened and irregular in shape, and the boundary of the lesion in the spinal cord was clear. After the abscess was formed, the enhanced CT scan showed a ring-shaped enhancement of the abscess wall.

MR manifestations: localized or diffuse banded hypointense on T_1WI and hyperintense on T_2WI can be seen on the plain scan of the spinal cord, and diffuse or patchy enhancement can be seen on the enhanced scan. After the combined abscess is formed, the enhanced scan shows the separable or circular enhancement of the abscess wall on T_1WI (Fig. 20.4).

Diagnostic Key Points

1. AIDS patients have a history of systemic or local infections, sudden paraplegia, urinary and fecal dysfunction, and symptoms such as high fever.
2. MRI showed banded hypointense on T_1WI in the thoracolumbar spinal cord and hyperintense on T_2WI. The enhanced scan showed ring-shaped or compartmental enhancement of the abscess wall.
3. The cerebrospinal fluid is cloudy in appearance, the number of white blood cells increases, mainly neutrophils, the protein content increases, the sugar and chloride content decreases, and the spinal canal is unobstructed. Bacterial culture shows the growth of *Staphylococcus aureus*.

Differential Diagnosis

1. Acute spinal epidural abscess in acute bacterial infections. Within 3–4 weeks of acute bacterial infection, the patient develops significant pain in the back of the

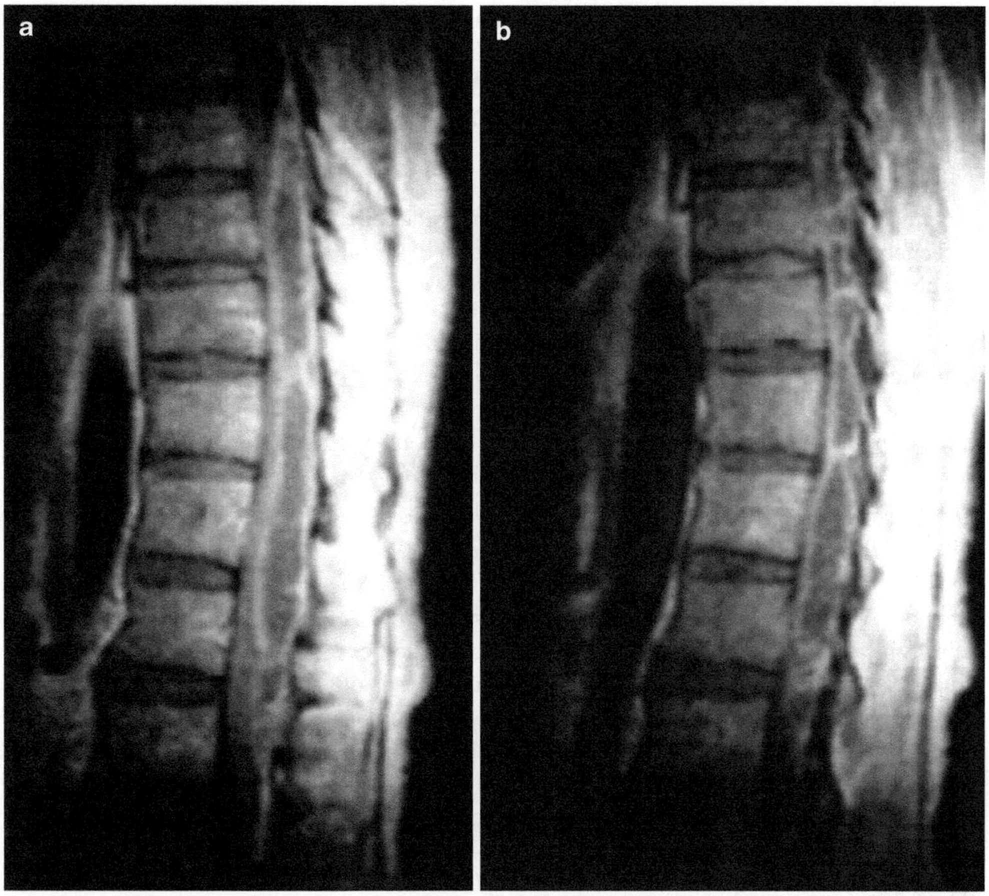

Fig. 20.4 AIDS-related *Staphylococcus aureus* infection of the spinal cord. (**a**, **b**) T_1WI strips of hypointense in the spinal cord of the thoracolumbar region, with an enhancement of the abscess wall in the spinal canal and compression of the spinal cord. (Image courtesy of Professor Li Hongjun, Beijing Youan Hospital, Capital Medical University)

lesioned segment, with inflammatory irritation of the nerve roots at the site of the lesion resulting in radicular pain and often transverse spinal cord damage within one to several days, manifesting as flaccid paralysis of the limbs, sensory deficits, and significant sphincter dysfunction. Lumbar puncture shows that the Quackenstedt test is positive, the appearance of the cerebral effusion is yellow, and the protein content is increased, which can be distinguished from the disease. MRI is the most reliable method for diagnosing extraspinal abscess. It can show infection of vertebral body, intervertebral space and soft tissue, compression and displacement of spinal cord, and the scope of the abscess.

2. Tuberculous myelitis is mainly caused by infection of *Mycobacterium tuberculosis* through blood or adjacent tissues, most commonly in the thoracolumbar spinal cord. Tuberculous myelitis has a slow onset and is more common in young adults. It often has a history of tuberculosis or contact history of tuberculosis patients. Most of it is secondary to tuberculous meningitis and vertebral tuberculosis. The clinical manifestations are staged spinal nerve root irritation pain, banding sensation, asymmetry and segmental sensory disturbance, hypoesthesia, and limb paralysis, and clinical manifestations are similar to spinal cord *Staphylococcus aureus* infection, tuberculous myelitis mostly involves the meninges, spinal cord, and nerve roots, mainly the pia mater, the dura mater is generally not involved, and *Staphylococcus aureus* infection can involve the entire thickness of the spinal membrane. Tuberculous myelitis MR shows single or multiple tuberculous granulomas, with enhanced thickening of the meninges and nerve roots, showing tubular or circular enhancement. It can be distinguished by related *Mycobacterium tuberculosis* laboratory examination, MR examination, and spinal cord *Staphylococcus aureus* infection.

Research Status and Progress

1. AIDS-related myelitis, spastic lower limb paralysis or paraplegia, should first undergo laboratory-related tests; currently, ELISA is commonly used to screen patient serum, and mainly monoclonal antibodies bound to specific antigens are used to detect pathogens in the tested materials by immunohistochemistry. According to research reports [5], the sensitivity, specificity, and positive and negative prediction rates of nucleic acid hybridization technology for detecting pathogens are all over 90%. Rapid enhanced tissue culture immunofluorescence technology (RET-CIF) is suitable for the detection of a large number of clinical specimens and has the character-

istics of rapidness, sensitivity, high separation rate, and time saving.
2. MRI is an ideal choice for the diagnosis of AIDS-related spinal cord lesions. MR can show the internal and external structures of the dura mater, as well as the size and scope of spinal cord lesions.
3. Spinal cord fMRI, MRS, DWI, DTI, MTR, and other new technologies provide new ideas for the diagnosis of spinal cord diseases.

20.1.2 Varicella-Zoster Virus Infection

Jianping Zhang and Guihua Jiang

20.1.2.1 Overview

Varicella-zoster viral myelitis is an acute inflammatory disease of the spinal cord caused by varicella-zoster virus (VZV) infection. Varicella-zoster virus is a double-stranded DNA neurotropic virus belonging to the alpha subfamily of herpesviruses. The virus spreads rapidly to all tissues and organs of the body and travels up the nerve fibers into the spinal cord to cause varicella-zoster myelitis. The cervical, thoracic, and lumbosacral segments of the spinal cord can all be affected, with the thoracic segment being the most common and showing clinical signs of spinal cord damage. The symptoms of varicella-zoster virus spinal myelitis are complex, with the rash being the first symptom, followed by acute spinal cord damage a few days or weeks later, usually with weakness of the limbs, sensory impairment, and autonomic damage. Asymmetrical signs and symptoms [6]. The pathogenesis is based on direct viral infection and/or immune-mediated nerve cell damage leading to demyelination; spinal cord infarction secondary to vasculitis; and spinal arachnoiditis [7].

The early diagnosis of varicella-zoster virus myelitis relies mainly on laboratory tests, which are slow to isolate and have a low positive rate, and are rarely used clinically. The current PCR technique has a high specificity and sensitivity and is widely used, especially the fluorescent quantitative PCR technique, which can rapidly detect latent and active infections and provide a reliable clinical basis for diagnosis.

20.1.2.2 Pathological Manifestations

The pathological changes of varicella-zoster viral myelitis are inflammatory and necrotic changes in the spinal cord tissue. The demyelination changes in the spinal cord tissue and the destruction of the normal nerve structure can be seen under the microscope, and the typical Cowdry type A inclusion bodies in the nucleus can be found.

20.1.2.3 Imaging

1. X-ray findings. X-ray plain films cannot detect myelitis. It has no diagnostic value for myelitis.
2. CT findings. Local thickening of the spinal cord, limited diagnosis of spinal cord diseases, mainly used to differentiate from tumorous lesions in the spinal canal.
3. MRI findings. The spinal cord is slightly thickened in one or more segments, with irregular T_1WI iso- or low-signal, T_2WI slightly high or high signal, single or multiple foci in the spinal cord, less than three vertebral segments in length, mostly incomplete transverse damage, swelling of the spinal cord in the segment, scattered T_1WI low, iso- and high-signal, T_2WI high signal in the spinal cord, poorly defined, and irregular MR enhancement. MR enhancement shows irregular patchy enhancement and adjacent spinal enhancement (Fig. 20.5). In the acute phase, DWI may show a high signal as one of its features.

20.1.2.4 Diagnostic Key Points

1. The patient has a typical history of varicella zoster rash infection in the clinic, with rash damage first and symptoms related to spinal cord damage later.
2. MR unscanned spinal cord was slightly thickened, and there were patches of low signal on T_1WI and high signal on T_2WI in the spinal cord. The MR-enhanced scan showed mild streak and patchy enhancement. Spinal cord lesions in the acute phase of the DWI sequence are obviously hyperintensive.
3. The white blood cell count and protein content of the cerebrospinal fluid were slightly increased or normal, and the cerebrospinal fluid was detected by PCR to show positive VZV-DNA and antibody positive.

20.1.2.5 Differential Diagnosis

1. Multiple sclerosis (MS) is an autoimmune disease characterized by white matter demyelination. Spinal cord MS mainly affects white matter. The clinical manifestations are related to the affected spinal cord. The clinical manifestations are complex and diverse, with recurrent attacks and progressive exacerbations as the main features. The MR of spinal cord MS showed long T_1WI, low-intensity or high-intensity patches on the posterior or lateral sides of the spinal cord.

   The boundary is not clear, and the range of the lesion is often less than two vertebral bodies. MR enhancement can be seen in the active phase, but not in the resting phase.
2. Acute disseminated encephalomyelitis is clinically mainly characterized by acute onset, rarely recurrent attacks, and mostly involves the brain parenchyma. The spinal cord is mostly characterized by patchy T_1WI with low signal, T_2WI with high signal, and enhanced MR scan.

20.1.2.6 Research Status and Progress

Positive varicella-zoster virus antibody in the cerebrospinal fluid of patients with herpes zoster viral myelitis is of diagnostic significance. The clinical basis is mainly based on the relationship between typical skin damage and spinal cord

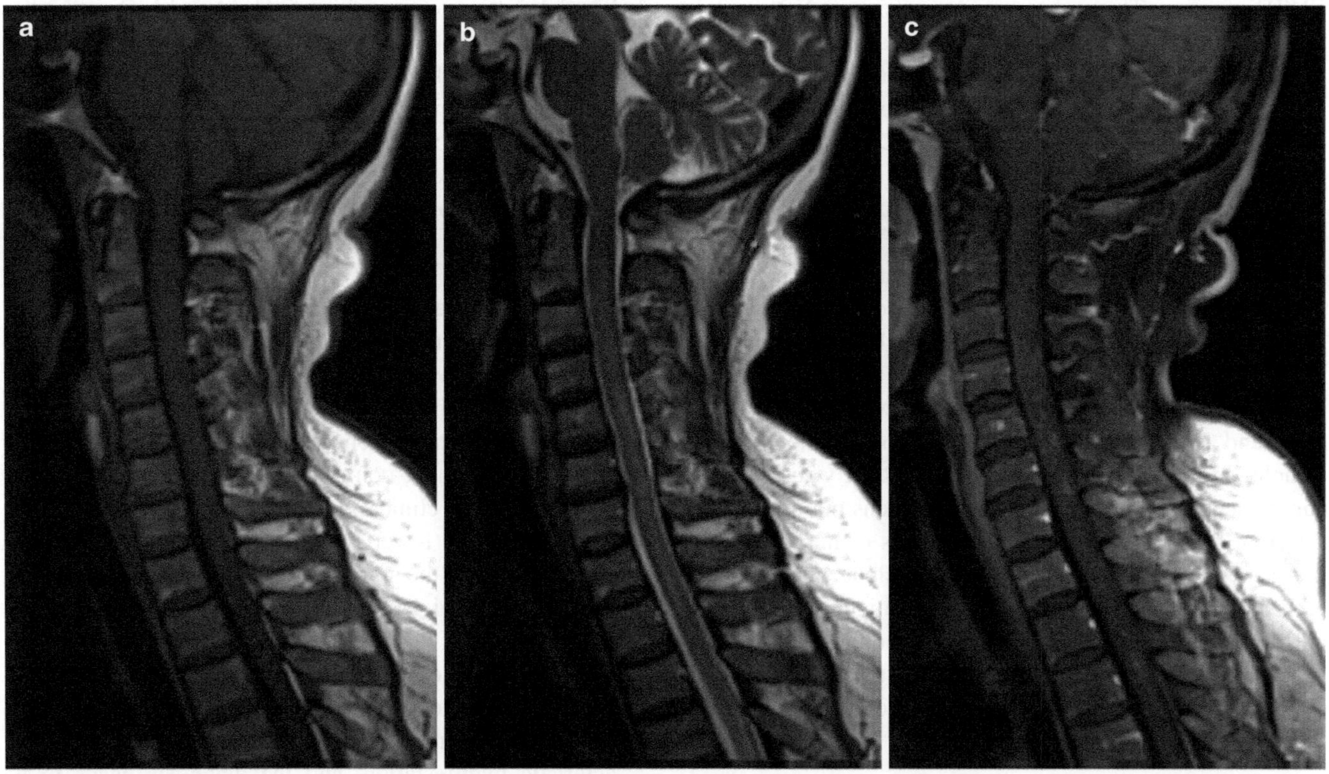

Fig. 20.5 Varicella-zoster virus infectious myelitis. (**a**, **b**) Punctate T_1WI low signal and T_2WI high signal along the long axis of the spinal cord at the level of the fourth to fifth cervical vertebrae (sagittal position); (**c**) Enhanced MRI showing punctate enhancement along the long axis of the spinal cord at the level of the fifth to sixth cervical vertebrae

damage, while patients without rash need help with imaging and laboratory examinations to confirm [8]. It is currently believed that a positive PCR-DNA test for herpes zoster in the cerebrospinal fluid is helpful for the diagnosis of patients without rash. MR examination provides important imaging evidence for herpes zoster viral myelitis. MR manifests as one or more segments of the spinal cord showing T_1WI with low signal, T_2WI with high signal, and a small number of discontinuous involvement of the cervical spinal cord and the full length of the thoracic spinal cord [9].

20.1.3 Enterovirus Infection

Jianping Zhang, Zongjun Zhang, and Guihua Jiang

20.1.3.1 Overview

Enteroviruses belong to the Picornaviridae family, including Enterovirus 71, Coxsackie virus, Echovirus, and poliovirus. Poliomyelitis virus is not described in this section; see Chap. 7 of this book. Enterovirus type 71 (entemvims 71, EV71) is highly neurotropic. The EV71 genome is a single-stranded positive-stranded RNA consisting of 7408 nucleotides, and the viral genome is infectious. The general symptoms of hand, foot, and mouth disease caused by EV71 are severe, and some patients will be accompanied by complications such as acute myelitis. In severe cases, death caused by central nervous system damage and neurogenic pulmonary edema will occur.

The main clinical manifestation of the corresponding acute myelitis caused by intestinal EV71 infection is acute flaccid paralysis (AFP), which is more common in children between 1 and 14 years of age. Most of them have a history of respiratory infection before the onset, and a few days later, sudden limb weakness and lesions are often involved. The anterior horn of the spinal cord causes acute flaccid paralysis of the muscles innervating the upper and lower limbs [6]. Humans are the only source of infection of EV71. They are often the most infectious within 1 week after the onset. The incubation period is 3–5 days on average. It can directly affect the nervous system through blood, lymph, and neuronal pathways, or through damage to the body. The immune system then aggravates the condition [10].

The routine diagnosis method of EV71 is virus isolation and culture, neutralization antibody detection, and immunohistochemistry. These methods are time-consuming and laborious and cannot meet the needs of processing a large number of samples at the same time during a virus epidemic. The PCR detection technology of EV71 is highly efficient and fast, and it has become an important means for rapid diagnosis of EV71. The prokaryotic expression product of the VP1 gene of EV71 is used as an antigen to diagnose

EV71 infection. The prokaryotic expression of VP1 protein is used as the detection antigen, which can detect both IgM in the serum of children with acute infection and IgG in the serum of patients who have been infected with EV71, and there is no cross-immune reaction with CA16 antiserum.

20.1.3.2 Pathological Manifestations

The pathological manifestations of EV71 infected myelitis are degeneration, necrosis, and thrombosis of the endothelial cells of small blood vessels in the spinal cord. Monocytes are infiltrated in a mantle form around the blood vessels, and there are no viral inclusion bodies. The ultrastructure shows the degeneration, vacuolization of nerve cells in the brainstem and spinal cord, and the formation of membranous vesicles in the mitochondria, and microRNA virus particles can be seen in some neurons. Viral antigens mainly exist in different brainstem nuclei, and processes of neurons in the brain stem nucleus and spinal cord include anterior horn cells and posterior horn cells. The viral antigens of the spinal cord nerve roots and the intestinal autonomic ganglia were also positive. Studies have shown direct pathological evidence that the virus enters the central nervous system through the peripheral nerves [11].

20.1.3.3 Imaging

MRI plain scan showed swelling and thickening of the cervical or thoracolumbar spinal cord, changes in the range and signal intensity of the cervical spinal cord and the anterior horn of the lumbar spinal cord. Myelitis is mainly located in the spinal cord and nerve roots around the spinal cord, with the anterior horn of the spinal cord. Involvement of cells and ventral nerve roots is common. In the anterior horn of the spinal cord, there are patches of slightly high signal or high signal on T_2WI (Fig. 20.6), T_1WI is slightly low or low signal, FLAIR is high signal, DWI is equal or slightly high signal, and ADC is slightly high signal. Transected spinal cord lesions are spotted, unilateral or bilateral anterior spinal horns are involved, sagittal lesions are striped or beaded (Fig. 20.7), and MR enhanced scan can show spinal anterior horn or spinal nerve root enhancement [12].

20.1.3.4 Diagnostic Key Points

1. A clear history of hand, foot, and mouth disease or herpetic angina, combined with clinical manifestations of myelitis.
2. MR plain scan of spinal cord local thickening and swelling, mainly from the thoracic segment to the lumbosacral segment below the affected spinal cord, followed by the cervical spinal cord. The lesions are mainly distributed in the anterior horn and ventral nerve roots of the spinal cord. The strips of T_1WI in the lesion are low signal. T_2WI is high signal, and DWI is slightly high or high signal. The enhanced scan showed no enhancement or slight enhancement in bars or dots.
3. The laboratory tests positive for IgM and IgG antibodies against VP1 in serum, and RT-PCR and fluorescence quantitative RT-PCR tests are positive.
4. Laboratory examination of the cerebrospinal fluid showed that the white blood cell count was significantly increased, the protein content was slightly increased, and the sugar and chloride content was normal. EV71 antibodies can be detected in the cerebrospinal fluid.

20.1.3.5 Differential Diagnosis

1. Poliomyelitis. Humans are the only host of poliovirus. The disease is mainly transmitted through fecal–oral infection. Poliomyelitis virus is a neurotropic virus that mainly invades the motor neurons of the anterior horn of the spinal cord. It is more common in the cervical and lumbar segments. The clinical manifestations are asymmetric flaccidity of the lower limbs (paralysis). In the acute or subacute phase, the spinal cord has obvious edema. MRI shows slightly high signal or high signal on T_2WI of the anterior horns of the spinal cord in the transverse position. T_2WI strip or linear high signal on the anterior edge of the spinal cord in the sagittal view. MRI shows that the bilateral anterior horn of the spinal cord involvement is a characteristic manifestation, and the diagnosis needs to be considered in combination with clinical symptoms, laboratory examinations, and imaging manifestations [13].
2. Guillain–Barré syndrome is an acute immune-mediated multiple demyelinating lesions. The clinical typical manifestations are loss of reflexes and ascending paralysis-type symmetrical limb weakness, with or without loss of sensation. Symptoms start from the hands and feet and gradually progress upward, from limbs to trunk within a few days, often induced by the reaction of antibodies produced by viral infectious diseases with myelin in the peripheral nervous system. The diagnosis of this disease mainly relies on clinical manifestations, neuroelectrophysiology, cerebrospinal fluid, and imaging examinations. MR shows that the spinal cord has no anterior horn disease or spinal nerve root enhancement, which is different from EV71-related acute flaccid paralysis.

20.1.3.6 Research Status and Progress

1. The diagnosis of enterovirus EV71 infection-related myelitis needs to be closely combined with clinical manifestations, a history of hand–foot–mouth disease and herpetic angina, and the manifestations of spinal cord damage with sudden acute flaccid paralysis.
2. Molecular biology detection methods have high sensitivity and specificity, including RT-PCR and fluorescence quantitative RT-PCR detection methods, of which fluorescence quantitative RT-PCR detection methods have 100% specificity.
3. Laboratory tests include serological neutralization test and ELISA detection method, detection of IgM and IgG antibodies against VP1 in the serum.

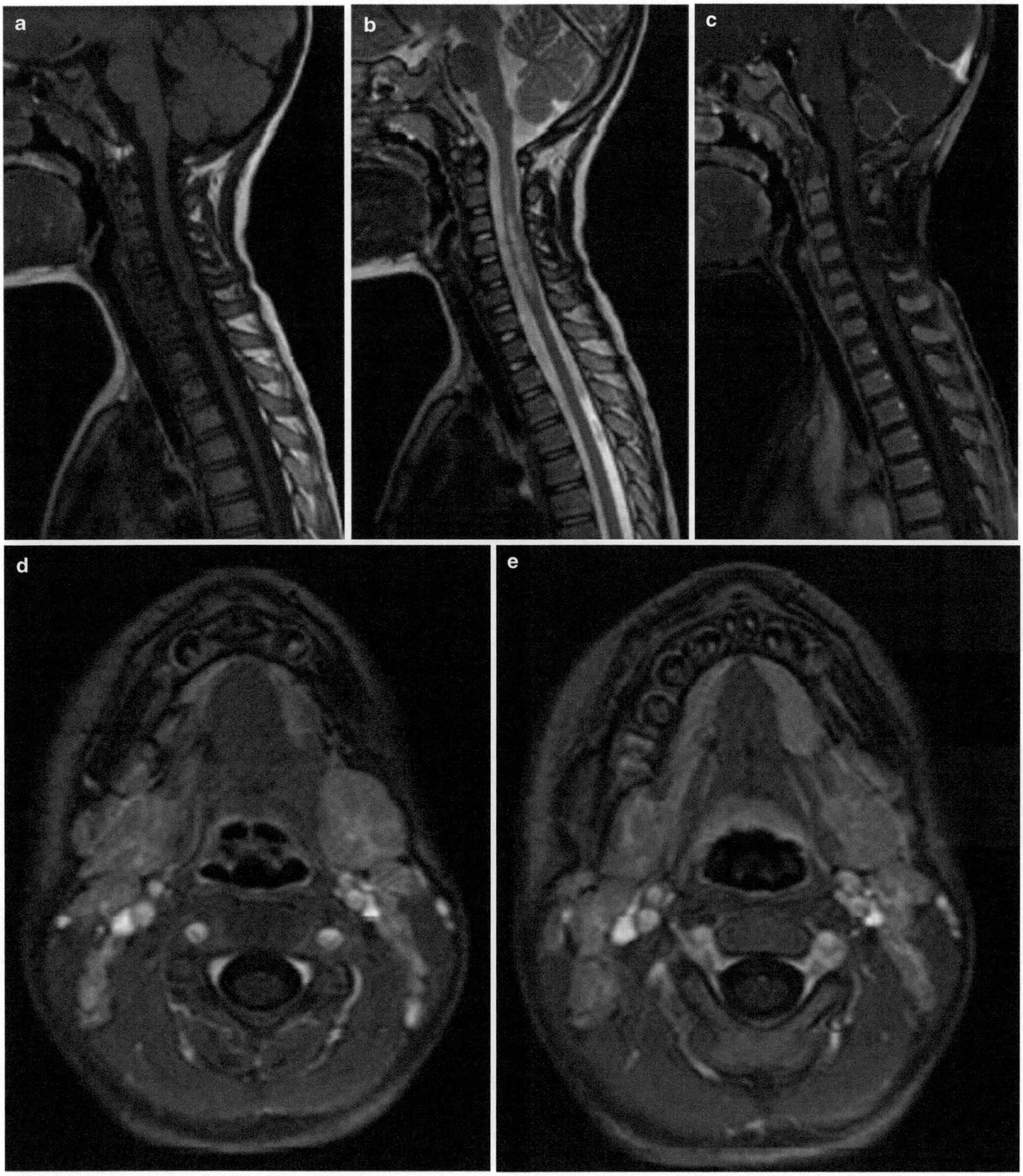

Fig. 20.6 EV71 infectious myelitis (1). (**a**) T_1WI plain scan showed 4–7 of the thickened cervical spinal cord with slightly low signal in stripes (sagittal view); (**b**) T_2WI lesions showed high signal in stripes (sagittal view); (**c**) MR enhancement showed mild lesion enhancement (sagittal position); (**d**, **e**) mild enhancement of the anterior horn of the spinal cord (transverse position)

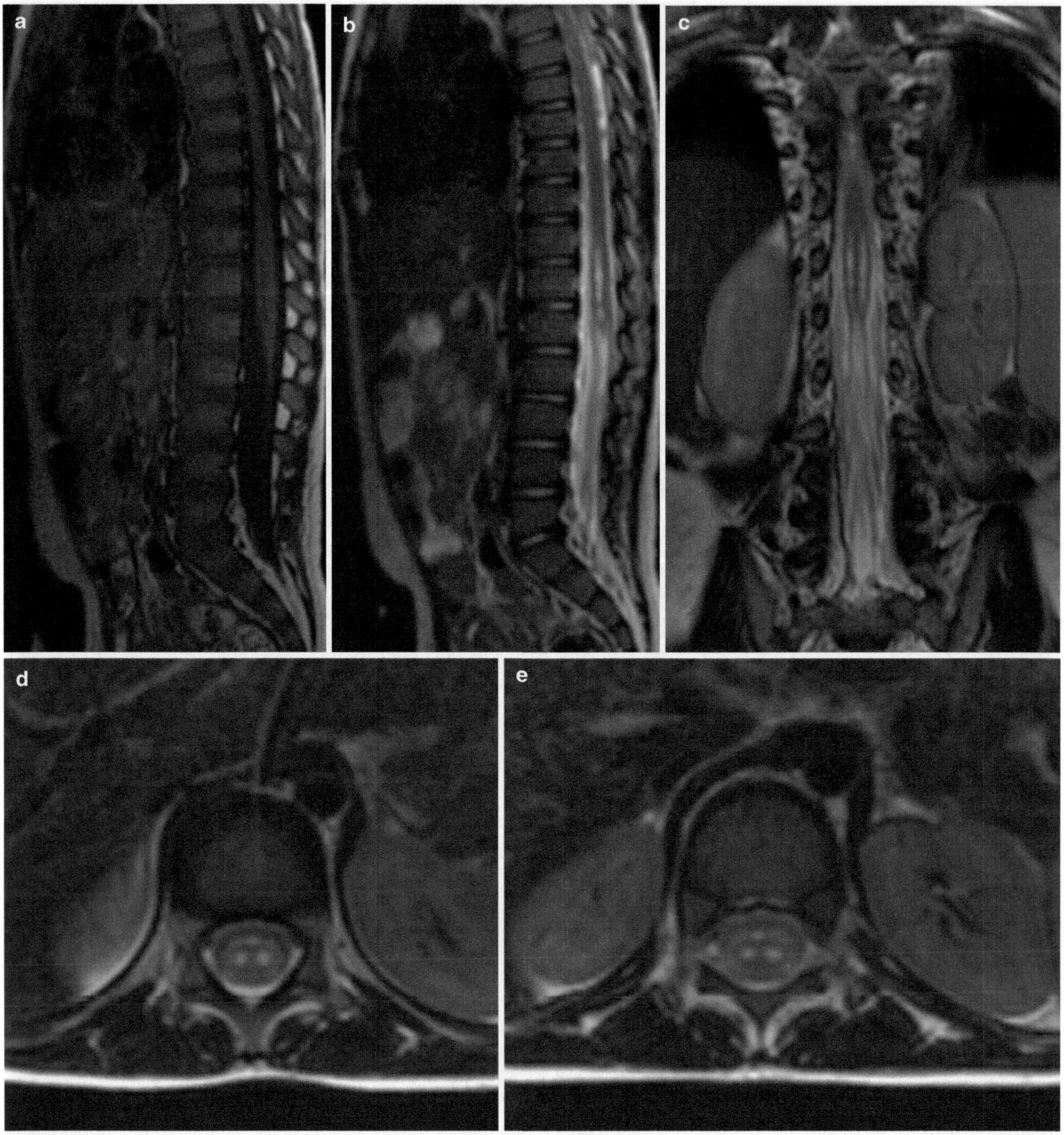

Fig. 20.7 EV71 infectious myelitis (2). (**a**) Thickened thoracolumbar spinal cord with low signal intensity on T_1WI, (sagittal view); (**b**, **c**) high signal intensity on T_2WI (sagittal and coronal); (**d**, **e**) symmetrical speckled high signal on T_2WI in the spinal cord signal (transverse position). (Picture provided by Zhao Xin, Director of the Third Affiliated Hospital of Zhengzhou University, thanks hereby)

4. Imaging examination: MRI can show early spinal cord lesions. MRI is the most sensitive method for evaluating enteroviral myelitis. It can observe the location, shape, scope, and extent of the lesion. Enterovirus EV71 infectious myelitis has characteristic changes, which mainly occur in the anterior horn of the spinal cord. MRI shows that T_2WI is more sensitive, and the effect of multi-directional observation combined with medical history is better. T_2WI/TRA and T_2WI/SAG should be used as routine scanning sequences. Provide reliable imaging evidence for disease evaluation and clinical treatment [14].

5. Electroneurophysiological examination can assess brainstem function and find spinal nerve roots, spinal cord, and brain lesions. The neuroelectrophysiological examination revealed a higher sensitivity to neurogenic damage. Electroneurophysiology combined with MR examination is more conducive to the detection of acute myelitis caused by spinal cord infection.

20.1.4 EB Virus Infection

Guihua Jiang, Jianping Zhang, and Qiang Liu

20.1.4.1 Overview

Epstein–Barr virus is the herpes virus-like particle that was first observed under an electron microscope when Epstein and Barr were studying Burkitt's lymphoma in 1963. Epstein–Barr virus is a double-stranded DNA virus that is universally susceptible to humans and belongs to the herpesvirus family (γ Subfamily), is a kind of herpes virus that loves human lymphocytes, also known as human herpesvirus type 4, and is also a carcinogenic virus. The source of infection is mainly patients and EB virus carriers. Humans are the host of Epstein–Barr virus infection and it is mainly spread through saliva. EB virus infection mainly lurks in B lymphocytes, mainly B lymphocytes. Studies have shown that EB virus can infect T lymphocytes, epithelial cells, and NK cells [15]. The body's immune response to EB virus includes humoral immunity and cellular immunity [16].

Epstein–Barr virus can cause a variety of neurological diseases, such as meningoencephalitis, encephalitis, myelitis, spinal radiculitis, cranial nerve and peripheral neuropathy, and polio-like syndrome. Epstein–Barr virus is related to a variety of diseases and can affect multiple systems and organs throughout the body. Also, 2–10% of acute primary EB virus infections are manifested as central nervous system infections. Based on their pathogenic diversity, it is believed that there are both direct EB virus invasion and nonspecific inflammatory reactions after infection. The virus can directly invade the nervous system, such as the axons in the meninges, brain and spinal cord, and peripheral nerves. Brain tissue damage can also be caused by immune-mediated CD8+ T lymphocytes directly producing toxins in the nervous system or by the deposition of antigen–antibody complexes. Central nervous system lymphoma caused by EB virus is another disease related to EB virus in the central nervous system. These diseases are especially common in immunodeficiency, including AIDS and organ transplant patients [17].

Clinical manifestations of EB virus infection of the nervous system: (1) acute EB virus encephalitis, clinical manifestations include fever, headache, vomiting, aphasia, localized muscle twitching, numbness or hyperesthesia, disturbance of consciousness, mental symptoms, manifestations of brain damage, and respiratory failure and may be combined with meningeal irritation; (2) acute EB viral myelitis, clinical manifestations include neck stiffness, changes in consciousness, weakened limb muscle strength, or muscle weakness [18].

Laboratory diagnosis of Epstein–Barr virus nervous system infection is mainly through PCR detection of serum and cerebrospinal fluid. Detection of Epstein–Barr virus DNA and RNA through PCR technology has become a direct method for early diagnosis. PCR technology can quickly detect very small amounts of viral DNA in cerebrospinal fluid and has the advantages of strong specificity, high sensitivity, speed, simplicity, and noninvasiveness [19].

20.1.4.2 Pathological Manifestations

The main pathological manifestation of EB virus is infectious myelitis in the spinal cord. There are a large number of inflammatory demyelination foci, inflammatory cell infiltration, inflammatory exudation around the venule, and a perivascular sheath composed of lymphocytes and monocytes.

20.1.4.3 Imaging

MR plain scan showed that the diseased spinal cord was thickened and swollen, and the spinal cord had scattered dots, strips, and other signals or low signal on T_1WI and high signal on T_2WI (Fig. 20.8). Gray matter is affected, the entire length of the spinal cord can be affected, the boundary is clear, and bilateral spinal nerve roots can be strengthened. The spinal cord may also be normal, and after 1–2 days, a re-examination will show myelitis lesions. Enhancement can be seen in irregular punctiform and patchy enhancement.

20.1.4.4 Diagnostic Key Points

1. He has a clear history of EB virus infection and clinical manifestations of acute myelitis.
2. MR plain scan showed thickening and swelling of the spinal cord, and there were strips of T_2WI hyperintensity, gray matter was involved, and bilateral spinal nerve roots were strengthened.
3. Laboratory examination of cerebrospinal fluid showed that the white blood cell count was significantly increased, mainly lymphocytes, protein, sugar, and chloride content were normal, and EBV-CA-IgM antibody positive could be detected in the cerebrospinal fluid.

20.1.4.5 Differential Diagnosis

Epstein–Barr virus infectious myelitis needs to be differentiated from myelic multiple sclerosis, spinal cord infarction, spinal cord tumors, and syringomyelia. Spinal cord multiple sclerosis lesions are located in the cervical and upper tho-

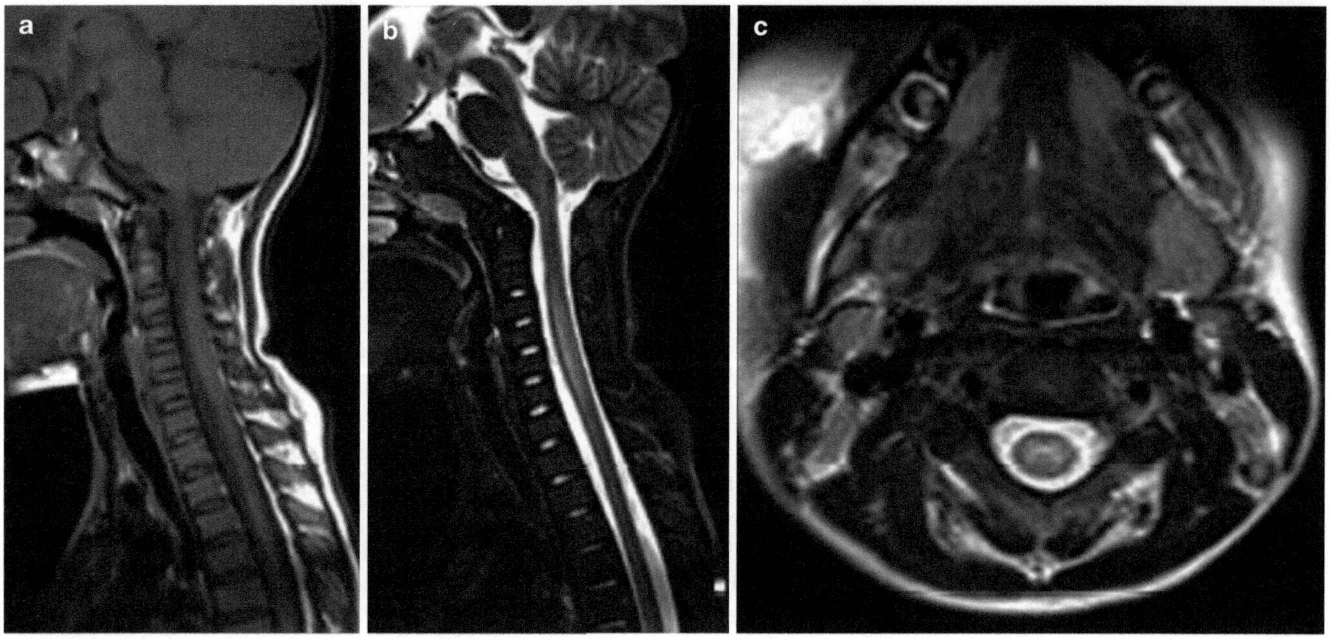

Fig. 20.8 Epstein–Barr virus infectious myelitis. (**a**) T_1WI shows thickening of the third to sixth cervical spinal cords, T_1WI shows isointensity or low signal (sagittal position); (**b**) T_2WI shows striped high signal (sagittal position); (**c**) T_2WI lesion shows high signal (transverse position)). (Picture provided by Zhao Xin, Director of the Third Affiliated Hospital of Zhengzhou University, thanks hereby)

racic segments. The posterior cord and lateral cord are prominent. They are multiple foci, with multiple occurrences of demyelination of the spinal cord ranging from new to old, with a relapse-remission process, and no clear history of infection. Local enhancement can be seen during the active period of the MR-enhanced scan. The MR manifestations of spinal cord infarction are similar to myelitis, with sudden clinical emergencies, no history of infection, and rapid clinical progress. Spinal cord tumors usually progress slowly, the spinal cord is thickened and irregular, and obvious space-occupying can be seen in the spinal canal. Syringomyelia is often secondary to spinal cord infarction, spinal cord tumors, and necrotizing myelitis in the later stage; MR showed uniform low signal on T_1WI and high signal on T_2WI. Partial separation was visible inside, which had obvious characteristics and could be distinguished from myelitis.

20.1.4.6 Research Status and Progress

Myelitis caused by Epstein–Barr virus infection is rarely reported, and it mostly occurs in preschool children. The pathogenic mechanism of Epstein–Barr virus is not fully understood. Current studies have shown that Epstein–Barr virus can directly invade the nervous system, such as the meninges, brain and spinal cord, and axons in multiple nerves. It can also be caused by immune-mediated CD8+ T lymphocytes producing toxins, directly entering the nervous system or depositing antigen–antibody complexes. Patients usually have a history of obvious prodromal fever and infection of the respiratory or digestive tract. Clinically, the main symmetry manifestations of flaccid paralysis of the limbs, the limbs are weak, the proximal end is heavier than the distal end, the tendon reflexes of the affected limbs are weakened or disappeared, the pathological signs are negative, and there is no sensory involvement. EB virus laboratory diagnosis is mainly through PCR detection in serum and (or) cerebrospinal fluid to directly search for the presence of the viral genome or its expression products (RNA, protein). It can be combined with imaging findings, clinical symptoms, and laboratory tests to make an early diagnosis of the disease [6].

20.1.5 Rabies Virus Infection

Guihua Jiang and Jianping Zhang

20.1.5.1 Overview

Rabies is an acute infectious disease caused by rabies virus (RV) infection with acute damage to the central nervous system. Rabies virus infectious myelitis is extremely rare [20]. The rabies virus belongs to the rabies virus genus of the Rhabdoviridae family. The rabies virus looks like a bullet with a diameter of 75–80 nm and a length of 175–200 nm. The outer layer is a dense envelope with many filamentous protrusions on the surface. The distal ends of the protrusions are mallet-shaped. The entire virus has a honeycomb hexagonal structure. The virus genome is a negative-strand single-stranded RNA. The main clinical manifestation of rabies is acute, progressive, and almost irreversible encephalomyelitis. Rabies virus invades the human body mainly through damaged skin or mucous membranes and multiplies in large numbers after reaching the dorsal root ganglion through nerve endings and then ascending to the cerebellum and spinal cord, causing acute inflammation of the cerebellum and spinal cord. Rabies virus cannot pass through intact skin. It enters the body through direct contact with wounds or mucous membranes. The most common way is bites or scratches by carnivorous animals such as dogs, cats, wolves, etc., carrying rabies virus, or transplantation of virus carriers. Humans are the ultimate host of rabies virus. Once human rabies develops, its mortality rate is 100%, and timely measures to prevent it are the only way to save lives. Clinically, the symptoms of the nervous system are more complex, divided into manic type and paralytic type. Manic type is common. Manic type is mainly manifested as mania, excitement, pharyngeal muscle spasm, limb paralysis, water fear, etc. The typical symptoms are water fear, wind fear, and salivation. The symptoms of rabies are characteristic [21]. Paralytic type is the early manifestation of spinal cord transverse damage such as progressive flaccid paralysis of the limbs and urinary and fecal dysfunction, without excitatory symptoms such as excitement and hydrophobia [22].

Rabies virus invades the human body on damaged skin or mucous membranes. It has a strong affinity for nerve tissue. The pathogenic process of rabies can be divided into three stages: in the first stage, the rabies virus reproduces in the local tissue of the wound; in the second stage, the rabies virus binds to the acetylcholine receptor of the neuromuscular junction, and the virus travels to the center along the axon of the peripheral nerve. After the nervous system spreads and enters the central nervous system to reach the dorsal root ganglia of the spinal cord, it will multiply in the body and then invade the spinal cord. The brain mainly invades the neurons of the cerebellum; in the third stage, the virus spreads from the central nervous system to the peripheral nerves and invades various tissues and organs, especially the salivary glands, tongue taste buds, and olfactory nerve epithelium. The spread of the virus to the vagus ganglia, sympathetic ganglia, and cardiac ganglia can cause dysfunction of the cardiovascular system and even sudden death.

In rabies virus pathogenic testing, the accuracy of virus isolation and culture diagnosis is relatively high, but it takes a long time, and it needs to be combined with immunofluorescence-specific detection. The immunofluorescence detection time is short, and the sensitivity and specificity are high. RT-PCR technology has low requirements for sample purity and can quickly detect rabies virus-specific nucleic acid sequences from brain tissue, cerebrospinal fluid, saliva, skin, and other tissues, and the results have high specificity and high sensitivity.

20.1.5.2 Pathological Manifestations

The pathological changes are mainly acute diffuse encephalomyelitis, especially the dorsal root ganglion and spinal cord, which are equivalent to the bite site. Under the microscope, the main manifestations are acute myelitis, nerve cell degeneration and necrosis, lymphocytes, and plasma around blood vessels. Cells infiltrate, forming a vascular cuff phenomenon. Negri bodies were detected in spinal cord nerve cells, posterior horn ganglion sympathetic ganglia, etc. Negri corpuscles are characteristic diagnostic indicators appearing in nerve cells and have diagnostic significance. They are colonies of rabies virus. They are round or quasi-circular. After staining, they are cherry red, with a diameter of 3–10 nm, neat edges, and one or two small spots resembling a cell nucleus, under the electron microscope, it can be seen that the Negri corpuscle contains baculovirus particles.

20.1.5.3 Imaging

Human rabies viral myelitis is mainly manifested as transverse myelitis, which is low signal on T_1WI and high signal on T_2WI. The spinal cord can be normal or slightly thickened, and enhanced scans can show enhancement or no enhancement (Fig. 20.9) [23].

20.1.5.4 Diagnostic Key Points

1. The patient has a history of bites or scratches from animals carrying rabies virus.
2. MR examination: T_1WI of the brain stem and spinal cord showed low signal performance, T_2WI slightly high signal or high signal.
3. Cerebrospinal fluid examination: Anti-rabies virus antibodies can be detected in the cerebrospinal fluid.

20.1.5.5 Differential Diagnosis

1. The main symptoms of tetanus are muscle rigidity and muscle spasm. In the early stage, the patient closed her teeth tightly and later showed a wry smile and reflexed horns, but she was not afraid of water. The muscles of tetanus patients are tonic and spasm, and muscle tone is high, while those of rabies patients are completely relaxed during the intermittent period. Rabies patients do not have their teeth closed, and water fear and difficulty swallowing are the most prominent symptoms. For spinal cord MR examination, there is no obvious abnormality in patients with tetanus, while obvious imaging changes can be seen in the spinal cord of patients with rabies, which provides a reliable diagnostic basis for early differential diagnosis.
2. Rabies-like hysteria. The patient suffers for a short period after being bitten by an animal. There is a feeling of tightness of the larynx within a period of time, unable to drink water and excitement, but not afraid of wind, salivation,

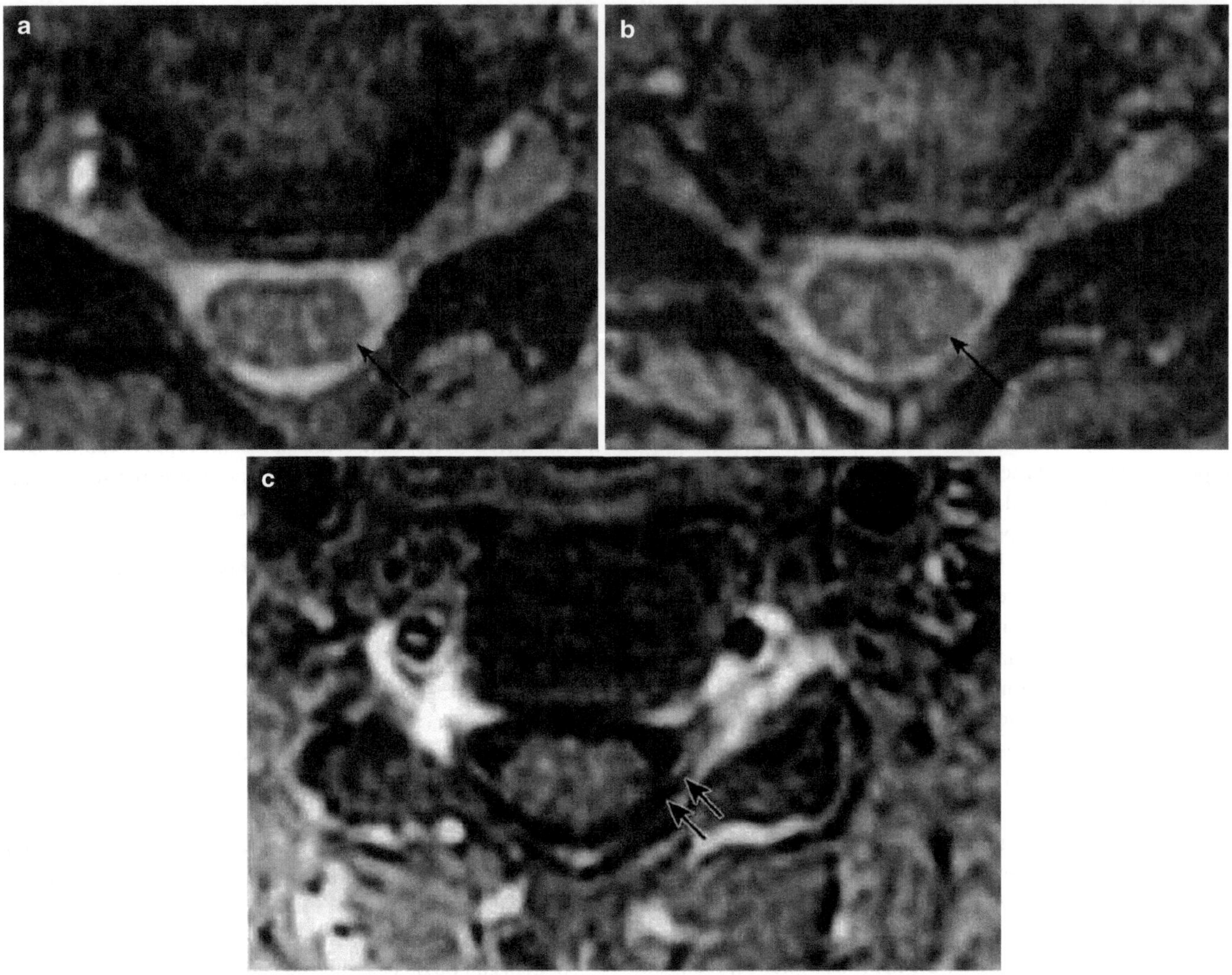

Fig. 20.9 Human rabies viral myelitis. (**a**, **b**) T_2WI in the spinal cord shows slightly high signal (transverse position); (**c**) the nerve root on the left side of the neck has mild to moderate enhancement. (Picture provided by Professor Li Hongjun, Beijing You'an Hospital, Capital Medical University, thanks hereby)

fever, and paralysis. Rabies virus antibody is negative. After suggestion, persuasion, and symptomatic treatment, it can often recover quickly. MR examination of the spinal cord has no abnormal findings, which can be distinguished from rabies.

20.1.5.6 Research Status and Progress

The rabies virus enters the local tissues from the wound and is transmitted to the central nervous system along the nerve axis. After reaching the dorsal nerve roots of the spinal cord, the virus multiplies in large numbers. Kind of neurological symptoms. According to clinical manifestations, rabies is divided into manic type and paralytic type. After humans are infected with rabies virus, the fatality rate is higher. MR examination can provide a strong basis for early diagnosis. MR can noninvasively display the changes in morphology and functional metabolism of the brain and spinal cord, which is of great value for early diagnosis.

20.2 Bacterial Infection of Spinal Cord and Spinal Canal

20.2.1 Epidural Abscess and Subdural Abscess

Hui Xing, Zhiqiang Xu, and Guihua Jiang

20.2.1.1 Overview

Intraspinal abscess is an acute purulent infection that can occur in the epidural space, subdural space, or spinal cord. Most intraspinal abscesses are secondary to infections in other parts, with skin sores or cellulitis being the most common. They can be caused by purulent infection of other tissues and organs, such as perirenal abscess, lung abscess, mastoiditis, ovarian abscess, and bacterial endocarditis, by systemic sepsis, or by skin sores and furuncles in corresponding or similar segments. Infections like spinal suppurative myelitis spread directly and occasionally in open injuries or cervical and lumbar punctures directly implanted with germs [24, 25]. Some people point out that it is difficult to find the primary lesion. The most common pathogenic bacteria is *Staphylococcus aureus*, and pneumococcus and streptococcus can also be seen. Pathogenic bacteria can enter the spinal canal through blood or lymphatic metastasis. During spinal examination or treatment, pathogenic bacteria are brought in by mistake. The epidural space starts at the foramen magnum and reaches the sacral vertebrae. The ventral dura mater is closely connected to the vertebral body. Only the epidural space is not obvious. When descending to the thoracic segment, the epidural space is wider and fat is full, with a rich blood vessel supply. Therefore, spinal abscesses caused by blood transfer mostly occur on the dorsal side of the middle and lower thoracic spine, followed by the lumbosacral segment, and the cervical and upper thoracic segments are rare. Intravertebral canal abscesses can be divided into spinal epidural abscess (SEA), spinal subdural abscess (SSA), and intraspinal abscess according to the different involved sites. Among them, the SEA is the most common, followed by the SSA and spinal cord. Internal abscesses are extremely rare [24]. The SEA is a purulent infection of the localized adipose tissue and venous plexus in the epidural space in the spinal canal, causing pus accumulation in the epidural space or proliferation of a large amount of granulation tissue, thus resulting in compression of the spinal cord. In addition, purulent inflammation of the spinal artery, spinal vein, and epidural venous plexus can cause spinal cord blood supply disorders and severe spinal cord dysfunction. Furthermore, the SEA is a neurosurgical emergency, and the spinal cord injury caused by it is usually sharp and serious. Without timely diagnosis and treatment, the disability rate and fatality rate are both high. While the incidence of SEA is relatively low, which, however, in recent years, has also increased year by year with the increase in intravenous use of illegal drugs and the continuous improvement of diagnostic techniques. The SEA can occur at any age and is more common in young adults, with more men than women. The SSA is a purulent infection in which pus accumulates between the subdural membrane and the arachnoid membrane. The onset is more rapid, and the early symptoms are often lack of specificity, with fever and headaches dominating.

The typical clinical manifestations of SEA are pain in the spine or back of the diseased segment, fever, and progressive neurological dysfunction. The SEA can be divided into four stages according to neurological symptoms, namely Stage 1: severe pain in the affected spine; Stage 2: pain in the nerve roots of the affected spine; Stage 3: motor weaknesses and sensory disturbances below the level of the affected spinal cord, and defecation dysfunction; and Stage 4: paralysis. As the disease progresses, patients may have motor weaknesses below the spinal cord level, sensory disturbances, and dysfunction of urination and defecation in the late stage, and may also suffer from sepsis or even death [26].

The clinical manifestations of intraspinal abscesses are related to factors such as the amount of pus, the location of the abscess, the degree of spinal cord edema, and personal physiques. A small number of patients have an insidious onset and mild symptoms. Neurological symptoms do not appear until a few months later. The white blood cell count in laboratory tests often rises. Cerebrospinal fluid examination showed increased white blood cell count and protein content, but it is not a specific manifestation of intraspinal abscess. The positive rate of cerebrospinal fluid bacterial culture is low, which is about 25%.

20.2.1.2 Pathological Manifestations

The SEA and the SSA can be divided into three types: acute, subacute, and chronic ones. The acute type is more common.

1. The acute stage pathological changes of acute spinal epidural abscesses and subdural abscesses include tissue congestion, exudation, a large number of white blood cell infiltration, adipose tissue necrosis, a large amount of pus accumulating in the epidural space, forming pocket pus of different sizes of cavities. Sometimes, the lesions can involve the papilla and arachnoid, causing increased blood vessel congestion.
2. As for subacute spinal epidural abscesses and subdural abscesses, there may be pus and granulomatous tissue in the epidural space.
3. In terms of chronic spinal epidural abscesses and subdural abscesses, the spinal epidural is granulation tissue with no signs of infection or obvious pus on the outside, but bacteria can sometimes be cultured.

Due to the increased pressure in the epidural space, pus can spread longitudinally, and the disease can involve several segments. Abscesses can compress the spinal cord. At the same time, due to inflammatory pathological changes, it can cause varying degrees of inflammation in the arachnoid and spinal cord parenchyma and hinder spinal venous return. Infectious thrombosis of the spinal cord artery aggravates the blood circulation disorder of the spinal cord, resulting in spinal cord edema, softening, and transverse lesions.

20.2.1.3 Imaging

1. Spinal epidural abscess
   (a) X-ray examination: X-rays of the spine are mostly unchanged. As X-ray imaging of the spine can show the upper or lower level of the spinal cord obstruction, but not the extent of the abscess, the level of sensory loss cannot be predicted, and the X-ray of the spinal cord photographic imaging cannot find the cause of the spinal epidural obstruction. In addition, spinal cord X-ray imaging is an invasive procedure, which may cause pain during the puncture, infection

at the puncture site, bleeding, arachnoiditis, and other complications. Myelography showed obstruction in the spinal canal and filling defect.

(b) CT: The appearance of the density of the epidural space is increased, while the normal blood vessels and nerves are blurred, and the boundary with the spinal cord is not clear, which can show bone destruction more clearly. The enhanced scan shows obvious ring enhancement of the abscess wall. Compared with X-ray examination, the changes in surrounding soft tissues can be observed. The CT scan showed a large number of epidural masses in the spinal canal next to the spinal canal.

(c) MRI: When the early stage of the lesion is mainly degeneration, liquefaction, and necrosis, it is manifested as hypointense on T_1WI and hyperintense on T_2WI in the epidural space; when the lesion is mainly granulation tissue hyperplasia, T_1WI shows hypointense and T_2WI shows slightly hyperintense; when there is the main fibrous tissue hyperplasia, T_1WI and T_2WI both show hypointense. In the middle and late stages of the disease, the hyperplastic granulation tissue and fibrous tissue constitute the wall of the abscess, with the latter as the main one. When there is a certain amount of hemosiderin around the abscess, a complete or partial low signal ring can be seen on T_2WI. The fat around the abscess partly or completely disappears due to inflammation. All spinal epidural abscesses are fusiform, while the upper and lower epidural space of the abscess widens, and the corresponding dural sac and spinal cord are compressed and shifted to the opposite side in an arc. The mature abscess has a lower signal area in the center on T_1WI. During the enhanced scan, the peripheral abscess wall showed ring-shaped enhancement, but there was no enhancement in the center, and the central hypointensity area was displayed more clearly. Abscesses in the immature stage are uniformly enhanced as a whole, and there is no low signal area in the center (Fig. 20.10).

2. Subdural abscess

(a) CT: The lesion is located in the subdural space between the subdural and arachnoid. The density can be slightly higher than that of the cerebrospinal fluid. The early enhancement is not obvious. After 1–3 weeks, the surrounding empyema is gradually enhanced, which may be accompanied by varying degrees of space effect.

(b) MRI: On T_1WI, the pus often shows a signal slightly lower than the spinal cord. It can also show a low signal when the pus is thin. The pus displays a high signal on T_2WI, and the signal is obviously high on DWI. The enhanced scan can clearly show the location of the lesion, the local space-occupying effect, and the spine, and the involvement of the surrounding tissues is of high diagnostic value; the wall around the abscess is markedly enhanced in an enhanced scan.

20.2.1.4 Diagnostic Key Points

1. The patient has a clear history of purulent bacterial infection and symptoms of spinal cord compression.
2. The SEA is located in the epidural space, mostly showing fusiform lesions, while the SSA is located in the subdural space, featuring CT with iso-density or slightly low-density, and T_1WI is characterized by iso-intensity or slightly low-intensity. The inside of the T_2WI lesion is high-intensity, and the surroundings are visible low signal abscess walls. Enhanced scanning showed obvious ring enhancement, and the internal pus had no enhancement; in typical cases, DWI pus showed high signal intensity.
3. Routine blood examination showed that white blood cell count, neutrophil ratio, erythrocyte sedimentation rate, C-reactive protein, and other inflammatory indicators increased, which were diagnostically significant [26].
4. Cerebrospinal fluid examination demonstrated an increase in the number of white blood cells and increased protein content. The positive rate of cerebrospinal fluid bacterial culture is low.

20.2.1.5 Differential Diagnosis

The SEA and the SSA can be differentiated based on whether the lesion is epidural or subdural. The SEA needs to be differentiated from metastases, lymphomas, and epidural hematomas; while the SSA needs to be differentiated from schwannomas, meningiomas, and arachnoid cysts.

1. **Intraspinal tumors:** Tumors in the spinal canal are easily affected due to their different locations. Extramedullary epidural lymphomas or metastases are common and need to be differentiated from the SEA. Lymphomas are mostly solid masses, featured with isodensity CT scans, isointensity T_1WI and T_2WI, uniform multiple signals, and mostly damaged adjacent bones. Enhanced scans usually show obvious uniform enhancement. The mature SEA abscess wall is circular, and enhancement can be differentiated based on the different enhancement characteristics. The overall SEA abscess in the immature stage is uniformly enhanced, and there is no low signal area in the center. The differential diagnosis should be combined with the history of the disease and the signal characteristics of the lesion. In addition to a clear history of the primary tumor, metastatic tumors are mainly caused by direct invasion of adjacent vertebral masses, often accompanied by multiple vertebral bone destruction. The SEA often has clear

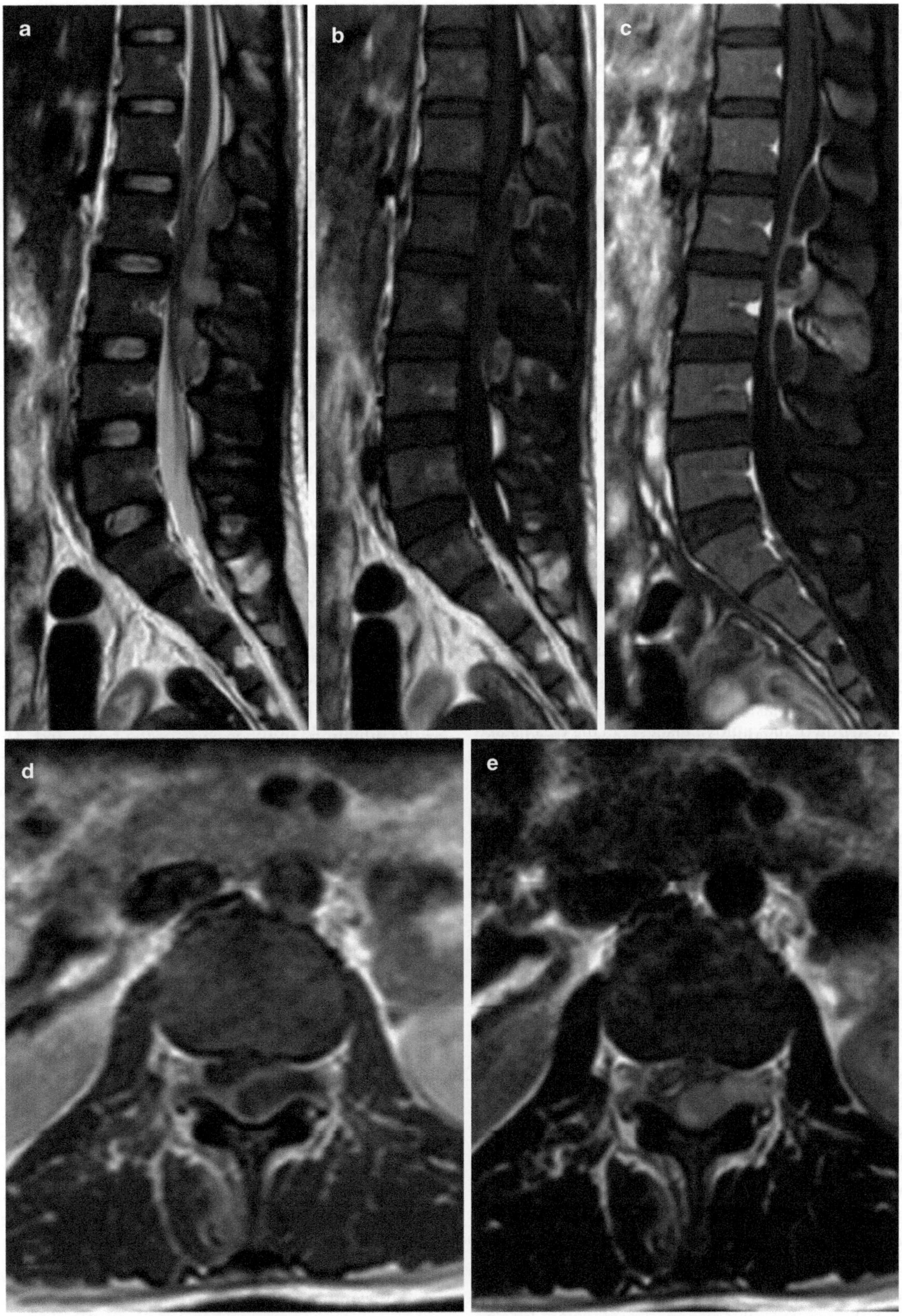

Fig. 20.10 Epidural abscess. (**a**) MRI plain scan: the first to fourth lumbar vertebral body level epidural T_2WI shows a fusiform slightly hyperintense, while the abscess wall displays hypointense (sagittal); (**b**) extradural lesions show slightly hypointense on T_1WI, while the wall of the abscess shows iso-hyperintense (sagittal); (**c**) the wall of the abscess shows obvious circular enhancement on the enhanced scan (sagittal); (**d**) the wall of the abscess is enhanced on the enhanced scan (horizontal axis); (**e**) the lesion is located in the epidural gap, the central pus presents hyperintense on T2WI, and the peripheral abscess wall presents iso-hypointense (horizontal axis)

purulent bacterial infections. The history of the disease was mostly fusiform, and the main body of the lesion was located in the epidural space. Extramedullary subdural schwannomas and meningioma are common and need to be differentiated from the SSA. Neurilemmomas are mostly cystic solid lesions, and the solid components of the tumor are significantly enhanced on enhanced scanning. The cystic components are ring-shaped enhancements on the cyst wall. The enhancement forms are often irregular and obviously different from the ring-shaped enhancement of typical abscesses. Therefore, it is easier to combine with the history of infection. Regarding identity, meningiomas are mostly solid subdural masses, with a wide basement connected to the adjacent dura mater. More uniformly, the enhanced scan shows the "spine tail sign," which is the obviously different annular enhancement of the abscess.

2. **Epidural or subdural hematoma:** Most patients have a history of trauma or vascular malformations, without a history of fever, and usually have a rapid onset. Hematoma has different imaging manifestations due to its different periods, and at the acute stage it manifests as hypointensity on T_1WI and hyperintensity on T_2WI and DWI; when the lesion is mainly granulation tissue hyperplasia, it manifests as hypointense on T_1WI and isointense or slightly hyperintense on T_2WI; when there is the main fibrous tissue hyperplasia, T_1WI and T_2WI are both show hypointensity. In the middle and late stages of the disease, the abundant macrophages on the abscess wall phagocytically produce paramagnetic substances, and a characteristic T_2WI low signal loop appears. During the enhanced scan, the wall of the abscess in the mature stage showed ring-shaped enhancement, without internal enhancement, and the whole lesion in the immature stage was uniformly enhanced. In summary, the differential diagnosis of epidural and subdural hematoma and the SEA/SSA should be combined with the medical history based on the characteristics of the lesion signal and enhancement characteristics. DWI examination can be conducive to the differential diagnosis when there are more pus components.

20.2.1.6 Research Status and Progress

Both CT and MRI can be used for the examination of spinal epidural abscesses and subdural abscesses. Due to its high sensitivity and noninvasiveness, MRI can infer the condition of spinal cord involvement and becomes the first choice for the diagnosis of intraspinal abscesses.

MRI examination has no radiation damage, and the ability to show normal anatomy and lesions is obviously better than CT. It shows that there are no dead angles in the anatomical structure and lesion area, thus being more conducive to the diagnosis and differential diagnosis of the disease and providing important information for the location, qualitative analysis, and even diagnosis of the disease. The functional imaging technology of MRI can play an important role in the diagnosis and differential diagnosis of intraspinal abscesses and postoperative evaluation. Abscesses show high signals on DWI, and MRS can detect specific metabolites. However, due to the relatively long MRI imaging time, poor display of calcification, and poor cortical bone structure, for patients with MRI contraindications and those who need more information about the disease, the CT examination can be further improved so as to assist in clinical diagnosis and treatment.

20.2.2 Pyogenic Myelitis and Intramedullary Abscess

Guihua Jiang, Yuanyuan Fang, and Zhiqiang Xu

20.2.2.1 Overview

Pyogenic myelitis and intramedullary abscess refer to acute purulent infections in the spinal cord, which mainly occur in children. The incidence is 25% in children under 5 years of age, and the ratio of male to female is 3:2. Spinal cord abscess can paralyze patients within a few hours to a few days. The delayed diagnosis will cause severe disability or even death [27]. Eighty percent of the infection are secondary to infections in other parts of the body, and 20% are primary lesions with an unclear source of infection. The most common pathogenic bacteria for spinal abscess are *Staphylococcus aureus*, and some gram-negative bacteria (such as streptococcus, actinomycetes, and proteus) can also cause disease. People with compromised immune function and intravenous drug abusers are at a higher risk. Moreover, 80% of spinal cord abscesses involve the thoracic spinal cord, most of which are single abscesses, and only 20% are multiple abscesses. Occasionally, they may affect most or the entire length of the spinal cord [28]. There are three ways of infection of purulent myelitis and spinal abscess: (1) direct bacterial cultivation caused by thoracic puncture and lumbar puncture; (2) blood-borne or lymphatic transmission; and (3) direct local infection spread.

The clinical manifestations of purulent myelitis and spinal abscess depend on the location of the abscess, which may include fever, nerve root pain, abnormal nerve function, etc. In the early stage, it can be manifested as pain in the distribution area of the involved spinal cord, or symptoms of spinal cord compression in a short period of time, which are manifested as motor, sensory, and sphincter dysfunction below the lesion level. According to clinical manifestations, spinal abscess can be divided into three types, namely, (1) acute type, where symptoms appear within 1 week; (2) subacute type, where symptoms appear within 1–6 weeks; (3) chronic type, where symptoms appeared over 6 weeks. The acute clinical manifestations are similar to those of acute transverse myelitis, whereas subacute and chronic spinal cord abscesses show a gradual process, similar to spinal cord tumors [29].

Spinal cord abscess is extremely rare in clinical practice. There are few relevant reports, and most of them are misdiagnosed cases. Magnetic resonance imaging (MRI) can provide a lot of important information for the diagnosis of the disease, which is of great value for the guidance of clinical treatment.

20.2.2.2 Pathological Manifestations

The occurrence and development of purulent myelitis and spinal abscess are a continuous process, which can be divided into three stages according to different pathological manifestations. (1) In the acute myelitis stage, spinal abscess of any type caused by any reason will initially cause localized suppurative myelitis, which lasts for 7–14 days, with localized inflammation, congestion, edema, and necrosis of the spinal cord, accompanied by venule inflammatory embolism. Under the microscope, polymorphonuclear cell infiltration around blood vessels can be seen. (2) In the pyogenic necrosis stage, myelitis continues to spread after 7–14 days; the softened necrotic area gradually expands and merges, which forms a larger abscess cavity, surrounding the new blood vessels, and a large number of connective tissue hyperplasia, and gradually forming an inconspicuous and irregular granulation tissue. Moreover, a large number of neutrophil infiltration can be seen under the microscope. (3) The stage of abscess wall formation lasts 3–4 weeks, which can be as short as 12–14 days, or as long as more than half a year. The abscess cavity is enlarged, and the surrounding connective tissues and glial cells significantly increase, therefore causing the abscess wall gradually thickened. The abscess wall can be classified into three layers under the microscope. The inner layer is a zone of inflammatory cells with infiltrating purulent exudate, granulation tissue, glial cells, a large number of new blood vessels, and neutrophils. The middle layer is a large number of fibrous connective tissues. The outer layer is constituted by hyperplastic glial cells, increased blood vessels, and infiltrating white blood cells [30].

20.2.2.3 Imaging

1. X-ray findings: Spinal cord X-rays are generally not significantly different, which often exhibit limited diagnostic value. Some cases may have local infections such as intervertebral disc or vertebral body inflammation.
2. Myelography performance: In the myelography, part of the spinal cord can be seen thickened, with or without displacement.
3. CT findings: CT can clarify the extent of the lesion and show the thickening of the spinal cord in the corresponding spine plane. The acute myelitis stage is manifested by the thickening of the spinal cord and hypodensity shadows with unclear borders in the spinal cord. Generally, there is no obvious enhancement or spot-like enhancement can be seen on the enhanced scan. In the stage of necrosis and abscess wall formation, the abscess cavity is iso-density or slightly hypodensity in the plain scan, with gas density or gas-liquid plane can be seen in part of the abscess cavity, and the abscess wall is generally iso-density. On the enhanced scan, there is no enhancement in the abscess at the stage of necrosis, but there may be slight enhancement at the periphery. At this time, the abscess wall is slightly thickened and uneven, and the outer edge is blurred. At the stage of abscess wall formation, the abscess wall is thin, smooth, and uniform, and obvious enhancement can be seen.
4. MRI findings: The MRI findings of spinal cord abscesses correspond to the disease progression.
   (a) Acute myelitis stage: In the early stage, the lesion shows blur boundary, irregular shapes and iso or slightly hypointense on T_1WI. On T_2WI, the central inflammation and peripheral edema are both hyperintense, and sometimes the signal of central inflammation can be slightly lower than that of the peripheral edema. The occupying effect is obvious. On Gd-DTPA enhanced scan, most of lesions do not show enhancement, and a few may show patchy or uneven enhancement when the blood-brain barrier is damaged. After the late necrotic area merges with each other, the early abscess formation shows hypointense in the central area on T_1WI, and hyperintense on T_2WI. There are thin and irregular ring lesions around it, which shows iso or slightly hyperintense on T_1WI and iso or slightly hypointense on T_2WI. Enhanced scan shows circular enhancement, which usually lasts for 30–60 min, and peripheral spinal cord edema persists [31].
   (b) Suppurative necrosis: The sign of spinal cord abscess formation is the appearance of the abscess wall. The abscess wall presents isointensity or slightly hyperintensity on T_1WI, and slight hypointensity on T_2WI. Pus presents hypointensity on T_1WI, and hyperintensity on T_2WI. Perifocal edema shows slight hypointensity on T_1WI, and slight hyperintense on T_2WI. On the Gd-DTPA enhanced scan, the abscess wall shows obvious ring enhancement, but the abscess cavity has no enhancement. The signal characteristics of the abscess wall may be related to collagen or hemorrhage. However, according to recent studies, it is more likely that the macrophages

distributed around the abscess engulfed paramagnetic free radicals to shorten the local T_1 and T_2 relaxation time. The pus of an abscess contains a large amount of protein components, which can cause local tissue to be viscous, thus limiting the diffusion of water molecules. The DWI sequence shows a characteristic hyperintensity [32].

20.2.2.4 Diagnostic Key Points

1. Pyogenic myelitis and intramedullary abscess usually occur in children with a clear history of purulent bacterial infection and symptoms of spinal cord compression.
2. Typical MR manifestations: In the acute myelitis stage, the diseases are manifested as blurred or irregularly shaped isointensity or slightly hypointensity on T_1WI. Central inflammation and peripheral edema both show hyperintensity on T_2WI. On Gd-DTPA enhanced scan, most of the lesions have no enhancement. Spinal cord abscess shows iso-intensity or slight hyperintensity of the abscess wall on T_1WI, and slight hypointensity on T_2WI. On Gd-DTPA enhanced scan, the abscess wall has obvious ring-like enhancement, and the pus shows hypointensity on T_1WI and hyperintensity on T_2WI. The perifocal edema displays slight hypointensity on T_1WI and slight hyperintensity on T_2WI. On Gd-DTPA enhanced scan, the pus shows no enhancement.
3. Abscess enhancement caused by special pathogenic factors may not follow the above rules and may have various shapes, even in flower-ring. There may be wall nodules, and the abscess walls can have different thicknesses and irregular inner and outer edges. It is easy to be mistaken for a malignant glial tumor.
4. Cerebrospinal fluid examination: The number of white blood cells increases, mainly neutrophils, and the protein content is high. The growth of pathogenic bacteria can be seen in bacterial culture.

20.2.2.5 Differential Diagnosis

For acute spinal cord abscess, it is easier to be diagnosed in combination with its typical clinical manifestations. For subacute and chronic intramedullary abscesses, the clinical manifestations are not typical, and imaging findings need to be differentiated from common intramedullary lesions such as non-suppurative myelitis, ependymoma, astrocytoma, and intramedullary dermoid cyst.

1. Non-suppurative myelitis: It is more common in other parts of the body after a viral infection or multiple sclerosis. MRI findings show swelling and thickening of the spinal cord. T_2WI shows multiple, patchy hyperintensities with unclear edges in the thickened spinal cord, and patchy enhancement can be seen during the active scanning phase.
2. Ependymoma: It is the most common intramedullary tumor. The clinical manifestations are mainly localized neck and back pain, dyskinesias, and paresthesias gradually appearing below the tumor segment. Tumors are mostly composed of solid parts and cystic parts. On plain T_1WI, the tumor shows heterogeneous iso or hypointensity, and on T_2WI, it mainly shows hyperintensity, with cystic degeneration, necrosis, and hemorrhage. On an enhanced scan, obvious enhancement can be seen in the solid part of the tumor while the cystic part shows no enhancement.
3. Astrocytoma: It is the most common intramedullary tumor in children. MRI findings show thickening of the spinal cord, with isointensity on T_1WI and hyperintensity on T_2WI, and cystic change and hemorrhage can also be seen. Enhanced scans mostly show mild enhancement, which can be manifested as focal or diffuse.
4. Intramedullary dermoid cyst: the MRI manifestations are diverse due to the mixed components of the lesion. The cystic components mainly show hypointensity on T_1WI, and hyperintensity on T_2WI, or mixed iso and hyperintense on T_1WI, and iso and hypointense on T_2WI. The envelope of the lesion is complete, with the boundary being clear. There is no obvious enhancement in the tumor on the enhanced scan, and line-like enhancement can be seen at the edge.

20.2.2.6 Research Status and Progress

Diffusion-weighted magnetic resonance imaging (DWI) can provide important information for the diagnosis and differential diagnosis of spinal cord abscess. The pus of bacterial spinal cord abscess is composed of a variety of inflammatory cells, bacteria, necrotic tissues, and a viscous liquid of protein. Due to the increases in cell viscosity, the diffusion of water molecules is significantly restricted, and the ADC value decreases. In the suppurative necrosis stage, because the abscess contains a large amount of protein in the pus, it can cause local tissue to be sticky and the diffusion of water molecules is limited. The DWI sequence shows a characteristic high signal. However, the abscess cavity of tuberculous abscess is formed by necrosis and liquefaction of caseous material, and its internal cell structure becomes less, so the diffusion of water molecules is accelerated, and the ADC value increases. DWI imaging only applies sensitive gradients in the three directions of the fiber bundles X, Y, and Z. It cannot fully and correctly evaluate the spread of different tissues in the three-dimensional space. Tissue anisotropy is often underestimated. Therefore, the effect of DWI on the diagnosis of spinal cord diseases is restricted. There are still deficiencies in further functional assessment and efficacy monitoring.

20.3 Tuberculosis Infection of Spinal Cord and Spinal Canal

Dan Zhang, Yulin He, and Jian Wang

20.3.1 Overview

Spinal tuberculosis is a non-suppurative inflammation of the spinal cord caused by *Mycobacterium tuberculosis*, with less incidence. It can be clinically manifested as tuberculous spinal meningitis, tuberculous granuloma, tuberculoma of the spinal cord, tuberculous abscess, etc. Because inflammation can spread to the spinal cord, meninges, and spinal nerve roots, the former is also called tuberculous spinal meningitis. Solitary tuberculoma of the spinal cord is very rare. There are three ways of infection of spinal cord tuberculosis: The primary disease is spread through the blood, through the cerebrospinal fluid, and invaded by tuberculosis lesions in adjacent organs. The most common cause is the direct spread of tuberculosis in adjacent organs, e.g., tuberculous meningitis spreads downward to the spinal cord or adjacent pyramids, and tuberculosis spreads into the spinal canal, etc. Other causes such as blood dissemination secondary to tuberculosis or tuberculosis primary to the spinal cord are rare [33]. In developed countries, the rising trend of tuberculosis in recent years cannot be excluded from the HIV epidemic. In fact, tuberculosis is often the first clinical manifestation of HIV infection. In the United States, the most risky infected population comes from immigrants from tuberculosis-endemic areas. Most of these immigrants are AIDS patients, homeless persons, drug abusers, alcohol addicts, etc.

20.3.2 Pathological Manifestations

Spinal tuberculosis is the most common in the thoracic segment, followed by the cervical and lumbar segments. The early stage of spinal cord tuberculosis is dominated by proliferative tuberculous granulomas, which are rich in inflammatory cells and less collagen fibers. As the course of the disease progresses, caseous necrosis can be seen inside the lesion, and inflammatory cells infiltrate around the lesion. At this time, the spinal cord is swollen and thickened, and those who involve the spinal membrane show thickening of the spinal membrane and adhesion. Pathologically, it can be seen that thick exudate accumulates and surrounds the spinal cord. Sometimes it can invade the spinal cord. It can involve arteries and cause inflammation, which can lead to spinal cord infarction. It can also form tuberculous granulomas, miliary nodules, or tuberculous abscesses [34]. Tuberculosis nodules are small and scattered white. Observed under the microscope, they are like nodules in other parts. They are composed of epithelial cells and some macrophages, lymphocytes, plasma cells, and connective tissue surrounded by a central caseous necrosis area. Severe cases may be accompanied by syringomyelia.

20.3.3 Imaging

1. Tuberculous spinal meningitis.
   (a) Spinal membrane manifestations: The affected spinal membrane is irregular patchy or strip-like thickening, isometric or on plain MRI, iso or slightly hyperintense on T_1WI, and hyperintense on T_2WI. The thickened spinal membrane after enhanced scanning is obviously abnormally enhanced.
   (b) Spinal cord manifestations: The affected spinal cord is obviously thickened and swollen. MRI plain scan shows isointense on T_1WI, while T_2WI shows slightly hyperintense, and the boundary is not clear. Most of them have no obvious enhancement on the enhanced scan (Fig. 20.11).
2. Tuberculous granulomas. As the course of the disease further develops, intramedullary tuberculosis nodules and granulomas form and manifest as iso or slightly hypointense on T_1WI and slightly hyper or hypointense on T_2WI. The lesions appear to have solid homogenous enhancement on the enhanced scan (Fig. 20.12).
3. Spinal tuberculoma. When tuberculous granuloma progresses further to the later stage, caseous necrosis occurs in the center of the lesion, forming a mature tuberculoma. When the center of the lesion is dominated by coagulation necrosis, the lesion contains a large amount of *Mycobacterium tuberculosis*, and T_1WI usually shows little hypointense or isointense solid nodules and T_2WI shows iso or hypointense, and there is usually no abnormal enhancement on the enhanced scan. If the inflammatory cells infiltrate around the mature tuberculoma, the lesion will show obvious ring enhancement after the enhanced scan, and the ring wall thickness can be uniform or uneven. The course of the disease further progresses. The epithelial cells, fibroblasts, macrophages, and proliferating glial around the lesion form an envelope, which display iso or slightly hypointense on T_1WI, and hypo or slightly hyperintense on T_2WI. The lesion

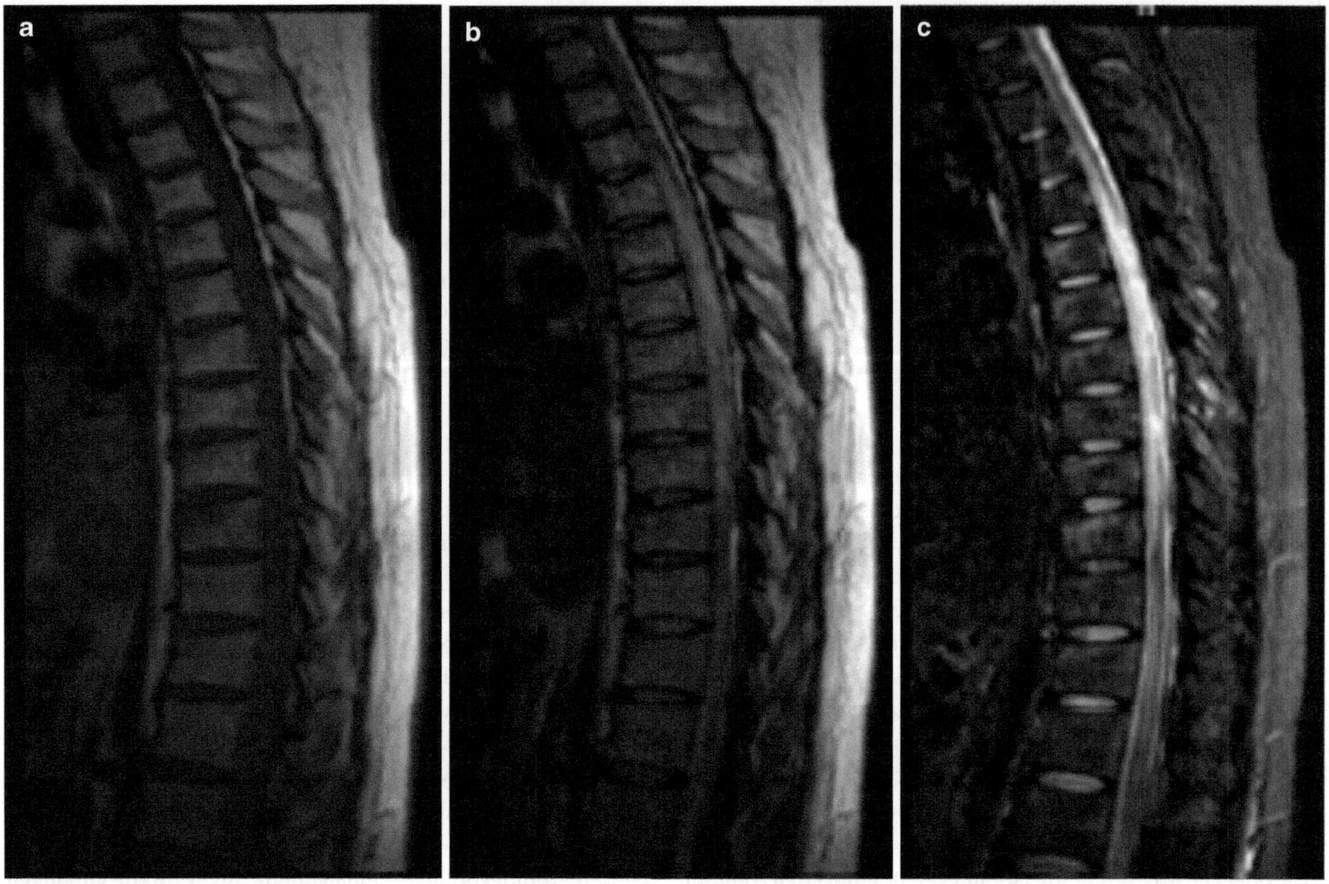

Fig. 20.11 Tuberculous myelitis. (**a**) The spinal cord is slightly thickened at the level of the third to tenth vertebrae, and strips of lesions can be seen, with a slightly hypointense on T_1WI; (**b**) the lesions on T_2WI show a strip of slightly hyperintense; (**c**) the lesions on the fat suppression sequence display hyperintense. (Picture provided by Dr. Wang Yan, Sixth People's Hospital of Xinjiang Uygur Autonomous Region, thanks hereby)

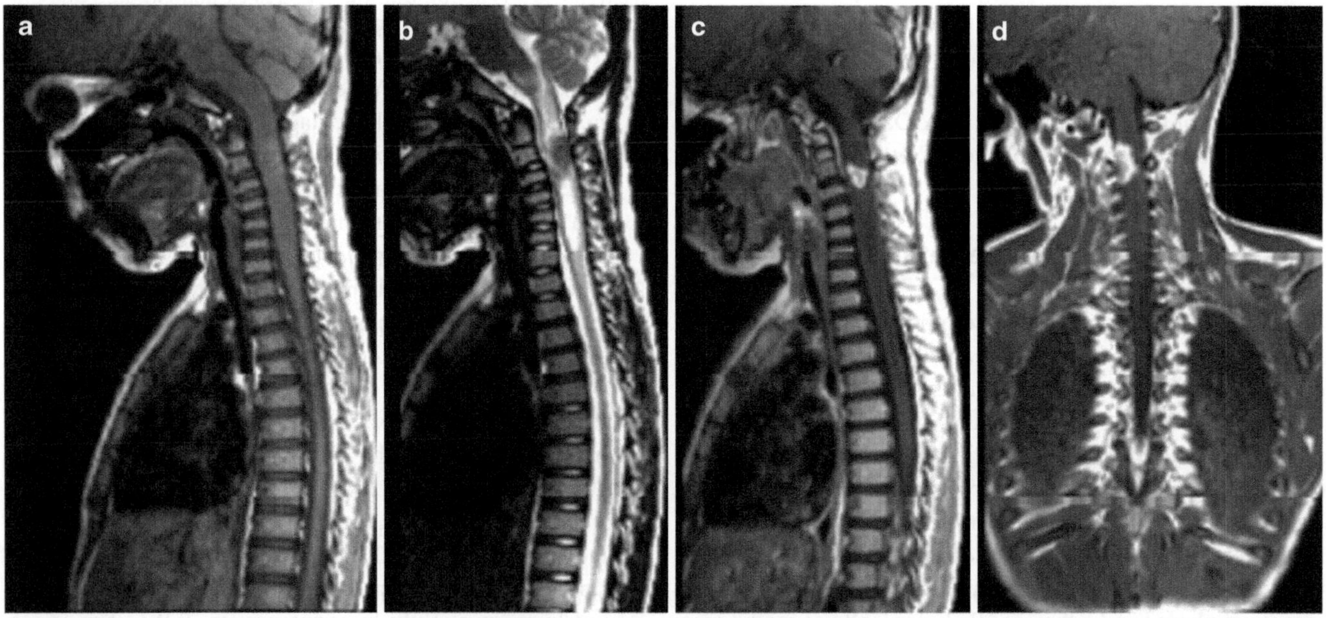

Fig. 20.12 Tuberculous granuloma of the spinal cord. (**a**) Localized thickening of the spinal cord in the second to seventh cervical vertebral body segments, irregular spinal cord lesions at the level of the second cervical vertebral body, manifest as iso/slightly hyperintense on T_1WI; (**b**) T_2WI shows slightly hypointense of the lesion with hyperintense edema around the lesion and syringomyelia; (**c**, **d**) T_1WI enhanced scan shows that the lesion is more uniform and with obvious solid enhancement (sagittal and coronal)

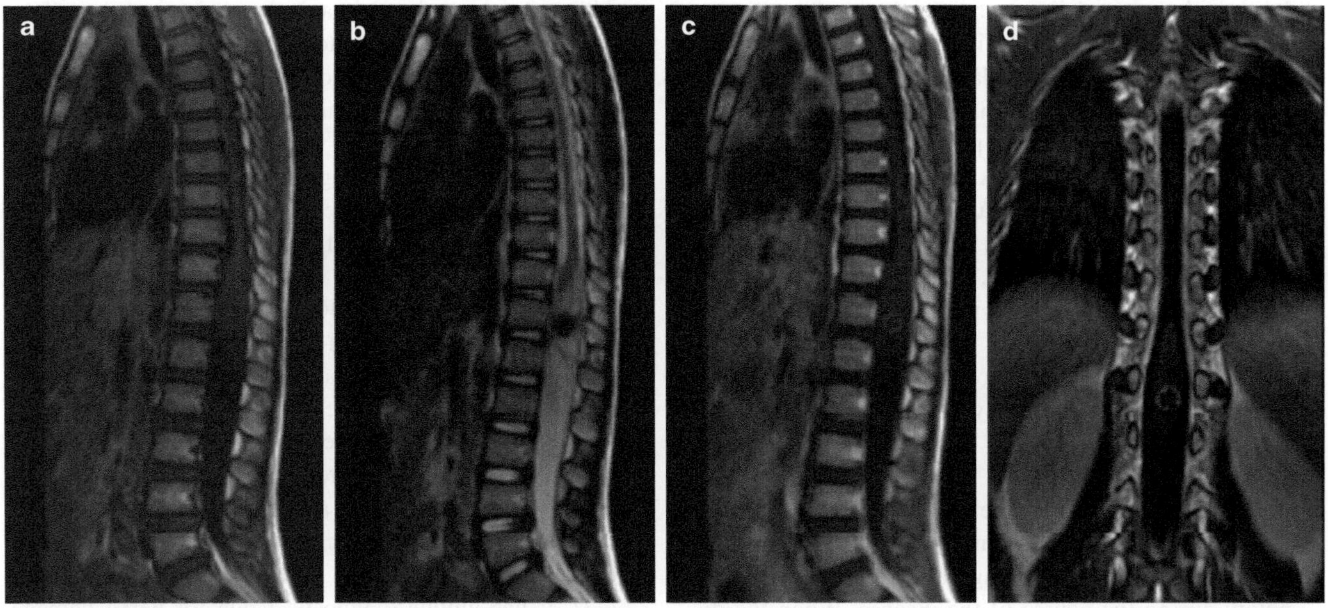

Fig. 20.13 Spinal tuberculoma. (**a**) The cone of the medulla is slightly thickened at the level of the 12th thoracic vertebra to the 1st lumbar vertebra, and a type of circular lesion is seen, with a slightly hypointense on T_1WI; (**b**) the lesion displays hypointense with clear boundaries on T_2WI; (**c**, **d**) the posterior lesion showed circular enhancement (sagittal and coronal) on enhanced T_1WI scan. (Picture provided by Dr. Wang Yan from the Sixth People's Hospital of Xinjiang Uygur Autonomous Region, thanks hereby)

envelope displays ring-like enhancement on the enhanced scan, and the thickness is relatively uniform [35, 36]. In summary, perilesion edema area and the center solid or liquid caseous matter showed no abnormal enhancement on the enhanced scan. Inflammatory cells or envelopes were enhanced to form a "target sign", which is a characteristic manifestation of mature tuberculoma (Fig. 20.13).

Miliary tuberculoma is a special type of tuberculoma, mostly secondary to miliary tuberculosis. Spinal cord lesions are diffusely distributed. The diameter of the lesions is usually ≤2 mm. It shows isointense on T_1WI, and slightly hyperintense or hypointense on T_2WI. On the enhanced scan, the lesions showed multiple miliary nodular enhancements, and some lesions showed small ring enhancements.

4. **Tuberculosis abscess.** When liquefaction necrosis occurs in the center of mature tuberculoma focus, tuberculosis abscess is formed, and the focus displays hypointense on T_1WI and hyperintense on T_2WI signal, and ring enhancement on the enhanced scan.

20.3.4 Diagnostic Key Points

1. Spinal tuberculosis: can be seen at any age, mainly seen in young people between 20 and 30 years old. The lesions usually occur in the cervical and thoracic spinal cord.
2. Meningeal tuberculosis: the spinal membrane is obviously thickened, surrounding or compressing the spinal cord. On the enhanced scan, the lesions in the sagittal view mostly present "tubular" enhancement, while the lesions in the axial view mostly present "circular" enhancement.
3. Tuberculous myelitis: The affected spinal cord is obviously thickened and swollen, and most of the lesions have no obvious enhancement on the enhanced scan.
4. Tuberculous granuloma of the spinal cord: the lesion showed nodular or circular enhancement on the enhanced scan; enhanced scan of miliary tuberculosis showed diffusely distributed miliary enhanced nodules in the medulla, with some small circular enhancements.
5. Cerebrospinal fluid acid-fast staining smear positive and cerebrospinal fluid culture of *Mycobacterium tuberculosis* can be diagnosed.

20.3.5 Differential Diagnosis

Patients with spinal cord tuberculosis have subacute or chronic spinal cord involvement and generally have a history of tuberculosis in the past. Combined with corresponding MRI and cerebrospinal fluid examinations, the diagnosis is not difficult [37]. Spinal tuberculosis and purulent myelitis, acute disseminated myelitis, multiple sclerosis, intramedullary tumors, and other imaging manifestations are sometimes similar, so they need to be distinguished from each other [38].

1. **Suppurative myelitis.** The disease progresses quickly. The typical pathological processes of spinal cord tubercu-

losis include exudation, organization, adhesion, etc. Active pulmonary tuberculosis or tuberculosis that occurs in other organs can be secondary to spinal cord tuberculosis, and the progress of spinal tuberculosis is relatively slow. The two have different performances in cerebrospinal fluid and blood-related examinations, antibiotic treatment response, etc., which can help distinguish them.

2. Acute disseminated myelitis usually secondary to other feelings in the spinal cord, infectious diseases, acute onset, and obvious clinical symptoms. It mostly occurs in the cervical-thoracic spinal cord. The spinal cord is slightly thickened. The lesions are not obvious on the T_1WI sequence and display hyperintense on T_2WI. On the enhanced scan, the lesions show patchy or strip-like enhancement [39, 40].
3. **Multiple sclerosis.** It frequently occurs in women aged 20–40, acute or subacute onset, sensitive to hormonal treatment, and symptoms aggravate and relieve alternately during the course of the disease. When the disease is in the acute phase, there is no obvious change in spinal cord morphology, and patchy abnormal enhancement can be seen in the spinal cord after the enhanced scan. When the disease progresses to the chronic phase, the spinal cord atrophy and the subarachnoid space widen [41].
4. **Intramedullary tumors** are more common in middle-aged and elderly people, and the disease progresses more slow, among which spinal cord metastases are rare and have other primary tumor lesions. Intramedullary tumors have obvious space-occupying effects. The spinal cord is locally thickened, and liquefaction and necrosis can be seen inside the lesion. On the T_2WI sequence, there are obvious hyperintensity edemas around the lesion, and some of them are combined with syringomyelia. On the enhanced scan, the lesion showed obvious circular or nodular enhancement, and the spinal membranes are mostly unaffected [42].

20.3.6 Research Status and Progress

Conventional X-ray examinations cannot show spinal cord lesions, and CT examinations cannot show subtle changes in spinal cord lesions. MRI examinations have a high resolution of soft tissue and can accurately display the location, size, and number of lesions from multiple levels and multiple planes and it is the best imaging method to examine spinal cord diseases. MRI plain scan can show the characteristic changes of spinal cord tuberculosis and the corresponding accompanying signs, such as thickening of the meninges and syringomyelia. Enhanced scanning and fat suppression technology can better display small lesions during the inspection process.

Although conventional imaging examinations can effectively reflect the scope and extent of spinal cord lesions, they provide limited information on spinal cord microstructure damage. With the continuous advancement of functional magnetic resonance imaging technology, such as diffusion tensor imaging (DTI) and magnetic resonance spectroscopy (MRS), more attention has been paid to the changes in the fine structure and biochemical function of the spinal cord.

1. Magnetic resonance myelography (MRM). It does not use contrast agents, which is safe and noninvasive. As a supplement to conventional MRI, it does not take much time, the post-image processing is also very convenient, and the imaging quality can fully meet the diagnostic requirements. It has been reported that the MRM images obtained by half-Fourier acquisition of fast spin echo sequences are more conducive to the observation of nerve roots, spinal ganglia, and postganglionic spinal nerves [43]. It has unique diagnostic value for nerve damage, arachnoid cysts, nerve root walking variation, and neurogenic tumors caused by intervertebral disc degeneration and various other reasons, and it is also helpful for the location of space-occupying lesions in the spinal canal.
2. **Diffusion-weighted magnetic resonance imaging (DWI).** The diffusion state of water molecules can provide more detailed and objective imaging information. In recent years, it has gradually been applied to the early diagnosis of spinal cord injury, multiple sclerosis and other spinal cord diseases, the evaluation of spinal cord function, and the observation of the efficacy of different treatment programs [44]. However, DWI cannot completely correctly evaluate the spread of different tissues in the three-dimensional space, and tissue anisotropy is often underestimated. Therefore, DWI is still insufficient for further functional evaluation and efficacy monitoring of spinal cord diseases.
3. **Magnetic resonance diffusion tensor imaging (DTI).** It has been considered a sensitive biological indicator for the diagnosis of spinal cord injury. DTI can distinguish between normal and damaged nerve bundles, distinguish glial scars, and locate the scar formation process. Glial scar is a physical and cellular barrier for the regeneration of axons after spinal cord injury. Therefore, DTI has potential advantages in evaluating the efficacy of cell therapy that reduces or inhibits scar formation.
4. Diffusion tensor tracking (DTT). It can visually display the change of white matter fiber bundles and the most effective methods to show live fiber bundles. This method vividly shows the three-dimensional morphology, spatial structure, and walking path of white matter fiber bundles, especially when the lesion invades the white matter of the brain, the role of imaging can be expanded from simple early diagnosis and assessment of lesion size to direct

comparison of lesions and important. The relationship between fiber bundles explains the clinical symptoms and evaluates the prognosis [45, 46]. Clinically, it can also be used to guide surgical operations. After surgery, the effect of surgery can be evaluated by observing the process of fiber bundle regeneration. However, DTT currently has certain limitations: DTT can only provide intuitive information and cannot perform quantitative measurement and statistical analysis; it cannot accurately determine the cause of damage to the fiber bundle.

5. Hydrogen proton spectroscopy (^{1}H-MRS). It is less commonly used in the evaluation of spinal cord disease.

20.4 Other Infections of Spinal Cord and Spinal Canal

20.4.1 Hydatid Disease in the Spinal Canal

Chunhui Jiang, Fei Wang, Jian Wang, and Luolin Yin

20.4.1.1 Overview

Hydatid disease is a zoonotic parasitic disease caused by the larvae of hydatid echinococcosis (hydatid), also known as echinococcosis. The adults of echinococcus are parasitic in the small intestines of canines (such as dogs, wolves, foxes, etc.), and the larvae can be parasitic in various parts of humans and various herbivorous animals (such as sheep, camels, etc.). Humans are infected by accidental eating of worm eggs. It is more common in the liver, followed by the lungs, and other organs may also be affected. The common types of echinococcosis in China are cystic echinococcosis caused by *Echinococcus granulosus* infection and alveolar echinococcosis caused by multilocular echinococcosis (alveolar hydatid) infection. Spine and spinal canal hydatid infections are more common with *Echinococcus granulosus*, and multilocular echinococcosis is extremely rare.

Hydatid disease in the spinal canal is mostly caused by the direct invasion of hydatid infection in the adjacent vertebral body, and it is rare in the spinal canal alone. Studies have reported that 25–84% of echinococcosis patients with neurological impairment can develop this disease [47]. The name of the disease has been reported in different literatures. It is also called hydatid disease invading the spinal canal, extramedullary subdural hydatid disease, spinal hydatid disease or hydatid cyst, intraspinal hydatid disease, etc. Currently collectively referred to as intraspinal hydatid disease, according to the relationship between the lesion and the spinal cord and dura mater, it is further divided into intramedullary echinococcosis and extramedullary echinococcosis. The latter is further divided into intradural echinococcosis and epidural echinococcosis. Early diagnosis of intraspinal echinococcosis is difficult. Therefore, patients with slow-progressive spinal cord compression and other organs of the body in echinococcosis endemic areas should be highly vigilant for the occurrence of this disease [48]. A negative serum immunological test for echinococcosis cannot rule out the disease.

20.4.1.2 Pathological Manifestations

The cysts of cystic echinococcosis are slightly white translucent cysts, which are filled with colorless and transparent cyst fluid, similar to cerebrospinal fluid. Observed under a light microscope, the cyst wall is divided into inner and outer layers. The inner cyst is the worm itself, and the outer cyst is the fibrous envelope formed by the host's immune response. There is only slight adhesion between the two, which contains blood vessels to supply nutrients. After the worm body dies, the cyst wall may be calcified. The inner capsule of the hydatid cyst is composed of a cuticle and germinal layer. The former is composed of germinal layer cell secretions without cell structure, and the latter is mainly composed of germinal cells, which have obvious reproductive ability, and groups of cells can sprout into the cyst cavity to form many pedicled fertile cysts, daughter cysts, and protoscoleces. The protoscoleces larvae are oval in shape, with four suction cups and apical processes visible. There are two loops of head hooks on the apical processes. When the apical process enters the body, it is oval, and when the apical process turns out from the body, it is pear shaped. The fertile cysts, daughter cysts, and protoscoleces free in the cyst fluid are collectively referred to as hydatid sand.

Blister echinococcosis is generally pale yellow or off-white nodules when observed with the naked eye, and the cut surface is spongy, like a solid tumor. Observed under a light microscope, unlike cystic echinococcosis, protosicular segments are rarely seen in the vesicles of cystic echinococcosis. Generally, only the stratum corneum is seen, and the stratum corneum is thin, and occasionally unicellular germinal layers are seen. Alveolar echinococcosis grows in the form of internal and external double germination. Multiple small verrucous protrusions can be seen on the wall of the mother sac, which gradually extend outward to form multiple small vesicles. The small vesicles continue to proliferate and aggregate to the outer periphery and gradually form solids. Sexual nodules or lumps. Vesicles of alveolar echinococcosis are mostly round, dendritic or fissure, surrounded by eosinophil infiltration, accompanied by typical granulation tissue formation and fibrous tissue hyperplasia.

20.4.1.3 Imaging

1. Intraspinal cystic echinococcosis
   (a) Intramedullary cystic echinococcosis: (1) CT findings, simple intramedullary cystic echinococcosis is extremely rare [49], and CT has great limitations in the display of spinal cord lesions, so CT examina-

tions is of little value in the diagnosis of intramedullary cystic echinococcosis. The CT findings of this disease are similar to hydatid cysts in the brain parenchyma. It is a round or oval cystic mass on the plain scan, with smooth and sharp edges, and uniform internal density, close to the density of the cerebrospinal fluid. When echinococcosis degenerates, the cyst wall may merge calcification and calcification of the cyst wall is a characteristic manifestation of echinococcosis cysts. Enhanced scanning cysts generally have no abnormal enhancement. When echinococcosis cysts are combined with infection, the cyst wall may have mild enhancement. (2) MRI manifested as single or multiple cystic space-occupying lesions with thin cyst wall and MRI showed cerebrospinal fluid-like signals. T_1WI shows hypointense and T_2WI shows hyperintense, surrounded by a continuous, uniform thickness of the cyst wall. The cyst wall displays slightly hypointense on T_2WI, which is its characteristic manifestation. Part of the lesions can also be separated. The cyst wall is generally not enhanced on the enhanced scan and may be slightly enhanced when combined with infection. Primary intramedullary cystic echinococcosis does not invade the vertebral body and paravertebral soft tissues.

(b) Extramedullary (subdural/extra) cystic hydatid disease: (1) X-ray examination shows generally no obvious abnormalities. X-ray examination shows poorly the structure of the spinal canal; even if echinococcosis cystic is combined with calcification, it is not easy to show. When extramedullary echinococcosis in the spinal canal involves adjacent vertebral bodies, polycystic and expansive bone destruction of the vertebral body may occur, local bone density is reduced, and the lesions are round or quasi-round irregular and transparent. The shadows have sharp boundaries, some are calcified, some are osteolytic destruction, slightly swelled, the edges are clear but irregular, and the vertebrae become flat, widened, or compressed into a wedge shape. Lesions can invade the pedicle and lamina of the vertebral arch causing the unclear structure of the pedicle. Generally, the intervertebral disc is mostly not invaded. This point can be distinguished from spinal tuberculosis. (2) The performance of spinal canal angiography, usually extramedullary cystic echinococcosis, has no specific manifestations on spinal canal imaging. When the echinococcosis cyst is large, it can block the corresponding segment of the spinal canal, and only a small amount of contrast agent passes through. The blood vessels around the cyst are compressed and displaced. (3) CT findings, cystic lesions can be seen in the spinal canal, with clear boundaries, epidural lesions are mostly fusiform, subdural lesions are mostly elliptical, CT value is similar to cerebrospinal fluid, spinal cord is pushed and displaced, and the cyst wall is merged. The calcification presents a complete or incomplete shell-like hyperdense shadow and if there is a partition in the capsule, it indicates the disease. Multiascus myeloderm cysts are characterized by the appearance of different numbers of small cysts in the large sac, forming the characteristic performance of a "cyst (ascus) inside the cyst (the mother sac)" or the cyst has a partition, and the density of the ascus is slightly lower than the density of the mother sac. (4) MRI showed that the spinal cord at the location of the lesion was significantly compressed and displaced, the epidural lesions were mostly fusiform with the adjacent subarachnoid space narrowed, and the subdural lesions were mostly elliptical with the adjacent subarachnoid space widened. The cyst fluid signal of simple cyst-type extramedullary cystic echinococcosis is similar to that of cerebrospinal fluid, and a continuous and uniform cyst wall can be seen at the edge of the lesion. Multi-ascus extramedullary cystic echinococcosis manifests as multiple ascuses of different sizes in the mother sac, which are arranged along the periphery of the mother sac and are shaped like "rose petals". Both the mother sac and the ascus sac fluid display hypointense on T_1WI, but the signal of the ascus sac fluid is lower than that of the mother sac, and the ascus wall is often unclear. The mother sac and ascus sac fluid display hyperintense on T_2WI, and the mother sac wall and ascus wall show slightly hypointense and with no enhancement on the enhanced scan. Co-infection can see ring enhancement. When the inner capsule ruptures, the inner capsule floats in the sac fluid, forming a "drifting band sign." Multiple small sacs and partitions can be seen in the large sac, which are characteristic of MRI, which is of diagnostic significance. In the sacral canal lesions, cauda equina adhesion can also be seen, and the boundary with the surrounding tissues is not clear. The lesions can grow along the intervertebral foramen, and adjacent vertebral bodies may have bone destruction and absorption [50].

2. Intraspinal alveolar echinococcosis

(a) Intramedullary alveolar echinococcosis: (1) CT findings, intramedullary alveolar echinococcosis is rare, the lesion is a dense mass or nodule of soft tissue, and punctate or granular calcification can be seen inside, which is the degeneration of the cyst wall in the small vesicle metamorphosis caused by calcium salt deposition, which is a characteristic manifestation of intramedullary echinococcosis on CT. Enhanced scans often show obvious irregular ring enhancement. (2) MRI manifestations, intramedullary alveolar echinococcosis is mostly caused by spinal alveolar echinococcosis invading into the intramedullary or the whole body multi-organ alveolar echinococcosis metastasizes, but rarely metastasizes to the intramedullary, and the primary intramedullary is even rarer. Intramedullary alveolar echinococcosis often presents as round or nodular solid lesions, which are isointense on T_1WI, and hypointense on T_2WI, and may contain small high-signal vesicles of varying sizes. The unique signal characteristics on T_2WI are similar to the characteristic manifestations of cerebral alveolar echinococcosis. On enhanced scanning, intramedullary alveolar echinococcosis usually shows ring-shaped and irregular-shaped edge enhancement (Fig. 20.14).

(b) Extramedullary (subdural/extra) alveolar echinococcosis: Extramedullary subdural alveolar echinococcosis is located on the inner side of the spinal canal with widening of the adjacent subarachnoid space. The extramedullary alveolar echinococcosis is located outside the dura mater in the spinal canal, and the adjacent subarachnoid space is narrowed, and the spinal cord is obviously compressed and displaced. The imaging findings of extramedullary alveolar echinococcosis are basically the same as those of intramedullary lesions.

20.4.1.4 Diagnostic Key Points

1. Patients with echinococcosis in endemic areas, history of contact with susceptible animals, or echinococcosis in other parts of the body.
2. The clinical manifestations have symptoms and signs of spinal cord compression.

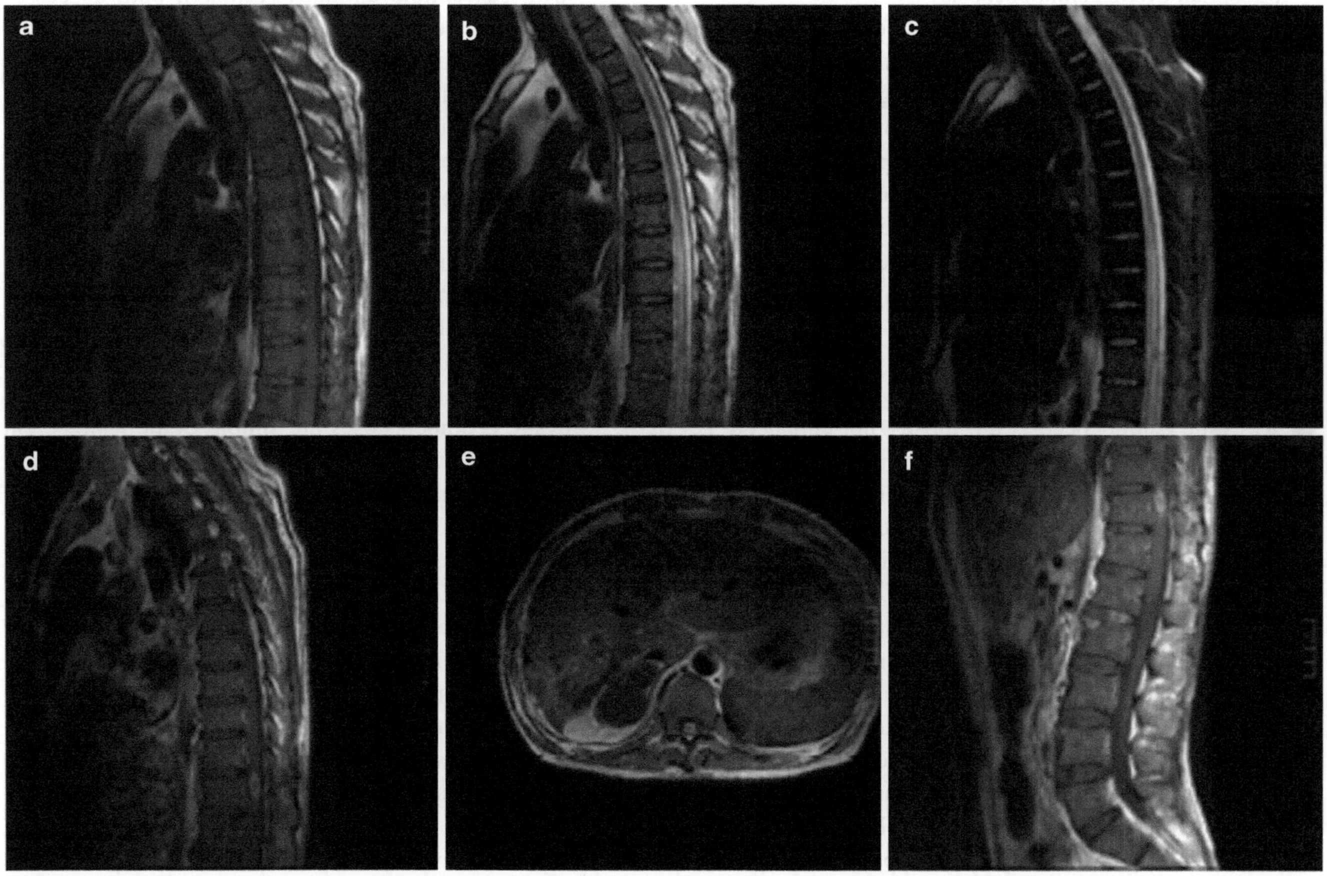

Fig. 20.14 Intramedullary alveolar echinococcosis. (**a**) T_1WI showed that nodular and other signal lesions can be seen in the spinal cord at the level of the 11th thoracic vertebral body, from the top of the lesion to the level of the 6th thoracic vertebral body, in the spinal cord from below to the level of the 1st lumbar vertebral body, there are strips of spinal cord edema and medulla. Syringomyelia lesions showed hypointense (sagittal view); (**b**) T_2WI showed that the 11th thoracic vertebral level intraspinal cord lesions displayed hypointense, and spinal cord edema and syringomyelia showed hyperintense (sagittal view); (**c**) fat suppression sequence, the 11th thoracic vertebral level of the spinal cord showed hypointense; (**d–f**) T_1WI enhanced scans showed that the 11th thoracic vertebral level of the spinal cord edge displays ring-like enhancement, and spinal edema and syringomyelia were not seen enhanced (thoracic spine sagittal position, thoracic spine axial position, lumbar spine sagittal position)

3. CT plain scan of cystic echinococcosis showed hypodense in the cyst cavity, with partitions visible inside, and calcification of the cyst wall; MR plain scan showed hypointense on T_1WI, and hyperintense on T_2WI. Multiple small cysts and partitions were seen in the large cyst. Its characteristic MRI manifestations have diagnostic significance. The lesion without enhancement or with slight enhancement of the cyst wall on the enhanced scan.
4. Alveolar echinococcosis on plain CT scan showed an isodense solid nodule or mass with calcification; MR T_2WI plain scan showed mixed signals dominated by hypointense, with multiple hyperintense vesicles of varying sizes inside and this is its characteristic performance. Lesion displays irregular ring-like enhancement on the enhanced scan.
5. Echinococcosis seroimmunology test is positive; negative cannot be ruled out of this disease.

20.4.1.5 Differential Diagnosis

1. Intraspinal cystic echinococcosis
   (a) Intramedullary cystic echinococcosis: it needs to be differentiated from angioreticuloma in the spinal cord, intestinal cysts, and syringomyelia [51]. (1) Angioreticuloma: It is a more common cystic solid space-occupying lesion in the spinal cord, usually manifested as "large cystic with nodules," that is, small solid nodules can be seen in large cystic lesions, while the cystic echinococcosis is only a simple cyst. On the enhanced scan, the solid part of the angioreticuloma manifests obvious nodular enhancement, and the cystic part could also show ring-like enhancement. However, enhanced scans of cystic echinococcosis are mostly not enhanced. (2) Intestinal cyst: It is a rare malformed cyst caused by congenital endoderm developmental disorder. It is mainly formed by the development of the remnant tissue of the neural bowel tube. It is more common in children. It is often associated with notochordal hypoplasia and longitudinal spinal cord malformation. Most intestinal cysts appear as round or oval cystic lesions with clear boundaries. Their signal characteristics depend on the content of the cyst, and most of them are similar to the cerebrospinal fluid signal. For example, when it contains more protein and intracystic hemorrhage, T_1WI may show hyperintense and T_2WI may show hypointense. The cyst fluid of hydatid cysts is mostly similar to the cerebrospinal fluid signal, and there are partitions in some lesions, and there are no adjacent ridge congenital malformations of the marrow. (3) Syringomyelia: It can be divided into congenital and acquired. The former is mostly accompanied by combined malformations such as inferior tonsillar hernia of the cerebellum, and the latter is mostly complications of trauma, tumor, inflammation, and so on. CT showed a hypodense cyst with a clear inner boundary of the spinal cord. The CT value was the same as that of the cerebrospinal fluid in the subarachnoid space. T_1WI showed hypointense, and T_2WI showed hyperintense. The essence of syringomyelia is the expansion of the central canal of the spinal cord, so the lesion has no obvious cyst wall and no partition inside the lesion. These can be distinguished from cystic echinococcosis.
   (b) Extramedullary (subdural/epidural) cystic echinococcosis: need to be differentiated from intraspinal abscess, schwannoma, and arachnoid cyst [51]. (1) Extramedullary subdural/extramedullary abscess: abscesses generally have a rapid onset and have a clear history of bacterial infection, while cystic echinococcosis generally has a slow onset, with a history of residence in endemic areas or a history of contact with susceptible animals. Although both abscesses and cystic echinococcosis have thicker cyst walls, the cyst walls of cystic echinococcosiss generally have no enhancement, while the cyst wall of abscesses can show obvious ring enhancement. In addition, the pus of an abscess shows a clear hyperintense on DWI, while the cyst fluid of an cystic echinococcosis generally displays hypointense on DWI. (2) Schwannoma: It is the most common extramedullary subdural space-occupying lesion, and the tumor is prone to cystic transformation and needs to be differentiated from extramedullary subdural cystic echinococcosis. Schwannomas are mostly cystic solid lesions, while cystic echinococcoses are simple cystic lesions. On enhanced scanning, the solid components of schwannoma are significantly enhanced, and the cystic components of the cyst wall are enhanced with ring-shaped, while cystic echinococcoses are mostly not. In addition, schwannomas can grow into the paravertebral soft tissues along the adjacent intervertebral foramen, forming a characteristic "dumbbell-like" appearance. The adjacent vertebral bone and paravertebral soft tissues are not violated, and they only show signs of compression and displacement. The extramedullary cystic echinococcosis in the spinal canal is mostly caused by the direct invasion of adjacent vertebral body. Therefore, the adjacent vertebral body and appendage bone can have obvious bone destruction, and the paravertebral soft tissue can also be invaded. (3) Arachnoid cyst: arachnoid cysts in the spinal canal are generally located under the extramedullary dura and are often irregular in shape, while hydatid cysts are mostly regular round-like masses with obvious cyst wall visible, while

arachnoid cysts are mostly displayed unclear due to the thin wall of the capsule. In addition, multi-ascus cystic echinococcoses have the characteristic performance of separation or "cysts in the cyst," combined with the history of residence in echinococcosis endemic areas or the history of contact with susceptible animals, and it is not difficult to identify.

2. Intraspinal alveolar echinococcosis
   (a) Intramedullary alveolar echinococcosis: need to be differentiated from astrocytoma, tuberculoma, and teratoma in the spinal cord. (1) Astrocytoma in the spinal cord: It is the most common primary tumor in the spinal cord. It usually manifests as thickening of the spinal cord, with irregular morphological space-occupying lesions. T_1WI shows hypointense and T_2WI shows slightly hyperintense. The signal is generally more uniform, and the typical feature of alveolar echinococcosis is that T_2WI mainly shows hypointense with multiple small hyperintense vesicles of varying sizes. Enhanced scanning showed uniform enhancement, while vesicular echinococcosis mostly showed circular enhancement. Identify the two with capital. (2) Tuberculoma in the spinal cord: The imaging findings of tuberculoma and alveolar echinococcosis are similar. Both are nodular lesions with internal calcification and mostly display hypointense on T_2WI, with enhanced scan showing circular enhancement. However, tuberculoma is usually caused by pulmonary tuberculosis or the spread of tuberculosis blood from other parts of the body and is often accompanied by signs of tuberculous meningitis. The alveolar echinococcosis is mostly secondary to hepatic alveolar echinococcosis, and adjacent vertebral bone can also be invaded, and the characteristic small vesicle structure different from tuberculosis can be seen on T_2WI. Combining the medical history, it is not difficult to distinguish between the two. (3) Teratoma in the spinal cord: It usually has a variety of components. In addition to visible calcified tissue, cystic tissue and adipose tissue can also be seen. The MR signal has various manifestations, and the enhanced scan of mature teratoma is mostly not enhanced. The vesicular hydatid disease does not contain fat components, and the enhanced scan can show circular enhancement to distinguish between the two.
   (b) Extramedullary (subdural/epidural) alveolar echinococcosis: need to be differentiated from neurogenic tumors and vascular malformations in the spinal canal. (1) Neurogenic tumor: It is the most common extramedullary subdural space, and the tumor is easy to merge with cystic transformation. If the tumor is mainly cystic, the enhanced scan can show circular enhancement, which needs to be differentiated from alveolar echinococcosis. However, the cysts of neurogenic tumors are generally larger and integrated as a whole, while the vesicles in alveolar echinococcosis have multiple minor lesions, and the imaging findings are different. In addition, although neurogenic tumors can grow along the intervertebral foramina to the paravertebral soft tissues, they do not invade the adjacent bone and soft tissues and only cause signs of compression. The alveolar hydatid disease is mostly caused by the direct invasion of adjacent vertebral echinococcosis. Therefore, the adjacent vertebral body and appendage bone may have obvious bone destruction, and the paravertebral soft tissue may also be invaded. (2) Vascular malformations: Vascular malformations in the spinal canal usually manifest as tortuous worm-like malformed vascular nests, which show a low-signal flow-empty effect on T_2WI, but there are no vesicles inside the lesion, and the enhanced scan is usually not enhanced. This point can be compared with Identification of alveolar hydatid disease.

20.4.1.6 Research Status and Progress

Intraspinal hydatid disease is a rare disease, and previous studies [52] mostly focused on morphology. In addition to magnetic resonance water imaging, other new functional technologies are rarely reported. Magnetic resonance water imaging technology can not only clearly show the tissue structure containing liquid but also outline the outline of the lesion, which has special advantages for the diagnosis of hydatid disease. Compared with conventional MRI, magnetic resonance hydroimaging technology can show the small ascus of cystic echinococcosis in the spinal canal, the small vesicles of alveolar echinococcosis, and other fine structures. It can also outline the lesion and show the extent of the lesion and show the relationship between the lesion and the adjacent structure of the spinal canal. The combined application of magnetic resonance hydroimaging technology and conventional MRI can increase the detection rate of hydatid disease in the spinal canal.

20.4.2 Lyme Disease

Rui Huang, Jianhua Ma, and Jian Wang

20.4.2.1 Overview

Lyme disease is a type of *Borrelia burgdorferi* (Bb) that uses ticks as a vector. The disease caused by infection is a zoonotic disease that can affect multiple organs and multiple systems. Most patients have a history of tick bites. The clinical manifestations of Lyme disease have certain characteristics. Usually, the skin is first affected and manifested as characteristic chronic migratory erythema, followed by symptoms of nerve, heart, and joint involvement.

The disease is widely distributed and spread all over the world, but it is mostly in the United States and European countries. It also occurs in Xinjiang, Heilongjiang, Jilin, and Henan in our country. The peak incidence of the disease is from May to September, and the people are generally susceptible. It is more common in people who enter or live in forests and rural areas. It is more common in young and middle-aged men. Among them, 10–15% of patients with *Borrelia burgdorferi* infection can affect the central nervous system, leading to Lyme neuroborreliosis (LNB). The most common clinical manifestations of Lyme disease of the adult nervous system are radiculitis and meningitis, followed by facial nerve palsy, and less common manifestations are meningoencephalitis, encephalomyelitis, cerebrovascular inflammation, and peripheral neuropathy [53].

The incubation period of Lyme disease is generally about 7 days, and the clinical manifestations are divided into three phases. Stage I: Mainly chronic migratory erythema, which occurs in limbs, groin area, and armpits and is often accompanied by fever, chills, headache, fatigue, nausea, vomiting, joint pain, and other nonspecific manifestations. Stage II: Mainly affects the nervous system and heart. Nervous system involvement is manifested as meningitis, radiculitis, meningoencephalitis, followed by myelitis, etc.; heart involvement is manifested as myocarditis, atrioventricular block, and pericardium. Stage III: Mainly involvement of joints. It occurs in large joints such as knee joints and hip joints and manifests as recurrent joint pain and swelling. Laboratory examination of Lyme disease: spirochetes can be separated from the patient's blood, cerebrospinal fluid and diseased tissues; using immunofluorescence assays, western blotting and other tests to detect anti-spirospiral antibodies in the patient's serum and cerebrospinal fluid can confirm Lyme disease diagnosis.

20.4.2.2 Pathological Manifestations

Within 3–32 days after the tick bite, the patient developed migratory erythema, and entered the first stage. It starts with red macules or papules, and after a few days or weeks, the lesion expands to the surroundings to form a clear round skin lesion, generally more than 5 cm in diameter. It can be seen under the microscope that there is lymphocyte infiltration in the superficial and deep blood vessels of the surrounding skin, including plasma cells, tissue cells and a small number of giant cells or neutrophils.

When spirochetes circulate with the blood to the central nervous system, it enters the second stage. Nervous system damage includes spinal cord nerve sheath fibrosis and focal demyelination changes. The severity of peripheral neuropathy may be related to the level of circulating immune complexes.

A few months after the occurrence of the disease, it enters the third stage, where multiple joints are involved and progress to chronic arthritis, which is a characteristic manifestation of this stage. The articular cartilage necrosis, degeneration, or atrophy can be seen under the microscope, and the synovial fluid shows villous hypertrophy, fibrin deposition, and a large number of monocyte infiltration. Sometimes multiple spirochetes are located in the blood vessel or surrounding part of the blood vessel to cause vasculitis obliterans, and burgdorferi can be found in synovial fluid culture.

20.4.2.3 Imaging

The imaging manifestations of Lyme disease of the spinal cord are diverse, including diffuse spinal cord lesions or granulomatous lesions, meningeal and (or) nerve enhancement, and vascular lesions, of which meningeal and (or) nerve enhancement are the most characteristic.

The preferred examination technique for the diagnosis of spinal cord Lyme disease is MRI. MRI usually manifests as swelling of the spinal cord. Diffuse abnormal signals can be seen in the spinal cord, often located in the center or front of the spinal cord, with long segmental distribution, with isointense or slightly hypointensity on T_1WI, and slightly hyperintensity on T_2WI. After enhancement, the spinal membranes or nerve roots are obviously abnormally strengthened, which can be nodular or diffuse enhancement [54].

20.4.2.4 Diagnostic Key Points

1. There is a history of residence in an infected area and a history of tick bites; the peak period of incidence is from May to September, and young and middle-aged men are prone to hair loss.
2. The clinical manifestations are chronic migratory erythema of the skin, and the corresponding manifestations of the nervous system, heart, and joint involvement.
3. MRI manifests as diffuse spinal cord lesions or granulomatous lesions, abnormal enhancement of the meninges and (or) nerves, and vascular lesions, of which abnormal enhancement of the meninges and (or) nerves is the most characteristic.
4. In laboratory tests, spirochetes can be isolated from the patient's blood, cerebrospinal fluid, and diseased tissues; the use of immunofluorescence assays, western blotting, and other tests to detect anti-spiraloid antibodies in the patient's serum and cerebrospinal fluid can confirm the diagnosis.

20.4.2.5 Differential Diagnosis

1. Multiple sclerosis (MS) is more common in young women, and there is no obvious cause before the onset of

the disease. It is characterized by a multi-phase disease course and recurrent episodes; while Lyme disease is more common in young men. Most of them have a history of tick bites before the onset, accompanied by chronic migratory erythema on the skin, and the corresponding manifestations of the nervous system, heart, and joint involvement. Spinal cord MS lesions are often located in the white matter area of the spinal cord, such as the posterior cord, lateral cord, subpial area, etc., and the general range is less than 2 vertebral body segments, the cross-sectional area of the lesion is less than 1/2 the area of the spinal cord, and the surrounding edema is generally mild and can be manifested as no enhancement or patchy abnormal enhancement on enhanced scan; while Lyme disease lesions are often located in the center or front of the spinal cord, showing long-segmental distribution. After an enhanced scan, the meninges or nerve roots are obviously abnormally enhanced. This is a characteristic enhancement of Lyme disease.

2. Acute disseminated encephalomyelitis (ADEM) is prevalent in children under 10 years of age. Most patients have a history of infection or vaccination a few weeks before the onset of disease; while Lyme disease is more common in young men and most of them have a history of tick bites before the onset, accompanied by chronic skin migratory erythema, the nervous system, heart, and joints are affected; ADEM spinal cord lesions are mostly located in the white matter of the spinal cord, and gray matter can also occur. They are focal or segmental, but most of them manifest the involvement of longer spinal cord segments (>3 vertebral body segments) and even the entire spinal cord. The spinal cord is generally not thickened and may not enhance or show patchy abnormal enhancement on enhanced scans, while Lyme disease lesions are often located in the center or front of the spinal cord, showing long segmental distribution. The spinal cord is swollen, and the meninges or nerve roots are obviously abnormally enhanced on the enhanced scan.

20.4.2.6 Research Status and Progress

With the development of new magnetic resonance technology, MRI has been helpful in the diagnosis of spinal cord Lyme disease in recent years. However, due to the lack of research reports on spinal cord Lyme disease, some new MRI technologies can provide potential applications for spinal cord Lyme disease. Value. DWI can detect the diffusion movement of water molecules in living tissues. Conventional MRI sequences have certain limitations in assessing the degree of spinal cord involvement, while DTI can quantitatively assess the damage of spinal cord fiber bundles. DTI can be used to study anisotropic tissues (such as white matter tracts), but it is more limited for isotropic tissues (such as gray matter tracts). Myelin water fraction (MWF) can evaluate the integrity of myelin sheath by detecting the water component incorporated in the myelin sheath, which can effectively improve the diagnosis rate of spinal cord lesions and better track the onset of the disease. Magnetization transfer imaging (MTI) transfers the magnetization state saturated with bound water in the tissue to free water, thereby reducing the signal intensity of bound water. Because bound water in the central nervous system is mainly related to myelin, lipids, and proteins, the signal reduction may indicate myelin sheath or axon damage.

20.4.3 Syphilitic Myelitis

Yuanyuan Fang, Zhiqiang Xu, and Guihua Jiang

20.4.3.1 Overview

Syphilis is a sexually transmitted disease caused by *Treponema pallidum*. Its incidence has been significantly reduced due to the widespread use of penicillin. However, in recent years, due to the spread and prevalence of sexually transmitted diseases, its incidence has rebounded. In developing and developed countries, the incidence of simultaneous *Treponema pallidum* and HIV infection is increasing. The neurological complications of these two infections occur occasionally. Changes in the patient's immune status may change syphilis from latent to active, leading to myelitis [55].

Syphilis is caused by *Treponema pallidum* infection. Four to 10% of early syphilis will appear neurosyphilis without antibiotic treatment or incomplete treatment, which refers to damage to the brain, meninges, and spinal cord. A set of characteristic clinical syndromes. The most common early-stage syndrome of neurosyphilis is syphilitic meningitis. Most patients present with asymptomatic meningitis, while syphilitic myelitis is extremely rare in the clinic, accounting for only 1.5% of all neurosyphilis cases [56, 57].

Syphilitic myelitis involving the meninges is also called syphilitic meningomyelitis. Because of the lack of specificity in clinical and imaging findings, it is easy to miss the diagnosis, which affects the timing and therapeutic effect of its treatment. The pathogenesis of syphilitic spinal meningitis remains unclear. The early manifestations are the weakness of the lower limbs, paresthesia, and sphincter dysfunction. If not being diagnosed and treated in time, it can further develop into lower limb paresis or paraplegia, and even irreversible paralysis in the later stage. Its clinical manifestations are also called Erb's spastic paraplegia (Erb's spastic paraplegia) [56, 57].

The first choice for the treatment of syphilitic myelitis is penicillin. For patients who are mildly allergic to penicillin, they can take an intravenous infusion of ceftriaxone or oral minocycline hydrochloride, whereas those who are severely allergic to penicillin need to receive the desensitization treatment of β-lactam antibacterial drugs before penicillin treatment. The treatment effect of most patients is good, but there are differences in the speed and degree of recovery [58].

Laboratory tests help the diagnosis of the disease, and cerebrospinal fluid examination is the key to the diagnosis of syphilitic myelitis. If the history of syphilis is unknown, the serum fluorescent *Treponema* antibody absorption test/*Treponema pallidum* gelatin particle agglutination test/enzyme immunoassay should be performed first to confirm whether *Treponema pallidum* is currently or previously infected. For patients with known syphilis, it is recommended that the lumbar puncture be performed for the detection of cerebrospinal fluid white blood cells and cerebrospinal fluid protein, as well as venereal disease research laboratory (VDRL) test and western blotting to detect *Treponema pallidum* IgM antibody. Cerebrospinal fluid VDRL test is specific for diagnosing neurosyphilis, but it is not sensitive. A positive test can confirm neurosyphilis.

20.4.3.2 Pathological Manifestations

In the pathological process of syphilitic myelitis, the thickening of the dura mater shows inflammatory changes, and it adheres to the arachnoid and pia mater, causing damage to the blood vessels and nerve roots of the spinal cord. *Treponema pallidum* from the spinal cord surface gradually invades the center of the spinal cord and finally leads to spinal cord degeneration and damage. The pathological manifestations are pale treponema and surrounding lymphocyte infiltration with gliosis [59].

20.4.3.3 Imaging

Syphilitic myelitis has a wide range of spinal cord lesions on MRI, usually involving long spinal cord segments and even the entire length of the spinal cord. T_2WI shows multiple hyperintensity (Fig. 20.15), but a few may have hypointense lesions. The enhanced scan shows two imaging manifestations, namely, the "candle tears sign" and the "reversal sign." "Candle tears sign" is manifested as focal enhancement of the superficial part of the spinal cord under the meninges, suggesting a pathological process in which the pale treponema invades from the surface to the center of the spinal cord. However, the "candle tears sign" is not a specific manifestation, which can also occur in neurosarcoidosis and tuberculous encephalomyelitis. "Reversal sign" refers to the enhanced part of the spinal cord parenchyma that shows isointensity or hypointensity on T_2WI. This sign is specific, but it does not occur often. The possible mechanism is the inflammatory response of the spinal cord parenchyma after the destruction of the blood–spinal cord barrier [60, 61]. After regular treatment, the above lesions can disappear completely [62, 63].

20.4.3.4 Diagnostic Key Points

1. Syphilis-positive patients show the clinical manifestations of bilateral corticospinal tract damage, including paralysis of the lower limbs, paresthesias, and sphincter disorders.
2. T_2WI findings reveal hyperintense lesions in the long-segment spinal cord, and the enhanced scan shows "candle tears sign" and/or "reversal sign."
3. A positive cerebrospinal fluid VDRL test can confirm the diagnosis, but a negative test still cannot rule out neurosyphilis.

20.4.3.5 Differential Diagnosis

Clinically, it is not difficult to make a diagnosis based on the manifestations of posterior root and posterior cord lesions of the spinal cord, specific Argyll-Robertson pupil with a his-

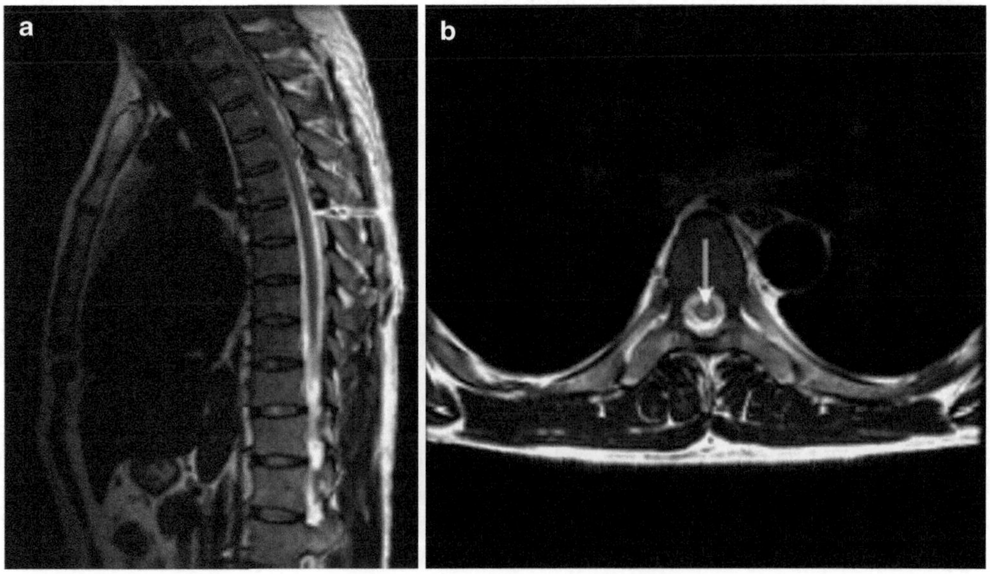

Fig. 20.15 Spinal neurosyphilis. (**a**, **b**) T_2WI showed patchy hyperintensity (arrows) in the thoracic spinal cord (sagittal, axial)

tory of syphilis infection, combined with specific serum and cerebrospinal fluid syphilis tests. However, it still needs to be differentiated from spinal cord infarction, demyelinating diseases, spinal cord tumors, and other diseases.

1. **Spinal cord infarction.** It is related to severe atherosclerotic disease, aortic dissection, or severe hypotension and is most commonly seen in Adam-kiewicz artery or anterior spinal artery occlusion. The anterior spinal artery supplies all gray matter (except for the posterior horn) and the corticospinal tract, so the central gray matter of the spinal cord is more prone to ischemic infarction than the peripheral white matter. This is different from syphilitic myelitis, which often involves the dorsal spinal cord.
2. **Spinal cord demyelination.** It may also have long spinal cord involvement and a variety of morphological enhancements, but spinal cord involvement is rare and usually coexists with intracranial lesions. Isolated spinal cord lesions are very rare.
3. **Spinal cord tumor.** The lesion is more limited, and the long-segment spinal cord involvement is rare. It can enhance variably on the enhanced scan.

20.4.3.6 Research Status and Progress

In recent years, with the development of new magnetic resonance technology, MRI has been helpful in the diagnosis of syphilitic myelitis. However, due to the lack of research reports on syphilitic myelitis, some new MRI technologies can provide potential application value for the disease. DWI can detect the diffusion movement of water molecules in living tissues. Conventional MRI sequences have certain limitations in assessing the degree of spinal cord involvement, while DTI can quantitatively evaluate the damage of spinal cord fiber bundles.

20.4.4 Human T-Cell Lymphoma Virus Type 1 Related Myelopathy/Tropical Spastic Paralysis

Guihua Jiang, Cong Huang, and Ning Xu

20.4.4.1 Overview

Human T cell lymphotropic virus type 1 (HTLV-1) is the first human retrovirus to be discovered. There are 10–20 million infected people. The vast majority of infected people are asymptomatic, lifelong virus carriers, and 5–10% of patients develop adult T-cell leukemia/lymphoma or HTLV-1 associated myelopathy/tropical spastic paralysis (HAM/TSP). HAM/TSP is a group of slowly progressing spinal cord diseases caused by HTLV-1 infection. The disease can occur at any age and is more common in adults. It is more common after 30 years of age. The peak is around 40 years old, with an average of 37 years old (6–75 years old). There are more women than men, and the ratio of men to women is about 1:2. The onset is insidious and progresses slowly. The basic feature is progressive spastic paraplegia, with obvious upper motor neuron damage and mild sensory and sphincter disorders. The main nervous system manifestations: (1) bilateral pyramidal tract damage, spastic paralysis of both lower limbs, increased muscle tone, lower limb hyperreflexia, ankle clonus, and positive pathological signs. The upper bound of the damaged pyramidal tract is unclear, but it is generally at the mid-thoracic level. In the late stage, there may be increased muscle tone of the upper limbs and tendon hyperreflexia, but there may be no changes in muscle strength. (2) Sensory disturbances, subjective sensory disturbances are more obvious than objective sensory disturbances, showing acupuncture-like pain, radiating downwards; deep sensory disturbances may be present. (3) The extrapyramidal system is damaged, and upper limb tremors may occur. There is no tremor when resting, but tremor when the arms are stretched forward (positional), with a frequency of 5–8 times per second. Oral prednisone can improve the tremor. (4) Autonomic nerve damage, bladder dysfunction is common, and frequent urination, poor urination, and urinary incontinence appear early; impotence and loss of libido often occur, and constipation appears later.

Gessain et al. [64] first detected HTLV-1 antibodies in serum and cerebrospinal fluid of tropical spastic paralysis (TSP) patients in 1985. In 1986, HTLV-1 antibodies were also found in the serum and cerebrospinal fluid of some patients with chronic myelitis in Jamaica, Colombia, and Martinique, and it was first pointed out that tropical spastic paralysis was caused by HTLV-1 infection. And it was confirmed in the serum and cerebrospinal fluid of patients with tropical spastic paralysis found in Jamaica. In 1986, Osame et al. [65] reported six cases of human T-lymphocyte virus type 1 with myelopathy (HAM) in Japan and believed that these cases were the same disease as the tropical spastic paralysis reported by Gessain. In 1988, WHO held a scientific research group meeting on "Human T Lymphocyte Virus Type 1 Infection and Associated Diseases" in Kagoshima, Japan. The research group believed that human T Lymphocyte Virus Type 1 associated with myelopathy and HTLV-1 positive tropical spastic paralysis is the same disease clinically and pathologically, and it is named "Human T Lymphocyte Virus Type 1 with Myelopathy/Tropical Spastic Paralysis (HAM/TSP)" at the same time. As of 2002, the literature reported about 20,000 HAM/TSP cases worldwide.

So far, the pathogenesis of HAM/TSP is unclear. It may be related to the following four situations. (1) Virus directly invades the nervous system and causes damage to the nervous system; (2) cellular immune response in the nervous system, HTLV-1 infection can promote the proliferation of peripheral lymphocytes without growth factors, and this self-proliferation response participates in HTLV-1 spontaneous growth of infected T lymphocytes; (3) injury to the nervous system through antibody-mediated immune response; (4) genetic factors [66].

Routine and biochemical examinations of cerebrospinal fluid can be normal, and acute T lymphocyte leukemia-like cells can be detected in peripheral blood, and lymphocytosis and protein increase may also be present. HTLV-1 antibodies appear in the cerebrospinal fluid, so the IgG index in the cerebrospinal fluid increases, and a monoclonal band specific to HTLV-1 appears. The disease responds well to glucocorticoid treatment.

20.4.4.2 Pathological Manifestations

Pathologically, it is mainly chronic spinal meningitis of polio and white matter caused by the immune response mediated by T lymphocytes, followed by axonal degeneration. In the later stage of the disease, the inflammatory activity of the spinal cord is reduced, but spinal atrophy is more obvious; the lesions are mostly located in the chest. In section, it can be seen that the corticospinal tract, spinocerebellar tract or lateral spinothalamic tract showed degenerative changes, accompanied by infiltration of peripheral blood vessels and parenchymal lymphocytes, as well as foamy macrophages, proliferating astrocytes and glial cells [67]. Extensive loss of myelin and axons, especially the corticospinal tract in the spinal cord. The most severely damaged part is the middle and lower thoracic spinal cord.

20.4.4.3 Imaging

HAM/TSP mainly affects the cervical spinal cord and thoracic spinal cord, especially the posterior columns on both sides, gray matter hind feet, and lateral columns; some cases can involve the brain parenchyma [68–71]. The MR manifestations of the spinal cord of HAM/TSP patients can be divided into three categories:

(1) Normal spinal cord manifestations; (2) spinal atrophy; (3) focal or diffuse hyperintensity on T_2WI with or without spinal cord swelling, 60% of patients on plain T_2WI showed abnormal hyperintensity, mostly located on both posterior columns. In the early clinical stage of HAM/TSP patients with rapidly progressing gray matter, hind feet, and lateral columns, abnormally hyperintensity on T_2WI can reflect the active inflammation of the spinal cord. Research by Yamamoto et al. [69] showed that in early HAM/TSP patients, the corticospinal tracts on both sides showed enhancement on the enhanced scan, which may be caused by the destruction of the blood–brain barrier in the bilateral corticospinal tracts during the active period of inflammation. Spinal cord atrophy is manifested in front and back directions, and white matter atrophy is the main form, especially in the lateral column [68]. The imaging findings of the spinal cord are related to the patient's course and prognosis. Unlike multiple sclerosis, spinal atrophy in HAM/TSP patients does not mean that the patient is more paralyzed or the immunotherapy is less effective, but the hyperintense of the spinal cord means the course of the disease. The progress is rapid and the response to immunomodulatory treatment is worse. The IgG antibody titer of the patient's cerebrospinal fluid increases.

20.4.4.4 Diagnostic Key Points

1. Mostly occur in middle-aged patients with insidious onset, longer course of disease, symptoms of progressive and symmetrical pyramidal tract damage, manifested by symptoms of spastic spinal palsy such as upper and lower extremity tendon hyperreflexia, positive pathological signs, normal mandibular reflex, absence of abdominal wall reflex, etc.
2. MRI plain scan showed swelling of the affected spinal cord with hyperintensity on T_2WI, mostly located in the posterior column of the spinal cord, gray matter hind feet, and lateral column; enhanced scan showed patchy enhancement; it may also be manifested as normal or atrophy of the spinal cord.
3. Blood and cerebrospinal fluid HTLV-1 antibodies are positive.

20.4.4.5 Differential Diagnosis

Slowly progressing spastic paralysis and mild sensory disturbances are the main manifestations of spinal cord lesions in the young and middle-aged. The T_2WI spinal cord on MRI shows abnormally high signals. At the same time, the positive HTLV-1 antibody combined with serum and cerebrospinal fluid may be considered for this disease. The differential diagnosis includes spinal cord changes caused by other reasons, such as multiple sclerosis, acute transverse myelitis, and subacute combined degeneration of the spinal cord.

1. Multiple sclerosis (MS) is the most common demyelinating disease in young and middle-aged women. It is characterized by the frequent spread of lesions and frequent remission and relapse in the course of the disease. The clinical manifestations are diverse, including limb weakness, hypoesthesia, ataxia, and other symptoms. Individual involvement of the spinal cord accounts for 8.6–29% of multiple sclerosis. The lesions mostly involve the lateral and posterior cords of the spinal cord. The cross-section is <1/2 the area of the spinal cord and the length is>3 mm, but <2 vertebral body segments. The edema is generally lighter. MRI manifestations vary with different stages. The active lesions mainly display hypointense on T_1WI, and hyperintense on T_2WI; DWI shows hyperintense. In the static phase, changes are not obvious on T_1WI and T_2WI shows slightly hyperintense, and DWI

shows isointense or hypointense. Most of the lesions had enhancement during the active phase of the enhanced scan, but no enhancement or mild enhancement was seen during the resting period or after hormone therapy. Enhancing lesions can be flaky, nodular, circular, semicircular, and arc shaped. The degree of enhancement is related to the destruction and repair of the blood–brain barrier. Nodular enhancement is a new lesion, while circular enhancement often indicates the reactivity of the old lesion. However, HAM/TSP are mostly progressive exacerbations without remission or seizures, and the appearance of a monoclonal band specific to HTLV-1 in the cerebrospinal fluid can be distinguished.

2. Acute transverse myelitis (ATM). It mainly involves cervical and thoracic spinal cord, or both at the same time. Typical lesions involve 3–4 vertebral body segments, and abnormal signals can extend beyond the level of clinically located signs. Characteristic performance is the enhancement or lack of acute sensory and motor function. On MRI, the diameter of the spinal cord is normal or slightly thickened, with hypointense on T_1WI and hyperintense on T_2WI.

   Laboratory tests can be identified.
3. Subacute combined degeneration (SCD) of the spinal cord is degeneration and disease of the central and peripheral nervous system caused by insufficient vitamin B12 intake, absorption, binding, transport, or metabolism. The lesions are mainly in the posterior cord and lateral cord of the lower cervical spinal cord, which are manifested as deep sensory deficits symptoms such as loss, sensory ataxia, and spastic paralysis. On T_2WI, the posterior cord or lateral cord of the spinal cord and the long-segment longitudinal band-like abnormal hyperintensity. The transverse T_2WI shows the posterior cord and the lateral cord symmetrically distributed hyperintense. The typical posterior cord involvement shows "inverted V sign" and "eight characters". Sign combined with laboratory vitamin B12 examination can be identified.

20.4.4.6 Research Status and Progress

1. The cerebrospinal fluid routine and biochemical examinations of HAM/TSP may be normal, and there may also be lymphocytosis and protein increase. HTLV-1 antibodies appear in the cerebrospinal fluid, the IgG index in the cerebrospinal fluid increases, and a monoclonal band specific to HTLV-1 appears.
2. The MRI manifestations of HAM/TSP are not specific and can be normal spinal cord manifestations or spinal cord atrophy. T_2WI manifests as focal or diffuse hyperintensity with or without spinal cord swelling.
3. The development and application of new technologies such as fMRI, MRS, DWI, DTI, and MRM of the spinal cord provide new ideas for the diagnosis of spinal cord lesions and provide more useful clinical information. However, there are currently few reports and further research is needed.

20.4.5 *Mycoplasma pneumoniae* Myelitis

Guihua Jiang, Cong Huang, and Ning Xu

20.4.5.1 Overview

Mycoplasma pneumoniae (MP) is a relatively common pathogen of community-acquired respiratory tract infections in children, which can cause multiple system diseases such as the respiratory system, nervous system, cardiovascular system, and blood system. Among them, *Mycoplasma pneumoniae* myelitis (MPM) is a serious complication of the nervous system caused by MP infection. It has been reported that 6–7% of mycoplasma infection patients have central nervous system symptoms [72, 73], which are specifically manifested as meningitis/meningoencephalitis, brain inflammation, ADEM and polyneuritis, etc. [74, 75]. It has been found that many central nervous system diseases are related to MP infection, of which encephalitis is the most common, accounting for more than 70%. Pathogenesis of its nervous system so far is still unclear, and three pathophysiological mechanisms have been proposed, namely direct infection, autoimmunity, and neurotoxicity [76].

MPM can occur at any age and mainly occurs in young people. There is no obvious gender difference. Most of the onset is sporadic. A few days or 1–2 weeks before the onset, symptoms such as fever, upper respiratory tract infection, and general malaise are common. Its clinical manifestations often described as ATM and ADEM. ATM is one of the most serious complications after mycoplasma respiratory tract infection, with an incidence rate of 1.34–8.2%. The lesions are often confined to several segments of the spinal cord. The thoracic spinal cord is most commonly involved. It is characterized by limb paralysis, conduction bundle sensory disorder, and defecation disorder of the area below the lesion [77]. The mechanism of ADEM caused by MP infection is still unclear. It may be that MP directly invades and causes cell damage. Its metabolites, proteases, hydrogen peroxide, and neurotoxins act on tissues and cause lesions in the corresponding parts. ADEM is usually with more than two scattered lesions, and its clinical symptoms are similar to ATM, manifested as sensory, motor, and autonomic dysfunction below the lesion. Cerebrospinal fluid white blood cell count will increase in 40–60% of cases. Cerebrospinal fluid MP-IgM is positive, but the positive rate is low. It is related to the fact that the antigen of MP and the nerve cells of the host share some common antigenic components. After infection, it will cause the activation of polyclonal B lymphocytes and the production of autoantibodies of the corresponding tissues, thereby forming an immune complex and causing immune damage to the nervous system. Serum MP-IgM is positive, but other viral and bacterial infections should be excluded.

20.4.5.2 Pathological Manifestations

MPM affects multiple segments of the spinal cord; the thoracic cord is the most common, followed by the cervical and lumbar spinal cords. ATM is mostly confined to one spinal segment, and multifocal fusion or multiple spinal cord scattered lesions are rare [77]. The macroscopic findings show severe swelling of the affected spinal cord, soft texture, and unclear boundaries between gray and white matter. The microscope showed gray and white matter necrosis, destruction of neurons, axons, and myelin sheaths, proliferation of astrocytes, perivascular lymphocyte infiltration, intramedullary and pia mater vasodilation, and hyperemia.

20.4.5.3 Imaging

There is no specific report on the imaging manifestations of MPM. MRI is mainly manifested as thickening of the spinal cord at the lesion site, multiple patchy and spot-like abnormal signals in the spinal cord, hypointense on T_1WI, and hyperintense on T_2WI with poor signal uniformity and the lesions can be fused. The lesions display patchy enhancement on the enhanced scan. In some cases, the spinal cord has no abnormal signals.

20.4.5.4 Diagnostic Key Points

1. Fever and respiratory tract, digestive tract. And other precursor infection symptoms may occur before the onset. The main symptoms are motor, sensory, and autonomic dysfunction below the diseased vertebral body.
2. MRI manifests as thickening of the spinal cord, multiple patchy, spot-like abnormal signals in the diseased spinal cord, hypointense on T_1WI, and hyperintense on T_2WI, the signal is not uniform, and the lesions can be fused. On the enhanced scan, the lesion showed patchy enhancement.
3. The cerebrospinal fluid white blood cell count will increase in 40–60% of cases. Cerebrospinal fluid examination is positive for MP-IgM, and the positive rate is low; serum MP-IgM is positive, but other viral and bacterial infections should be excluded.

20.4.5.5 Differential Diagnosis

Diagnosis of MPM is relatively difficult, and MP-IgM positive in serum or cerebrospinal fluid is of certain significance. Combined with the patient's history of prodromal infection, this disease must be taken into consideration. It is mainly differentiated from diseases that cause acute paralysis of the limbs, such as spinal metastases or spinal tuberculosis, spinal cord hemorrhage, multiple sclerosis, spinal cord infarction, etc.

1. Spinal metastases are manifested as bone resorption destruction and spinal canal stenosis, which compresses the spinal cord and causes spinal cord injury, but the intervertebral space is still clear, and it is more common in elderly patients. The diagnosis can be made with the history of tumors.
2. Spinal tuberculosis. It manifests as bone resorption and destruction, involvement of intervertebral discs resulting in narrowing of the intervertebral space, and cold abscess formation in the paravertebral area and inside and outside the spinal canal. Patients are often accompanied by systemic toxic symptoms such as hypothermia and emaciation.
3. Spinal cord hemorrhage. It is mainly caused by spinal cord trauma or vascular malformation. The diagnosis is confirmed when the cerebrospinal fluid from the lumbar puncture is hemorrhagic, and there is severe back pain, paraplegia, and sphincter dysfunction.
4. Multiple sclerosis (MS). It is the most common demyelinating disorder in young and middle-aged women and is characterized by multiple focal spreads and a disease course that often alternates between remission and relapse. The clinical manifestations are diverse and may include limb weakness, hypesthesia, ataxia, and other symptoms. Individual involvement of the spinal cord accounts for 8.6–29% of multiple sclerosis. The lesions mostly involve the lateral and posterior cords of the spinal cord. The cross-section is less than 1/2 the area of the spinal cord, and the length is greater than 3 mm, but less than 2 vertebral body segments. The edema is generally mild. MRI manifestations vary with different stages. The active lesions mainly display hypointense on T_1WI and hyperintense on T_2WI; DWI shows hyperintense. In the static phase, changes on T_1WI are not obvious and T_2WI shows slightly hyperintense, and DWI displays isointense or hypointense. Most lesions have enhancement during the active phase of the enhanced scan, but no enhancement or mild enhancement is seen during the resting period or after hormone therapy. Enhancing lesions can be flaky, nodular, circular, semicircular, and arc-shaped. The degree of enhancement is related to the destruction and repair of the blood–brain barrier. Nodular enhancement is a new lesion, while circular enhancement often indicates the reactivity of the old lesion. Combined with the clinical manifestations of patients, it can be distinguished from MPM. Before MPM, there are fever, respiratory, digestive, and other pro-infection symptoms. The clinical features are mainly paralysis of the limbs below the lesion level, sensory disturbances of the conduction bundle, and defecation disorders.
5. Spinal cord infarction is very rare, the onset is more rapid, and it is more common in the thoracic spinal cord and

cervical spinal cord may also be affected. A typical MRI manifests as hyperintense on T_2WI with an "eagle eye sign" in the axial view, and a discontinuous pencil-like hyperintensity in the anterior part of the aqueduct in the sagittal view.

20.4.5.6 Research Status and Progress

1. Diagnosis of MPM is relatively difficult. Patients with pre-infection and corresponding clinical signs should first undergo serum and cerebrospinal fluid examinations. Serological examination is still the main diagnostic method used by clinicians to determine mycoplasma infection, but there are large differences in sensitivity and specificity, especially the poor specificity of IgM testing. At present, there is no sensitive and specific gold-labeled serological examination method. IgM antibodies rise shortly after an acute infection and may last for 6 months. IgG antibodies will increase in just a few weeks and will continue for several months.
2. MRI is the preferred imaging examination for MPM. It can scan multiple parameters and multiple sequences and accurately display the location of the lesion, the extent of the lesion, and the enhancement mode. Sagittal display with T_2WI and STIR is optimal. The application of MRI functional imaging in spinal cord lesions is gradually increasing, but the application in *Mycoplasma pneumoniae* myelitis needs further research.
3. X-ray or CT examination can be performed to understand the condition of the lungs and provide an important basis for the diagnosis of lesions.

20.5 Noninfectious Inflammatory Diseases of the Spinal Cord and Spinal Canal

20.5.1 Chronic Spinal Radiculitis

Guihua Jiang, Cong Huang, and Zongjun Zhang

20.5.1.1 Overview

Chronic spinal radiculitis is a general term for spinal nerve root degeneration and/or chronic inflammation caused by various reasons. The disease can affect any segment of the spinal nerve root, of which the cervical thoracic and lumbosacral segments are the most common, also known as chronic cervical thoracic radiculitis and chronic lumbosacral radiculitis.

The spinal nerves emanate from the spinal cord in a total of 31 pairs: 8 pairs of cervical nerves, 12 pairs of thoracic nerves, 5 pairs of lumbar nerves, 5 pairs of sacral nerves, and 1 pair of caudal nerves.

The first to seven pairs of cervical nerves exit the spinal canal through the intervertebral foramen above the corresponding vertebral body, while the eighth pair of cervical nerves exit the spinal canal through the intervertebral foramen below the seventh cervical vertebra. The thoracic and lumbar nerves exit the spinal canal through the intervertebral foramina below the corresponding vertebral body. The first to fourth pairs of sacral nerves exit through the corresponding anterior sacral foramen and posterior sacral foramen and the fourth pair of sacral nerves and the pudendal nerve exit the sacral canal through the sacral fissure. All spinal nerves are composed of anterior and posterior roots of the corresponding segment merging in the intervertebral foramen. All spinal nerves are mixed nerves and each spinal nerve contains both motor and sensory fibers. The anterior roots are primarily motor and the posterior roots are primarily sensory.

There are many causes of spinal radiculitis [78–80]. Intramembranous radiculitis is mainly caused by infection, poisoning, nutritional disorders, etc.; extramembranous radiculitis is mainly caused by muscle and transverse process trauma and inflammation. The lesions in the inner segment are mostly bilateral and extensive, while the lesions in the outer segment are mostly unilateral and more limited.

Patients often have a slow onset, often caused by cold, coughing, defecation, etc., or their symptoms aggravate. The posterior nerve root is damaged, manifested by radiation pain and numbness within the innervation range, such as intercostal neuralgia caused by thoracic radiculitis. Damage to the anterior nerve root is manifested as motor neuron paralysis in different degrees in the distribution area, such as muscle atrophy, muscle weakness, and tendon reflexes. Sacral nerve root damage can also be manifested as atonic bladder and sexual dysfunction. When the disease involves the arachnoid membrane, it is called meningeal-radiculitis, and if it also involves the spinal cord, it is called spinal cord-meningeal-radiculitis, which can produce symptoms of spinal arachnoiditis [81, 82]. Cerebrospinal fluid examination showed a slight increase in lymphocytes. The muscles in the damaged area mainly showed denervation electromyogram changes, and the peripheral nerve motor and sensory conduction speed slowed down. The latency of sensory nerve-evoked potentials is prolonged, and electromyography is an important examination method to clarify the disease.

20.5.1.2 Pathological Manifestations

Gross observation of nerve root manifests hypertrophy in general and observation under the microscope shows the vasodilation and hyperemia of the spinal pia mater and the infiltration of inflammatory cells around the blood vessels with demyelination changes [83].

20.5.1.3 Imaging

1. **X-ray.** Although it does not show the spinal nerve roots, but shows the physiological curvature of the spine, the

continuity of serial lines, and it shows degenerative changes such as vertebral osteophytes and bony redundancy.

2. **CT.** It shows more clearly the bony condition of the vertebral body and small joints, whether the intervertebral disc is compressing the nerve roots, whether the spinal canal is narrowed, and whether the anterior and posterior longitudinal ligaments are calcified.
3. MRI shows spinal nerve root hypertrophy, which displays hypointense on T_1WI and hyperintense on T_2WI. Enhanced scan may have mild to moderate enhancement.

20.5.1.4 Diagnostic Key Points

1. There are clear clinical symptoms, such as lumbosacral pain, numbness and muscle weakness, muscle atrophy, and tendon reflexes or disappearance.
2. CT showed vertebral bone hyperplasia, osteophyte formation, spinal canal, intervertebral foramina, and lateral recess stenosis; MRI showed thickening and hypertrophy of spinal nerve roots, T_1WI showed hypointense, and T_2WI showed hyperintense with mild to moderate enhancement on the enhanced scan.
3. Lymphocytes can be slightly increased in the cerebrospinal fluid examination. EMG shows denervation changes, and the peripheral nerve motor and sensory conduction velocity slow down. Sensory nerve-evoked potentials often indicate a prolonged incubation period.

20.5.1.5 Differential Diagnosis

Chronic spinal radiculitis can often be diagnosed based on clinical manifestations, corresponding neurological signs, and imaging findings. In addition to asking for a detailed medical history, biochemical examinations, electromyography examinations, etc. should be performed. Chronic spinal radiculitis needs to be differentiated from cervical spondylosis and lumbar spondylopathy, spinal cord tumors, acute myelitis, and spinal cord compression.

1. Cervical spondylosis and lumbar spondylosis are more common in middle-aged and elderly patients. However, there are manifestations of dizziness or spinal cord involvement with the Spurling sign (knock on the top of the head or pressure from the top of the head to the neck can cause increased pain in the upper limbs). Imaging examination can show whether there is vertebral hyperosteogeny, osteophytes, intervertebral foramina stenosis, etc., and determine whether the posterior longitudinal ligament and ligamentum flavum are thickened and intervertebral disc degeneration.
2. Spinal cord tumors have a slow onset and are progressively worsening. Early symptoms are often limited. Lumbar puncture can show subarachnoid obstruction, the number of cells is often normal, and the amount of cerebrospinal fluid protein is often increased. Imaging examination can clearly show spinal cord lesions and surrounding conditions.
3. Acute myelitis has a rapid onset, showing a transverse spinal cord injury symptoms and signs. MRI can show spinal cord edema and thickening, T_1WI shows isointense or slightly hypointense, and T_2WI shows hyperintense, with enhanced scan showing patchy enhancement.
4. Spinal cord compression can occur acute and chronic spinal cord compression symptoms, including nerve root symptoms, sensory disturbances, dyskinesias, and spinal membrane irritation. Imaging examination can clarify the specific situation.

20.5.1.6 Research Status and Progress

1. X-ray examination and CT can show the bone quality, especially the bone quality of the facet joints. A variety of post-processing methods of CT (VRT, CPR, MPR, etc.) can more clearly show the bone condition around the nerve root, whether the lateral recesses and intervertebral foramina are stenoses.
2. MRI. In addition to conventional scans, MRI can also be used for neuroimaging (MRN), which can clearly show the nerve root alignment and signal changes, with the best coronal display. The brachial plexus and lumbosacral plexus nerves have been investigated more frequently, such as diffusion-weighted imaging with background suppression (DWIBS), three-dimensional fast spin-echo (SPACE), and water-fat separation techniques for nerve imaging, but there is no imaging technique that can visualize the nerve entirety. The STIR sequence is significantly more sensitive to water alteration than the spin-echo sequence and is more effective in visualizing brachial plexus injury. It is also insensitive to magnetic field inhomogeneities and can effectively suppress fat signals around the mandible, upper chest, neck, and brachial plexus nerve. However, the STIR technique itself has a low signal-to-noise ratio (SNR), so free breathing and multiple signal averaging techniques can be used to improve the SNR.
3. MRI functional sequences, such as DWI and DTI, have a certain effect on the MRN of the lumbosacral plexus. DWI is used to evaluate the random microscopic motion of water molecules in the tissue, that is, Brownian motion. DWI has the advantage of suppressing background structures and blood flowing in blood vessels, thereby selectively highlighting high-signal nerves. DTI is an extension of DWI, which considers and measures anisotropic diffusion (biological tissues are highly anisotropic). DTI can provide useful neural structure information. However, DWI and DTI have a relatively low spatial resolution, may be time-consuming, and may have image distortion, which cannot be ignored in imaging of fine structures such as local nerves.

4. Spinal cord hydroimaging (MRM). As an additional sequence of conventional MRI, it does not take much time, and the post-image processing is also very convenient, and the imaging quality can fully meet the diagnostic requirements, without the use of contrast agents, and is safe and noninvasive. MRM images are more conducive to the observation of nerve roots, spinal ganglia, and postganglionic spinal nerves. As a supplement to conventional MRI imaging techniques, it has unique diagnostic value for nerve damage caused by intervertebral disc degeneration and various other reasons, nerve root walking variation, and neurogenic tumors and is used to locate space-occupying lesions in the spinal canal.

20.5.2 Sarcoidosis Myelitis

Guihua Jiang, Cong Huang, and Hongyan Chen

20.5.2.1 Overview

Sarcoidosis, also known as Boeck sarcoid tumor, also known as Schaumann's benign lymphogranulomatosis and Besnier frostbite-like lupus, is a non-caseating necrotizing epithelial cell granulation inflammatory disease, the cause is not clear, and young people are often affected, mainly invading the lung parenchyma, and involving multiple organs of the whole body, such as lymph nodes, skin, joints, eyes, liver, kidney and heart, etc. The clinical symptoms are relatively hidden, and the patient will eventually die suddenly due to complete atrioventricular block and/or congestive heart failure, and even sudden death as the first symptom. The global annual incidence of sarcoidosis is 10–20 per 100,000. The central nervous system and symptomatic patients account for 5–15% of patients with sarcoidosis, and the autopsy detection rate is about 25%; the pia mater at the bottom and the third ventricle area are commonly affected areas [84, 85]. Sarcoidosis involving the spinal cord is very rare, accounting for 0.4–1% of all nodules [86]; arachnoid lymphocyte infiltration and non-caseating formation of granuloma-like granulomas is a characteristic of central nervous system involvement. Non-caseating granulomas are mainly composed of epithelial cells, giant cells, lymphocytes, and other mononuclear cells, sometimes accompanied by fibrous tissue reactions. Nodular lesions can be along the perivascular space violation of spinal cord substance.

The clinical symptoms and signs are nonspecific and vary according to the location of the granuloma. Common symptoms include weight loss, fever, discomfort, fatigue, and joint pain, as well as spot or papule-like rashes. In addition, it can also affect the eyes, manifesting as uveitis and visual impairment. Patients with sarcoidosis with swollen paratracheal lymph nodes and certain acute peripheral arthritis, uveitis, and erythema nodosa are called acute sarcoidosis or Laeffgren syndrome, while uveitis with mumps and facial nerve palsy is called Heerfordt syndrome. The manifestations of sarcoidosis of the nervous system are diverse, depending on the location of the disease and the extent of the disease [86]. The manifestations of early spinal cord lesions are relatively rare. The symptoms of spinal cord lesions are similar to those of multiple sclerosis, such as paresis, paresthesias, and nonspecific signs of myelopathy.

The advanced stage of activity can be manifested as leukopenia, anemia, and increased red blood cell sedimentation rate. Serum angiotensin-converting enzyme (SACE) activity increases in the acute phase, which is meaningful for prompting the diagnosis. Elevated levels of soluble interleukin-2 receptor (sIL-2R) and interleukin-2 receptor (IL-2R) in serum have important implications for the diagnosis of sarcoidosis. Decreased plasma albumin and increased blood calcium, serum alkaline phosphatase, and serum uric acid can be seen. In addition, in some patients, α1-antitrypsin, β2-microglobulin (β2-MG), serum adenosine dehydrogenase (ADA), fibronectin (Fn), and lysozyme can be elevated, and it has certain reference significance in the clinic.

20.5.2.2 Pathological Manifestations

The disease is a chronic non-caseating granulomatous disease of unknown cause. Non-caseating granuloma is mainly composed of epithelial cells, giant cells, lymphocytes, and other mononuclear cells, sometimes accompanied by fibrous tissue reactions. Nodular granuloma grows around the blood vessels, accompanied by lymphocyte infiltration, which forms subarachnoid granuloma nodules. These granulomas are attached to the adventitia of blood vessels and extend to the parenchyma along the perivascular space.

20.5.2.3 Imaging

Sarcoidosis myelitis is mainly diagnosed by MRI, which mainly manifests as leptomeninges enhancement, dura mater enhancement, local spinal cord swelling and thickening with T_2WI showing hyperintense (may be focal or diffuse), and an enhanced scan showing spots lamellar or diffuse intramedullary enhancement; DWI showed iso or slightly hyperintense, and the ADC value was slightly increased; most of the lesions exceeded three vertebrae; vertebral bone marrow enhanced on the enhanced scan. Lesions can involve any segment of the spinal cord, the cervical spinal cord is the most common, followed by the thoracic spinal cord, conus, and cauda equina [87–96]. Junger et al. [91] divided the MRI manifestations of sarcoidous myelitis into four stages, which roughly corresponded to the stages of the histological evolution of the disease. Phase 1 corresponds to early inflammation in which MRI-enhanced scans show enhancement of the "line-like" leptomeninges along the surface of the spinal cord. The second stage is spinal cord parenchymal involvement, secondary to soft meningitis, progressing along the perivascular space, local spinal cord swelling and thickening; T_2WI shows hyperintense and MRI-enhanced scan shows that the lesion can be enhanced or not, and the disease can develop concentrically and diffuse enhancement lesions appear. The third stage is the reduction of intramedullary focal and multifocal inflammatory lesions, the thickened spinal cord returns to its normal shape, and the residual localized lesions or multiple focal abnormal enhancements after spinal cord injury can be seen inside. The fourth stage is the chronic stage (the period when inflammation subsides), and the size of the spinal cord returns to normal or shrinks, without enhancement on the enhanced scan.

Zalewski et al. [97] reported the enhancement pattern of spinal sarcoidosis in nine cases with subacute onset (4 weeks) and myelitis as the first manifestation, mainly manifested as long-segment traverse T_2WI hyperintensity and dorsal subpial enhancement with the central canal enhancement. The axial view shows that the posterior subpial crescent-shaped layered enhancement combined with central canal enhancement leads to a bifurcation at the tip of the lesion resembling a trident head, so central canal enhancement and "Trident sign" in subacute myelitis should be considered as myelitis.

20.5.2.4 Diagnostic Key Points

1. Chest CT showed signs of pulmonary sarcoidosis.
2. MRI findings: Plain scan shows local swelling and thickening of the spinal cord. The enhanced scan shows patchy or diffuse intramedullary enhancement, with line-like enhancement at the edge. The diagnosis can be made based on the characteristics of intramedullary enhancement and pia mater enhancement. In addition, neurosarcoidosis should be considered in the case of central canal enhancement and "trident sign" in subacute myelitis.
3. Laboratory examination: Leukopenia, anemia, and rapid erythrocyte sedimentation rate may occur in the active stage; the activity of serum angiotensin-converting enzyme (SACE) increases in the acute stage; the soluble interleukin-2 receptor in the serum (SIL-2R) and interleukin-2 receptor (IL-2R) are elevated.

20.5.2.5 Differential Diagnosis

The clinical manifestations of sarcoidial myelitis are nonspecific, most of which are accompanied by intracranial and body lesions, and those with isolated spinal cord involvement are rare, but MRI is typically manifested as spinal cord swelling and thickening, intramedullary patchy enhancement, and adjacent spinal pia mater enhancement, combined with increased SACE activity and increased sIL-2R and IL-2R can prompt the diagnosis. This disease is mainly differentiated from intramedullary tumors, multiple sclerosis, acute transverse myelitis, and spinal cord infarction.

1. Intramedullary tumors have a slow onset, no obvious cause or symptoms, and progressive aggravation. MRI plain scan can accurately detect spinal cord lesions, intramedullary tumors and localized thickening of the spinal cord, with slightly hypointense on T_1WI, and slightly or obvious hyperintense on T_2WI, with uneven signals.
2. Multiple sclerosis occurs most often in young and middle-aged women. Common demyelinating diseases are characterized by the frequent spreading of the lesions, frequent remission and relapse in the course of the disease, and various clinical manifestations, including limb weakness, hypoesthesia, ataxia, and other symptoms. Only the spinal cord is involved in 5–24%of patients, and 60% of the lesions are located in the cervical spinal cord. Multiple sclerosis of the spinal cord usually involves the lateral and posterior cords of the spinal cord and usually does not involve the gray matter junction. The cross section is <1/2 of the area of the spinal cord, and the length is >3 mm, but <2 vertebral body segments and edema is generally mild. The morphology of the spinal cord remains unchanged. On MRI, T_1WI mostly shows isointense, and T_2WI shows hyperintensity. In symptomatic patients, plaque enhancement occurs in more than 50% of patients and enhancement rarely occurs during the inactive phase of the disease. In addition, 6–14% of patients have spinal cord swelling, and 2–40% of patients have spinal cord atrophy.
3. Acute transverse myelitis is characterized by acute sensation with motor function enhanced or absent. On MRI, the diameter of the spinal cord is normal or slightly thickened, with hypointense on T_1WI, and hyperintense on T_2WI, with varied enhancement. It mainly involves the cervical spinal cord and thoracic spinal cord, or both. Typical lesions involve 3–4 vertebral body segments. Abnormal signals can extend beyond the level of clinically located signs. The prognosis of acute transverse myelitis changes greatly, and it can recover in a few weeks or months. MRI mainly manifests as the disappearance of abnormal signals and the spinal cord morphology returns to normal or spinal cord atrophy occurs.
4. Spinal cord infarction is very rare, accounting for 1% of infarcts, mainly because the spinal cord has very rich collateral circulation, it is more common in the thoracic spinal cord, and the cervical spinal cord can also be affected. Anterior spinal artery syndrome is the most common type of spinal cord infarction. One-third of patients present with radiation-like pain. The typical imaging manifestations are "eagle eye sign" or "snake eye sign", which present symmetrical hyperintensity of the anterior horns of the gray matter of the spinal cord on axial T_2WI image. Acute infarction manifests as hyperintense on DWI with hypointense on ADC.

20.5.2.6 Research Status and Progress

1. Patients with sarcoidial myelitis have increased SACE activity and sIL-2R and IL-2R are elevated.
2. MRI is the first choice for sarcoidial myelitis. The main manifestations are local swelling and thickening of the spinal cord, which manifest hyperintense on T_2WI (may be focal or diffuse), and with patchy or diffuse intramedullary enhancement, and soft spinal membrane enhancement and dura mater can also enhanced; DWI shows normal or slightly increased signal with slightly increased ADC value, and the range of enhancement lesions is wide, most of which are more than three vertebrae. Because most of the patients are accompanied by intracranial and body diseases, when the spinal cord imaging examination fails to confirm the diagnosis, it is possible to understand the patient's lungs, skin, salivary glands, or intracranial conditions, which can help confirm the diagnosis.
3. The diagnosis is mainly based on biopsy.

20.5.3 Paraneoplastic Myelopathy

Cong Huang, Hongyan Chen, and Guihua Jiang

20.5.3.1 Overview

Paraneoplastic syndromes (PSs) are a group of neurological symptoms and signs caused by malignant tumors through remote effects. They are not caused by tumor metastasis or direct invasion, nor are they caused by infection, ischemia, or metabolic disorders and are mainly caused by malignant tumors, such as lung cancer, ovarian cancer, etc., which can cause remote effect and appear as central nervous system gray matter inflammation and neurodegeneration [98, 99]. When the distant organs affected by the tumor are in the nervous system, it is called neurological paraneoplastic syndrome (PNS), which can affect any part of the nervous system, and the central nervous system is affected by diffuse gray encephalopathy, cerebellar degeneration, cancerous myelopathy and limbic encephalitis, etc.; when involving the peripheral nervous system, it manifests as polyneuropathy and compound mononeuritis; when involving the neuromuscular junction, it manifests as myasthenia gravis, neuromuscular rigidity, and dermatomyositis/polymyositis.

If the distant effect of the tumor appears in the spinal cord, it is called paraneoplastic myelopathy (PM) [100]. The incidence of PM is low, and the cause is still unclear. At present, it is believed that the occurrence of PM is mainly related to autoimmunity [101]. Clinicians attach great importance to PM mainly based on the following three points: one is that PM can often cause severe and long-lasting neurological deficits; the other is that PM can indicate that the body may have a tumor in the hidden stage; and the third is that early diagnosis can gain more time for tumor treatment and neurological recovery. The main diagnosis is based on the detection of anti-neuronal antibodies in the serum and cerebrospinal fluid of PM patients. At present, the main antibodies related to this syndrome can be detected in the patient's serum and cerebrospinal fluid, namely anti-neuronal nuclear antibody type 1 (anti-Hu antibody), Purkinje cell cytoplasmic antibody (anti-Yo antibody), and anti-neuronal antibody skeleton protein antibody (anti-Ri antibody), anti-dual carrier protein IgG antibody, brain failure response modulator protein-5-IgG (CRMP-5-IgG) antibodies, cancer-related retinopathy (CAR) antibodies, and anti-voltage-gated calcium channel antibodies are highly specific for suggesting PS or tumors and are also an important basis for the diagnosis of PM [102, 103].

The main clinical manifestations of PS spinal cord injury are necrotizing myelopathy and subacute motor neuron disease [100, 101]. (1) Necrotizing myelopathy: there is no specific type of primary tumor, but it often occurs in lung cancer, lymphoma, prostate cancer, thyroid cancer, and breast cancer. Most of them have subacute onset and gradually develop into complete transverse spinal cord injury. The patient's first symptom was asymmetrical weakness of the lower limbs, followed by paraplegia, incontinence, sensory disturbances, etc., but there was no pain. Patients can die within days or weeks. The clinical symptoms appear before the tumor is discovered or during the remission period of the tumor. Cerebrospinal fluid examination showed increased monocytes and protein. The pathological manifestations are mainly transverse mass necrosis of the affected spinal cord. PM mainly affects polio and/or white matter. Myelin and axons can also be involved, but inflammatory reactions are rare. (2) Subacute motor neuron disease: The cause of the disease is not clear. It may be a secondary infection due to the long-term use of immunosuppressants, which reduces the immune function of the body. The pathology is similar to polio, but the polio virus cannot be isolated. This disease usually starts after 40–50 years of age, with a long course and slow progress. It is often accompanied by Hodgkin's disease or other malignant lymphomas. It usually starts after the diagnosis of malignant tumors, and the symptoms of neurological damage mostly appear in the tumors. In the remission phase, the clinical manifestations are mainly subacute progressive weakness of the lower limbs without pain, and the upper limb involvement is generally relatively mild. The clinical symptoms of this disease are mostly without cranial nerve motor nucleus involvement. Electromyography shows denervation potentials, and some patients may have mild paresthesias. In cerebrospinal fluid examination, 77% of patients had lymphocytosis, 92% of patients had elevated cerebrospinal fluid protein, and 81% of patients had positive autoantibodies [104]. The pathological manifestations are deletion and degeneration of the anterior horn cells of the spinal cord. At the same time, the white matter of the spinal cord can also be seen with lamellar demyelination changes, and the posterior cord lesions are more obvious.

20.5.3.2 Pathological Manifestations

The pathological characteristics of PM vary widely. The pathology of necrotizing myelopathy is mainly transverse large-scale necrosis of the spinal cord, which mainly affects the gray matter of the spinal cord. Myelin and axons may also be involved, but inflammatory reactions are rarely seen. The pathological changes of subacute motor neuron disease are degenerative changes of the anterior horn cells of the spinal cord. The white matter of the spinal cord can also be seen in the form of demyelination changes. The posterior cord of the spinal cord is the most obvious, and the lateral cord is without lesions. There is generally no inflammatory response in the spinal cord.

20.5.3.3 Imaging

1. The diseased segment of the spinal cord is obviously swollen, and the gray matter (motor pathway) is extensively and symmetrically involved in the spinal cord, and the lateral cord (25%), posterior cord (20%), and central gray matter (20%) are mainly symmetrically involved [104].
2. T_2WI showed multiple patchy or diffuse heterogeneous hyperintensities in the medullary of the diseased segment, with fusion and with or without enhancement on the enhanced scan. In a recent series of case studies, 65% of patients showed hyperintensity on T_2WI, and 70% of patients presented with a long-stage spinal cord injury of more than three vertebral segments [104].
3. Approximately 50% of patients with spinal cord can always show no abnormalities [98].

20.5.3.4 Diagnostic Key Points

1. There is a clear history of tumors.
2. Local swelling and thickening of the spinal cord can be seen on MRI plain scan, patchy or diffuse hyperintense can be seen on T_2WI, and the enhanced scan is abnormally enhanced.
3. Specific antibodies can be seen in serum and cerebrospinal fluid, such as anti-Hu antibodies, anti-Yo antibodies, anti-Ri antibodies, cancer-related retinopathy antibodies, and anti-voltage-gated calcium channel antibodies. They are highly specific for suggesting PS or tumors and are important basis for diagnosing PM. Cerebrospinal fluid examination showed lymphocytosis in 77% of patients and increased cerebrospinal fluid protein in 92% of patients.

20.5.3.5 Differential Diagnosis

1. Radiation myelopathy. For patients with a clear tumor, if there is a manifestation of spinal cord injury, PM should be considered. Because PM symptoms are symmetrical and the level of spinal cord damage rises rapidly, combined with no history of radiotherapy, it can be distinguished from radiation myelopathy.
2. Spinal cord compression caused by epidural metastasis. PM should be considered if there is no back pain or percussion pain in the spine area, which can be distinguished from spinal cord compression caused by epidural metastasis.
3. Spinal cord subacute combined degeneration (SCD) is the degeneration and disease of the central and peripheral nervous system caused by the ingestion, absorption, binding, transport, or metabolism of B12. The lesions are mainly in the posterior cord and lateral cord of the lower cervical spinal cord, which are manifested by symptoms such as deep sensory loss, sensory ataxia, and spastic paralysis. MRI T_2WI showed abnormally hyperintense in the posterior cord or lateral cord with long longitudinal bands of the spinal cord. Axail T_2WI showed symmetrically distributed hyperintense in the posterior cord and the lateral cord. The typical posterior cord involvement showed "inverted V sign" and character "八" sign; due to the different locations of the lesions, it can be manifested in various forms, as well as "dot sign" and character "小"sign. The shorter the course of the disease, the higher the probability of enhancement. The old lesions are mainly fibrous hyperplasia and generally without enhancement. Combined with laboratory vitamin B12 examination can confirm the diagnosis.
4. Neuromyelitis optica (NMO) is a severe immune-mediated idiopathic demyelination and necrosis disease, mainly involving the optic nerve and spinal cord. MRI of the acute phase mainly manifests as swelling of the spinal cord in more than three spine segments with increased signal on T_2WI, mainly involving the central axon, and more than 70% of the lesions are confined to the central gray matter, which can be punctate, butterfly or "H" shape with enhancement on the enhanced scan. Extensive spinal cord atrophy in the chronic phase (the marginal atrophy involves more than three adjacent complete spinal segments, and the tail is adjacent to a spinal cord segment), with or without focal or diffuse T_2 signal changes, may be accompanied by the formation of syringomyelia. Combined with the changes and symptoms of the patient's optic nerve, the diagnosis can be confirmed.
5. Compressive myelopathy. The clinical manifestations are caused by compression of the spinal cord with subacute or chronic spinal cord symptoms. The cause is mostly severe spinal stenosis caused by a herniated disc. In a few

cases, tumors or tumor-occupying lesions can also cause spinal cord compression. MRI T_2WI shows hyperintense in the spinal cord at the compression level, without enhancement on the enhanced scan.

20.5.3.6 Research Status and Progress

1. PM may be an independent spinal cord lesion or other neurological lesions; about 60% of patients are women, with a median age of 62 years (37–79 years); about 2/3 of patients with spinal cord symptoms appear in tumor diagnosis forward. The diagnosis of PM is mainly based on the patient's clinical manifestations and related serum and cerebrospinal fluid antibody tests. Typical clinical manifestations are the most important basis for diagnosis. Serum or cerebrospinal fluid-specific antibodies can diagnose PM and suggest potential tumor properties. Anti-Hu antibodies are related to paraneoplastic encephalomyelitis and small cell lung cancer; anti-Yo antibodies are related to paraneoplastic cerebellar degeneration and reproductive system or gynecological tumors; anti-Ri antibodies are associated with breast cancer.
2. MRI is the preferred imaging examination method for spinal cord lesions. First, it can confirm whether there is a lesion in the spinal cord. Second, the location, scope, and cross-sectional involvement of the spinal cord lesions are understood, such as involving gray matter or white matter, anterior, posterior or lateral positions, symmetrical or not, and enhancement patterns.
3. The development and application of new technologies such as fMRI, MRS, DWI, DTI, and MRM of the spinal cord provide new ideas for the diagnosis of spinal cord lesions.

20.6 Infection of the Meninges (Spinal Meningitis)

Guihua Jiang, Cong Huang, and Yulin He

20.6.1 Overview

Spinal meningitis mainly includes spinal dura materitis (hypertrophic spinal pachymeningitis), leptomeningitis of spinal cord, and spinal arachnoiditis. This section mainly introduces hypertrophic spinal pachymeningitis.

Hypertrophic spinal pachymeningitis (HSP) is a rare disease that presents with limited or diffuse dural thickening in combination with inflammatory fibrosis [105, 106]. The first stage of HSP was described by Charcot and Joffy in 1869 and was divided into three stages: stage 1 is intermittent radicular pain that may progress to persistent pain; stage 2 is characterized by limb weakness and muscle atrophy; and stage 3 is characterized by muscle dysfunction and spastic paralysis of the limbs, manifested by paralysis, incontinence, and respiratory distress secondary to intercostal muscle and diaphragm paralysis [106]. It is more common in adults and is slightly more common in men than in women. Cases without a clear etiology are called idiopathic HSP, and some are secondary to infections (e.g., tuberculosis, syphilis, fungal infections, etc.), tumor dissemination or metastasis, autoimmune diseases (nodal disease, rheumatoid arthritis, Wegener's granulomatosis, etc.), metabolic diseases, trauma, intrathecal steroids, spinal anesthesia, myelography, etc. [107–117], 15 16].

HSP has an insidious onset and is often seen as a chronic infection, but it can also be acute and develop rapidly, peaking 2–5 days after onset. The main manifestations are symptoms caused by compression of the spinal cord and nerve roots [111, 112]. As the compression progresses, the spinal cord may soften and develop a cavity. The extent of dural thickening is variable and can involve one or more vertebral levels, with cervical and thoracic dural involvement being the most common first symptoms. Laboratory tests are not specific, but some may show increased erythrocyte sedimentation rate, elevated C-reactive protein, significantly elevated cerebrospinal fluid protein, and normal or high cerebrospinal fluid pressure [111, 113]. In a study by Kupersmith et al. [114] on the relationship between cerebrospinal fluid proteins and dural hypertrophy, it was found that the more extensive the dural thickening, the higher the cerebrospinal fluid protein content.

20.6.2 Pathological Manifestations

The thickened dura mater of HSP has a significant proliferation of fibrous tissue components, most of which also have chronic inflammatory cells such as neutrophils, plasma cells, and lymphocytes, in addition to some vascular inflammatory changes such as necrotizing granulomas.

20.6.3 Imaging

MRI showed obvious thickening of the dura mater, and the dorsal side was significantly thicker than the ventral side. The axially hyperplastic dura mater showed a regular or irregular crescent shape, and the epidural showed a band-like or fusiform increase. The cause of the fat signal is currently unclear. Thickened spinal dura mater usually shows hypo or isointensity on T_1WI, while T_2WI shows obvious hypointensity (Fig. 20.16), which is a characteristic feature, mainly because the thickened dura mater is a fiber with less water content. T_2WI signal is significantly reduced in some cases. In addition, the edge of T_2WI in some cases shows hyperintense, which represents the infiltration of inflammatory cells around the dura; the enhanced scan of the thickened dura is significantly enhanced or not enhanced (Fig. 20.16). Significant enhancement may be caused by a large number of inflammatory cells infiltrating the thickened dura mater, resulting in the proliferation of small blood vessels within it, or by leakage of contrast into the enlarged fibrous tissue spaces, or, if enhancement is not significant, it may indicate that the hypertrophic dura mater is dominated by collagen fibrillation. In addition, FDG PET/CT in immunoglobulin G4 (IgG4)-associated hypertrophic dural meningitis of the spinal cord shows increased FDG uptake in the lesion [113–117].

20.6.4 Diagnostic Key Points

1. Clarify whether there is a special medical history, such as infection/tumor dissemination or metastasis, autoimmune diseases (sarcoidosis, rheumatoid arthritis, Wegener's granulomatosis, etc.), metabolic diseases, trauma, intrathecal steroids, spinal cord anesthesia, myelography, etc.
2. MRI findings: the dura mater is obviously hyperplasia and hypertrophy, and the dorsal dura mater is thicker than the ventral dura mater, and the axial position shows a regular or irregular crescent shape. T_1WI showed iso or hypointense, T_2WI showed obvious hypointense, which is more characteristic, and significantly enhanced or not enhanced.

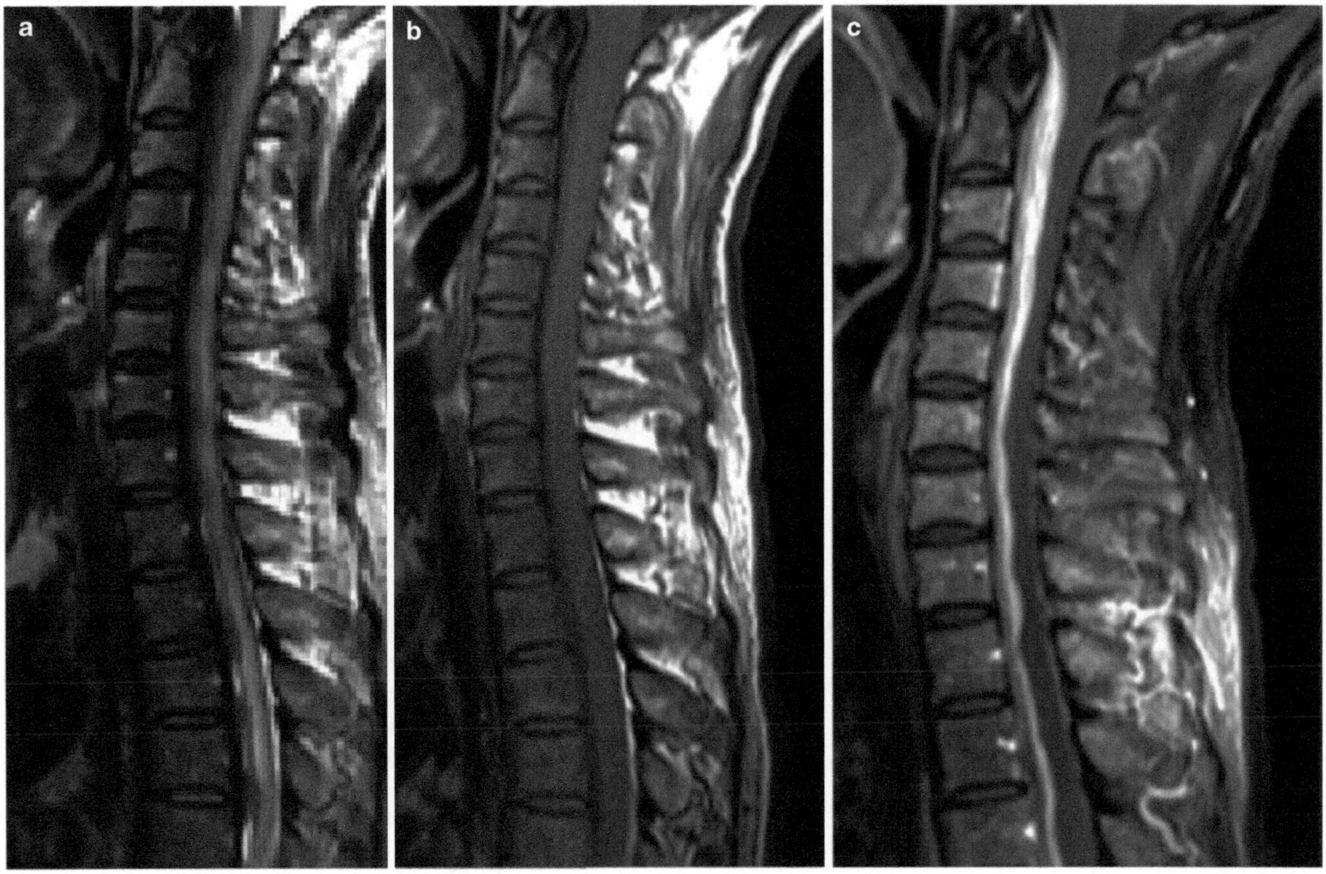

Fig. 20.16 IgG_4-related hypertrophic spinal arachnoiditis. (**a**) T_2WI shows uneven thickening of the ventral dura mater of the spinal cord from the first cervical vertebrae to the sixth thoracic vertebral body segment, showing hypointense, spinal canal stenosis, spinal cord compression, and increased signal (sagittal view); (**b**) on T_1WI, the above-mentioned lesions are unclear (sagittal view); (**c**) enhanced T_1WI shows obvious uniform enhancement of the ventral thickened dura mater, and no abnormal enhancement of the dorsal dura mater (sagittal view). (Image courtesy of Zhang Lihua, Peking University Third Hospital)

3. FDG PET/CT showed increased FDG uptake in the lesion.
4. Laboratory tests are mostly nonspecific, and a small number of them may have increased red blood cell sedimentation rate, increased C-reactive protein, significantly increased cerebrospinal fluid protein, and normal or high cerebrospinal fluid pressure.

20.6.5 Differential Diagnosis

MRI of HSP showed regular or irregular crescent-shaped abnormal signal shadows in the periphery of the dura. T_1WI showed iso or hypointense, and T_2WI showed obvious hypointense with obvious enhancement, and should mainly differentiate with meningiomas, lymphomas, meningeal membranes metastasis, and epidural hematoma.

1. Meningiomas are relatively rare and occur more often in the cervical spine, followed by the thoracic spine, rarely involving the lumbar spine, and are mostly manifested as calcification and thickening of the dura mater with extradural soft tissue masses, which are more limited and have a wide base connected to the dura mater. Most of the dura mater will form a "C" shape to surround the dural sac with enlargement of the adjacent intervertebral foramen, while HSP calcification is relatively rare and the thickened dura mater mainly compresses the dural sac while "C" shape formation, which surrounds the dural sac, is rare, and the foramen is rarely enlarged. The spinal meningioma lesion is isointense on T_1WI and slightly hyperintense on T_2WI and is more limited in extent than HSP and rarely exceeds ten vertebral bodies.
2. Lymphoma is relatively rare and can be primary or secondary. Most patients present with persistent or intermittent low back pain with weakness in both lower limbs, and the pain is generally severe. The lesion showed hypointense on T_1WI, and T_2WI presents iso or slightly hyperintense, which often leads to the destruction of bone resorption in adjacent vertebral bodies and appendages.
3. Metastatic tumors have a clear history of tumors; the dura mater is mostly localized thickening, T_1WI shows isointensity, and T_2WI shows hyperintensity; enhanced scan is dominated by uneven nodular enhancement, which can involve the spinal cord and vertebral body at the same time.
4. Epidural hematoma has a rapid onset, most of which have clear violent history of trauma or use of anticoagulant drugs. In the early stage, it manifests as epidural hypointensity, crescent-shaped or band-shaped lesions, limited or extensive scope, most of which are accompanied by thickening or displacement of the dura, and no enhancement is seen on the enhanced scan.

20.6.6 Research Status and Progress

1. HSP laboratory tests are mostly nonspecific, and a small number may have increased erythrocyte sedimentation rate, increased C-reactive protein, increased cerebrospinal fluid protein, and normal or high cerebrospinal fluid pressure.
2. MRI examination of soft tissue has a high resolution, multi-parameter, multi-sequence imaging and can accurately display the location, size and number of lesions from multiple levels and multiple planes. It is the primary examination for this disease. It can clarify the location, scope, enhancement method, and surrounding structure of the disease. Hyperplasia and hypertrophy of the dura mater showed iso or hypointense on T_1WI, while T_2WI showed obvious hypointense, which is more characteristic. It may be with or without significant enhancement. The diagnosis can be made in combination with the patient's medical history.
3. DWI can provide more detailed and objective imaging information by reflecting the diffusion state of water molecules. It provides more useful information for the diagnosis and differential diagnosis of HSP.
4. FDG PET/CT showed increased FDG uptake in the lesion.

References

1. Li H, Wu H, Sun J, et al. MRI manifestations of AIDS combined with cervical spinal cord Toxoplasma infection (report of 3 cases). Radiol Pract. 2009;24(9):931–4.
2. Ma L, Yang H, Xu X, et al. Metabonomics study of glial cells infected by herpes simplex virus type 1. Chin J Histochem Cytochem. 2017;26(2):134–41.
3. Zeng Q, Dong J, Meng Y, et al. Epidemiological research progress of human cytomegalovirus infection. Shandong Med. 2017;57(12):110–2.
4. Li H. Practical AIDS imaging. Beijing: People's Medical Publishing House; 2012.
5. Xu J, Guo N, Liu M. Value of enzyme-linked immunoassay screening for HIV antibodies in HIV diagnosis. Int J Virol. 2016;23(1):53–6.
6. Feng X. Modern medical imaging, vol. 1. Shanghai: Fudan University Press; 2016.
7. Yang R, Wang Y, Dai X. Varicella-zoster virus myelitis: 1 case report and literature review. Chin J Clin Neurosci. 2008;16(5): 509–11.
8. Hung CH, Chang KH, Kuo HC, et al. Features of varicella zoster virus myelitis and dependence on immune status. J Neurol Sci. 2012;318(1/2):19–24.
9. Zhu J, Lin A, Wu X, et al. Clinical analysis of 7 cases of herpes zoster myelitis. Chin J Nerv Ment Dis. 2017;43(11):672–5.
10. Liu W, Zhang Q, Cao X. Research progress on the mechanism and treatment of central nervous system injury caused by enterovirus EV71 infection. J Chengdu Med Coll. 2016;11(2):257–62.
11. Xing JJ, Liu D, Shen S, et al. Pathologic studies of fatal encephalomyelitis in children caused by enterovirus 71. Am J Clin Pathol. 2016;146(1):95–106.

12. Fu H, Zou Y. Clinical analysis of enterovirus 71 infection of hand, foot and mouth disease with acute flaccid paralysis. J Clin Pediatr. 2012;30(4):347–50.
13. Peng B, Du Z, Li X, et al. The evolution and prognosis of non-polio enterovirus 71-related acute flaccid paralysis from clinical and magnetic resonance imaging. Chin J Pediatr. 2012;50(4):255–60.
14. Ren Q, He L, Liu Z, et al. Clinical and MRI analysis of enterovirus 71 infection of hand, foot and mouth disease with acute flaccid paralysis. J Med Imaging. 2014;24(4):567–70.
15. Miao Y, Lin L, Jin Y, et al. Analysis of clinical characteristics of 60 cases of adult EB virus infection. Chin J Clin. 2015;43(10):37–40.
16. Gong S, Li J, Zhang W, et al. Six children with EB virus infection-related myelitis. Chin J Pract Pediatr Clin Med. 2016;31(22):1741–4.
17. Ma F, Liu Q, Cui X, et al. Research progress on EB virus infection-related diseases in children. Armed Police Med. 2015;26(7):736–40.
18. Zhang M, Yang M. Research progress of EB virus encephalitis in children. Med Rev. 2010;16(16):2444–6.
19. Xiao J, Yao J, Cheng L. Clinical testing methods for EB virus infection-related diseases. Mod J Integr Tradit Chin Western Med. 2011;20(28):3634–6.
20. Li H. Practical imaging of infectious diseases. Beijing: People's Medical Publishing House; 2016.
21. Tian Z, Meng Q, Zhang J. A case of rabies encephalomyelitis. Chin J Coal Ind Med. 2013;16(3):447–8.
22. Liang C, He B, Yang G, et al. A case report of paralytic rabies. Chin Trop Med. 2007;7(6):928.
23. Kumar VA, Nirdesh J, Kumar GL, et al. Atypical rabies with MRI findings: clue to the diagnosis. BMJ Case Rep. 2011;10(5):1–3.
24. Babic M, Simpfendorfer CS, Berbari EF. Update on spinal epidural 1 2 abscess. Curr Opin Infect Dis. 2019;32(3):265–71.
25. Zhang H, Wang R, Song S, et al. MRI signs of suppurative spinal infection. Radiol Pract. 2010;25(2):189–92.
26. Noori SA, Gungor S. Spinal epidural abscess associated with an epidural catheter in a woman with complex regional pain syndrome and selective IgG3 deficiency: a case report. Medicine (Baltimore). 2018;97(50):e1327.
27. Fareed S, Nashwan AJ, Abu JS, et al. Spinal abscess caused by Salmonella bacteremia in a patient with primary myelofibrosis. Am J Case Rep. 2017;18:859–64.
28. Bakhsheshian J, Kim PE, Attenello FJ. Intramedullary cervical spinal cord abscess. World Neurosurg. 2017;106:1049.e1–2.
29. Liu F, Liu H, Li L, et al. MRI diagnosis of spinal cord abscess (1 case report and literature review). J Pract Radiol. 2008;24(5):584–6.
30. Liu F, Liu H, Li L, et al. MRI diagnosis of intramedullary abscess: one case report and literatures review. J Pract Radiol. 2008;5:584–6.
31. Esenwein SA, Horch C, Meindl R, et al. Intramedullary abscess of the spinal cord-a rare pathology. Case report, therapeutic regimen and review of the literature. Zentralbl Neurochir. 2003;64(2):80–5.
32. Bartels RH, Gonera EG, van der Spek JA, et al. Intramedullary spinal cord abscess. A case report. Spine (Phila Pa 1976). 1995;20(10):1199–204.
33. Yang Y, Wang X, You C, et al. Four cases of spinal cord intramedullary tuberculoma. Chin J Surg. 2004;42(19):1215–6.
34. Wang GC, Wu SW. Spinal intramedullary tuberculoma following pulmonary tuberculosis: a case report and literature review. Medicine (Baltimore). 2017;96(49):e8673.
35. Dai H, Wen D, Peng L, et al. MRI findings of spinal tuberculoma. Guangdong Med. 2013;34(4):593–5.
36. Xu G, Han D, Qiao Y, et al. MRI manifestations of spinal tuberculoma. In: Chinese Medical Equipment Association CT Engineering Technical Committee 2012 Academic Conference, p. 117–22.
37. Peng J, Luo TY, Lv FJ, et al. MRI in diagnosis and differential diagnosis of intraspinal tuberculoma, metastasis and neurofibromatosis. Chin J Med Imaging Technol. 2011;27(4):702–5.
38. Dai H, Peng L, Zhang T, et al. MRI manifestations of spinal cord tuberculosis. Chin J Clin Med Imaging. 2012;23(10):751–3.
39. Wu A, Zhang L, Zhang B, et al. Comparison of MRI images of deep gray matter lesions in the brain of acute disseminated encephalomyelitis, multiple sclerosis and optic neuromyelitis. Chin J Neuromed. 2013;12(9):919–22.
40. Ma L, Yu S. Brain MRI manifestations of acute disseminated encephalomyelitis. Chin J Radiol. 2000;34(8):515–7.
41. Li S, Li P. MRI diagnosis of spinal cord multiple sclerosis. Chin J Radiol. 1997;31(5):322–5.
42. Ren ZQ, Wang XH, Wang JA, et al. Diagnostic and differentially diagnostic effects of low field MR for spinal metastases and spondylocace. Chin J Med Imaging Technol. 2002;18(11):1144. 1145
43. Peng Y, Li C. Application of MR imaging technology in the nerve roots and ganglia of the lumbosacral region. Imaging Res Med Appl. 2018;2(17):94–5.
44. Chen N, Qin W, Li K. Technical characteristics and clinical application of spinal cord diffusion imaging. J Med Imaging. 2006;16(6):635–9.
45. Fujiyoshi K, Konomi T, Yamada M, et al. Diffusion tensor imaging and tractography of the spinal cord: from experimental studies to clinical application. Exp Neurol. 2013;242:74–82.
46. Chang Y, Jung TD, Yoo DS, et al. Diffusion tensor imaging and fiber tractography of patients with cervical spinal cord injury. J Neurotrauma. 2010;27(11):2033–40.
47. Cavus G, Acik V, Bilgin E, et al. Endless story of a spinal column hydatid cyst disease: a case report. Acta Orthop Traumatol Turc. 2018;52(5):397–403.
48. Du G, Wang Y, Liu B, et al. Two cases of spinal hydatid disease. Chin J Neurosurg. 2007;23(7):532.
49. Zhang Z, Fan J, Dang Y, et al. Primary intramedullary hydatid cyst: a case report and literature review. Eur Spine J. 2017;26(S 1):107–10.
50. Yin M, Zang J, Liu J, et al. MRI diagnosis of 1 case of intraspinal hydatid disease in the lumbosacral region. Chin J Med Imaging. 2004;12(3):240.
51. He X, Lu J. Diagnosis and differential diagnosis of intraspinal cystic lesions. Chin Med Imaging Technol. 2003;19(6):773–4.
52. Eljebbouri B, Gazzaz M, Elmostarchid B. Unknown case: part 2: vertebral and spinal cord hydatidosis. Spine (Phila Pa 1976). 2013;38(26):2302.
53. Lindland ES, Solheim AM, Andreassen S, et al. Imaging in Lyme neuroborreliosis. Insights Imaging. 2018;6:1–12.
54. Makhani N, Morris SK, Page AV, et al. A twist on Lyme: the challenge of diagnosing European Lyme neuroborreliosis. J Clin Microbiol. 2011;49(1):455–7.
55. Tohge R, Shinoto Y, Takahashi M. Longitudinally extensive transverse myelitis and optic neuropathy associated with syphilitic meningomyelitis and human immunodeficiency virus infection: a case report and review of the literature. Intern Med. 2017;56(15):2067–72.
56. Liu Z, Dong H, Zhang C, et al. A case of syphilitic meningomyelitis. J Brain Nerv Dis. 2016;24(9):573–7.
57. Lu H, Jiao L, Liu Z, et al. Two cases of syphilitic myelitis with long-segment myelopathy and literature review. Chin J Neurol. 2016;49(12):967–9.
58. Hu H, Yan X, Guo X, et al. Clinical and imaging analysis of syphilitic myelitis (with 2 case reports and literature review). J Apoplexy Neurol Dis. 2015;32(9):797–802.
59. He D, Jiang B. Syphilitic myelitis: magnetic resonance imaging features. Neurol India. 2014;62(1):89–91.
60. Siu G. Syphilitic meningomyelitis. J Am Osteopath Assoc. 2017;117(10):671.

61. Kikuchi S, Shinpo K, Niino M, et al. Subacute syphilitic meningomyelitis with characteristic spinal MRI findings. J Neurol. 2003;250(1):106–7.
62. Weiner MF, Silver JR. Historical review: suspension therapy for the treatment of tabes dorsalis. Eur Neurol. 2014;72(3/4):163–72.
63. Chiver-Stainer L, Fischer U, Hauf M, et al. Syphilitic myelitis: rare, nonspecific, but treatable. Neurology. 2009;72(7):673–5.
64. Gessain A, Vernant JC, Maurs L, et al. Antibodies to human T-lymphotropic virus type-I in patients with tropical spastic paraparesis. Lancet. 1985;2(8452):407–10.
65. Osame M, Usuku K, Izumo S, et al. HTLV-1 associated myelopathy, a new clinical entity. Lancet. 1986;1(8488):1031. 1032
66. Cartier L, Ramírez E, Galeno H. HTLV-1 tax gene on the etiological identification of tropical spastic paraparesis. A clinical, serological and polymerase chain reaction (PCR) study in 72 patients. Rev Med Chil. 1999;127(8):945–52.
67. Liu W. Research progress on human T-cell leukemia virus type 1 tax protein. Foreign Med Blood Transfus Hematol. 1998;21:241–3.
68. Puccioni-Sohler M, Gasparetto E, Cabral-Castro MJ, et al. HAM/TSP: association between white matter lesions on magnetic resonance imaging, clinical and cerebrospinal fluid findings. Arq Neuropsiquiatr. 2012;70(4):246–51.
69. Yamamoto F, Yamashita S, Yamamura A, et al. Abnormal spinal MRI findings in human T-cell lymphotrophic virus type I-associated myelopathy. Clin Neurol Neurosurg. 2009;111(7):624–8.
70. Silva MTT, Araújo A. Spinal cord swelling in human T-lymphotropic virus 1-associated myelopathy/tropical spastic paraparesis: magnetic resonance indication for early anti-inflammatory treatment? Arch Neurol. 2004;61(7):1134. 1135
71. Yukitake M, Takase Y, Nanri Y, et al. Incidence and clinical significances of human T-cell lymphotropic virus type I-associated myelopathy with T2 hyperintensity on spinal magnetic resonance images. Intern Med. 2008;47(21):1881–6.
72. Guleria R, Nisar N, Chawla TC, et al. Mycoplasma pneumoniae and central nervous system complications: a review. J Lab Clin Med. 2005;146(2):55–63.
73. Narita M, Matsuzono Y, Togashi T, et al. DNA diagnosis of central nervous system infection by mycoplasma pneumoniae. Pediatrics. 1992;90(2):250–7.
74. Tsiodras S, Kelesidis TH, Kelesidis I, et al. Mycoplasma pneumoniae-associated myelitis: a comprehensive review. Eur J Neurol. 2006;13(2):112–24.
75. Zhang Z, Chen R, Chen S. Research progress of Mycoplasma pneumoniae infection involving the nervous system. Chin J Pract Nerv Dis. 2017;20(22):112–6.
76. Bitnun A, Richardson SE. Mycoplasma pneumoniae: innocent bystander or a true cause of central nervous system disease? Curr Infect Dis Rep. 2010;12(4):282–90.
77. Csábi G, Komáromy H, Hollódy K. Transverse myelitis as a rare, serious complication of Mycoplasma pneumoniae infection. Pediatr Neurol. 2009;41(4):312–3.
78. Zhao X, Li L, He J, et al. Acute disseminated cerebrospinal nerve root neuritis. Chin Med Guide. 2011;9(30):354–6.
79. Freilich D, Swash M. Diagnosis and management of tuberculous paraplegia with special reference to tuberculous radiculomyelitis. J Neurol Neurosurg Psychiatry. 1979;42(1):12–8.
80. Agrawal MM, Mahajan RS, Bilimoria FE, et al. Myelitis: a rare neurological complication of herpes zoster. Indian J Dermatol. 2016;61(6):687–9.
81. Last AR, Hulbert K. Chronic low back pain: evaluation and management. Am Fam Physician. 2009;79(12):1067–74.
82. Wadia NH, Dastur DK. Spinal meningitides with radiculomyelopathy. J Neurol Sci. 1969;8(2):239–60.
83. Kobayashi S, Yoshizawa H, Yamada S. Pathology of lumbar nerve root compression. Part 2: morphological and immunohistochemical changes of dorsal root ganglion. J Orthop Res. 2004;22(1):180–8.
84. Delaney P. Neurologic manifestations in sarcoidosis: review of the literature with of 23 cases. Ann Intern Med. 1977;87(3):336–45.
85. Wiederholt WC, Sieker RG. Neurological manifestations of sarcoidosis. Neurology. 1965;15(12):1147–54.
86. Christoforidis GA, Spickler EM, Recio MV, et al. MR of CNS sarcoidosis: correlation of imaging features to clinical symptoms and response to treatment. Am J Neuroradiol. 1999;20(4):665–9.
87. Greco A, Steiner RE. Magnetic resonance imaging in neurosarcoidosis. Magn Reson Imaging. 1987;5(1):15–21.
88. Nesbit GM, Miller GM, Baker HL Jr, et al. Spinal cord sarcoidosis: a new finding at MR imaging with GD-DTPA enhancement. Radiology. 1989;173(3):839–43.
89. Kelly RB, Mahoney PD, Cawley KM. MR demonstration of spinal cord sarcoidosis: report of a case. Am J Neuroradiol. 1988;9:197–9.
90. Waubant E, Manelfe C, Bonafe A, et al. MRI of intramedullary sarcoidosis: follow-up of a case. Neuroradiology. 1997;39(5):357–60.
91. Junger SS, Stern BJ, Levine SR, et al. Intramedullary spinal sarcoidosis: clinical and magnetic resonance imaging characteristics. Neurology. 1993;43(2):975–82.
92. Soni N, Bathla G, Pilenahalli-Maheshwarappa R. Imaging findings in spinal sarcoidosis: a report of 18 cases and review of the current literature. Neuroradiol J. 2019;32(1):17–28.
93. Kobayashi S, Nakata W, Sugimoto H. Spinal magnetic resonance imaging manifestations at neurological onset in Japanese patients with spinal cord sarcoidosis. Intern Med. 2013;52(18):2041–50.
94. Kasliwal MK, Harbhajanka A, Nag S, et al. Isolated spinal neurosarcoidosis: an enigmatic intramedullary spinal cord pathology-case report and review of the literature. J Craniovertebr Junction Spine. 2013;4(2):76.
95. Weidauer S, Wagner M, Nichtweiß M. Magnetic resonance imaging and clinical features in acute and subacute myelopathies. Clin Neuroradiol. 2017;27(4):417–33.
96. Roy K, Tripathy P, Senapati A, et al. Intradural extramedullary sarcoidosis case report and review of literature. Asian J Neurosurg. 2010;5(1):87.
97. Zalewski NL, Krecke KN, Weinshenker BG, et al. Central canal enhancement and the trident sign in spinal cord sarcoidosis. Neurology. 2016;87(7):743–7.
98. Flanagan EP, Keegan BM. Paraneoplastic myelopathy. Neurol Clin. 2013;31(1):307–18.
99. Flanagan EP, McKeon A, Lennon VA, et al. Paraneoplastic isolated myelopathy: clinical course and neuroimaging clues. Neurology. 2011;76(24):2089–95.
100. Graber JJ, Nolan CP. Myelopathies in patients with cancer. Arch Neurol. 2010;67(3):298–304.
101. McKeon A, Pittock SJ. Paraneoplastic encephalomyelopathies: pathology and mechanisms. Acta Neuropathol. 2011;122(4):381–400.
102. Sillevis SP, Grefkens J, de Leeuw B, et al. Survival and outcome in 73 anti-Hu positive patients with paraneoplastic encephalomyelitis/sensory neuronopathy. J Neurol. 2002;249(6):745–53.
103. Pittock SJ, Kryzer TJ, Lennon VA. Paraneoplastic antibodies coexist and predict cancer, not neurological syndrome. Ann Neurol. 2004;56(5):715–9.
104. Gummadavelli A, Motelow JE, Narayanan NS. Clinical reasoning: a 64-year-old woman with progressive quadriparesis. Transverse myelitis (TM). Neurology. 2013;81(12):e89–94.
105. Sylaja PN, Cherian PJ, Das CK, et al. Idiopathic hypertrophic cranial pachymeningitis. Neurol India. 2002;50(1):53–9.

106. Chen Z, Huang G, Xu B, et al. Clinical analysis of hypertrophic dura materitis. Med Rev. 2017;23(20):4154–7.
107. Lu HT, Li MH, Hu DJ, et al. Hypertrophic cranial pachymeningitis accompanied by inflammation of the nasopharygeal soft tissue. Headache. 2009;49(8):1229–31.
108. Yamakita N, Hanamoto T, Muraoka N, et al. Hypopituitarism and diabetes insipidus with localized hypertrophic pachymeningitis (Tolosa-Hunt syndrome) associated with Hashimoto thyroiditis. Am J Med Sci. 2004;327(1):38–43.
109. Lowden MR, Gill D. Teaching neuro image: idiopathic hypertrophic spinal pachymeningitis. Neurology. 2009;72(5):27–32.
110. Hsu HT, Hsu SS, Chien CC, et al. Teaching neuro image: idiopathic hypertrophic spinal pachymeningitis mimicking epidural lymphoma. Neurology. 2015;84(9):e67–8.
111. Li X, Zhao J, Wang Q, et al. The clinical features of 17 cases of hypertrophic dura mater. China Clin J Bed Immun Allergy. 2015;9(4):287–91.
112. Wang Y, Jiang C, Nie Y. Analysis of the clinical and imaging characteristics of hypertrophic dura mater. J Stroke Neurol Dis. 2017;34(1):39–42.
113. Zhang L, Yuan H. Comparative analysis of images between hypertrophic spondylitis and epidural meningioma. Chin J Radiol. 2016;50(2):143–5.
114. Kupersmith MJ, Martin V, Heller G, et al. Idiopathic hypertrophic pachymeningitis. Neurology. 2004;62(5):684–94.
115. Tao X, Huang L, Xiao X. MRI diagnosis of idiopathic hypertrophic spondylitis. Chin J Radiol. 2003;37(7):665.
116. van der Pol CB, Chakraborty S, Cofe I, et al. Case 216: hypertrophic spinal pachymeningitis. Radiology. 2015;275(1):303–7.
117. Ranasinghe MG, Zalatimo O, Rizk E, et al. Idiopathic hypertrophic spinal pachymeningitis. J Neurosurg Spine. 2011;15(2):195–201.

Complications Associated with Post-surgical Infection

21

Wensheng Wang, Jun Guo, Mingwang Zhu, Dabiao Deng, and Lijuan Gao

Neurosurgical CNS infections refer to infectious diseases of the skull and spinal canal secondary to neurosurgical disease or requiring neurosurgical management; sometimes, early diagnosis is difficult and diagnostic imaging can provide an important diagnostic basis. Post-neurosurgical infections are predominantly bacterial, including post-neurosurgical epidural abscesses, subdural pus, brain abscesses, meningitis, and ventriculitis; cranial infections are due to cranial trauma, ventricular and lumbar pool external drainage, shunts, and implant-related meningitis or ventriculitis. This chapter focuses on postoperative infections and chemical meningitis to provide valuable imaging information for clinical diagnosis.

21.1 Post-surgical Infection

Wensheng Wang, Jun Guo, and Mingwang Zhu

21.1.1 Overview

Postoperative infection is a rare and, in severe cases, life-threatening complication after neurosurgery, with an incidence of less than 1%, usually seen at 1–2 weeks postoperatively. Infection often begins at the cutaneous margin and spreads to the skin, skull, meninges, extracerebral space, and brain parenchyma, eventually manifesting as scalp infection, bone flap infection, meningitis, infected extracerebral effusion, encephalitis, and brain abscess [1].

Most infections after craniotomy are intracranial, and scalp incision infections are quite rare. Scalp infections are seen as redness, swelling, or pus overflow from the scalp, and the source of infection can sometimes be traced to the bone flap, which can also develop from superficial wound infections, with the two being mutually beneficial. The skull is a flat bone, consisting of an outer plate, a plate barrier, and an inner plate; the plate barrier has a loose structure, and within it are plate barrier veins, which anastomose into a network; the separated bone flaps are inactive because the blood supply is blocked, and bacteria can easily nourish in the loose plate barrier and spread [2].

Infected extracerebral effusion, also known as infected extracerebral pus, is usually the result of wound infection, bone flap infection, or postoperative complications of meningitis; the pus accumulation is usually encapsulated and can be followed by encephalitis and brain abscess. Encephalitis is the initial stage of septic brain parenchymal infection. When an abscess forms, necrosis may appear in the center of the lesion, and the lesion consists of liquefied necrotic and inflammatory tissue fragments surrounded by a very thin envelope, which may thicken slightly as the disease progresses and the abscess is completely encapsulated. Depending on the location and extent of inflammation, patients may also show signs and symptoms of meningeal irritation, increased intracranial pressure, and local neurological impairment.

21.1.2 Pathological Manifestations

When the bone flap is infected, the sparse plate barrier is susceptible to bacterial colonization and spread. Pathological examination may show fibrous tissue hyperplasia, fibrosis, inflammatory cell infiltration, and a small number of degenerated degenerative cells in the bone marrow cavity.

Encephalitis is the initial stage of septic brain parenchymal infection and is characterized by limited inflammation,

W. Wang (✉) · J. Guo · D. Deng
Guangdong Sanjiu Brain Hospital, Guangzhou, China

M. Zhu
Capital Medical University Sanbo Brain Hospital, Beijing, China

L. Gao
The First Affiliated Hospital of Xinjiang Medical University, Urumqi, China

H. Li et al. (eds.), *Radiology of Infectious and Inflammatory Diseases - Volume 1*,
https://doi.org/10.1007/978-981-99-0039-8_21

congestion, edema, and necrosis of brain tissue with small venous inflammatory emboli and meningeal reactions. Perivascular polymorphonuclear cell infiltration was seen microscopically. As the disease continues to progress, encephalitis continues to spread and the softened necrotic areas of the brain gradually expand and fuse to form larger pus cavities surrounded by irregular granulation tissue, the latter consisting mainly of new blood vessels and large amounts of connective tissue. A large infiltration of neutrophils was seen microscopically. Eventually, the abscess wall continues to thicken with a marked increase in surrounding connective tissue and the proliferation of neuroglial cells. Microscopically, the abscess wall consists of three layers of structures. The innermost layer consisted of purulent exudate and granulation tissue with massive neovascularization and neutrophil infiltration; the middle layer consisted mainly of massive fibrous connective tissue; and the outer layer consisted mainly of neuroglial proliferation with brain tissue edema, increased vascularization, and leukocyte infiltration.

21.1.3 Imaging

The purpose of imaging is to detect deep infections such as bone flap infections, infected extracerebral effusions, meningitis, or inflammation of the brain. Clinically, patients often have fever and other signs of toxicity.

1. Scalp infections. Intracranial infections account for the majority of post-craniotomy infections, while the probability of infection is relatively low in clinical practice due to the rich blood supply to the scalp. Scalp infections commonly occur when contaminants or foreign bodies are not removed or are incompletely removed after cranial injury. The earliest CT and MR manifestations of superficial surgical site infection are dural line thickening, indistinct borders, and striated or nodular enhancement on enhancement (Fig. 21.1). Histologically, these signs are associated with edema, inflammation, and granulation tissue proliferation along the meningeal capitellar complex.
2. Bone flap infection. On CT, it was manifested as multiple patchy or spotted laminar osteolytic changes, corresponding skin thickening, increased subcutaneous fat density, and subcapsular tendinous or extracerebral effusion, especially as the number of postoperative days continues to increase and the amount of effusion increases, which may support the diagnosis of infection. On MRI, upper bone flap infection causes altered signal in the bone marrow of the plate barrier, T_1WI shows decreased signal, fat suppression T_2WI signal is increased, and the enhanced scan shows homogeneous enhancement.
3. Infected extracerebral effusion. Epidural abscess on CT shows a fusiform fluid density under the cranial plate, with an enhanced scan showing dural thickening and marked enhancement at the inner edge of the effusion. Subdural empyema shows crescentic fluid density on CT, often slightly above the cerebrospinal fluid, located in the cerebral convexity or distributed along the cerebral falx, with enhanced scans showing medial edge enhancement, often with occupying effects, edema, and significant diffuse enhancement of the adjacent brain surface. CT can detect most dural cavity infections. On MRI, the signal intensity of epidural abscess or subdural empyema is lower than brain parenchyma and higher than cerebrospinal fluid on T_1WI. Whether T_1WI or T_2WI, the signal intensity of postoperative infected pus accumulation is lower than that of chronic phase hematoma, and the peripheral enhancement on enhanced scan is more obvious than that of hematoma due to the evident peri-abscess envelope hematoma. The DWI sequence shows restricted pus diffusion in epidural abscess or subdural empyema, with hyperintensity on high b values ($b = 1000$) of images and hypointensity on the image of "ADC"(Fig. 21.2). But the false positive rate for postoperative DWI diagnosis of epidural abscess is about 47%and the false negative rate for subdural empyema is about 29%, so the detection rate is not high.
4. Encephalitis and brain abscess.
   (a) Encephalitis. CT plain scan shows a patchy hypodense shadow in the operative area. MRI shows iso or hypointense on T_1WI and hyperintensity on T_2WI, with indistinct borders. After Gd-DTPA enhancement, the lesion shows mild patchy enhancement in the early phase. There is no significant restriction of water molecule diffusion during the encephalitis phase, which shows isointensity.
   (b) Brain abscess. In the early phase of brain abscess envelope formation, on CT plain scan, the envelope is annularly iso or slightly hyperdense, with thin walls, smooth inner edges, and hypodense within the envelope. After enhancement, the envelope is annularly enhanced, usually with a thin annular wall on the side of the ventricle. In the early envelope stage of brain abscess, the hypodense area in the envelope (brain necrosis area) is hyperintense relative to the gray matter on T_2WI, surrounded by a thick and irregular ring with slightly hyperintense on T_1WI. This ring is iso or hypointense on T_2WI, and the enhanced scan shows nodular or ring-like enhancement. When necrotic foci appear in the brain parenchyma, their diffusion is restricted with reduced ADC value, and the necrotic area shows a significant hyperintense on the DWI sequence. In the late enve-

Fig. 21.1 Postoperative scalp infection. (**a**) Postoperative CT plain scan showing soft tissue swelling of the scalp in the right occipital operative area; (**b**) postoperative 1 month later CT plain scan showing increased soft tissue swelling of the scalp in the right occipital area compared with before

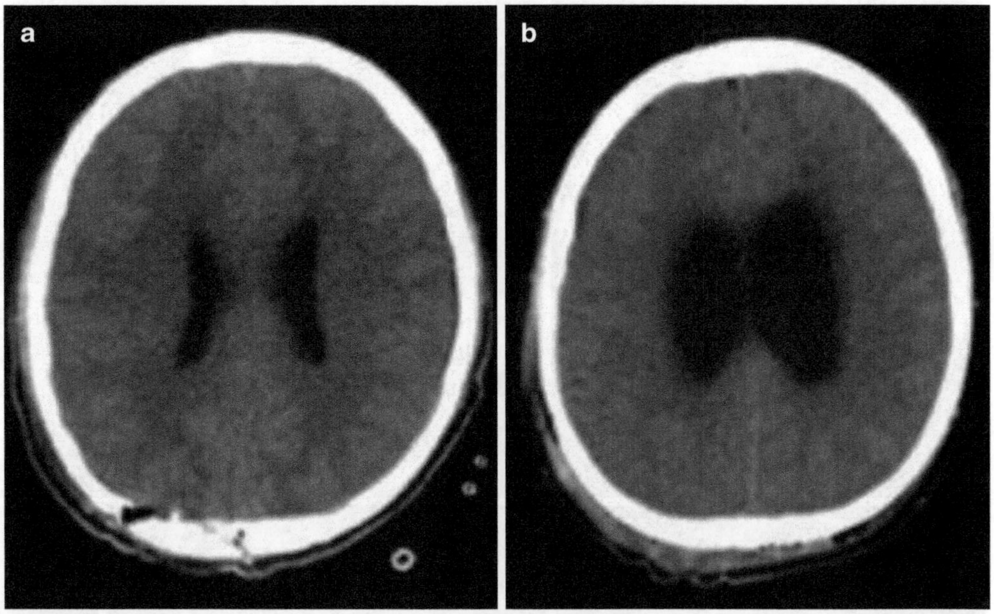

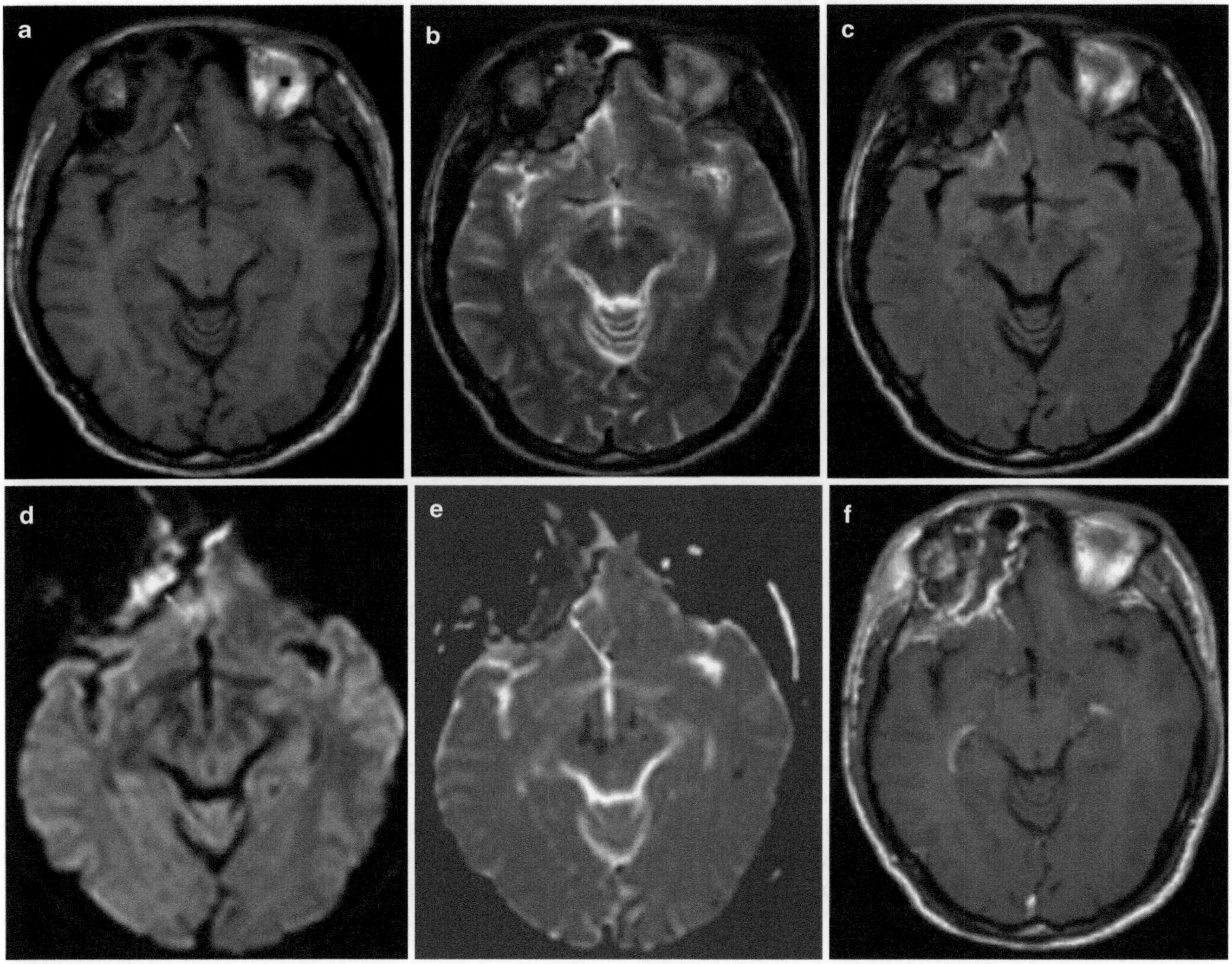

Fig. 21.2 Postoperative pus accumulation under the bone flap. Arcuate lesion visible under the right frontal bone flap 5 years after traumatic brain injury. (**a**) T_1WI shows the lesion as isointense with interspersed strips of hypointense; (**b**) T_2WI shows the lesion as predominantly slightly hyperintense with a ring-shaped hypointense envelope visible in the periphery; (**c**) FLAIR sequence shows the lesion is predominantly isointense (arrow), with small patchy hyperintense edematous bands visible in the adjacent brain parenchyma; (**d**) DWI sequence shows pus is hyperintense. (**e**) ADC map shows pus is hypointense; (**f**) T_1WI enhanced scan shows that lesion is ring-like enhancement, and adjacent dura is thickened and significantly enhanced

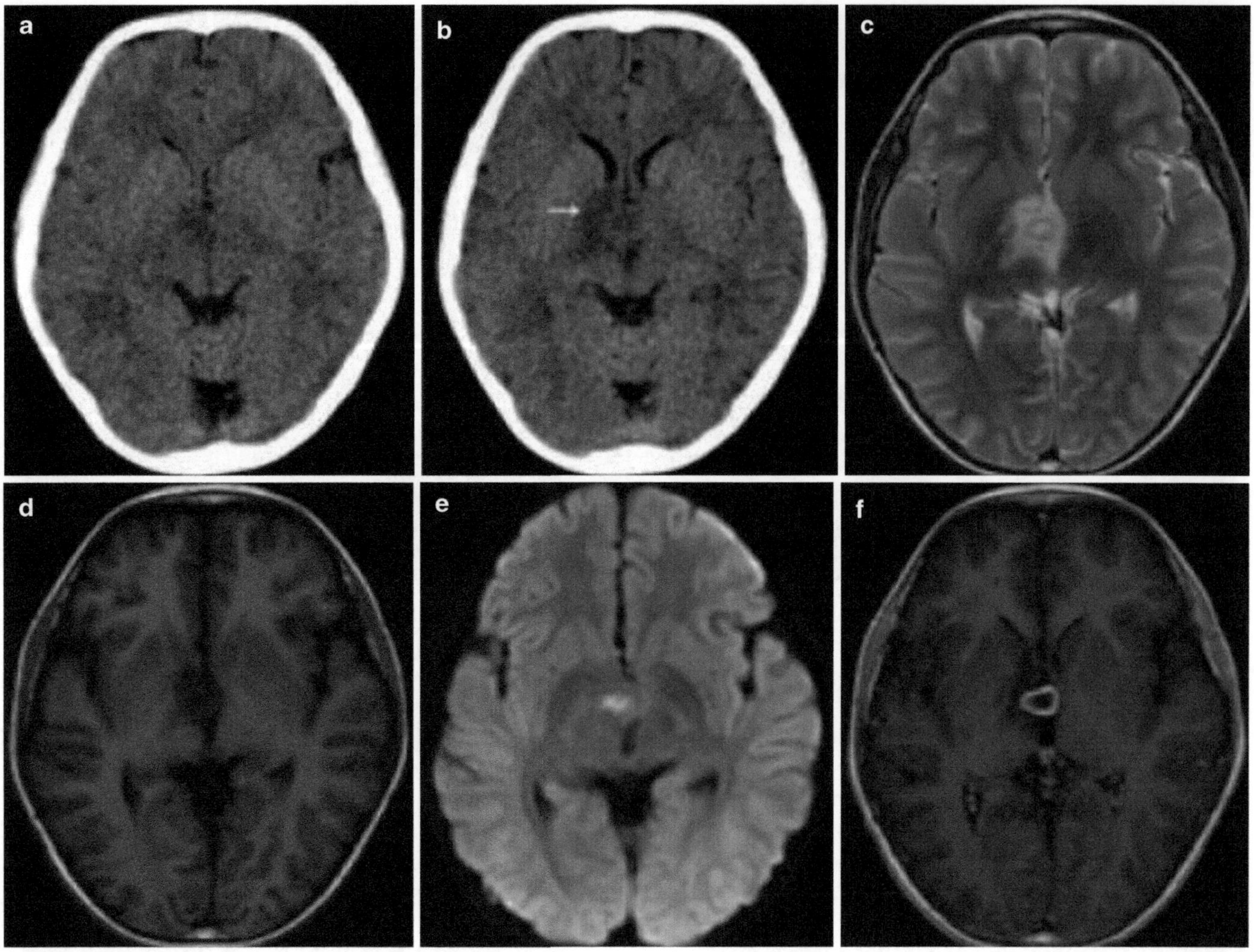

Fig. 21.3 Postoperative brain abscess. Postoperative right thalamic malformation tumor. (**a**) Day 1 CT plain scan shows no abnormality; (**b**) Day 10 CT plain scan after surgery, new sheet hypodense shadow appears around the right thalamus surgical area (arrow); (**c**) T_2WI shows hyperintense of pus in the center of the lesion, hypointense of abscess wall, and hyperintense of edema zone is seen around the lesion; (**d**) T_1WI shows hypointense of pus and isointense of abscess wall; (**e**) DWI shows the pus is hyperintense. (**f**) T_1WI enhanced scan shows the abscess wall is ring-like enhancement with a smooth inner wall

lope stage of brain abscess, the envelope is significant enhancement with a slightly thicker annular wall (Fig. 21.3). After effective treatment, the abscess cavity may gradually shrink. Some authors believe that progressive reduction in the diameter of the enhanced ring is the only reliable criterion for determining the healing phase of an abscess [2]. The abscess is no longer enhancement after complete healing. Some abscesses may become calcified during healing. In the brain, parenchymal infections of all stages are accompanied by perifocal edema and occupying effects, which may gradually decrease as the abscess matures.

21.1.4 Diagnostic Key Points

1. Clear surgical history; mostly clear cause of infection such as postoperative cerebrospinal fluid nasal leak and ear leak.
2. The earliest CT and MRI at the superficial site of surgery show linear thickening of the dura, indistinct borders, and striated or nodular enhancement on enhanced scans.
3. Bone flap infection with multiple patchy or patchy osteolytic changes on CT with or without fragmented bone fragments or subcapsular tendinous and/or epidural abscess or granulomatous tissue growth.

4. Infected subdural fluid is isodense on CT, iso or hyperintense (relative to cerebrospinal fluid) on T_1WI, and iso or hypointense on T_2WI; encapsulated pseudomembranes and septa show significant enhancement after enhanced scan; pseudomembranes encapsulated by undrained pus may calcify in the chronic phase.
5. Encephalitis CT plain scan shows a patchy hypodense shadow in the surgical area, with mild patchy enhancement within the lesion at the early stage (untreated postoperative 7 days) on the enhanced scan.
6. Brain abscesses in parenchymal brain infections. The envelope is a very thin hypointense ring on T_2WI with a clear border and is significantly enhanced on T_1WI with a smooth edge.
7. Cloudy cerebrospinal fluid, cerebrospinal fluid leukocytes >10 × 10^6/L, positive cerebrospinal fluid bacteriology (gold standard).

21.1.5 Differential Diagnosis

1. Postoperative scalp infection. It should be distinguished with postoperative scalp swelling and scalp effusion, etc. In the early postoperative period, scalp swelling at the surgical site is usually a nonspecific change that is usually slowly absorbed over several weeks. Scalp effusion is usually aseptic and consists of a mixture of cerebrospinal fluid with blood or its degradation products. On CT, postoperative scalp infection and postoperative scalp swelling are both hyperdense, while scalp fluid is hypodense; on MRI, postoperative scalp infection and postoperative scalp swelling are inhomogeneous hypointense on T_1WI, and hyperintense on T_2WI with abnormal enhancement in scalp infection but not in scalp swelling after enhancement. Scalp effusion is hypointense on T_1WI, hyperintense on T_2WI, and no enhancement after enhancement. If the scalp swelling persists for a prolonged period or worsens, it should suggest wound or bone flap infection, pus accumulation, distended hematoma, and cerebrospinal fluid leak.
2. Bone flap infections. It should be compared to simply inactive bone flaps and changes after radiation therapy, etc. After several years, inactivated bone flaps become heterogeneous density on CT and the borders between the bone cortex and the barrier space are ill-defined, with piebald appearance. Similar bone changes can also be seen after radiation therapy. Clinically, the distinction between infected bone flaps and simply inactive bone flaps and changes after radiation therapy is based primarily on symptoms and signs of bone flap infections.
3. Encephalitis. It should be distinguished from aseptic postoperative reactions, brain swelling, brain infarcts, and tumor remnants. Although all of them are hypodense occupying lesions in the surgical area on CT plain scan, the differentiation between them is usually not very difficult when combined with clinical symptoms and the enhanced presentation of cerebritis. Sometimes, a short period of periodic CT or MRI (after enhancement) reviews may be required to identify brain parenchymal infection. In the absence of an early postoperative CT or MRI baseline examination, it is often difficult to differentiate a thick-walled abscess with ring-like enhancement from a residual tumor in the late postoperative period.

21.1.6 Status and Progress of Research

1. Magnetic resonance diffusion-weighted imaging (DWI). The thick pus in the abscess is composed of inflammatory cells, microorganisms, and proteins, which are strongly adsorbed to water molecules, resulting in restricted diffusion, with ADC values being reduced, and DWI shows significant hyperintense with reduced ADC values. Some studies have shown that DWI is not applicable to exclude the diagnosis of postoperative abscesses, 40% of diagnosed postoperative abscesses do not show diffusion restriction, and ADC values are higher in postoperative abscesses than in spontaneous brain abscesses, possibly because of the patient's reduced postoperative cellular immune response and the fact that surgical intervention and/or the underlying pathological process disrupts normal anatomy, resulting in impaired blood supply and the formation of ineffective cavities in which both cell and protein concentrations are decreased, with a decrease in diffusion restriction, and correspondingly DWI signal decreases. The longer the time interval is between surgery and abscess drainage, the lower the ADC value performances, probably because with the prolongation of the time interval, the abscess matures and a large number of inflammatory cells, through marginal collection, excursion, and chemotaxis, accumulate to the lesion location and then cell density reaches the threshold required for DWI signal change [3–5].
2. Hydrogen proton spectrum imaging (^{1}H-MRS). It can be used as an important complementary imaging method to conventional MRI and DWI. The central necrotic region of the abscess lacks normal brain tissue metabolites, so the NAA peak, the Cho peak, and the Cr peak are absent. Brain abscess pus cavity tissue is hypoxic and necrotic, Lac and/or Lip peaks appear, pathogenic microorganisms in the pus and (or) multinucleated leukocytes in the pus secrete large amounts of protein hydrolases that hydrolyze proteins to form a variety of amino acid (AA, 0.9 ppm) substrates, which are detectable by using ^{1}H-MRS when AA substrates accumulate locally to a certain concentration, so AA is considered as a characteristic marker of septic abscesses [2, 6].

3. Magnetic resonance perfusion imaging (PWI). The area of maximum relative cerebral blood volume (rCBV) in brain abscesses appears consistent with the area of enhancement, whereas brain tumors, especially gliomas and metastases, often appear inconsistent [7]. Chan et al. [8] concluded that rCBV values are significantly different between brain abscesses and brain tumors, and the rCBV values in brain abscesses are lower in brain abscesses than those in brain tumors, due to the fact that the cystic wall of tumors is rich in vascular, and the local blood–brain barrier is disrupted, whereas the abscess wall of mature abscesses are composed of collagen fibers.

21.2 Chemical Meningitis

Wensheng Wang, Dabiao Deng, and Lijuan Gao

21.2.1 Overview

Chemical meningitis (chemical meningitis) is a disease characterized by aseptic meningitis that usually appears in some patients after neurosurgery and is generally thought to be a result of postoperative hemorrhage, surgical manipulation, cystic tumor contents, protein denaturation of brain tissue after electrocoagulation of brain tissue, placement of artificial materials, bone debris, etc., which irritates the subarachnoid space and produces large amounts of inflammatory cytokines thereby inducing an inflammatory response similar to bacterial meningitis, such as dermoid cyst ruptures spontaneously and cholesterol particles enter the subarachnoid space, symptoms causing symptoms of meningeal irritation [9–15]. Tumor resection or other intracranial surgery, which causes massive blood accumulation, can also cause an inflammatory response and make inflammatory cytokines enter the cerebrospinal fluid. This inflammatory cascade response may result from a disruption of the blood–brain barrier. However, the pathogenesis of aseptic meningitis remains elusive because the symptom of fever still exists after the blood in the cerebrospinal fluid has been cleared. Chemical meningitis can also be triggered by vaccination, application of drugs, systemic inflammatory diseases, and tumors. Chemical meningitis is associated with the entry of nonbacterial irritants into the subarachnoid space (e.g., blood, dermoid cyst, methotrexate intravenous drip) [16]. Cerebrospinal fluid examination in such patients may reveal increased white blood cells and protein and decreased glucose, but negative bacterial cultures. Chemical meningitis can lead to meningeal fibrosis and dense adhesions of the pia mater to the arachnoid. It usually appears 3–7 days after surgery, while chemical meningitis caused by intrathecal drug injection usually occurs 12–24 h after intrathecal injection. Patients may have clinical symptoms such as fever, headache, nausea, vomiting, and epilepsy. The concept of chemical meningitis was first introduced as a result of his finding that patients with brain tumors developed nonfluctuating fever after surgery, and that fever reappeared after postoperative absorption of fever. The acute clinical presentation and standard laboratory tests of chemical meningitis are not easily distinguishable from bacterial meningitis.

21.2.2 Pathological Manifestations

Aseptic chemical meningitis causes pathological changes generally in the form of meningeal fibrosis and dense adhesions of the soft meninges to the arachnoid membrane; if intracranial dermatomal cysts rupture spontaneously and craniopharyngiomas rupture and leak causing chemical meningitis pathological changes, necrotic material and a few neutrophils are seen microscopically [12].

21.2.3 Imaging

1. CT Findings. The CT findings vary depending on the contents entering into the subarachnoid space in surgical injury or in the early postoperative period. If the content is lipid component (e.g., craniopharyngioma, epidermoid cyst, or dermoid cysts), CT plain scan may show line-like slightly hyperdense in the cerebral sulcus around the operation area; in middle and late-stage, CT may have no apparent positive sign; if the content is protein-rich fluid (e.g., enterogenous cyst), CT may have no apparent positive sign. After enhancement, the meninges may be without enhancement or may be localized or diffuse enhancement of the meninges.
2. MRI Findings. MRI findings are different according to the contents spilling into the subarachnoid space; if it is a lipid component, MRI may show patchy or speckled hyperintense on T_1WI, hyperintense on T_2WI, and hypo-intensity on fat suppression sequence; if it is protein-containing liquid, the signal varies according to the concentration of protein-containing. For low concentration, T_1WI shows hypointense, while T_2WI shows hyperintense; for moderate concentrations, both T_1WI and T_2WI show hyperintense; for high concentrations, T_1WI shows hyper-intensity, while T_2WI shows hypo-intensity. If it is blood, the MRI findings vary depending on the component and period. After enhancement, the meninges may be without enhancement or may be localized or diffuse enhancement of the meninges. But meningeal enhancement is generally located around the surgical area in post-craniotomy patients. MRI can detect the lesion earlier than CT and show the details and scope of the lesion more clearly, so MRI has a higher diagnostic accuracy than CT. In the late stage of chemical meningitis, meningeal adhesions, ventricular dilatation, and effusion may be seen.

21.2.4 Diagnostic Key Points

1. A definite history of surgery or intrathecal drug injection is seen, most often after the rupture of a cerebral epithelioid cyst, with clinical manifestations of hyperthermia, cervical tonicity, convulsions, and coma.
2. At the early stage of post-surgery, localized or diffuse meningeal enhancement may be seen after enhancement. If the lipid component of an associated craniopharyngioma, epidermoid cyst, or dermoid tumor enters the subarachnoid space, MR shows hyperintense on T_1WI and T_2WI, hypointense on fat suppression sequence; CT plain scan shows fat density; cholesteatoma (epidermoid cyst) shows hyperintense on DWI sequence; if symptoms such as intracranial meningeal irritation signs and recurrent fever are present, the etiologic diagnosis of chemical meningitis is supported.
3. Cerebrospinal fluid examination. White blood cell count is mildly elevated; bacterial and fungal culture results are negative. Cerebrospinal fluid bacterial smear and culture is the gold standard for differentiation and diagnosis of bacterial meningitis and aseptic meningitis.

21.2.5 Differential Diagnosis

1. Bacterial meningitis. Most patients had a negative CT examination after enhancement. And enhanced MRI examination is significantly more sensitive than CT. Imaging findings of bacterial meningitis and chemical meningitis can be very similar, and the distinction between them primarily relies on the clinical history and cerebrospinal fluid examination.
2. Pia mater tumor metastases, choroid plexus tumors, embryonal tumors, and gliomas have a tendency to metastasize with meningeal dissemination. These tumors may show meningeal enhancement similar to chemical meningitis for months or years after resection, but the former is often accompanied by nodular meningeal enhancement, and repeated cerebrospinal fluid examinations may be abnormal. Tumor cells can occasionally be found in the cerebrospinal fluid. Meningeal biopsy is required when identification is difficult.

21.2.6 Status and Progress of Research

1. *FLAIR sequence enhancement:* According to the studies, the FLAIR sequence enhancement with a low concentration of contrast agent was superior to conventional T_1WI enhancement for the detection of meningeal lesions at an early stage. The main imaging finding is hyperintense in the cerebral sulcus. This can be used as an important complementary imaging method for the early detection of postoperative meningeal lesions [17].
2. *DWI:* Cholesteatoma (epidermoid cyst) has markedly restricted diffusion and is characterized by hyper-intensity on DWI. Combined with clinical manifestations of meningeal irritation and recurrent fever, it can support the etiological diagnosis of chemical meningitis.

References

1. Buang SS, Haspani MS. Risk factors for neurosurgical site infections after a neurosurgical procedure: a prospective observational study at hospital Kuala Lumpur. Med J Malaysia. 2012;67(4):393–8.
2. Shen T, Chen X. Neuroimaging. Shanghai: Shanghai Science and Technology Press; 2004. p. 964–6.
3. Kawaguchi T, Sakurai K, Hara M, et al. Clinico-radiological features of subarachnoid hyperintensity on diffusion-weighted images in patients with meningitis. Clin Radiol. 2012;67(4):306–12.
4. Lotan E, Hoffmann C, Fardman A, et al. Postoperative versus spontaneous intracranial abscess: diagnostic value of the apparent diffusion coefficient for accurate assessment. Radiology. 2016;281(1):168–74.
5. Liu H, Zhao J. Diffusion-weighted imaging in the diagnosis and differential diagnosis of brain abscess. Imaging Res Med Appl. 2018;2(18):64–6.
6. Lummel N, Koch M, Klein MN, et al. Spectrum and prevalence of pathological intracranial magnetic resonance imaging findings in acute bacterial meningitis. Clin Neuro Radiol. 2016;26(2):159–67.
7. Cha S, Knopp EA, Johnson G, et al. Intracranial mass lesions: dynamic contrast-enhanced susceptibility-weighted echo-planar perfusion MR imaging. Radiology. 2002;223(1):11–29.
8. Chan JHM, Tsui EYK, Chau LF, et al. Discrimination of an infected brain tumor from a cerebral abscess by combined MR perfusion and diffusion imaging. Comput Med Imaging Graph. 2002;26(1):19–23.
9. Wang L, Chang XN, Fu C, et al. An enterogenous cyst with atypical pathological findings and chemical meningitis. Springerplus. 2016;5(1):1993.
10. Hadden D, Allen I. Chemical meningitis due to rupture of a craniopharyngioma cyst. J R Soc Med. 2004;97(12):585–6.
11. Wen B, Cheng J, Zhang Y, et al. Ruptured intracranial epidermoid cyst MRI diagnosis. Radiol Pract. 2013;28(1):34–7.
12. Yoshua E, Keith K, Bhattacharjee MB, et al. Traumatic rupture of an intracranial dermoid cyst: case report and literature review.: Surg Neurol Int. 2013;4(1):80.
13. Shen T, Chen X. Neuroimaging. Shanghai: Shanghai Science and Technology Press; 2004.
14. Forgacs P, Geyer CA, Freidberg SR. Characterization of chemical meningitis after neurological surgery. Clin Infect Dis. 2001;32(2):179–85.
15. Sanchez GB, Kaylie DM, O'Malley MR, et al. Chemical meningitis following cerebellopontine angle tumor surgery. Otolaryngol Head Neck Surg. 2008;138(3):368–73.
16. Ding X, Deng J, Xia Y, et al. Intrathecal methotrexate causes severe chemical meningitis analysis of four cases of membranitis. China Drugs Clin. 2007;7(9):711–2.
17. Yu L, Zhang H, Ma X, et al. CUBE T_2FLAIR sequence in meningitis lesions. J Pract Med Imaging. 2016;17(4):282–4.

GPSR Compliance

The European Union's (EU) General Product Safety Regulation (GPSR) is a set of rules that requires consumer products to be safe and our obligations to ensure this.

If you have any concerns about our products, you can contact us on ProductSafety@springernature.com

In case Publisher is established outside the EU, the EU authorized representative is:

Springer Nature Customer Service Center GmbH
Europaplatz 3
69115 Heidelberg, Germany

Batch number: 10731524

Printed by Printforce, the Netherlands